D1711757

The Stigma of Mental Illness - End of the Story?

Wolfgang Gaebel • Wulf Rössler
Norman Sartorius
Editors

The Stigma of Mental Illness - End of the Story?

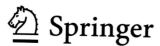
Springer

Editors
Wolfgang Gaebel
Department of Psychiatry and Psychotherapy
Heinrich-Heine-University
LVR-Klinikum Düsseldorf
Düsseldorf
Germany

Norman Sartorius
Association for the Improvement of Mental
Health Programmes
Geneva
Switzerland

Wulf Rössler
Psychiatric University Hospital
University of Zurich
Zurich
Switzerland

ISBN 978-3-319-27837-7   ISBN 978-3-319-27839-1   (eBook)
DOI 10.1007/978-3-319-27839-1

Library of Congress Control Number: 2016938229

Springer Cham Heidelberg New York Dordrecht London
© Springer International Publishing Switzerland 2017

Printed on acid-free paper

This Springer imprint is published by Springer Nature
The registered company is Springer International Publishing AG
The registered company address is: Gewerbestrasse 11, 6330 Cham, Switzerland

Contents

Introduction... xv
Wolfgang Gaebel, Wulf Rössler, and Norman Sartorius

Part I Stigma and Discrimination: Different Perspectives

1 On Revisiting Some Origins of the Stigma Concept as It Applies to Mental Illnesses.. 3
Bruce G. Link and Heather Stuart

2 Stigma and Stigmatization Within and Beyond Psychiatry........ 29
Asmus Finzen

3 Structures and Types of Stigma................................ 43
Lindsay Sheehan, Katherine Nieweglowski, and Patrick W. Corrigan

4 Stigma in Different Cultures................................. 67
Mirja Koschorke, Sara Evans-Lacko, Norman Sartorius, and Graham Thornicroft

5 Disorder-specific Differences............................... 83
Claire Henderson

6 Who Is Contributing?.. 111
Alexandre Andrade Loch and Wulf Rössler

7 Discrimination and Stigma.................................. 123
Dzmitry Krupchanka and Graham Thornicroft

8 The Influence of Stigma on the Course of Illness............ 141
Harald Zäske

9 Changes of Stigma over Time................................ 157
Georg Schomerus and Matthias C. Angermeyer

10 The Viewpoint of GAMIAN-Europe............................ 173
Pedro Manuel Ortiz de Montellano

11 The Role of Family Caregivers: A EUFAMI Viewpoint......... 191
Bert Johnson

12 **Stigma, Human Rights and the UN Convention
    on the Rights of Persons with Disabilities**...................... 209
    Peter Bartlett

Part II **"Fighting" Stigma and Discrimination: Programs in Different
         Parts of the World**

13 **Opening Doors: The Global Programme to Fight Stigma
    and Discrimination Because of Schizophrenia**.................. 227
    Heather Stuart and Norman Sartorius

14 **Fighting Stigma in Canada: Opening Minds Anti-Stigma
    Initiative**.. 237
    Shu-Ping Chen, Keith Dobson, Bonnie Kirsh, Stephanie Knaak,
    Michelle Koller, Terry Krupa, Bianca Lauria-Horner, Dorothy Luong,
    Geeta Modgill, Scott Patten, Michael Pietrus, Heather Stuart,
    Rob Whitley, and Andrew Szeto

15 **Like Minds, Like Mine: Seventeen Years of Countering
    Stigma and Discrimination Against People with Experience
    of Mental Distress in New Zealand**........................... 263
    Ruth Cunningham, Debbie Peterson, and Sunny Collings

16 **Australian Country Perspective: The Work of** *beyondblue*
    and SANE Australia... 289
    Georgie Harman and Jack Heath

17 **ONE OF US: The National Campaign for Anti-Stigma
    in Denmark**.. 317
    Johanne Bratbo and Anja Kare Vedelsby

18 **The Time to Change Programme to Reduce Stigma
    and Discrimination in England and Its Wider Context**.......... 339
    Claire Henderson, Sara Evans Lacko, and Graham Thornicroft

19 **See Change: The National Mental Health Stigma
    Reduction Partnership in Ireland**............................ 357
    Kahlil Coyle, Sorcha Lowry, and John Saunders

20 **See Me: Scotland Case Study**................................ 379
    Judith Robertson

21 **The German Mental Health Alliance**......................... 405
    Astrid Ramge and Heike Becker

22 **Stigma in Midsize European Countries**...................... 417
    Alina Beldie, Cecilia Brain, Maria Luisa Figueira, Igor Filipcic,
    Miro Jakovljevic, Marek Jarema, Oguz Karamustafalioglu,
    Daniel König, Blanka Kores Plesničar, Josef Marksteiner,
    Filipa Palha, Jan Pecenák, Dan Prelipceanu, Petter Andreas Ringen,
    Magdalena Tyszkowska, and Johannes Wancata

Contents

vii

Part III "Fighting" Stigma and Discrimination: Strategic Considerations

23 **Fields of Intervention** 435
Richard Warner

24 **Strategies to Reduce Mental Illness Stigma** 451
Nicolas Rüsch and Ziyan Xu

25 **"Irre menschlich Hamburg" – An Example of a Bottom-Up Project** 469
Thomas Bock, Angela Urban, Gwen Schulz, Gyöngyver Sielaff, Amina Kuby, and Candelaria Mahlke

26 **Illness Models and Stigma** 485
Andreas Heinz

Part IV "Fighting" Stigma and Discrimination: Commentaries

27 **What Has Proven Effective in Anti-Stigma Programming** 497
Heather Stuart

28 **What Has Not Been Effective in Reducing Stigma** 515
Julio Arboleda-Flórez

29 **Closing Mental Health Gaps Through Tackling Stigma and Discrimination** 531
Sue Bailey

Part V Overcoming Stigma and Discrimination: Recent Programmatic and Contextual Approaches

30 **Improving Treatment, Prevention, and Rehabilitation** 537
Wolfgang Gaebel, Mathias Riesbeck, Andrea Siegert, Harald Zäske, and Jürgen Zielasek

31 **Stigma and Recovery** 551
Elizabeth Flanagan, Anthony Pavlo, and Larry Davidson

32 **Stigma and the Renaming of Schizophrenia** 571
Toshimasa Maruta and Chihiro Matsumoto

33 **Trialogue: An Exercise in Communication Between Users, Carers, and Professional Mental Health Workers Beyond Role Stereotypes** 581
M. Amering

34 **Empowerment and Inclusion: The Introduction of Peer Workers into the Workforce** 591
Geoff Shepherd and Julie Repper

35 Targeting the Stigma of Psychiatry and Psychiatrists............. 613
    Ahmed Hankir, Antonio Ventriglio, and Dinesh Bhugra

36 Exemplary Contribution of Professional Scientific Organizations:
    The European Psychiatric Association........................ 627
    Marianne Kastrup, Andreas Heinz, and Danuta Wasserman

37 Addressing Stigma: The WHO Comprehensive Mental
    Health Action Plan 2013–2020.............................. 635
    Shekhar Saxena

Erratum E1

Conclusion and Recommendations for Future Action 641
Wolfgang Gaebel, Wulf Rössler, and Norman Sartorius

Index 651

Contributors

Michaela Amering Department of Psychiatry and Psychotherapy, Medical University of Vienna, Vienna, Austria

Matthias C. Angermeyer Department of Public Health, University of Cagliari, Cagliari, Italy

Julio Arboleda-Flórez Department of Psychiatry, Queen's University, Kingston, ON, Canada

Sue Bailey Academy of Medical Royal Colleges, London, UK

Peter Bartlett Department of Law and Social Sciences, Faculty of Social Sciences, University of Nottingham, Nottingham, UK

Heike Becker Department of Psychiatry and Psychotherapy, Medical Faculty, Heinrich-Heine-University, LVR-Klinikum Düsseldorf, Düsseldorf, Germany

Alina Beldie Department of Psychiatry Middelfart, Region of Southern Denmark, Middelfart, Denmark

Dinesh Bhugra Institute of Psychiatry, King's College London, London, UK

Thomas Bock Center for Psychosocial Medicine, University Medical Center Hamburg Eppendorf, Hamburg, Germany

Irre menschlich Hamburg e.V., Center for Psychosocial Medicine, University Medical Center Hamburg Eppendorf, Hamburg, Germany

Cecilia Brain Institute of Neuroscience and Physiology, Department of Psychiatry and Neurochemistry, Sahlgrenska Academy, University of Gothenburg, Gothenburg, Sweden

Johanne Bratbo The National Campaign for Anti-stigma in Denmark, Danish Committee for Health Education, Copenhagen, Denmark

Shu-Ping Chen Centre of Health Services and Policy Research, Mental Health Commission of Canada, Ottawa, ON, Canada

Sunny Collings Dean's Department, University of Otago, Wellington, New Zealand

Patrick W. Corrigan Institute of Psychology, Illinois Institute of Technology, Chicago, IL, USA

Kahlil Thompson Coyle See Change and Shine – Supporting People Affected by Mental Ill Health, Dublin, Ireland

Ruth Cunningham Department of Public Health, University of Otago, Wellington, New Zealand

Larry Davidson Department of Psychiatry, Yale University School of Medicine, New Haven, CT, USA

Keith Dobson Department of Psychology, University of Calgary, Calgary, AB, Canada

Sara Evans-Lacko Institute of Psychiatry, Psychology and Neuroscience, King's College London, London, UK

Maria Luisa Figueira Department of Psychiatry, University of Lisbon, Lisbon, Portugal

Igor Filipcic Department of Psychiatry, University Hospital Center Zagreb, Zagreb, Croatia

Asmus Finzen Berlin, Germany

Elizabeth Flanagan Department of Psychiatry, Yale University School of Medicine, New Haven, CT, USA

Wolfgang Gaebel Department of Psychiatry and Psychotherapy, Medical Faculty, Heinrich-Heine-University, LVR-Klinikum Düsseldorf, Düsseldorf, Germany

Ahmed Hankir Department of Psychiatry, Carrick Institute for Graduate Studies, Cape Canaveral, USA

Georgie Harman *beyondblue*, Hawthorn, VIC, Australia

Jack Heath SANE Australia, South Melbourne, VIC, Australia

Andreas Heinz Department of Psychiatry and Psychotherapy, Charité – Universitätsmedizin Berlin, Berlin, Germany

Claire Henderson Institute of Psychiatry, Psychology and Neuroscience, King's College London, London, UK

Miro Jakovljevic Department of Psychiatry, University Hospital Center Zagreb, Zagreb, Croatia

Marek Jarema 3rd Department of Psychiatry, Institute of Psychiatry and Neurology, Warsaw, Poland

Bert Johnson EUFAMI (European Federation of Associations of Families of People with Mental Illness), Leuven, Belgium

Oguz Karamustafalioglu Psychiatry Department, Sisli Etfal Teaching and Research Hospital, Istanbul, Turkey

Marianne Kastrup Centre for Transcultural Psychiatry, Psychiatric Centre Copenhagen, Copenhagen, Denmark

Bonnie Kirsh Department of Occupational Science and Occupational Therapy, University of Toronto, Toronto, ON, Canada

Stephanie Knaak Department of Community Health and Epidemiology, Mental Health Commission of Canada, Ottawa, ON, Canada

Michelle Koller Centre for Health Services and Policy Research, Queen's University, Kingston, Canada

Department of Community Health and Epidemiology, Mental Health Commission of Canada, Ottawa, ON, Canada

Daniel König Clinical Division of Social Psychiatry, Department of Psychiatry and Psychotherapy, Medical University of Vienna, Vienna, Austria

Mirja Koschorke Department of Health Service and Population Research, Institute of Psychiatry, Psychology and Neuroscience, King's College London, London, UK

Terry Krupa School of Rehabilitation Therapy, Queen's University, Kingston, ON, Canada

Dzmitry Krupchanka Institute of Psychiatry, Psychology and Neuroscience, King's College London, UK

Amina Kuby Center for Psychosocial Medicine, University Medical Center Hamburg Eppendorf, Hamburg, Germany

Bianca Lauria-Horner Department of Psychiatry, Dalhousie University, Halifax, NS, Canada

Bruce G. Link Department of Epidemiology, Columbia University, New York, NY, USA

Alexandre Andrade Loch Laboratory of Neuroscience (LIM-27), Institute of Psychiatry, School of Medicine, University of São Paulo, São Paulo, Brazil

Sorcha Lowry See Change and Shine – Supporting People Affected by Mental Ill Health, Dublin, Ireland

Dorothy Luong Department of Occupational Therapy, University of Toronto, Toronto, ON, Canada

Candelaria Mahlke Center for Psychosocial Medicine, University Medical Center Hamburg Eppendorf, Hamburg, Germany

Josef Marksteiner Department of Psychiatry and Psychotherapy A, LKH Hall, Hall in Tirol, Austria

Toshimasa Maruta Health Management Center, Seitoku University, Matsudo City, Chiba Prefecture, Japan

Chihiro Matsumoto Department of Psychology, Rikkyo University, Tokyo, Japan

Geeta Modgill Mental Health Commission of Canada, Ottawa, ON, Canada

Hans-Jürgen Möller Department of Psychiatry and Psychotherapy, Medical Center of the University of Munich, Munich, Germany

Anne-Maria Möller-Leimkühler Department of Psychiatry and Psychotherapy, Medical Center of the University of Munich, Munich, Germany

Pedro Manuel Ortiz de Montellano[†] GAMIAN-Europe (Global Alliance of Mental Illness Advocacy Networks-Europe), Brussels, Belgium

Katherine Nieweglowski Institute of Psychology, Illinois Institute of Technology, Chicago, IL, USA

Filipa Palha Association Encontrar+se (Association to Support Persons with Severe Mental Disorders), Education and Psychology, Portuguese Catholic University, Lisbon, Portugal

Scott Patten Departments of Community Health Sciences and Psychiatry, Mental Health Commission of Canada, Ottawa, ON, Canada

Anthony Pavlo Department of Psychiatry, Yale University School of Medicine, New Haven, CT, USA

Jan Pecenák Clinic of Psychiatry, Faculty of Medicine, University Hospital, Bratislava, Slovakia

Debbie Peterson Social Psychiatry and Population Mental Health Research Group, University of Otago, Wellington, New Zealand

Michael Pietrus Mental Health Commission of Canada, Ottawa, ON, Canada

Blanka Kores Plesničar University Psychiatric Hospital Ljubljana, Ljubljana-Polje, Slovenia

Dan Prelipceanu Department of Psychiatry, Carol Davila Medicine and Pharmacy University, Bucharest, Romania

Astrid Ramge German Mental Health Alliance, Berlin, Germany

Julie Repper ImROC Programme, Centre for Mental Health, London, UK

Mathias Riesbeck Department of Psychiatry and Psychotherapy, Medical Faculty, Heinrich-Heine-University, LVR-Klinikum Düsseldorf, Düsseldorf, Germany

Petter Andreas Ringen Specialized Inpatient Department, Gaustad, Division for Mental Health and Addiction, Oslo University Hospital, Oslo, Norway

Judith Robertson "See Me", Scottish Association for Mental Health, Glasgow, Scotland

Wulf Rössler Psychiatric University Hospital, University of Zurich, Zurich, Switzerland

Nicolas Rüsch Clinic for Psychiatry II, Section Public Mental Health, University of Ulm, Ulm, Germany

Norman Sartorius Association for the Improvement of Mental Health Programmes, Geneva, Switzerland

John Saunders See Change and Shine – Supporting People Affected by Mental Ill Health, Dublin, Ireland

Shekar Saxena Department of Mental Health and Substance Abuse, World Health Organization, Geneva, Switzerland

Georg Schomerus Department of Psychiatry, University of Greifswald, Greifswald, Germany

Gwen Schulz Center for Psychosocial Medicine, University Medical Center Hamburg Eppendorf, Hamburg, Germany

Beate Schulze Research Unit for Clinical and Social Psychiatry, University of Zurich, Zürich, Switzerland

Lindsay Sheehan Institute of Psychology, Illinois Institute of Technology, Chicago, IL, USA

Geoff Shepherd Department of Health Services and Population Research, Institute of Psychiatry, University of London, London, UK

ImROC Programme, Centre for Mental Health, London, UK

Andrea Siegert Department of Psychiatry and Psychotherapy, Medical Faculty, Heinrich-Heine-University, LVR-Klinikum Düsseldorf, Düsseldorf, Germany

Gyöngyver Sielaff Center for Psychosocial Medicine, University Medical Center Hamburg Eppendorf, Hamburg, Germany

Heather Stuart Centre for Health Services and Policy Research, Queen's University, Kingston, ON, Canada

Department of Public Health Sciences, Mental Health Commission of Canada, Ottawa, ON, Canada

Andrew Szeto Department of Psychology, University of Calgary, Calgary, AB, Canada

Graham Thornicroft Institute of Psychiatry, Psychology and Neuroscience, King's College London, London, UK

Magdalena Tyszkowska 3rd Department of Psychiatry, Institute of Psychiatry and Neurology, Warsaw, Poland

Angela Urban Irre menschlich Hamburg e.V., Center for Psychosocial Medicine, University Medical Center Hamburg Eppendorf, Hamburg, Germany

Anja Kara Vedelsby The National Campaign for Anti-stigma in Denmark, Danish Committee for Health Education, Copenhagen, Denmark

Antonio Ventriglio Department of Clinical and Experimental Medicine, University of Foggia, Foggia, Italy

Johannes Wancata Clinical Division of Social Psychiatry, Department of Psychiatry and Psychotherapy, Medical University of Vienna, Vienna, Austria

Richard Warner[†] Mental Health Center of Boulder County, Colorado Recovery, Boulder, CO, USA

Danuta Wasserman Department of Public Health Sciences, NASP, Karolinska Institutet, Stockholm, Sweden

Rob Whitley Department of Psychiatry, McGill University, Montréal, QC, Canada

Ziyan Xu Department of Psychiatry II, University of Ulm, Ulm, Germany

Harald Zäske Department of Psychiatry and Psychotherapy, Medical Faculty, Heinrich-Heine-University, LVR-Klinikum Düsseldorf, Düsseldorf, Germany

Jürgen Zielasek Department of Psychiatry and Psychotherapy, Medical Faculty, Heinrich-Heine-University, LVR-Klinikum Düsseldorf, Düsseldorf, Germany

Introduction

Wolfgang Gaebel, Wulf Rössler, and Norman Sartorius

There has always been a stigma around mental illness. But looking back to the last two centuries, which roughly cover the era of modern psychiatry, it was only for the last 60 years that the term stigma has developed from a quite undefined concept to a broadly used, well-described conception backed with facts from hundreds of scientific studies. In turn, the term stigma has become so popular that it became part of the everyday language.

Denying mental illness, as it was popular during the times of antipsychiatry, is possibly an under-researched area of stigma. But stigma research in general has been a reaction of established psychiatry to antipsychiatry. Stigma research is rooted in social sciences, dealing with all kinds of social influences on the onset and course of mental illnesses. Surprisingly, stigma impacts on all areas of psychiatry starting with the disease model and diagnostic concept and the subsequent illness course, self-stigma and structural stigma, stigma in different disorders up to stigma through professionals. Stigma is in various forms prevalent in all cultures. Potentially everybody might be contributing to the stigma of mental illness.

During the last half of the twentieth century, a dramatic institutional development has taken place. While the first half of the twentieth century was dominated by large and remote asylums, grossly neglected by public and health policy, there has been a significant increase in outpatient facilities and consecutively a likewise increase in patients. Today we know from epidemiology that about 40 % of the general population receive a lifetime diagnosis of a mental disorder (though only about one-third to one-half of these people receive treatment). Thus, everywhere everybody knows a person with a mental disorder. Nonetheless there have been almost no changes in levels of stigmatization in the general population in spite of the fact that a person we know and feel close to, i.e., a spouse, a relative, a friend, a colleague or a neighbour, might be affected from a mental disorder. And even worse, whenever something happens in the world where a mentally ill person may be involved, the level of stigma in the general population increases.

One almost might get the impression that the fears associated with mental illnesses are deeply rooted in mankind, obviously more or less unchangeable and all efforts in vain. Most likely the best anti-stigma campaign would be to find a 'cure' against mental illness. This eventually could be possible if we address clearly illness entities. But this is not the case with mental illness. We find almost all symptoms of mental illnesses on a continuum and the majority of symptoms are below the threshold of a psychiatric diagnosis.

There have been activities to change the name of schizophrenia, a disorder strongly associated with stigma because of its assumed dangerousness and unpredictability. This has happened in Japan and other Asian countries. There have been other efforts directed to the affected persons themselves like strengthening the recovery process and empowering the patients as well as the caregivers to take responsibility for their treatments. Users and caregivers have their own voice today. Further there have been efforts to bring together users, caregivers and providers of care to increase the mutual understanding. And there are efforts to promote the inclusion of the affected in the society. Far too much the institutional development has favoured the exclusion of the affected in the community. And finally there are promising programmes to reduce self-stigma.

Many campaigns and programmes have been conducted all over the world aiming at a change of societal attitudes – and ultimately behaviours – towards the mentally ill. These activities have been a powerful tool to direct the public's and specific target groups' attention to stigma, discrimination and prejudice of mentally ill persons.

Much has been published on the stigma of mental illness in recent years – including books on theoretical and practical issues, on 'lessons learned' and how to 'fight' stigma and discrimination (e.g. Arboleda-Flórez and Sartorius 2008; Corrigan et al. 2011; Gaebel et al. 2005; Stuart et al. 2012; Thornicroft 2006).

Why then another compendium like this one?

Although our understanding of mental illness has improved and we have numerous new options for the treatment of mental illnesses and a multitude of awareness campaigns and public information have taken place, the stigma of mental illness is still the main obstacle to the development of mental health services and a heavy burden for all touched by mental illness, people who have them, their families, mental health workers, mental health services and treatment methods. There is no 'end of the story' of fighting stigma in sight. During the last few decades, we have learned a lot from the various anti-stigma activities all over the world and our intention was to bring together knowledge and experience in the field, to make it more easily available for those who will continue to work on the prevention and reduction of stigma and for those who will want to learn more about the successes and failures in this field of work in recent years.

A book with a scope like this one – a 'reader' – can only be selective both in the choice of topics and authors. Documents from a broader field of international agencies have not been acquired due to space restriction. Intentionally, overlap among the chapters was not avoided in keeping the individuality of contributions and for the sake of separate readability of the chapters, most of which are referenced in the recommendations section in the final chapter.

Entitled *The Stigma of Mental Illness: End of the Story?*, this book is organized in seven chapters, each giving an overview on some of the above core developments and actions. This "Introduction" is followed by Part I including analyses of stigma and discrimination from different perspectives – ranging from history, science and human rights to views by patients' and family members' organizations (see Chaps. 1, 2, 3, 4, 5, 6, 7, 8, 9, 10, 11 and 12). Part II presents a representative selection of current programmes and views on 'fighting' stigma and discrimination, covering programmes in different parts of the world (see Chaps. 13, 14, 15, 16, 17, 18, 19, 20, 21 and 22), followed by strategical considerations in Part III (Chaps. 23, 24, 25 and 26) and evaluative commentaries in Part IV (Chaps. 27, 28 and 29) with a focus on what has proven effective or not. Part V presents some new approaches to overcoming stigma and discrimination (see Chaps. 30, 31, 32, 33, 34, 35, 36 and 37) such as improving treatment; accepting and promoting the concept of recovery; renaming of schizophrenia; promoting the trialogue of contacts between mental health workers, families and mentally ill people; empowerment; and inclusion. It also presents notions about the reduction of the stigma associated with psychiatry and psychiatrists and describes the contribution of regional scientific associations or global health organizations like the WHO. The final chapter summarizes the current situation, draws conclusions and presents recommendations for future action.

We hope that this book will help in developing anti-stigma programmes and influence the way in which we interact with those affected by the illness and their families and contribute to a better understanding of our profession.

We want to thank all the authors for their excellent contributions. We also thank Susanne Schaller for coordinating the manuscript handling and corresponding with the authors and Philip Barclay-Steuart for conducting the final editing process. Finally, we thank the publisher, in particular Corinna Schäfer, Dr. Sylvana Freyberg, and Wilma McHugh, for their flexible preparation for publishing.

References

Arboleda-Flórez J, Sartorius N (2008) Understanding the stigma of mental illnes: theory and interventions, 1st edn. Wiley, West Sussex

Gaebel W, Möller H-J, Rössler W (2005) Stigma – Diskriminierung – Bewältigung: Der umgang mit sozialer ausgrenzung psychisch kranker, 1st edn. Kohlhammer, Stuttgart

Corrigan PW, Roe D, Tsang HWH (2011) Challenging the stigma of mental illness: lessons for therapists and advocates, 1st edn. Wiley, West Sussex

Stuart H, Arboleda-Flórez J, Sartorius N (2012) Paradigms lost: fighting stigma and the lessons learned. Oxford University Press, New York

Thornicroft G (2006) Shunned: discrimination against people with mental illness. Oxford University Press, New York

Part I

Stigma and Discrimination: Different Perspectives

On Revisiting Some Origins of the Stigma Concept as It Applies to Mental Illnesses

1

Bruce G. Link and Heather Stuart

Background

It is difficult to imagine a more successful concept than that of stigma. Over the past six decades, it has enjoyed a meteoric rise, moving from an obscure term to one that is evident not only in academic work but in common parlance. It has been applied to a massive number of circumstances ranging from race and ethnic differences to incarceration, sexual minority status, psoriasis, incontinence, and many more. In these circumstances, it has been useful to describe and help explain the shame, social awkwardness, rejection, misunderstanding, and exclusion that people in these situations experience. The concept has been elaborated to help bring to light different aspects of this complex array of circumstances, and researchers have developed a large set of measures to assess those processes. It has been used by those who have felt the afflictions of stigma to identify the psychosocial processes involved and thereby to muster resistance to them. Among all of the circumstances that are stigmatized, one of the most prominent and most studied has been that of mental illness. This chapter provides a selective history of the origins and development of the stigma concept as it pertains to mental illnesses.

We begin with a brief assessment of the growth of the stigma concept and some empirical indicators of that growth. Next we use Goffman's formative work to mark

B.G. Link (✉)
Department of Epidemiology, Columbia University, 722 West 168th Street, Room 1609, New York, NY 10032, USA
e-mail: bgl1@columbia.edu

H. Stuart
Centre for Health Services and Policy Research, Queen's University,
21 Arch Street, Room 324B, Abramsky Hall, Kingston, ON K7L 3N6, Canada

Department of Public Health Sciences, Mental Health Commission of Canada,
Ottawa, ON, Canada
e-mail: heather.stuart@queensu.ca

© Springer International Publishing Switzerland 2017
W. Gaebel et al. (eds.), *The Stigma of Mental Illness - End of the Story?*,
DOI 10.1007/978-3-319-27839-1_1

four periods in the history of the concept: (1) a pre-Goffman period with an emphasis on attitudes and beliefs; (2) the contributions of Goffman's books, *Asylums* (1961) and *Stigma* (1963); (3) a post-Goffman era spanning the period of 1966 through roughly 1999 that included the partial resolution of the labeling debate, the introduction of social psychological experiments, an intense focus on mass media, and the spread of research to Germany and around the world; and (4) the current era of stigma research that has blossomed over the last 15 years or so. As other chapters will undoubtedly cover the evidence accumulated in the last identified era (1999–current day), the focus of this chapter will be on the other three. The potential value of this exploration is fourfold. First, it may be of intrinsic interest to those who are currently engaged in stigma-related research to know what their forebears were thinking about a concept that is currently so dear to them. Second, as we shall see, many of the concepts and issues we currently probe were at the very least foreshadowed in this earlier work. Returning to that work can deepen an understanding of the intellectual roots of our ideas and also help us avoid dead ends and blunders that these earlier researchers brought to light. Third, because the task of these earlier researchers was to map out the conceptual terrain of stigma, there is a strong tendency toward a depth of thought in much (but not all) of this earlier research. This is helpful for rethinking current concepts and highlights that, in some instances, novel thoughts put forward in the past have not been adequately represented in current research. Fourth, looking back provides a platform for recognizing intellectual accomplishments. In the ongoing effort to understand stigma, current research has developed a multilevel conceptualization with designs and measures that fit concepts at these multiple levels.

Two major caveats attend these four claims of potential usefulness. First, the current chapter will be unable to fully deliver on any of them, as they require a return to a careful reading of some of these earlier works. Instead, the goal only can be to provide some examples that might entice the reader to return to selected earlier works. Second, tracing intellectual history is a skill in and of itself and one that these writers cannot and do not claim to possess. The hope is that the chapter might provide a starting point that could entice someone trained specifically in the tracing of ideas to take up.

Some Indicators of the Growth of the Stigma Concept

Before Goffman's book, *Stigma: Notes on the Management of Spoiled Identity*, the term stigma was used in the social sciences to mean something quite close to its current meaning, but was used much less frequently than it is today. A Google Scholar search for the period 1900–1960 returns numerous scientific articles using the term "stigma," but almost all of these refer to botany (the receptive apex of the pistil of a flower) or other biological phenomena (a small mark, spot, or pore) rather than to social science meanings of the term. A Google Scholar search in the current era reveals something entirely different, with the social science meaning of the term ascendant and being applied to a vast array of stigmatizing circumstances. Another indicator of the large increase in interest is the number of published articles with the word "stigma" in the title or abstract. In 1980 the number stood at 19 for Medline and 14 for PsycINFO, but rose dramatically by the end of the century to 114 for Medline and 161 for PsycINFO in 1999 (Link and Phelan 2001). Incredibly, by 2010 the numbers were more than five times as high as in 1999: 758 for Medline and 851 for PsycINFO. Of course, not all of these referred to mental illness stigma but many did, and there is no doubt that this trend concerning stigma in general has also applied to mental illness stigma in particular. Based on these indicators at least, it seems that the stigma concept has enjoyed a tremendous growth in popularity over the years.

The Stigma Concept Before Goffman

Early Use of the Stigma Concept

The term stigma originates in early Greece where it signified a tattoo or mark that may have been used for decorative or religious purposes, but also as a mark to brand slaves and other undesirables. A sharp stick, termed a *stig*, was used to make the tattoo, hence the origin of the word *stigma* and its subsequent association with a mark or brand of shame. The early Greeks did not brand or stigmatize their mentally ill, but there is evidence that mental illnesses were associated with shame, loss of face, and humiliation. By the early nineteenth century, stigmata were firmly and negatively associated with mental illnesses, and important scholars of the day suggested that individuals who were "mentally defective" could be identified by morphological stigmata such as pointed ears, stunted growth, and cranial abnormalities. Because mental illnesses were considered to be the result of a hereditary taint, their management was viewed as a social rather than a medical problem. As a result, they became inextricably tied to other forms of degeneration, which conferred a broader stigma of moral incapacity to anyone labeled as such (Stuart et al. 2012). Despite these historical roots and presaging a debate about the consequences of labeling that would rage some 60 years later, Haslett (1899) denied labeling (certification) effects in a letter to the *British Medical Journal* by commenting:

> I cannot agree that certification has any of the disadvantages you mention-namely, that the doctor charges double fees, that the patient is doomed to lead a single and isolated life afterwards, and that a ban is cast upon the sisters and brothers. Surely if a depressed girl is placed in the house of a doctor, the fact of two medical certificates and a reception order having been first obtained (in no wise a public proceeding) cannot **attach a stigma of reproach** to the patient and her friends for the rest of their days. The suggestion is absurd. (Haslett 1899, p. 314)

Interestingly, the editors commented on Haslett's letter that they were "surprised to find disputed" the fact that there is a "social ban connected with being certified." Aside from presaging the entire theme of the labeling debate of the 1960s, it is clear that the term "stigma" was in use in the area of the mental illnesses as far back as this.

Explicit Conceptual Explorations of the Mental Illness Stigma Concept Before Goffman

The first article we located that began to explicate the stigma concept emerged from the Laboratory for Social and Environmental Studies at the National Institute of Mental Health in the United States that was headed at the time by sociologist John Clausen. It was in this unit where Goffman, as a fellow, conducted the ethnographic work that led to his book *Asylums* (1961). Stigma was on the minds of the small but enormously generative group at the Laboratory for Social and Environmental Studies, especially in the context of qualitative studies they were undertaking concerning wives of men who were hospitalized for mental illness. In light of that, one of the team members, Charlotte Green Schwartz (1956), authored a paper entitled "The Stigma of Mental Illness." She indicated that stigma had "two connotations: first, that in the minds of others the person is set apart – that is, different from the so-called normal person; second that he is set apart by a 'mark' which is felt to be 'disgraceful,' or even 'immoral,' by which he can be judged to be 'inferior'" (Schwartz 1956, p. 7). The second paper prior to Goffman that highlighted and defined stigma was authored by John and Elaine Cumming (1965) and carried the title "On the Stigma of Mental Illness." While it was published after Goffman's book, a footnote to the paper indicates that the report was "completed before the appearance of Erving Goffman's *Stigma* (Goffman 1963), no attempt will be made to relate the two different, but probably not incompatible, approaches to the problem" (Cumming and Cumming 1957; p. 135). The theme of Cumming and Cumming's exploration of stigma was "loss" – the loss of something essential and valuable. In the case of hospitalization for mental illness, Cumming and Cumming's claim was that what was "lost" was "in general, social competence and, in particular, predictability or reliability…" (p. 136). To our knowledge, the theme of stigma as "loss" has not been explicitly taken up in subsequent research, although the notion is clearly present when, for example, Link and Phelan (2001) identify "status loss" as a key component of stigma. Similarly, Yang and colleagues (2006) indicate that at its core stigma threatens "the *loss* or diminution of what is most at stake" for an actor in a given cultural context. In addition to its focus on loss, the Cumming and Cumming paper contains another significant premonition of subsequent research. The empirical portion of the paper reports on results of two stigma scales, one that includes items reflecting "a sense of shame or inadequacy" and is called "self-stigma" and a second that captures an "expectation of discrimination" called "situation stigma." Of course the self-stigma scale corresponds to Corrigan and Watson's (2002) highly influential identification of "self-stigma" as reflecting the internalization of public stigma. Similarly, the focus of the second scale on expectations of discrimination closely corresponds to the core concepts and measures associated with "modified labeling theory" (Link 1987; Link et al. 1989). Unfortunately, the Cumming and Cumming's scales were not presented in their original publication as it would be of great interest to determine how their measures might correspond to measures being used today.

Attitudes Toward Mental Illnesses in the 1950s and 1960s

Although the word stigma was rarely used in describing them, the major studies of attitudes in the 1950s covered content that is now subsumed under stigma research. Additionally, these studies introduced major methodological approaches to studying stigma that are still in use today. For example, the classic study by Cumming and Cumming (1957) entitled "Closed Ranks" focused on stereotypes about mental illnesses and was one of the first large-scale studies to incorporate a social distance scale in its repertoire. At the same time, the actual word "stigma" is mentioned only twice in the entire manuscript and does not appear in the index. We have chosen to describe a selection of these studies to indicate their contributions and continued utility.

Star's 1950 Nationwide Study in the United States

Dr. Shirley Star was a social and clinical psychologist who cut her teeth as part of the US contingent of social scientists called upon during World War II to support the war effort. As such, she contributed to the famous manuscript, *The American Soldier* (Stouffer et al. 1949), and in particular to work on the mental health aspects of combat and its aftermath. In 1949 she wrote a proposal to conduct a nationwide study of attitudes toward mental illnesses among approximately 3,500 respondents. She did the jockeying that was necessary at the time to procure the handsome sum of $25,000 from the National Institute of Mental Health. She later procured funds from foundations (Commonwealth, Field) and additional funds from NIMH to raise the approximately $84,000 spent on the study. At the time, the issue of open- versus close-ended questions in survey research had not been settled. Star produced a hybrid with enormous amounts of data from open-ended questions that she then developed meticulous codes to capture. The result was something like a 3,500-person qualitative study of enormous complexity. That, and what may have been a perfectionist streak on Star's part, likely contributed to the fact that the results of this amazing study were never fully published. The only accounts are mimeographed documents (a pre-Xerox form of copying) taken from talks she presented and interim reports she wrote.

The study made many contributions of which we will highlight three. First, Star introduced the highly influential methodological innovation of constructing vignette descriptions of people with mental illnesses as a means of gauging public reactions to such illnesses. Star created six vignettes describing conditions that mental health professionals at the time deemed mental illnesses and then asked the subjects in her study whether, among other things, they thought the described person had some kind of mental illness or not. One of the major findings of the study was that only one of the vignettes, the one describing frank psychosis (paranoid schizophrenia) with violence, was deemed to be a mental illness by a majority of the US public. The "Star Vignettes" as they came to be called were then picked up by other investigators and inserted into studies of the general public. With time a fairly consistent pattern of "increased recognition" of the vignettes as mental illnesses emerged causing some to be optimistic about changing public knowledge and attitudes (Lemkau and Crocetti 1962). The Star Vignettes gained even greater value when sociologist Derek Phillips had the creative insight to use them in a survey experiment, keeping the descriptions identical, but randomly varying the help source the person chose to address their condition. His finding that the persons described in the vignette faced increasing rejection (a social distance scale) as they were described as utilizing no help, utilizing help from a clergyman, doctor, psychiatrist, or mental hospital, was the first to bring the power of the experimental method to the study of labeling and stigma. The innovation of using vignettes, whether those of Star or newer ones modeled on hers, has had an enormous impact on the field of stigma research. Vignettes have been used to track changes in attitudes over time in the United States (Pescosolido et al. 2010) and Germany (Angermeyer and Matschinger 2005a, b) and to implement survey experiments to test the impact of labels (e.g., Link et al. 1987) and attributions of causes for the mental health conditions (e.g., Corrigan et al. 2003; Phelan et al. 2005). In a review of 62 population-based attitude surveys conducted between January 1990 and December 2004, 30 used vignettes as a stimulus (Angermeyer and Dietrich 2006), indicating they have become a stable in stigma research.

A second major contribution was Star's use of multiple methods to triangulate evidence regarding public conceptions and stigma. As already mentioned, she mixed close- and open-ended questions allowing her to gather information on both the quantitative response and the person's reason for giving that response. Additionally, she knew that people had very different ideas about what mental illness was and therefore withdrew from asking fixed format questions about "mental illness" recognizing that people would be answering questions about different things. Instead she asked an open-ended question: "Of course everybody hears a good deal about physical illness and disease, but now, what about the ones we call mental or nervous illness? When you hear someone say that a person is 'mentally ill' what does that mean to you?" By coding the verbatim responses (after appropriate probes), she was able to gauge what people thought of when they thought about mental illnesses. But of course, she also wanted to know whether people would think about mental illnesses as mental health professionals conceptualized them. Her vignettes describing such cases allowed her to do that. Certainly, she could not have imagined that her multi-method approach might be held out as an example by the next generation of stigma researchers – she was just trying to tackle an important problem in the best way she knew how. But that is really the point and it is still true today. Almost every question of importance demands a triangulation of evidence. The fact that such triangulation was evident in this early and very influential study is an important reminder to the field that should be heeded whenever possible. Moreover, the finding that people understand and stigmatize "mental illnesses" in different ways should be a lesson to present-day survey researchers, many of whom persist in measuring attitudes toward mental illnesses in general, rather than discrete disorders such as depression or schizophrenia.

A third contribution of this study comes in the content of the ideas that it generated. Star's multi-method approach resulted in a data structure that allowed her to assess not only what people thought mental illness was, but also how they came to a judgment about the issue. In her estimation, there are three essential features people used in deciding whether a behavior was mental illness or not. First was what she called an "almost complete loss of cognitive functioning" or in brief "a loss of reason" (Star 1955; p. 5). If a person knew what they were doing, they did not have mental illness. Second and almost a required consequence of the loss of reason, mental illness involves a loss of self-control to the point that a person is not responsible for his/her acts. Third, to be deemed mental illness, the behavior needs to be inappropriate – that is, neither reasonable nor expected in the situation at hand. Put another way, in order for it to be deemed "mental illness," behavior needs to be incomprehensible, even after a concerted effort to find a rational reason for that behavior. There is a depth to this analysis, and while the public has likely changed somewhat since she wrote in the 1950s, one wonders whether such an analysis might still apply to the public's view of psychosis. And if it did, and if people think of mental illness/psychosis as a loss of reason, a loss of control and predilection to engage in inappropriate and incomprehensible behavior, we might understand why they stigmatize psychosis/mental illness. Although Star did not use the word "stigma," she clearly described components of the concept by concluding that, for the general public, "mental illness is a very threatening and fearful thing" as it involves a "loss of what they consider to be the distinctively human qualities of rationality and free will, and there is a kind of horror in dehumanization," and mental illness is "something that people want to keep as far from themselves as possible" (p. 6). To our knowledge, this reasoning about how people think about mental illness has not been taken up as thoroughly and effectively as it might have been given its auspicious beginning in Star's work (but see Rosenberg 1984 for a prominent exception). This is unfortunate because it might have protected us from some prominent dead ends we have experienced in our efforts to address stigma. Consider for a moment that Star was correct and people conceptualize mental illness as loss of reason, loss of control, and engagement in inappropriate and incomprehensible behaviors; then how does telling them that this is an "illness like any other" change the circumstances that trouble them? How does telling them that the source of the unreason and lack of control and incomprehensibility is buried in genes, chemical imbalances, or defective brain circuitry relieve them of their concerns? The answer to these rhetorical questions is that these messages do not respond to public conceptions and would be unlikely to mitigate stigma. The fact that population-based studies have supported the conclusion that these approaches have failed (Pescosolido et al. 2010; Angermeyer and Matschinger 2005a) raises the question of whether Star, if she could return to the stage of the living, might tell us "I told you so." The main message for the current generation of stigma scholars is the potential value of revisiting Star's reasoning to see if it is apt in the current era (we suspect it is – at least for psychosis) and, if it is, to use it wisely in constructing evidence-informed approaches designed to reduce stigma.

Cumming and Cumming Effort to Change Attitudes (1952–1953)

Elaine Cumming, a sociologist, and her husband, John Cumming, a psychiatrist, had absorbed some of the information about public attitudes toward mental illnesses and decided, with a true public mental health spirit, to set out to change them. This public health spirit is all the more remarkable because the public health principles on which their work was founded were at odds with the mental health treatment system in the asylum era at the time, when mental illnesses were considered to be chronic and largely untreatable. They devised a quasi-experimental design that would allow inference about their efforts by choosing an intervention town that they dubbed Blackfoot and a control town they called Deerville. The two towns were located on the plains of Saskatchewan, Canada, far enough away from each other to avoid contamination of intervention effects, but similar enough to provide a useful comparison (John Cumming grew up in the province – a fact that may have led to the selection of the towns). Cumming and Cumming constructed a 6-month intervention to reduce social distance toward the mentally ill and improve citizens' sense of social responsibility for the management of mental illnesses. At the time, like most Canadians of the day, Blackfoot residents felt little social responsibility for the plight of the mentally ill and remained happily uninformed about the nature of mental illnesses and their treatments. Despite deplorable conditions in mental hospitals of the day, the public had an unshakeable belief in the effectiveness of mental hospitals, believing that they offered the "finest treatment available." The Cummings recognized that these relatively immovable ideas would not be receptive to the usual didactic methods or mass media interventions, so they relied on small group interactions and personal communications. Their program was fluid, taking advantage of community events that could be platforms for stigma reduction. These included films, radio shows, newspaper releases, and group discussions focusing on three themes: (1) the range of behavior that might be considered normal is broader than many believe, (2) mental health problems have causes that can be identified and related behaviors addressed, and (3) normal and abnormal behaviors reside on a continuum with no sharp demarcation point between the two. The intervention failed in two senses. First, the pre-/post-intervention assessments showed no evidence of hypothesized changes and no differences between the experimental and control towns in social distance or social responsibility. Second, Blackfoot residents, although initially very friendly, eventually became hostile and rejected the intervention both passively by withdrawing from participation and actively by, for example, asking that no more films about mental illness be shown to their group. In fact the mayor of the small town informed one of the study interviewers that the community had had "too much of this sort of thing" and indicated that "the sooner you leave the better" (Cumming and Cumming 1957, p. 44). The overall experience led Cumming and Cumming to use the term *Closed Ranks* in the title of their book to describe how the citizenry of Blackfoot banded together to maintain distance from the troubling concept of mental illness and the research team. These disappointing results reverberated throughout the public health community, perhaps leading to a general sense of nihilism about the possibility of reducing stigma through educational interventions, and another large-scale attempt to reduce stigma was not repeated in Canada for almost 40 years.

Looking back at the many things that Cumming and Cumming's vanguard effort gave us, we emphasize two: (1) the incorporation of social distance measures in research on mental illnesses and (2) a dramatic foreshadowing of the difficulties associated with interventions that try to change attitudes toward mental illnesses. The concept of "social distance" was developed in the context of the Chicago school of sociology in the United States to capture the willingness of different race/ethnic groups to comingle in the dense and rapidly changing urban neighborhoods of the city they studied (Park 1924). The first measure of the concept was developed by Bogardus (1926) to quantify social distance sentiments associated with race/ethnicity. To our knowledge, the first time a social distance measure was used to gauge behavioral intentions toward people with mental illnesses was in the context of Cumming and Cumming's study that was conducted in 1952–1953 and published in 1957. In Google Scholar searches for the terms "mental illness" and "social distance scale," we found no reference to a social distance scale predating the Cumming and Cumming study. Cumming and Cumming developed their social distance measure based on items they borrowed from an apparently unpublished attitude scale that they report having received from a man named Neil Agnew who worked at the Department of Health in Saskatchewan at the time. They used items from that scale, added items of their own, conducted scaling analyses (Guttman scaling), and came up with an eight-item scale to use in their own work to determine whether attitudes had changed in the experimental as opposed to the control community. Shortly thereafter, Whatley (1959) also published an eight-item social distance scale based on a study he conducted among 2001 residents of Louisiana in the United States in 1956. The relationship between the Cumming and Cumming and Whatley scales, if any, is unclear as neither study cites a prior published source for the scale they used. While the domain of content of the two scales is very much the same, there is no overlap in the specific items included suggesting that each research team independently constructed their own scale to measure social distance. Given the extremely widespread subsequent use of social distance scales in research on the stigma of mental illnesses, Cumming and Cumming's first use (1952–1953) and first publication (Cumming and Cumming 1957) of such a scale represent an enormous and lasting contribution to the field.

A second major contribution of the Cumming and Cumming study lies in lessons learned from their failed effort to change public attitudes/stigma. Two lessons stand out. First, the Cummings' subsequent critical appraisal and thematic analysis of interview data showed that their original assumptions had badly missed the mark. The town's people accepted a much wider spectrum of "normal" behavior than did the mental health educators who were trying to teach them to be more tolerant of abnormality. Second was the assumption that the lay population was ignorant of the social and biological causes of abnormal behaviors and needed professional advice in this regard. The population was already quite knowledgeable about mental illnesses, and this knowledge did not correspond to greater tolerance (a lesson that many anti-stigma literacy programs have since failed to appreciate). Finally, their most important message, that there was an arbitrary line between normality and abnormality, was entirely unacceptable to the residents who saw a sharp distinction between the mentally ill (those who had been hospitalized in a mental hospital) and the mentally well (most everybody else, regardless of the frequency and severity of any symptoms they may have had). Although the Cummings had appreciated the scope of the task before them, they had significantly underestimated the intensity of public prejudices and the immutability of stigmatizing views. Most importantly, however, they failed to empirically validate their theory of change and their educational messages *before* the program was initiated. Indeed, Cumming and Cumming (1957) were self-critical about the amount of theorizing they did before their experiment, advising "it is impossible to think too hard *before* such an experiment" (emphasis in the original). In their closing statement, they summarized their main mistake with reference to Kurt Lewin's now-famous epigram: "that there is nothing so practical as a *good theory*" (Cumming and Cumming 1957, p.158). While more recent efforts to change public stigma have at times involved theories as to why change should be expected, we could go much further toward enacting the model of theory *combined with intervention* that Cumming and Cumming emphasized. Too often our current efforts seem to be motivated by a shallow and unexamined assumption that what is wrong with public attitudes are inaccurate perceptions (myths) that need to be replaced with more accurate ones or that changes in knowledge or attitudes will naturally give way to the desired changes in behaviors. Rarely are such efforts motivated by a deeper evidence-informed theory as to why people might hold the beliefs they hold and how they might be affected by the message they have been delivered. Even research concerning our most reliable change agent – contact with persons who have a mental illness – often fails to specify a theory as to why or how such contact would change attitudes. Briefly put, the field of intervention research in the area of mental illness stigma would advance more rapidly if the Cumming and Cumming model of intervention *with theory* were more broadly implemented.

Second, the Cumming and Cumming study exemplifies how difficult it is to change public attitudes – one cannot just develop "enlightened" messages and deliver them to a public who will absorb them in intended ways. People believe things for reasons, the Cummings learned, and in their case, the messages delivered conflicted with values and beliefs that the residents of Blackfoot held dear. Current research has shown that education and contact interventions have positive effects, at least in the short run, on knowledge, attitudes, and beliefs of participants exposed to such interventions (Corrigan et al. 2012). This suggests that some progress has been made, at least in comparison to Cumming and Cumming's failed attempt to change attitudes. But at the population level, most evidence suggests either no change over time in core aspects of stigma such as stereotypes and social distance (e.g., Angermeyer and Matschinger 2005a, b; Pescosolido et al. 2010) or an actual move to worsening of beliefs in the domain of perceived dangerousness of people with mental illnesses (Phelan et al. 2000). It is interesting to note that D'Arcy and Brockman revisited the Blackfoot community 20 years after the Cumming's failed experiment. They used the identical study design and survey instruments to determine if stigmatizing attitudes had improved over time. Despite the substantial mental health reforms and liberalization of public attitudes that had occurred during this time, D'Arcy found that public attitudes toward the mentally ill and knowledge about psychiatric symptoms had changed little over the ensuing quarter century (D'Arcy and Brockman 1976).

This population-level intransigence harkens back to Cumming and Cumming's failure to change attitudes and thus to lessons learned from their study. It is not just ignorance or bad messaging, but rather people believe things for reasons, and even if those reasons make little sense or are unfair, if we fail to address such reasons, we can expect attitudes to change only in the short term and to be very difficult to alter at the population level. This last point coheres very nicely with Shirley Star's views on this issue (see above), which, although written 60 years ago, could be regarded as wise council for stigma researchers of today.

> I think that we must all soberly recognize that when we talk about the long-run aims of mental health education, we are talking about bringing about a veritable revolution in people's ideas about some very fundamental questions. This kind of change can occur, and I am certainly not here today to offer councils of despair, doubt or defeat. I would only suggest that fundamental changes are slowly and painfully achieved; usually far too slowly to satisfy the people who are laboring to bring them about. Perhaps by facing squarely the enormity of the task, we will all be more proud of, or at the very least, less disappointed and disillusioned by the relatively small changes that can be achieved in any one year or even five. (Star 1955, p. 9)

The Opinions About Mental Illness Scale (OMI)

The OMI was developed in the early 1960s by Cohen and Struening (1962, Struening and Cohen 1963) and has been used with some regularity ever since. Cohen and Struening (1962) sought the "adequate conception and objective measurement of attitudes toward mental illness" (p. 349) through a multidimensional scale. The OMI was developed in two large psychiatric hospitals based on the responses of 1,194 hospital workers. When the 70 items were factor analyzed, five dimensions were identified: (1) authoritarianism, that obedience to authority is critical and that people with mental illness are an inferior class requiring coercive handling; (2) benevolence, a kindly, paternalistic view of people with mental illnesses supported by humanism and religion rather than science; (3) mental hygiene ideology, the idea that mental illness is an illness like any other and that a rational, professional approach to people with mental illnesses is crucial for adequate treatment; (4) social restrictiveness, that the activities of people with mental illnesses should be restricted in domains such as marriage, voting, childbearing, jobs, and parenting; and (5) interpersonal etiology, the idea that mental illnesses arise from interpersonal experiences, particularly the lack of a loving home environment. In a subsequent paper (Struening and Cohen 1963), the original 70 items were reduced to 51 by retaining only items with mental illness content.

Among the reasons the OMI is of interest to current-day stigma researchers are three we will highlight. First, while some of the original items include outdated terms like "mental patient," small changes have allowed many of the items to be carried forward to current research. One way this happened is that in the late 1970s and early 1980s, Taylor and Dear (1981) published an instrument they called the Community Attitudes Toward Mental Illness (CAMI) scale. This scale relied heavily on the OMI seeking to reproduce three of its factors (authoritarianism, benevolence, and social restrictiveness) and therefore either incorporated many OMI items directly or reworded them to capture the same content. Thus, when current researchers use the CAMI (or some derivative of the CAMI), they simultaneously draw upon the pathbreaking research of Cohen and Struening's OMI. For example, the recent evaluation of England's "Time to Change" on public stigma (Evan-Lacko et al. 2013) included at least five items taken directly from the OMI and many others derived from the concepts introduced by the OMI. This long arm of the OMI has to some large extent been hidden, a fact that reveals that we have depended more on this pioneering work than we know.

Second, the OMI provides a potential lesson, or at least an option, for developing scales in the current era. While question writers are frequently advised to make their questions simple, direct, and clear, when this generally good advice gets translated to action, the questions that emerge are all too often uninspiring, boring, and pedestrian. When this happens, nothing is triggered inside the respondent that might be captured by the measurement process. In contrast the items in the Cohen and Struening scale have a poignancy and complexity aimed at supplying a stimulus that affects the respondent and provides something potent to react to. For example, one item reads, "Even though patients in mental hospitals behave in funny ways, it is wrong to laugh about them." In this item, the respondent needs to think about the circumstance of people with mental illness doing things that seem silly, funny, or out of place and then wonder whether "laughing" might be okay. Another item reads, "All patients in mental hospitals should be prevented from having children by a painless operation." In this instance, Cohen and Struening have added the phrase "by a painless operation" to what could have been a straightforward item "All patients in mental hospitals should be prevented from having children." The "painless operation" phrase gives someone responding the possibility to endorse something very restrictive but with a "nice person" lilt. The procedure is, after all, "painless." There could be disadvantages to this approach, as introducing complexity also introduces the possibility that people respond to different aspects of the complexity provided rather than to the same stimulus. At the same time, items that are simple minded, boring, and prosaic can leave the respondent inattentive and disconnected from the task at hand – factors that can also induce error and promote social desirability bias. In many ways, the Cohen and Struening's measure ends up a really nice balance between these two poles and therefore a model that current researchers might do well to emulate.

A third contribution of the OMI is its breadth of coverage and foreshadowing of themes that would subsequently emerge in stigma research. To take just one example, consider Link and Phelan's (2001) identification of co-occurring components of labeling, stereotyping, setting apart into "us" and "them" categories, status loss, and discrimination. Interestingly Cohen and Struening's measure builds in items that assess these components. The linking of labels (mental hospital patient) to stereotypes is prominent, for example, in items such as "People who are mentally ill let their emotions control them: normal people think things out" and "People who were once patients in mental hospitals are no more dangerous than the average citizen." The notion of separation into "us" and "them" is evident in items such as "A heart patient has just one thing wrong with him, while a mentally ill person is completely different from other people" and "There is something about mental patients that makes it easy to tell them from normal people." In addition, status loss ("To become a patient in a mental hospital is to become a failure in life") and an inclination to discriminate ("Anyone who is in a hospital for mental illness should not be allowed to vote") are also items in the OMI. Thus, in enacting their mission of providing "an adequate conception and objective measurement of attitudes toward mental illness," Cohen and Struening captured what others would much later propose to be "essential" features of stigma. For current-day researchers, this presaging is likely, as it is for us, both humbling in the sense that these earlier researchers already had in mind what we would later "discover" and also confirming in the sense that these earlier researchers saw the same things that we see.

Other Pre-Goffman Scholars

Of course this pre-Goffman period included scholars other than those we have highlighted, and a longer history would delve into their work and seek to understand its development more thoroughly. Worthy of mention, for example, would be the work of Clausen and Yarrow (1955) on wives' reactions to the unfolding illnesses of their husbands, Freeman and Simmon's (1963) studies of family attitudes and the return of patients from hospitals to community settings, Jum Nunnally's (1961) semantic differential studies of stereotypes about mental illnesses, and George Brown's (1962) explorations of "expressed emotion." Of particular note, however, would be the role of John Clausen who, as mentioned above, headed the Laboratory for Social and Environmental Studies at the National Institute of Mental Health in the United States. He created the context in which the studies of families were produced and where Charlotte Schwartz produced her pre-Goffman exploration of stigma (see above). Further it was John Clausen that Shirley Star turned to when she needed funds to implement her pathbreaking 1950 US nationwide study; Clausen also wrote a foreword that contextualized the results of the Cumming and Cumming monograph, and it was Clausen who provided the young Irving Goffman both with funds to support his work and access to Saint Elizabeth's Hospital to implement it. The field certainly would have started without him but perhaps not as strongly and as thoughtfully as it did.

Goffman's Contributions

As we can tell from our foray into some of the work that proceeded Goffman, there was a rich intellectual climate for him to draw upon. People were thinking about what we now call stigma, conducting research relevant to it, even laying out fledgling explorations of the concept itself. But the term, though in use, was not widely so, and no one had conceptually mapped the domain that could link all the disparate insights that were available to create a robust stigma concept. This is what Goffman did. He mapped the stigma concept, creating for the rest of us an extremely useful tool for interpreting and understanding this facet of human behavior. And he did it with his inimitable style, turning his wry eye to these phenomena in ways that made them poignant and salient for his readers. It is impossible to know, but if we imagine the full range of social science concepts, and ask ourselves why some have been more successful than others, one wonders whether the success of the stigma concept might partly be explained by the especially auspicious launch it received in Goffman's exceptionally talented hands.

Goffman was born in Alberta, Canada, the son of a tailor, and came to sociology only after first trying chemistry and filmmaking. He received his Ph.D. from the University of Chicago based on an ethnography he undertook in the remote Hebrides Islands of Scotland. His dissertation formed the basis for what became his first book *The Presentation of Self in Everyday Life* (1956). It is a natural precursor to his conceptualization of stigma as its focus was on how people sought to construct a social self in interactions with others, how they jockeyed for an image they preferred, and how they were sometimes blocked by others from making claims they could not sustain. Stigma fit right into this agenda and represented a further development of Goffman's interests in selves in social interaction. Because we assume most readers have familiarity with Goffman's Stigma, we will not elaborate here in detail, but instead summarize it briefly.

Goffman (1963, p. 3) provided a definition of stigma that almost everyone at least tips their hat to as an attribute that is "deeply discrediting" and reduces its bearer "from a whole and usual person to a tainted discounted one." But his essay did much more than this of course. It laid out types of stigma: what Goffman (1963, p. 4) called (1) "abominations of the body – the various physical deformities," (2) "blemishes of individual character" (mental illness, addiction, criminality), and (3) "tribal stigma of race, nation, and religion." Goffman's book (p. 41) also strongly introduced the concept of concealment in discussions of the concepts of "discredited" and "discreditable." And his work put forward the idea of stigma coping via concealment, educating others, withdrawing to groups that are unlikely to discriminate, and embracing the label to fight its stigmatizing consequences – essentially becoming what some people now call a "prosumer" (a "professional" consumer). Finally, Goffman identified what he called "courtesy stigma" or the tendency to stigma to travel from the stigmatized person to individuals connected by professional, marriage, and other family relationships. Although Goffman outlined various forms of stigma, he recognized that mental illnesses were among the most deeply discrediting of all stigmatized conditions – where the stigma associated with them could reduce someone from a whole person to one who was irredeemably tainted. In *Asylums*, Goffman (1961) was highly critical of mental hospitals for their anti-therapeutic and stigmatizing effects and along with contemporaries such as Laing (1960), Scheff (1966), Rosenhan (1974), Foucault (1975), and Szasz (1974, 1977) reinforced the notion that the negative and stigmatizing consequences of mental illnesses were more a result of the way in which psychiatry was organized, than the illnesses themselves. Together, these authors ushered in a worldview that was deeply distrustful of organized psychiatry and mental health systems. All of these concepts have had long arms with associated bodies of research. These and many other concepts from Goffman speak to his very important legacy in research on stigma.

The Post-Goffman Era: 1966–1999

Among the many developments following the publication of Goffman's book, we identify five occurrences as particularly important for the modern field of mental illness stigma: (1) the emergence and partial resolution of the labeling debate, (2) the development of social psychological theory and experimentation, (3) the beginnings of stigma research in the European context, (4) the emergence of a focus on the media as a source of negative attitudes, and (5) a dramatic move toward a global context for stigma research. While some part of this period has been called a "lull" in stigma research (Pescosolido 2013), a close examination of the intellectual and programmatic steps taken during this time identifies it as anything but a lull.

The Labeling Debate

Subsequent to its introduction by Goffman and others, stigma played a central role in the so-called labeling debate that emerged during the 1960s and early 1970s. Scheff (1966) constructed a formal labeling theory of mental illness that located the origin of stable mental illness in societal reactions, including stigmatizing reactions. The theory is called "labeling" theory because of the centrality it gave to the social definition of deviant behaviors. The debate concerning the role of labeling in mental illness involved both informal labeling processes (e.g., spouses labeling of their partners) and official labeling through treatment contact (e.g., psychiatric hospitalization). In Scheff's (1966) theory, the act of labeling was strongly influenced by the social characteristics of the labelers, by the person being labeled, and by the social situation in which their interactions occurred. He asserted that labeling was driven as much by these social factors as it was by anything that might be called the symptoms of mental illness. Moreover, according to Scheff, once a person is labeled, powerful social forces come into play to encourage a stable pattern of "mental illness." Stigma was a central process in this theory as it "punished" people who sought to shed the identity of mental illness and return to normal social roles, interactions, and identities.

Critics of the theory, especially Walter Gove, took sharp issue with Scheff's characterization of the labeling process. Gove argued that labels are applied far less capriciously and with many fewer untoward consequences than claimed by labeling theorists (Gove 1975). For some period between the late 1970s and early 1980s, professional opinion swayed in favor of the critics of labeling theory. Certainly the dominant view during that time was that stigma associated with mental illness was relatively inconsequential. Gove, for example, concluded that "… stigma appears to be transitory and does not appear to pose a severe problem" (Gove 1982, p. 290), and Crocetti et al. (1974) concluded, "former patients enjoy nearly total acceptance in all but the most intimate relationships." Moreover, when a group of expert stigma researchers was summoned to the National Institute of Mental Health in 1980 to review evidence about the issue, the term "stigma" was intentionally omitted from the title of the proceedings. Apparently, the argument that behaviors rather than labels are the prime determinants of social rejection was so forcefully articulated that the editors of the proceedings decided that stigma was not an appropriate designation when "one is referring to negative attitudes induced by manifestations of psychiatric illness" (Rabkin 1980, p. 327). It was within this context that the so-called modified labeling theory (described in some detail below) emerged in response to the then dominant anti-labeling, stigma-dismissing stance that characterized the field at the time.

Modified Labeling Theory

In the 1980s, Link and his colleagues developed a "modified" labeling theory that derived insights from the original labeling theory, but stepped away from the claim that labeling is a direct cause of mental illness (Link 1982, 1987; Link et al. 1989). Instead the theory postulated a process through which labeling and stigma jeopardize the life circumstances of people with mental illnesses, harming their employment chances, social networks, and self-esteem. By creating disadvantage in these domains and others like them, people who have experienced mental illness labels are put at greater risk of the prolongation or reoccurrence of mental illness. The modified labeling theory also provided an explanation as to how labeling and stigma might produce these effects and how key concepts and measures could be used in testing the explanation with empirical evidence.

The theory begins with the observation that people develop conceptions of mental illness early in life as part of socialization (Angermeyer and Matschinger 1996; Scheff 1966; Wahl 1995). Once in place, people's conceptions become a lay theory about what it means to have a mental illness (Angermeyer and Matschinger 1994; Furnham and Bower 1992). People form expectations as to whether most people will reject an individual with a mental illness as a friend, employee, neighbor, or intimate partner and whether most people will devalue a person with a mental illness as less trustworthy, intelligent, and competent. These beliefs have an especially poignant relevance for a person who develops a serious mental illness, because the possibility of devaluation and discrimination becomes personally relevant. If one believes that others will devalue and reject people with mental illness, one must now fear that this rejection will apply personally. The person may wonder, "Will others look down on me, reject me, simply because I have been identified as having a mental illness?" Then, to the extent that it becomes a part of a person's worldview, that perception can have serious negative consequences that affect self-confidence, social relationships, employment, and other life domains.

Aspects of the theory have since been tested with a broader range of outcomes, in different samples, by different investigators, and often using longitudinal data. These studies generally showed that the perceived devaluation-discrimination measure is associated with outcome variables including quality of life (Rosenfield 1997), self-esteem (Link et al. 2001, 2008; Livingston and Boyd 2010; Wright et al. 2000), social networks (Link et al. 1989; Perlick et al. 2001), depressive symptoms (Link et al. 1997; Perlick et al. 2007), treatment adherence (Sirey et al. 2001), and treatment discontinuation (Sirey et al. 2001).

Labeling as a "Package Deal"

Evidence from modified labeling theory and other approaches to labeling, stereotyping, and rejection strongly suggests that negative consequences associated with labeling are experienced by many people. At the same time, evidence from a voluminous body of research indicates that a variety of psychotherapies and drug therapies can be helpful in treating many mental illnesses. Given this, existing data simply do not justify a continued debate concerning whether the effects of labeling are positive or negative – clearly they are both. Rosenfield (1997) was the first to bring this point to light in a single study. She examined the effects of both treatment services and stigma in the context of a model program for people with severe mental illnesses. She showed that both the receipt of services (specific interventions that some people in the program receive and others do not) and stigma (Link's 1987 measure of perceived devaluation and discrimination) are related – in opposite directions – to multiple dimensions of a quality-of-life measure. Receipt of services had positive effects on dimensions of quality of life, such as living arrangements, family relations, financial situation, safety, and health, whereas stigma had equally strong negative effects on such dimensions. This insight and the empirical evidence to support it were critically important to resolving the labeling debate, certainly not for the strongest proponents of one or the other position but for the field in general as one could begin to study the origins of stigma without getting stuck in "either"/"or" conundrums associated with the labeling debate.

While it is sometimes claimed that the labeling debate raged was never resolved and ended up being a waste of time, the forgoing rendition of what transpired provides a much more congenial assessment. There was an approximation of a Hegelian thesis (Scheff 1966), antithesis (Gove), and synthesis (modified labeling theory) involved. Interestingly, this was precisely Scheff's intent when he constructed the first salvo in his provocative statement. Drawing on the philosopher of science Alfred North Whitehead who saw scientific conflict not as a disaster but as an opportunity, Scheff (1966) wrote: "In the present discussion of mental illness, the social system model is proposed not as an end in itself, but as an antithesis to the individual system model. By allowing for an explicit consideration of these antithetical models, the way may be cleared for synthesis, a model which has the advantages of both the individual and the social system models, but the disadvantages of neither" (Scheff 1966, p. 27). It may not have worked out quite as smoothly or as productively as planned, but something close to the hoped for scenario did occur. As such, the labeling debate, and at least its partial resolution, provides a potentially useful example for modern-day stigma researchers of the value of constructing and testing alternative hypotheses as an approach to refining knowledge.

Social Psychological Approaches to Stigma in the 1960s

The idea that stigma might be usefully studied in the laboratory is one that modern-day researchers take for granted. For many, the social psychological experiment is their main method, and a large portion of current-day research is based on findings from such experiments. Shortly after Goffman's work was published, Amerigo Farina of the University of Connecticut in the United States begin a pathbreaking program of mainly experimental research on the stigma of mental illness. His work explored many aspects of stigma and the social context in which the stigma occurred. For example, his work compared mental illness stigma to the stigma of homosexuality, varied whether the target of the experiment was the stigmatized person or the person who might enact the stigma, and implemented experiments both in college laboratories and in real-life settings such as department stores and psychiatric hospitals. To gain some purchase on this very large contribution, we briefly describe only a few of the many studies he implemented. Although Phillips (1963) had conducted a field experiment (see above), Farina was the first to bring the social psychology experiment to bear in mental illness stigma. In an initial study, Farina and Ring (1965) randomly assigned one of a pair of undergraduates to believe either that the other in the pair was "normal" or had been mentally ill. The participants were then assigned a joint task followed by questionnaire. It was found that when a co-participant was labeled mentally ill, the other subject in the pair preferred to work alone rather than with labeled person, blamed the labeled person for inadequacies in the joint performance, and saw the labeled person as more unpredictable, less able to get along with others, less able to understand others, and less able to understand himself. Described in the current era, the results of this experiment might seem unsurprising, but in the era shortly following Goffman's conceptual mapping of the concept, it provided some of the strongest empirical evidence of stigma and its consequences. In subsequent experiments, Farina and colleagues deepened their examination of stigma by focusing on the role of the stigmatized person. Farina et al. (1971) had individuals who had been hospitalized for mental illness interact with a person they believed might be a prospective employer. Participants were randomly assigned to believe either that their interviewer knew of their hospitalization or that no such information was conveyed. Subjects who believed they had been labeled behaved in less socially attractive ways and were judged less favorably by their interviewers than subjects who were not told they had been labeled. This, along with studies using a similar design (e.g., Farina et al. 1968), indicated the importance of expectations of rejection and processes that operate through the stigmatized person, ideas that foreshadowed modified labeling theory (Link et al. 1989) and self-stigma (Corrigan and Watson 2002).

In addition to the intriguing content explored, Farina's pathbreaking research at least foreshadowed and likely directly shaped much modern-day research on stigma. His work showed how the classic social psychological experiment might be usefully exploited to understand facets of stigma and its consequences for interpersonal relations. It was a theory-driven program of research with multiple experiments following one from the other with each one designed to elaborate on the one before it. The experiments brought the power of randomization to enhance internal validity and also frequently involved some mild deception that helped insure that participants' responses were not driven by experimenter-induced expectancies. Additionally, Farina embedded tasks in his protocols that allowed him to understand the influence of stigma processes on behavioral performance. Finally, and here we might wish that he had even greater influence on the field, Farina mixed the participant pool being studied to include not only college students (the standard standby for social psychological experiments) but also patients from mental hospitals, department store workers, and others. Following Farina and colleagues' auspicious use of social psychology in the study of stigma, seminal papers began to emerge in the 1980s (Sibicky and Dovidio 1987; Crocker and Major 1989) that incorporated an emerging social cognition theory into stigma theory, thereby leading to Corrigan and Penn's (1999) transformational paper entitled "Lessons from Social Psychology on Discrediting Psychiatric Stigma."

The Emergence of Stigma Research in the European Context

In the current era, as other chapters in this book will undoubtedly bring to light, stigma research is extremely strong in the European context. This was not always so. Of course all trends have multiple influences and determinants, but two apparent seeds in this impressive movement seem to reside in Matthias Angermeyer's program of research on stigma and in Norman Sartorius' conceptual engagement of the stigma concept and in his programmatic advocacy aimed at doing something about it. We identify these two scholars as initiators because their articles appeared relatively early and because citations in those articles did not identify precursors in the European context.

Angermeyer, a scholar whose early research focused on family context and gender differences in schizophrenia, published his first article on stigma entitled "Stigmatisierung psychisch Kranker: stadt versus Land" (Angermeyer et al. 1985). Shortly following this came a second study concerning some unintended stigma-related consequences of locating people with mental illnesses in settings where they were integrated with people with physical health problems (Angermeyer et al. 1987). But Angermeyer's influence grew even more dramatically when, just a short time later, he began to conduct multiple relatively large-scale population studies of the attitudes of the general public in Germany. The first survey was conducted in 1990, a time that just happened to precede a widely reported assassination attempt in which a woman described as having schizophrenia stabbed a candidate for chancellor with a butcher's knife. Another survey began only 2 weeks after this attack. Later, in a second attack, a man described as having schizophrenia shot and partially paralyzed the German Secretary of the Interior. As chance would have it, this occurred just 1 month before a third survey led by Angermeyer went into the field. This set of circumstances constructed one of the strongest natural experiments linking violent acts and their reporting by the media to attitudes toward people with schizophrenia. In addition to this very important set of findings, Angermeyer and colleagues' studies spoke to many additional issues of significant public health importance such as public trust in drug treatments for mental illnesses (Angermeyer et al. 1993), differences in attitudes toward treatment via psychotherapy as opposed to drugs (Angermeyer et al. 1993), what help-seeking strategies the public preferred (Angermeyer and Matschinger 1996), the role of contact with people with mental illnesses in mitigating stigmatizing attitudes (Angermeyer and Matschinger 1997), differences in attitudes between the former eastern and western parts of Germany (Angermeyer and Matschinger 1999), and many others. Additionally as Angermeyer and colleagues conducted more and more surveys, the possibility to examine time trends over the decade 1990–2001 emerged. In two very important papers, Angermeyer and Matschinger (2005a, b) showed that seemingly propitious changes in beliefs about the causes of disorders and in attitudes toward help seeking and the use of medications were not followed, as expected, by changes in desired social distance. In essence the program of research undertaken by Angermeyer and colleagues had three importance consequences. First, it brought a strong tradition of stigma research to Europe eventually creating what might be called a Leipzig School of stigma research that has since been carried on by many other younger scholars in Germany and elsewhere. Second, his studies showed the value that consistently strong survey research could have for understanding issues critical to public mental health. Third, and finally, it demonstrated the critical importance of surveillance of public conceptions over time as a means of judging whether and to what extent our efforts to change public opinions have been successful. His pathbreaking innovations in this regard have subsequently been taken up in both the United States (Pescosoldio et al. 2010) and England (Evans-Lacko et al. 2013).

A Focus on the Media

As research on public attitudes accumulated, interest in the sources of such attitudes also grew. Although many contributed to the emerging research on the depiction of mental illnesses in the mass media (see especially Nancy Signorielli 1989), Otto Wahl's work is perhaps the best known in this area. Beginning with a paper published in the once very popular weekly US magazine *TV Guide* entitled "Six TV Myths about Mental Illness," Wahl (1976) began a career studying the media depiction of mental illnesses. An early paper (Wahl and Roth 1982) enlisted raters to watch 385 prime-time television shows on five channels in February 1981 and rate their content. Wahl and Roth (1982) found that as many as one third of the programs touched on themes related to mental illness suggesting that the public was indeed frequently exposed to media messages. Coders were also asked to identify characters who were explicitly labeled as having a mental illness and to then rate how they were portrayed using 10 positive (e.g., poised, clever) and 10 negative (dangerous, unpredictable) codes. Wahl and Roth (1982) found that, in 9 % of the TV programs watched, a character was portrayed as a person with a mental illness and that the most common descriptive adjectives were "active," "confused," "aggressive," "dangerous," and "unpredictable." Wahl and colleagues continued to pursue research on portrayals of mental illnesses including an experimental assessment of the impact of a film portrayal of mental illness on viewers (Wahl and Kaye 1992), depictions in periodicals (Wahl and Kaye 1992), the print media (Wahl 1996), and even an examination of how generations of college students might be influenced by depictions of schizophrenogenic parents in abnormal psychology textbooks (Wahl 1989). What Wahl is best known for, however, is his 1997 book *Media Madness*. *Media Madness* makes it clear that the general public is bombarded with media depictions and that inaccuracies in such depictions vary from relatively minor misrepresentations and inaccuracies to sensational and horrendous stereotypes. Counterbalancing public health messages are generally a drop in the bucket in comparison and are often viewed with some suspicion because viewers recognize that the messages are intended to persuade. In contrast, media depictions are often embedded in dramas with no apparent attempt to "teach" or "persuade" and as such are less likely to be subject to critical evaluation of their truth value (Wahl 1997). The enormous impact of the book came in large part because of Wahl's extensive and detailed documentation of media portrayals. The reader is exposed to the actual media depictions and can see the relation between those detailed descriptions and Wahl's conclusions about the stereotyping of people with mental illnesses. Wahl's pathbreaking research has established media portrayals as one of the most important sources of public attitudes, suggested the importance of intervening to change such portrayals, and taught current-day social marketers what they are up against as they attempt to use the media to improve attitudes.

The Global Spread of Research and Action Addressing Stigma

Norman Sartorius' great contributions to the understanding of mental illness stigma can be partially captured by designating him the global "ambassador" of the concept. Sartorius is widely known for his extensive contributions to psychiatric epidemiology in general and to his World Health Organization studies of the course of schizophrenia in particular. In the mid-1990s, he turned a substantial portion of his attention to stigma, identifying it as a critical problem that called for a well-reasoned public mental health approach aimed at doing something about it. One arm of his "ambassador role" was directed toward his own profession of psychiatry. The title of his 1998 article published in *The Lancet*, "Stigma: what can psychiatrists do about it?" signaled this ambassadorial role (Sartorius 1998). It was a clarion call to psychiatrists to stand up to the substandard treatment people with mental illnesses experience around the world. His call asked psychiatrists to (1) interrogate their own attitudes and seek to improve them, (2) become advocates for people facing prejudice and discrimination, (3) shift their focus from symptoms only to helping people with mental illnesses enhance their quality of life, (4) keep their gaze fixed on instances in which stigma might be evident, and (5) keep open minds so as to learn from others about the best ways to address stigma. Heeding his own call, Sartorius (1997) sought to enact these principles through what became his second and even more impressive and impactful ambassadorial role – bringing a global focus to addressing the stigma of mental illnesses. As the then president of the World Psychiatric Association, Sartorius spearheaded a global program to fight the stigma associated with schizophrenia. The *Open the Doors* program engaged people in at least 20 countries with each site enacting local activities using key principles underlying the program (Sartorius and Schulze 2005). Of course it is hard to fully know the precise influence of this massive dissemination effort on the frequency or impact of stigma experienced by people with a mental illness or their family members, and it is clear that the effort to address stigma has been globalized. In 2005, members of the *Open the Doors* program established a scientific section within the World Psychiatric Association dedicated to stigma and mental health. The section has successfully cosponsored seven international stigma conferences. Stigma section members also contribute the scientific content to world congresses and international meetings and have made major contributions to the scientific literature. Indeed, a large part of the growth of applied stigma-related literature in the health sciences has been a result of the work of Stigma section members and their students. Thus, building capacity for evidence-based interventions has been an important legacy of this global initiative.

A key lesson learned from the *Open the Doors* global program was that anti-stigma interventions had to resonate with local communities. Subsequently, new theoretical approaches that attend to cultural variation, such as Lawrence Yang and colleagues' (2007) focus on "what matters most" in local cultural context, have emerged, massive public stigma surveys have been undertaken in multiple countries around the world (Pescosolido et al. 2013; Thornicroft et al. 2009), and clusters of outstanding researchers are now situated across the globe. Although we cannot trace every strand of influence, there is no doubt that the efforts of Sartorius and those he enlisted in his projects played a significant role in this global expansion.

In sum, if we consider the posing and partial resolution of the labeling debate, the uptake of stigma research within the social psychology framework of theory and experimentation, the intense examination of media influences, and the spread of strong research to Germany and then around the world, the post-Goffman period from 1966 to 1999 is anything but a "lull" as it was deemed to be by Pescosolido (2013). Instead, it was an enormously productive period where core issues were worked out, new conceptual and methodological paradigms set in place, and an active worldwide mental health initiative conceived and implemented.

Conclusion

We end by returning to the four ways that we hoped an examination of the history of the stigma concept might be helpful: (1) that such a foray might be of intrinsic interest to current stigma researchers, (2) that it would be enlightening and useful to see a foreshadowing of current concepts and approaches in these earlier studies, (3) that the initial task of mapping the domain of mental illness stigma induced some of these early researchers to deep thought which is both interesting to engage in its own right and in some instances potentially respiriting with respect to concepts we have left unexamined for too long, and (4) that by looking back we might gain some purchase on what we have achieved in the more recent era. With respect to the first three ambitions for the chapter, we hope the reader can conclude that they have at least been partially achieved.

The fourth goal has not been fulfilled, but having examined some part of the history of stigma research, we are at least in a position to consider the current era with that history in mind. We choose to do so by implementing a mind experiment. Implicitly we have been looking back essentially engaging in an intellectual conversation with the past. What if we were to imagine the early pioneers – Star, Cumming and Cumming, Farina, and Goffman – doing to us what we just did to them? What would they conclude about our contributions? First, we imagine them being awestruck and overwhelmed by the sheer volume of the research that currently exists. We might also imagine that they would view some part of this massive production to be a bit too cookie cutter inspired, formulaic, and sometimes dull. While it is true that we chose a select cadre investigator from the past, nevertheless their work is characterized by a depth of thought that we imagine they would want to see from us. Second, we imagine them respectfully reminding us that we had dropped several lines of intriguing investigation that they put forward (e.g., Star's examination of the process the public engages in deciding what mental illness is), missed learning from some of their mistakes (the need for more theory to be tightly attached to interventions), or forgot approaches to writing good items that might help avoid the stock, insipid fare that sometimes makes it into journals. But most of all, we think they would be deeply impressed – impressed by new and useful concepts, theories, population surveillance strategies, and concerted efforts to address public and self-stigma. They would greatly appreciate the growing global involvement as well as the concomitant emphasis on cultural differences in the experience of stigma. Additionally, they would likely admire the multilayered conceptualization that has developed including everything from macro-level structural stigma to microlevel assessment of implicit biases. Finally, they would be amused by our fits-and-starts efforts to reduce stigma and remind us that they had warned us so many years ago that it would not be easy. At the same time with the long sweep of time in their purview, we imagine they would see more progress than we see – the field has brought to light many aspects of the problem, people from policy makers to movie stars are on the issue, and the people who are disadvantaged by stigma have tools to communicate about and potentially resist what oppresses them. In taking a broad view, there seems to be something of a social movement underway that might, like other health-related social movements, produce slow but steady progress. Certainly our observers from the past would be hoping with us that this might prove to be true.

References

Angermeyer MC, Dietrich S (2006) Public beliefs about and attitudes towards people with mental illness: a review of population studies. Acta Psychiatr Scand 113:163–179

Angermeyer MC, Matschinger H (1996) Public attitude towards psychiatric treatment. Acta Psychiatr Scand 94(5):326–336

Angermeyer MC, Matschinger H (1997) Social distance towards the mentally ill: results of representative surveys in the Federal Republic of Germany. Psychol Med 27(01):131–141

Angermeyer MC, Matschinger H (1999) Lay beliefs about mental disorders: a comparison between the western and the eastern parts of Germany. Soc Psychiatry Psychiatr Epidemiol 34(5):275–281

Angermeyer MC, Matschinger H (2005a) Causal beliefs and attitudes to people with schizophrenia trend analysis based on data from two population surveys in Germany. Br J Psychiatry 186(4):331–334

Angermeyer MC, Matschinger H (2005b) Have there been any changes in the public's attitudes towards psychiatric treatment? Results from representative population surveys in Germany in the years 1990 and 2001. Acta Psychiatr Scand 111(1):68–73

Angermeyer MC, Classen D, Majcher-Angermeyer A, Hofman J (1985) Stigmatisierung psychisch Kranker: stadt versus Land. Psychother Psychosom Med Psychol 35(3–4):99–103

Angermeyer MC, Link BG, Majcher-Angermeyer A (1987) Stigma perceived by patients attending modern treatment settings: some unanticipated effects of community psychiatry reforms. J Nerv Ment Dis 175(1):4–11

Angermeyer MC, Held T, Görtler D (1993) Pro and contra: psychotherapy and psychopharmacotherapy attitude of the public. Psychother Psychosom Med Psychol 43(8):286–292

Bogardus ES (1926) Social distance in the city. Proc Publ Am Sociol Soc 20:40–46

Brown GW, Monck EM, Carstairs GM, Wing JK (1962) Influence of family life on the course of schizophrenic illness. Br J Prev Soc Med 16(2):55–68

Clausen JA, Radke Yarrow M (1955) Mental illness and the family. J Soc Issues11(4):3–5

Cohen J, Struening EL (1962) Opinions about mental illness in the personnel of two large mental hospitals. J Abnorm Soc Psychol 64(5):349

Corrigan PW, Penn DL (1999) Lessons from social psychology on discrediting psychiatric stigma. Am Psychol 54(9):765

Corrigan PW, Watson AC (2002) The paradox of self-stigma and mental illness. Clin Psychol: Sci Pract 9(1):35–53

Corrigan P, Markowitz FE, Watson A, Rowan D, Kubiak MA (2003) An attribution model of public discrimination towards persons with mental illness. J Health Soc Behav 44:162–179

Corrigan PW, Morris SB, Michaels PJ, Rafacz JD, Rüsch N (2012) Challenging the public stigma of mental illness: a meta-analysis of outcome studies. Psychiatr Serv 63(10):963–973

Crocetti GM, Spiro HR, Siassi I (1974) Contemporary attitudes toward mental illness. University of Pittsburgh Press, Pittsburgh

Crocker J, Major B (1989) Social stigma and self-esteem: the self-protective properties of stigma. Psychol Rev 96(4):608

Cumming E, Cumming J (1957) Closed ranks; an experiment in mental health education. Cambridge MA: Harvard University Press

D'Arcy C, Brockman J (1976) Changing public recognition of psychiatric symptoms? Blackfoot revisited. J Health Soc Behav 17:302–310

Evans-Lacko S, Henderson C, Thornicroft G (2013) Public knowledge, attitudes and behaviour regarding people with mental illness in England 2009–2012. Br J Psychiatry 202(s55):s51–s57

Farina A, Ring K (1965) The influence of perceived mental illness on interpersonal relations. J Abnorm Psychol 70(1):47

Farina A, Allen JG, Brigid B, Saul B (1968) The role of the stigmatized person in affecting social relationships1. J Pers 36(2):169–182

Farina A, Gliha D, Bourdreau LA, Ale JG, Sherman M (1971) Mental illness and the impact of believing others know about it. J Abnorm Psychol 77(1):1

Foucault M (1975) Madness and civilization. New York: Routledge

Freeman HE, Simmons OG (1963) The mental patient comes home. Wiley, New York

Furnham A, Bower P (1992) A comparison of academic and lay theories of schizophrenia. Br J Psychiatry 161(2):201–210

Goffman E (1959) The presentation of self in everyday life. New York: Anchor Books

Goffman E (1961) Asylums: essays on the social situation of mental patients and other inmates. New York: Anchor Books

Gove WR (1975) The labelling of deviance: evaluating a perspective. Wiley, New York

Gove WR (1982) Deviance and mental illness, vol. 6. Sage Publications

Handfield WJ (1899) Lunacy law and borderland cases. Br Med J. 1:314

Laing RD (1960) The divided self: an existential study in sanity and madness. Harmondsworth Penguin

Lemkau PV, Crocetti GM (1962) An urban population's opinion and knowledge about mental illness. Am J Psychiatry 118(8):692–700

Link B (1982) Mental patient status, work, and income: an examination of the effects of a psychiatric label. Am Sociol Rev 47:202–215

Link BG (1987) Understanding labeling effects in the area of mental disorders: an assessment of the effects of expectations of rejection. Am Sociol Rev 52:96–112

Link BG, Phelan JC (2001) Conceptualizing stigma. Annu Rev Sociol 27:363–385

Link BG, Cullen FT, Struening E, Shrout PE, Dohrenwend BP (1989) A modified labeling theory approach to mental disorders: an empirical assessment. Am Sociol Rev 54:400–423

Link BG, Struening EL, Rahav M, Phelan JC, Nuttbrock L (1997) On stigma and its consequences: evidence from a longitudinal study of men with dual diagnoses of mental illness and substance abuse. J Health Soc Behav 38:177–190

Nunnally JC (1961) Popular conceptions of mental health: their development and change. Holt, Rinehart, & Winston, Oxford

Park RE (1924) The concept of social distance. J Appl Sociol 8(5):339–344

Perlick DA, Rosenheck RA, Clarkin JF, Sirey JA, Salahi J, Struening EL, Link BG (2001) Stigma as a barrier to recovery: adverse effects of perceived stigma on social adaptation of persons diagnosed with bipolar affective disorder. Psychiatr Serv 52(12):1627–1632

Perlick DA, Miklowitz DJ, Link BG, Struening E, Kaczynski R, Gonzalez J, Manning LN, Wolff N, Rosenheck RA (2007) Perceived stigma and depression among caregivers of patients with bipolar disorder. Br J Psychiatry 190(6):535–536

Pescosolido BA (2013) The public stigma of mental illness what do we think; what do we know; what can we prove? J Health Soc Behav 54(1):1–21

Pescosolido BA, Martin JK, Long JS, Medina TR, Phelan JC, Link BG (2010) "A disease like any other"? A decade of change in public reactions to schizophrenia, depression, and alcohol dependence. Am J Psychiatry 167(11):1321–1330

Pescosolido BA, Medina TR, Martin JK, Scott Long J (2013) The "backbone" of stigma: identifying the global core of public prejudice associated with mental illness. Am J Public Health 103(5):853–860

Phelan JC (2005) Geneticization of deviant behavior and consequences for stigma: the case of mental illness. J Health Soc Behav 46(4):307–322

Phelan JC, Link BG, Stueve A, Pescosolido BA (2000) Public conceptions of mental illness in 1950 and 1996: what is mental illness and is it to be feared? J Health Soc Behav 41:188–207

Phillips DL (1963) Rejection: a possible consequence of seeking help for mental disorders. Am Sociol Rev 28:963–972

Rabkin JG, Gelb L, Lazar JB (1980) Attitudes toward the mentally Ill: research perspectives: report of an NIMH workshop, January 24–25, 1980. US Department of Health and Human Services, Public Health Service, Alcohol, Drug Abuse, and Mental Health Administration, National Institute of Mental Health, Division of Scientific and Public Information

Rosenberg M (1984) A symbolic interactionist view of psychosis. J Health Soc Behav 25:289–302

Rosenfield S (1997) Labeling mental illness: the effects of received services and perceived stigma on life satisfaction. Am Sociol Rev 64:660–672

Rosenhan DL (1974) On being sane in insane places. Clin Soc Work J 2:237–256

Sartorius N (1997) Fighting schizophrenia and its stigma. A new World Psychiatric Association educational programme. Br J Psychiatry 170(4):297–297

Sartorius N (1998) Stigma: what can psychiatrists do about it? Lancet 352(9133):1058–1059

Sartorius N, Schulze H (2005) Reducing the stigma of mental illness: a report from a global association. Cambridge University Press, Cambridge

Scheff TJ (1966) Being mentally ill: a sociological study. Chicago: Aldine

Schwartz, C.G. (1956). The stigma of mental illness. Journal of Rehabilitation, 22:7–29

Sibicky M, Dovidio JF (1986) Stigma of psychological therapy: stereotypes, interpersonal reactions, and the self-fulfilling prophecy. J Couns Psychol 33(2):148

Signorielli, N. (1989). The stigma of mental illness on television. Journal of Broadcasting and Electronic Media 33:325–331.

Sirey JA, Bruce ML, Alexopoulos GS, Perlick DA, Friedman SJ, Meyers BS (2001) Stigma as a barrier to recovery: perceived stigma and patient-rated severity of illness as predictors of antidepressant drug adherence. Psychiatric services 52(12):1615–1620

Stouffer SA, Lumsdaine AA, Lumsdaine MH, Williams RM Jr, Smith MB, Janis IL, Star SA, Cottrell LS Jr. (1949) The American soldier: combat and its aftermath. Studies in social psychology in World War II, vol. 2 Princeton: Princeton University Press

Struening EL, Cohen J (1963) Factorial invariance and other psychometric characteristics of five opinions about mental illness factors. Educ Psychol Meas 23:289

Stuart H, Arboleda-Flórez J, Sartorius N (2012) Paradigms lost: fighting stigma and the lessons learned. New York: Oxford University Press

Szasz TS (1974) The myth of mental illness: foundations of a theory of personal conduct. New York: Pell

Szasz TS (1977) Psychiatric slavery: when confinement and coercion masquerade as cure. Syracuse, NY: Syracuse University Press

Taylor SM, Dear MJ (1981) Scaling community attitudes toward the mentally ill. Schizophr Bull 7(2):225–240

Thornicroft G, Brohan E, Rose D, Sartorius N, Leese M, INDIGO Study Group (2009) Global pattern of experienced and anticipated discrimination against people with schizophrenia: a cross-sectional survey. Lancet 373(9661):408–415

Wahl O (1976) Six tv myths about mental illness. TV Guide. 13:4–8

Wahl OF (1989) Schizophrenogenic parenting in abnormal psychology textbooks. Teach Psychol 16(1):31–33

Wahl OF (1996) Schizophrenia in the news. Psychiatr Rehabil J 20(1):51

Wahl OF (1997) Media madness: public images of mental illness. Rutgers University Press

Wahl OF, Kaye AL (1992) Mental illness topics in popular periodicals. Community Ment Health J 28(1):21–28

Wahl OF, Lefkowits JY (1989) Impact of a television film on attitudes toward mental illness. Am J Community Psychol 17(4):521–528

Wahl OF, Roth R (1982) Television images of mental illness: results of a metropolitan Washington media watch. J Broadcast Electron Media 26(2):599–605

Yang LH, Kleinman A, Link BG, Phelan JC, Lee S, Good B (2007) Culture and stigma: adding moral experience to stigma theory. Soc Sci Med 64(7):1524–1535

Stigma and Stigmatization Within and Beyond Psychiatry

2

Asmus Finzen

In the past decades, awareness has grown that stigmatization is a heavy burden for people with psychosis and their relatives. The suffering because of the stigma, prejudices, defamation, and accusations becomes a second illness. Therefore, if psychiatry wants to treat successfully, it has to deal also with the stigmatization of its patients. Meanwhile, it is doing so not only on an individual level. Numerous national psychiatric professional associations, relative's groups, and self-help organizations for people who have experienced illness are attempting—sometimes in large-scale campaigns—to have a positive influence on the general public's perception of mentally ill people and psychiatry. These efforts are taking place under the generic term "de-stigmatization." De-stigmatization is a made-up word that is not found in any dictionary. Like "de-hospitalization," it signals hope and ambivalence at the same time.

If we want to evaluate whether the attempt to "de-stigmatize" mentally ill people is promising, we first have to consider the term "stigma" from a sociological perspective, which is not very familiar in psychiatry. We will thereby determine that stigmatization is by no means a problem that affects primarily mentally ill people, also not primarily ill people with "disreputable" illnesses (Sonntag 1977). Stigmatization is a ubiquitous societal phenomenon. It affects numerous groups of people who are excluded or can expect to be excluded. The sociological perspective puts a different perception in the forefront of the discussion about stigmatization: stigma management or overcoming stigma. It is more modest in its demands and concentrates on enabling stigmatized people to overcome their personal stigma and to "heal" their damaged identity (Goffman 1963).

The term "stigma" is not included in the German language "Dictionary of Psychiatry and Medical Psychology" (*Wörterbuch der Psychiatrie und medizinischen Psychologie*) published by Peters in 1999. Its meaning remains a mystery

A. Finzen
Stephanstr. 61, 10559 Berlin, Germany
e-mail: asmus.finzen@t-online.de

© Springer International Publishing Switzerland 2017
W. Gaebel et al. (eds.), *The Stigma of Mental Illness - End of the Story?*,
DOI 10.1007/978-3-319-27839-1_2

to us even after a glance at an everyday dictionary. The "Etymological Dictionary of the German Language" (*Etymologische Wörterbuch des Deutschen* 1995) proves to be more helpful:

> Stigma. 'trait, (degrading) characteristic, scar'. Lat. *stigma*. Originates from Greek *Stígma*, 'puncture, brand, mark burned into the skin, mark.' Greek *Stizein*, stab, pierce, tattoo, brand (related to prick and stab). Beginning of the 17th century adopted into German in its meanings 'sign burned into slaves and criminals as an insult, brand' and (Medieval Latin) 'one of the five wounds of Christ.' Metaphorical use since the second half of the 19th century 'mark, characteristic, mark of shame,' in medicine 'sign of disease'.......... [author's translation]

Only the *Duden* "Dictionary of Foreign Words" (*Das Fremdwörterbuch* 1990) leads us to the meaning of the word that we have in mind when we talk about stigma and stigmatization:

> 'Conspicuous sign of a disease' (med.). ....brand someone, denounce, assign characteristics to someone that are valued negatively by society, mark someone in a discriminatory way (sociol.). [Author's translation]

When we use the term stigma, we are indeed referring to its sociological meaning.

Goffman and Stigma

The American sociologist Erving Goffman devoted one of his early—now classical—books to the problem of stigmatization: *Stigma: Notes on the Management of Spoiled Identity* (1963). According to Goffman,

> The Greeks originated the term stigma to refer to bodily signs designed to expose something unusual and bad about the moral status of the signifier. The signs were cut or burnt into the body and advertised the bearer was a slave, a criminal, or a traitor—a blemished person, ritually polluted, to be avoided, especially in public places. (Goffman 1963)

Today the term is "widely used in something like the original literal sense, but is applied more to the disgrace itself than to the bodily evidence of it" (Goffman 1963). However, so far science has made hardly any attempts to describe the structural preconditions of stigma or even just to provide a definition of the term. Goffman's desire is to sketch "some very general assumptions and definitions."

In the following, I will adhere closely to Goffman's ideas because everything—almost everything—that has been spoken and written about stigma in recent sociology and psychiatry derives from him, if it is well founded, even if he is not named as the source.

Through the concept of stigma, i.e., damage to the social identity, he shows that many people who behave in a socially deviating way or who are condemned to an existence that deviates from the usual are concerned with far more than adhering to or violating rules and norms. Rather, they are concerned with the question of their social and personal identity and how these can be incorporated into their specific social environment—they are concerned with their "own life" in the complex environment of a large social society.

Wherever we live, whether we are aware of it or not, we have certain ideas about how people should behave, how they should live, what they should be like:

> When a stranger comes into our presence, then, first appearances are likely to enable us to anticipate his category and attributes, his 'social identity' ... because personal attributes such as 'honesty' are involved, as well as structural ones, like 'occupation.' We lean on these anticipations that we have, transforming them into normative expectations, into righteously presented demands. (Goffman 1963)

Goffman refers to these expectations as assigning a "virtual social identity." In contrast, the "actual social identity" contains those attributes and characteristics that a person actually has at his disposal. Aspirations and reality differ from each other. Such is everyday life from a social and sociological perspective. But there are differences that are accepted without difficulty and can be integrated and those for which it is impossible:

> ... in the extreme, a person who is quite thoroughly bad, or dangerous, or weak. He is thus reduced in our minds from a whole and usual person to a tainted, discounted one. Such an attribute is a stigma, especially when its discrediting effect is very extensive; ... It constitutes a special discrepancy between virtual and actual social identity. (Goffman 1963)

Incompatibility and Relativity of Attributes

Goffman adds that not all undesirable attributes are stigmatized, but only those that are incompatible with our view of what an individual should be:

> The term stigma, then, will be used to refer to an attribute that is deeply discrediting, but it should be seen that a language of relationship, not attributes, is really needed. An attribute that stigmatizes one type of possessor can confirm the usualness of another, and therefore is neither creditable nor discreditable as a thing in itself. (Goffman 1963)

In this context, Goffman gives the example of a college education: In some jobs in America, it is a flaw not to have one, and it is better to conceal this deficiency. In other jobs, however, it is better to conceal a college education so as not to be seen as a failure or outsider.

Goffman differentiates three "grossly different types" of stigma: the "abominations of the body," "blemishes of individual character perceived as weak will," that are "inferred from a known record of, for example, mental disorder, imprisonment, addiction, alcoholism, homosexuality, unemployment, suicidal attempts and radical political behavior. Finally there are the tribal stigma of race and religion, these being stigma that can be transmitted through lineages and equally contaminate all members of a family" (Goffman 1963).

All these examples have the same sociological attributes. The people concerned, whom we would otherwise have accepted without difficulty into our society, have an attribute that we cannot accept under any condition that causes us to consider as obsolete all their other qualities that we like about them: They have a stigma. They have "an undesired differentness from what we had anticipated." Essentially, we believe that people with a stigma are "not quite human." Therefore, we discriminate them and reduce their life chances "effectively, if often unthinkingly."

> We construct a stigma-theory, an ideology, to explain his inferiority and account for the danger he represents ... We use specific sigma terms such as cripple, bastard, moron in our daily discourse as a source of metaphor and imagery, typically without giving thought to the original meaning. We tend to impute a wide range of imperfections on the basis of the original one .... (Goffman 1963)

Traditions of Stigmatization

The exclusion of stigmatized people is by no means a privilege of modern society. It goes far back in history and is, as Müller (1996) presents in great detail in his book *The Cripple*, widespread throughout humanity. "Already God-fearing King David (approx. 1004–965 BC) hated the 'blind and lame' to his core" (Müller 1996, Book of Samuel 5: 8).

We know about the "fear of cripples" in ancient times, also in ancient medicine (Finzen 1969). Plato takes a clear stance in his late work, *Laws*: Not only should incorrigible beggars be cast out and criminals be put to death or banished. Also "disease carriers" who appear incurable must be exterminated. "Only healthy (i.e. 'pure' in the traditional understanding) general beings are viable." (Müller 1996) [Author's translation].

Throughout the Middle Ages, criminals were branded; lepers were furnished with special coats, bells, and rattles; a cross-shaped tonsure was shaved on the heads of the mentally ill (possessed); prostitutes had to wear unearthly colors; and Jews had to carry yellow patches on their garments. "The fear of coming too close to the evil and being fatally burned by its touch ran deep" (Müller 1996) [Author's translation].

The reformation did not change the situation at all:

> Churchgoers were undeterred, particularly because they at once gained a bold advocate in the great reformer Martin Luther. Misshapen children, he decided, should at best be killed straight after birth; after all, they had only limited life expectancy and until then would only uselessly 'gorge and souse'; generally, drowning seems to have been the preferred method. (Müller 1996) [Author's translation]

One has to remember what a long way we came in the twentieth century. Noteworthy, however, is how little we learnt from it. Genocide and ethnic cleansing marked the last century and the first decade of this century. In normal everyday life, people in wheelchairs are molested, people of a different skin color are bullied, mentally disabled people are ridiculed, and mentally ill people are discriminated against. It starts at preschool and continues at school, in the pub, in social groups, in soccer stadiums, and in political parties.

Roots of Stigmatization

All of the above is a consequence of stigma. And it is a dangerous illusion to believe that the social phenomenon of stigmatization can be abolished. If stigma is omnipresent, if it is just as common in simple societies as in complex ones and in historical times as in the present, then we have to ask ourselves whether the stigmatization of certain individuals with certain physical, mental, or social attributes is not a societal necessity. We have to ask ourselves whether the labeling and marginalization of "different people" is not a prerequisite for the maintenance of actual social identity and "norms."

There is much to suggest that this is the case. We can find supporting arguments in an essay by the American ethnomethodologist Harold G. Garfinkel (1956), for example, on the *Conditions of Successful Degradation Ceremonies*. According to this essay, the maintenance and promotion of the own identity requires that one identifies with members of one's own community; distinguishes oneself from others; if in doubt, excludes these others, particularly if they are seen to be different; and in any case understands the own identity as the better one, the superior one. This is promoted by social mechanisms that Garfinkel calls "degradation ceremonies." Such social rituals are necessary to ensure social coherence. An indispensable feature of social organizations is the ability to generate feelings of shame among its members. The possibility of removing identity is one of the sanction mechanisms of all social groups. It is a sociological axiom that is lacking only in "completely demoralized societies" (Garfinkel 1956). I will return to this topic in the last section.

This is not the place to clarify why that is the case. To ensure social solidarity, however, it appears to a certain extent imperative to promote and reward desired behavior and to mark, brand, and, in the worst case, ban undesirable behavior. Undesirable social behavior in its mildest form is simply "social deviation," in a more pronounced form is criminal or mentally disturbed, and in the worst case is a breaking of taboos, treason, or violence, an attack on the society that threatens its existence.

Whether a person's deviating behavior is classified as harmless or as dangerous to public safety is primarily a question of interpretation. Degradation rituals or ceremonies serve to promote this interpretive process. And whether someone is tolerated as an outsider or burned as a witch, receives therapy as a mentally ill person, or is murdered, as in the Third Reich, or—as was not unusual in historical societies—simply banished depends on the social leeway, the flexibility of the society, and its capacity for tolerance.

No matter what, stigma remains.

The Process of Stigmatization

The process and experience of stigmatization differ, depending on the type of stigma. But all stigmatized people have a similar experience. They have to acknowledge that they are different from other people, from "normal people." They have to learn to deal with that knowledge. The stigmatization and dealing with it becomes part of their biography. It contributes to the formation of their identity and leads, as Goffman writes, to a "damaged identity." He describes the path there as a "career." Thus, he readopts the term "moral career," which he coined in *Asylums* (1961) for the development of a long-term patient in an institution. The term "career" implies a development that can be influenced by the person concerned and became common in medical sociology in the 1970s (e.g., Uta Gerhardt 1986).

People with a stigma have similar life experiences "regarding their plight" and have "similar changes in conception of self—a similar 'moral career' that is both cause and effect of commitment to a similar sequence of personal adjustments" (Goffman 1963). However, this development differs depending on whether someone has a stigma at birth, becomes ill with a stigmatizing illness (or develops stigmatizing deviating behavior) in the course of his life, or is born into a society of stigmatized people, be they stigmatized for religious, national, or "racial" reasons.

Types of Stigma

Stigma at Birth

Numerous stigmas are present at birth: cleft lip and cleft palate (Uhlemann 1990), deafness and blindness, cerebral palsy (spastic paralysis) and mental disability, or red hair. Affected people have to—and can—learn from early childhood on to live with the disability and the reaction of their environment. Often, however, they only gradually start to perceive the stigma of their disability when dealing with "normal" children and adults. However, not all that rarely the realization of their disability happens abruptly, for example, when entering preschool or school. Until then, a protective environment can succeed in the child seeing himself "as a fully qualified ordinary human being, of normal identity …" (Goffman 1963).

The stigmatized person is avoided; he cannot find any friends, and if he does find some, often they do not want to be seen with him in public. He is rejected, ridiculed. He cannot find employment, also none that he could do just as well as others. He is made to feel useless and superfluous. He feels like an outsider, and he is.

Stigma Through Illness

If the stigma appears only later in life, the "individual has thoroughly learned about the normal and the stigmatized long before he must see himself as deficient. Presumably he will have a special problem in reidentifying himself, and a special likelihood of developing disapproval of self" (Goffman 1963). Goffman gives the example of an ill person with a colostomy:

> When I smelled an odor on the bus or subway before the colostomy I used to feel very annoyed. I'd think that the people were awful, that they didn't take a bath … I used to think that they might have odors from what they ate. I used to be terribly annoyed … So naturally, I believe that the young people feel the same way about me if I smell. (Goffman 1963)

There are many examples of physical disabilities that distort people: deformation of the head, loss of eyes or nose, primary diseases of the skin and burns, and in former decades most commonly the cleft lip and cleft palate. But mental illnesses also belong to this group, even if the disabilities they cause are not visible to everyone. Affected people are confronted with a special situation: They themselves have grown up with the reservations and prejudices about mentally ill people that predominate among "normal people." Accordingly, they—and their relatives—inevitably develop a disapproval of themselves. They do that all the more, the more pronounced the societal prejudices toward their illness are, the stronger they are rejected, ostracized, excluded, or ridiculed in their everyday lives. In this way, the stigma becomes a second illness, which can be just as much of a burden as the first illness and can become the primary obstacle to recovery.

Outsider: The Stigma of Affiliation

The stigma being affiliated with "different" social groups is certainly the most common type of stigma. In this context, "different" means nothing else than social differentness from the perspective of the assessing bodies. Such differences can be political, religious, or "racial." Their roots may lie in centuries-old mentalities. But they can also develop relatively quickly on the basis of radical social change.

The Indian caste system is an example of a tradition-bound societally desired and sanctioned stigmatization of the lowest caste, in particular of the so-called untouchables. Traditional Indian society had no doubt that their social "order" was all right. There was no doubt, even among the victims of this system of isolation and marginalization.

In Christianity, not only were non-Christians objects of marginalization. In the course of the centuries, secessions occurred time and again that were accompanied by violent conflicts, marginalization of dissenters through discrimination and stigmatization up to physical annihilation. Accordingly, the wars of the Middle Ages and early Modern Age were wars of religion. Similar developments characterize Islam. The most important schism of the Sunni and Shia in the seventh century has repercussions to the present day. At their core, the current conflicts in the Near East are wars of religion, even though enormous material and political conflicts also play a role.

The approach to Judaism has the longest stigmatizing tradition in our consciousness, since the expulsion of the Jews by the Romans and the beginning of occidental social life. In addition to integration, over the course of two millennia, there were repeated discrimination and marginalization, persecution of Jews, and, most recently, in the Third Reich, the attempt at the obliteration of what until the end of the Third Reich was called the Jewish "race."

This type of stigma has many similarities with the other types. But there is one decisive difference: The members of the stigmatized minority are physically and mentally "normal." They have better prerequisites for overcoming stigma, because they are healthy and because they live in a group of similarly stigmatized people. The fact that this is useless under extreme conditions has been proven by the fate of the Jews and the

Sinti and Romani people, homosexuals, and the many others who were suppressed and tormented in the Third Reich. The thematization of groups and of the belonging to such groups usually develops over a long time. But there are also exceptions. In the United States, for example, the persecution of citizens and immigrants in the McCarthy era resulted within a few years in the marginalization of thousands, people who until then had been of good standing, with all the characteristics of stigmatization. After September 11, 2001, the general suspicion of people belonging to the Islamic religious community led within months to marginalizations that previously had not been present. In Europe, Turks, Iraqis, Iranians, Pakistanis, Afghans, and others suddenly became Muslims, and the general suspicion of Islamism was applied to them all. And whenever hostile or even warlike conflicts occurred, the processes of marginalization were effectively involved. The change in the perception of Russians—all Russians—after the occupation and annexation of the Crimean Peninsula by the Russian government quickly led to an enemy image that had not been present for decades. People who tried to understand the development ran into the danger of being regarded as traitors and being taken into collective punishment as "Putin understanders."

One parallel to the second group of stigmatized people shall be mentioned: It occurs when the stigma, as is the case with numerous ill people, arises only later in life, for example, in the case of emigration or fleeing into a foreign country, a different culture.

Stigmatized People: Discredited and Discreditable

In the case of many people with physical disabilities, people with deformations, blind or deaf, and dumb people, the stigma becomes apparent as soon as we are in contact with them. Everyone can see that they are obviously marked and perhaps discredited. Stigma carriers also exist, however, whose "otherness" is not recognizable at first look. This is true for numerous members of stigmatized social groups: Often someone is not readily recognizable as a Jew or Muslim, protestant or catholic in the diaspora. These people are not discredited but discreditable. Mentally ill people are a good example here. Mentally ill people are both: They are discredited and discreditable. An inner circle of people, larger or smaller, knows that they are ill. Others can see it, e.g., because of extrapyramidal motor side effects of their medications. But most people are not aware of it. Mentally ill people, therefore, are a good model example for the situation of people who are not obviously stigmatized.

When people who know about the mentally ill person's illness meet them, they update the image of mentally ill people that they have internalized in the course of their own socialization. They have more or less pronounced prejudices, fear of their alleged unpredictability, their dangerousness. But in any case they are on guard. The matter-of-course social dealings with "normal people" are suspended. The basic trust in the reliability of social expectations that one usually has when dealing with other people is shaken. The social distance that the healthy maintain from mentally ill people is greater than the distance they maintain from people who are not known to have a mental disorder. Studies by Angermeyer and Siara (1994a) make this clear.

The average citizen is prepared to accept mentally ill people as neighbors or work colleagues. The situation is more difficult where greater proximity is concerned, for instance, as a subtenant, family member through marriage, or—understandably—in the supervision of young children (Angermeyer und Siara 1994b). The same study demonstrated how social distance grows when things happen that are appropriate for strengthening the reservations about mentally ill people. In Angermeyer's study, these events were the attempted assassinations of the German politicians Lafontaine and Schäuble in 1990 and the broad media coverage about them. Hoffmann-Richter et al. (1998) have shown in several studies that the media coverage about people with schizophrenia in newspapers and magazines has a negative tone also in everyday life, independent of extraordinary events. Thus, the local section of newspapers reports almost exclusively about schizophrenia in association with violent crimes, while information about the illness itself is extremely rare.

The awareness of reservations and prejudices results in many mentally ill people and their relatives trying to conceal the illness. This is possible if the illness is completely or largely overcome. But it has consequences, because concealing part of one's own identity is a burden. Goffman describes this as follows:

> The issue is not that of managing tension generated during social contacts, but rather that of managing information about his failing. To display or not to display; to tell or not to tell; to let on or not to let on; to lie or note to lie; and in each case, to whom, how, when, and where. (Goffman 1963)

In other words, mentally ill people who conceal their disorder live under constant tension and worry about being discovered—discredited. But not only that: While the "normal people," prejudices aside, maintain a certain degree of tactfulness toward people they know to be mentally ill, "secretly" ill people experience time and again that reservations and prejudices are expressed ruthlessly in informal conversations. Thus, they are confronted with such prejudices in an intensity that they would usually not have to bear if they revealed their illness. Moreover, they cannot expect people to make the allowances for them that they do for known mentally ill people if they have residual symptoms: reduced drive, depressivity, and general vulnerability. In other words, concealing the illness may solve some problems, but it exacerbates others. If a mentally ill person does not reveal himself,

> … it is not that he must face prejudice against himself, but rather that he must face unwitting acceptance of himself by individuals who are prejudiced against persons of the kind he can be revealed to be. Wherever he goes his behavior will falsely confirm for the other that they are in the company of what in effect they demand but may discover they haven't obtained, namely, a mentally untainted person like themselves. By intention or in effect the ex-mental patient conceals information about his real social identity, receiving and accepting treatment based on false suppositions concerning himself. (Goffman 1963)

Mentally ill people and people with a history of mental illness do indeed need to communicate with other people about their illness, their treatment, and the associated problems. A social life in a world of deception can be extremely burdensome and can promote a relapse. Nevertheless, finding people beyond the closest family circle who they can trust without fear of being abused or rejected is apparently one of the most difficult social challenges for people recovering from mental illness. An error of judgment can result in exactly what they want to avoid: being discredited by making their stigma visible and being betrayed by further divulgence of their secret.

Stigmatized people react differently to societal marginalization. People who are disabled from birth have a good chance of developing a high level of social competence—if their environment allows them to. For centuries, marginalization and isolation were the most widespread societal reactions to their otherness. This forced them into a marginal existence in which they had little chance to develop and substantiate themselves. In recent times, in particular times of inclusion, their chances for a life within society have significantly improved. Mentally ill people find themselves in a dilemma because of their stigmatization. One of their main problems is that while they were healthy they shared the prejudices against mentally ill people. Often they rightly feel excluded and devalued, as long as they are unable to recognize that such prejudices were wrong and still are. To achieve this, they need advice and support, if possible right from the beginning.

The groups of people who are physically and mentally healthy but stigmatized for social, religious, or racialist reasons find themselves in a fundamentally different situation. They usually live in groups together with other people who are stigmatized for the same reasons. They can talk about their fate. They can discuss how to deal with it and search for ways to maintain their identity, at best without it being damaged. This takes place through close integration and the development of a special group feeling. From within the group, it is then possible to develop defense strategies. One path, which was adopted time and again particularly by excluded groups in the diaspora, is the conviction of being something special, in extreme cases a "chosen" group or selected people. That conviction helps the affected people. But it can also become dangerous if the excluding society reacts to it with aggression and a lack of understanding. Throughout history there have been riots against such groups, in the worst case pogroms, physical obliteration of the parties concerned. Such events are particularly common in times of war. The murder of 10,000 Muslims in Srebrenica is only one example of such a terrible development in the recent past.

Stigmatization, Marginalization, and Social Solidarity

Some social axioms cannot be touched without endangering social solidarity. One of these axioms is affiliation—affiliation to the family, business, municipality, country, globalized world and also subgroups (sports clubs, self-help groups, religious communities, and German-Turkish or German-Kurdish community). Rules apply to each of these groups—social norms and expectations. In each of these groups, the members have their position, their individual status.

However, a societal group organizes itself; one of the most important elements is its borders. Within these borders, certain norms and values are valid that cannot be violated without punishment. They regulate qualifying for membership. One can be born into the group or attain membership. Everyone is a member of several such groups. This is more the case in the increasing social complexity of modern society than in traditional societies.

Also in multicultural societies, however, simultaneous membership in certain groups is impossible. The German-Turkish and German-Kurdish communities mentioned above may be an example for such a case. The barriers of a group can be easily penetrable, such as in leisure groups or on the lower levels of companies. But they can also be insurmountable, such as in the mafia, where orientation beyond the borders can all too easily be interpreted as betrayal and be punished with death.

Whatever such a societal group looks like, its members have to be capable of recognizing and adhering to the rules, norms, and values. It is one of the basic pre-requisites of human coexistence that the members of a group can rely on the predict-ability of the other members' behavior. This is why deviating behavior is met with sanctions, whether or not it was intentional or unintentional. And this is why the violation of central rules and values is punished by exclusion. In extreme cases, the degradation ceremonies then take effect that Garfinkel (1956) understands primarily as procedures to secure social borders against existential threats to social solidarity.

Stigmatization has a lot to do with protecting borders and making them visible. Stigma carriers visibly do not belong. They are marked, stricken, and branded. Their signs reveal, as Goffman writes about the source of the stigma, "something unusual and bad about the moral status of the signifier." The Islamic sharia has, so to speak, rescued the tradition of physical punishments from antiquity into modern times. The Nazis branded the Jews by forcing them to wear a yellow star.

Modern society also has its strict boundaries between those who belong and those who do not. It is no longer the lepers who are cast out but the homeless. The members of "fringe groups" are the ones who are more or less excluded: certain foreigners, asylum seekers, members of "sects" and certain radical religious com-munities, people with a sexual orientation other than heterosexual, radical dissi-dents, people with physical or mental disabilities, people with a deformed physical appearance, and mentally ill people.

The extent and rigorousness of the exclusion and marginalization differ. But one cannot imagine a society that refrains from such marginalizations. Certainly, the attitude toward homosexuality has changed. An issue of the German newspaper *Frankfurter Allgemeine Zeitung* from 1999 (No. 202, p. 7) contained two articles about homosexuals as officers and priests that made it clear that the stigmatization was still present. There is little to suggest that much has changed since then. And in our fast-moving times, when prejudices and reservations about one group are dis-mantled, new ones will be established against another group.

They are apparently subliminally present, always and everywhere, against cripples, mentally deficient people, "gypsies," Jews, and mentally disturbed people. Prejudices and resentments toward these people seem to be deeply rooted in Western people. And that fact demands our vigilance. Even if it is undisputed in sociology that borders are essential for the survival of social entities, the exclusion and exploitation of certain fellow human beings to "mark the boundaries" are a dangerous matter.

Social Exploitations and Prejudices

We should not, however, indulge in the illusion that we can fundamentally change this situation. We can try to mitigate particularly dangerous and irrational prejudices through targeted information and image advertising and, in individual cases, even to overcome them. In the past, the example of the mentally ill (Cumming and Cumming 1957) and also that of the Jewish population has shown time and again that such well-meant campaigns can also arouse resentments. In the end, fears—often irrational fears—are what maintains the stigmatization, and irrationality cannot be abolished through information and knowledge enhancement.

Meeting a physically deformed person can easily become a threat to one's own physical identity; meeting a person marked by a severe physical illness confronts one with the sometimes painstakingly compensated anxiety about one's own illness and death. The anxiety associated with meeting mentally disabled and mentally ill people ultimately originates from the widespread fear of "losing one's mind." Such anxieties are reflected in "social representations" (Moscovici 1961; Flick 1995), in internal images that one acquires over the course of one's life in a mixture of knowledge and feelings and that changes only very gradually, if at all. Meeting people who seem strange to us can also trigger anxieties or lead to defensive reactions. This is especially true in emotionally heated situations during political or religious conflicts, particularly if there have already been hostilities and the general situation appears threatening.

Social representations are not simple everyday knowledge. They are knowledge combined with ideological sometimes mythical and emotional beliefs and in the case of illnesses primarily fear. Nowadays, new age concepts become involved. In this context, efforts at persuasion therefore have to be also efforts at building relationships. Only if personal conviction is present can trust be built up, the social representations of those involved be stimulated and thus changed, and—in the end, not at the beginning—their knowledge be newly constituted. We experience time and again that this is far from unpromising, even in severely prejudiced conflicts. But this process needs persistence and time.

Final Remarks

Stigma and stigmatization are not problems specific to psychiatry but rather are ubiquitous. Anywhere where there are prejudices, where discrimination takes place, stigmatization will also be present. Stigmatization is prevalent everywhere where people are pressured, devalued, damaged in their identity, or excluded from society because of their cultural or ethnic affiliation, their religious denomination, or their illness attributes. The classical Goffman division of stigma into three types on the basis of social and cultural affiliation, stigma through illness, and stigma at birth can still serve as a tool today. The stigma of the mentally ill is an anomaly because, in contrast to most of the other kinds of stigmatization, it is usually not visible. Thus, it can be concealed. But nevertheless it exerts its destructive force on the people concerned. They have to worry constantly about being discovered or betrayed and looking like a fraud.

The ways of combating or overcoming the consequences of stigma differ, depending on the type of stigmatization. People who are excluded or persecuted because they belong to a minority group use their group affiliation for solidarity and perhaps also to put up resistance. They develop methods in their group to defend themselves against the social and cultural devaluation by others. People with stigma at birth, for example, through physical disfigurement, learn—at least in the best case—to deal with the stigma from childhood onward: but only in the best case, for instance, if the familial social environment or the societal conditions support them. On the one hand, people with stigma acquired through illness have the chance to develop a healthy, strong identity before the outbreak of the illness and to defend themselves accordingly. On the other hand, until that time they have lived in a world in which they have shared the prejudices that are now directed against them. And now, they may use these prejudices, which they do not immediately discard when they become ill, against themselves. In this context, one speaks of self-stigmatization. This phenomenon represents an approach for a third party to help overcome the stigma. This refers to individual help that should start right at the beginning of the stigmatizing illness.

Wherever there is stigmatization, attempts are made to reduce or even abolish it through influencing the social community. In the past decades, such so-called anti-stigma campaigns have been undertaken for mentally ill people almost everywhere in the world. Opinions differ on how successful they have been. However, there is some indication that the attempt to change societal attitudes is an arduous path that is destined to fail if the society itself favors intolerant attitudes and behaviors. On the other hand, societal development that favors tolerance and inclusion is also possible. Whenever attempting to reduce stigmatization, we should pay special attention to such societal tendencies and use them for our anti-stigma work.

Literature

Angermeyer MC, Siara CS (1994a) Effect of assassination attempts on Lafontaine and Schäuble on public opinion about psychiatric patients. Part 1: 1990 development. [In German]. Nervenarzt 65:41–48

Angermeyer MC, Siara CS (1994b) Effects on assassination attempts on Lafontaine and Schäuble on public opinion about psychiatric patients. Part 2: 1991 development. [In German]. Nervenarzt 65:49–56

Cumming E, Cumming J (1957) Closed ranks. An experiment in mental health education. Harvard University Press, Cambridge, MA

Duden (1980/2007/2010) Fremdwörterbuch. Mannheim: Duden-Verlag

Finzen A (1969) The doctor, the patient and society. Gustav Fischer, Stuttgart

Flick U (1995) Psychologie des Sozialen. Repräsentationen in Wissen und Sprache. Rowohlr, Reinbeck

Garfinkel H (1956) Conditions of successful degradation ceremonies. Am J Sociol 61:420–424

Gerhardt U (1986) Patientenkarrieren. Suhrkamp, Frankfurt/Main

Goffman E (1961) Asylums. Essay on the social situation of mental patients and other inmates. Anchor Books, Garden City

Goffman E (1963) Stigma. Notes on the management of spoiled identity. Prentice-Hall, Englewood Cliffs

Hoffmann-Richter U (2000) Psychiatrie in der Zeitung. Urteile und Vorurteile. Edition Das Narrenschiff im Psychiatrie-Verlag, Bonn

Hoffmann-Richter U, Alder B, Finzen A (1998) "Vermischte Meldungen". Ein kriminogenes Leiden. Die Schizophrenie im Lokalteil der Neuen Zürcher Zeitung. Krankenhauspsychiatrie 9:110–115

Moscovici S (1961) La psychoanalyse, son image et son public. Presses Universitaires Française, Paris

Moscovici S (1984) The phenomena of social representations. In: Farr RM, Moscovici S (eds) Social representations. Cambridge University Press, Cambridge, pp 3–69

Müller KE (1996) Der Krüppel. CH Beck, München

Peters UH (1999) Wörterbuch der Psychiatrie und Medizinischen Psychologie. 5. Auflage. Urban & Schwarzenberg

Sonntag S (1977) Illness as metaphor. Farrar, Strauss and Giroux, New York

Uhlemann T (1990) Stigma and normality. Vandenhoeck & Ruprecht, Göttingen

Structures and Types of Stigma

3

Lindsay Sheehan, Katherine Nieweglowski,
and Patrick W. Corrigan

Stigma is a complex phenomenon described by the intersection of structures and types. In this chapter, we describe components of these structures, which largely derive from social psychological research, and types, which reflect mechanisms of stigma and mental illness. This includes a discussion of stigma as experienced by family members and more implicit forms of stigma. These constructs sometimes vary by mental illness so this chapter summarizes research in this area as well (Box 3.1).

Information Box 3.1: A Brief Overview on Stigma
- Stigma is comprised of three social-cognitive structures: stereotypes, prejudices, and discrimination.
- Three common stereotypes of mental illness are dangerousness, incompetence, and permanence, which can often result in discriminatory behaviors against the individual.
- Mental illness stigma includes the following types: public stigma, self-stigma, label avoidance, structural stigma, and courtesy stigma.
- The stigma of mental illness varies depending on diagnosis, symptoms, visibility, and multiple group membership.

L. Sheehan (✉) • K. Nieweglowski • P.W. Corrigan
Department of Psychology, Illinois Institute of Technology, 3300 S Federal St,
Chicago, IL 60616, USA
e-mail: lsheehan@iit.edu; knieweg1@hawk.iit.edu; corrigan@iit.edu

© Springer International Publishing Switzerland 2017
W. Gaebel et al. (eds.), *The Stigma of Mental Illness - End of the Story?*,
DOI 10.1007/978-3-319-27839-1_3

Social Psychological Structures

In his seminal work, sociologist Erving Goffman (1963) described stigma as comprised of (a) tribal identities (race, ethnicity), (b) abominations of body (physical abnormalities), and (c) blemishes of individual character (e.g., mental illness, addiction). Since Goffman's era, social psychology has contributed to the understanding of stigma on ethnicity, gender, sexual orientation, and health conditions through the application of the social-cognitive model. This model is useful in explaining the process of stigma development for people with mental illness in particular. According to the social-cognitive model (Table 3.1), stereotypes, prejudice, and discrimination are components of stigma formation. Stereotypes are public attitudes (e.g., "Most people think women are bad drivers"), prejudice is the emotional reaction resulting from agreement with public attitudes ("Yes, women *are* clueless when it comes to driving- and I'm nervous to ride with them"), and discrimination is the behavior that results from stereotypes and prejudices (e.g., female drivers are not hired at the same rate as males). For stigma to occur, the public must first identify difference and then label the difference between themselves and the stigmatized group (Link and Phelan 2001). In some stigmatized groups, such as blacks and females, group membership is readily apparent. In the case of mental illness, social cues such as eccentric appearance, the presence of symptoms, or overt labeling ("I know that guy; he's bipolar") provide the foundation from which the cognitive-behavioral process unfolds. When a person is identified as a member, or potential member, of a stigmatized group, stereotypes associated with that group are activated, and the person is labeled as a group member. Stigma occurs when the cultural environment dictates that label as negative and when there is a distinction between the stigmatized and the stigmatizer ("She's a woman and won't be able to handle

Table 3.1 A matrix for understanding stigma

	Public stigma	Self-stigma	Label avoidance	Structural stigma
Stereotype (cognitive)	People with mental illness are violent	People with mental illness are incompetent	People with mental illness are "psycho"	People with mental illness are lazy
Prejudice (affective)	Landlord feels scared of Bob because he has a mental illness	I am a person with mental illness and therefore incompetent. Who would want to date me?	I have a mental illness and am ashamed to be seen as "psycho"	I feel disgusted by Joann; if she really wanted a job, she could try harder
Discrimination (behavior)	Landlord won't rent apartment to Bob	I think "why try" and stop looking for a relationship	I don't tell my boss I need time off to see a therapist for fear I will lose my job	Funding cuts for employment programs in mental health

this truck like us men") (Link and Phelan 2001). This results in the loss of status and opportunity for the stigmatized group in the form of discrimination.

Stereotypes and Prejudice

Although stereotypes may facilitate information-processing speed and provide social information (Bodenhausen and Richeson 2010), stereotypes are often not based in fact and change over time within a particular culture (Angermeyer et al. 2014b). For example, many in the USA are familiar with the stereotype that women are bad drivers. Statistically, however, females are less likely than males to be involved in vehicle accidents and engage in less risky driving practices (Insurance Institute for Highway Safety 2013; Li et al. 1998). At one time, Irish-Americans were viewed as lazy, unintelligent, and alcoholic and were discriminated against in housing and employment. Today, Irish-Americans are seen in a much more favorable public light. Likewise, stereotypes about mental illness are overgeneralization about the group that vary by cultural context (Pescosolido et al. 2008).

Whereas stereotypes are thoughts based on public opinion, prejudice occurs when people endorse the stereotype and experience negative affective reactions to the stigmatized person. We may be aware that people generally believe women are bad drivers but may disagree with that stereotype and therefore do not stigmatize. However, if we endorse the stereotype of women as bad drivers, when we get in the car with a woman, we may feel scared or annoyed. Similarly, if we agree with the stereotype that people with depression are lazy, we may blame them for their illness, get angry, and deny them our social support. Prejudice thus links the stereotype with the discriminatory behavior. To fully provide a basis for understanding stigma, we will examine mental illness specific stereotypes and prejudice in the categories of dangerousness, incompetence, and permanence (see Fig. 3.1).

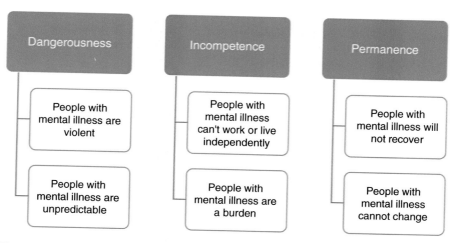

Fig. 3.1 Common stereotypes of mental illness

Dangerousness Among the most prominent and problematic stereotypes applied specifically to people with mental illness are those of dangerousness or unpredictability ("Those people with schizophrenia can become violent at any moment and go on a shooting rampage") (Broussard et al. 2012; Link et al. 1999; Haywood and Bright 1997). When landlords endorse the stereotype of a person with schizophrenia as dangerous, they may be afraid to have such a person as a tenant and may deny their rental applications. Research shows that the stereotype of people with mental illness as dangerous impacts how willing the public is to have people with serious mental illness as friends, neighbors, and colleagues (Angermeyer and Matschinger 2005). Exaggerated media portrayals of people with mental illness are implicated in the development and exacerbation of this stereotype (Vahabzadeh et al. 2011; Haller et al. 2006; Stout et al. 2004; Michalak et al. 2011). When someone with schizophrenia commits a violent crime, news organizations may selectively report the event, focusing on the mental health diagnosis of the person over the crime itself (Angermeyer and Schulze 2001). This strengthens the connection between schizophrenia and violence in the mind of the public and further promotes the stereotype of dangerousness. The public views people with mental illness as much more dangerous than the research suggests they actually are; other factors such as age, gender, and ethnicity are in fact stronger predictors of violence than mental illness status (Corrigan et al. 2004). Additionally, those with mental illness are more likely to be victims of violent crime than perpetrators of violence (Choe et al. 2008).

Incompetence Another commonly endorsed stereotype of mental illness is that of incompetence ("That bipolar guy should not be making his own decisions! He doesn't know what he's doing") (Pescosolido et al. 2013). Endorsement of the incompetence stereotype can lead family members or care providers to assume a paternalistic role and behave in a controlling or coercive manner by unnecessarily assuming guardianship, payeeship, or other decision-making roles. People with mental illness are denied access to more independent living options when assumed that they are not competent to live on their own. Similarly, in the workplace, employees with mental illness endure teasing, hostile attitudes, and comments insulting their cognitive abilities (Jenkins and Carpenter-Song 2009).

Permanence and Constancy Finally, mental illnesses are viewed by the public as severe and chronic ("Those people with schizophrenia never really recover – it's just a downward spiral") (Hayward and Bright 1997). When the public see mental health conditions as unchangeable, there may be less emphasis on rehabilitation, treatment, and recovery. Independent living opportunities may be forgone in favor of long-term treatment models such as nursing homes and institutions because of this mind-set. When we see mental illness as unchangeable, we may be more prone to categorize those with a psychiatric diagnosis as different – and justify different behavior toward them. Those who conceptualize mental illness as biologically based, and thus less changeable, may be at greater risk for displaying stigma toward people with mental illness (Schomerus et al. 2014).

Moderators of Stigma Development

Additional variables moderate the development and expression of stigma. Goffman (1963) first suggested visibility as an important factor. Those people who are visible because of personal appearance or self-identification will be more closely associated with stigma's effects. We discuss the concept of visibility further in our section on label avoidance. Controllability, fear, and familiarity also contribute to stigma expression and are discussed below (Bos et al. 2013; Corrigan et al. 2001).

Controllability and Responsibility Controllability refers to the extent to which group membership and its prejudice is under the person's agency. For example, lung cancer is generally perceived as high in controllability under the assumption that lung cancer is caused by preventable smoking behavior. In contrast, breast cancer is viewed as less controllable (Mosher and Danoof-Burg 2007). When the public believes that serious mental illness results from personal weakness (and thus is more controllable), they are more likely to stigmatize (Jorm and Griffiths 2008). Similar to controllability, those who are perceived as somehow responsible for the stigmatizing condition are also judged more harshly (Corrigan and Watson 2005). Blame and shame are results of public opinions that people with a psychiatric diagnosis choose their condition or could achieve recovery if they just took their medication or tried to work harder on treatment goals. Weiner (1995) distinguishes between onset and offset responsibility. Whereas onset responsibility refers to how responsible the person is for the development of condition or group membership, offset responsibility is how well they are able to manage recovery. People with obesity, for example, are seen as having both high onset and offset responsibility; therefore, they may be more stigmatized than other conditions in which onset and offset responsibilities are lower (Malterud and Ulriksen 2011).

Fear Groups associated with dangerous-related stereotypes, such as those with drug addiction and mental illness, tend to experience greater stigma (Janulis et al. 2013). When the dangerous stereotype is agreed with and applied to someone, fear will result. Fear then translates into stigma (Corrigan et al. 2002). For example, social distance measures show research participants who report fear of people with schizophrenia are less willing to have someone diagnosed with schizophrenia as a neighbor, friend, or romantic partner (Corrigan et al. 2002).

Familiarity Members of the public who know someone with mental illness or have personal experiences themselves with psychiatric problems generally have more positive attitudes toward those with mental illness desire lower levels of social distance (Corrigan et al. 2001; Broussard et al. 2012). Familiarity is defined as experience and knowledge related to mental illness and occurring on a continuum. Those with lived experience with depression will have higher familiarity than those who have an acquaintance with the disorder or who have done reading on the subject. The link between familiarity and social distance is important when designing anti-stigma interventions, as familiarity can be fairly easily enhanced.

Discrimination

Discrimination occurs when overt behaviors reflect stereotypes and prejudice in ways that limit or devalue the stigmatized group members. In the female driver example, women may be discouraged or prohibited from pursuing careers in the transportation industry or be subject to snide comments from male passengers. Attitudes and biases influence behaviors directed toward people with mental illness as well (Stull et al. 2013). Discriminatory behavior applied to those with mental illness is divided into three categories: avoidance and withdrawal, segregation, and coercion (see Table 3.2). We examine these three categories of stigma in detail and discuss the concept of interactional discrimination.

Avoidance and Withdrawal Avoidance and withdrawal may impact people in employment, housing, school, health care, and public space. Employers will not hire, landlords will not rent, and schools will deny admission or fail to provide appropriate support services. When someone with a visible mental illness walks down the sidewalk or sits down on the bus, people may cross the street or move to another seat, distancing themselves from that person. Avoidance and withdrawal are driven largely by the fear stereotype ("I don't want that person with mental illness threatening my tenants or shooting up my workplace"). Avoidance may also be driven by annoyance or disgust. In one large international survey, over half of those with schizophrenia felt that others avoided them because of their diagnosis (Harangozo et al. 2014). Neighbors do not want a mental health center or group home located in their area, because it will blight their community and bring down property values. Supervisors can deny reasonable employment accommodations, threaten to fire the employee, and withhold opportunities for advancement when someone discloses a mental illness or goes through a period of hospitalization while employed (Russinova et al. 2011). People with mental illness also experience discrimination within the health-care system, suffering from disparities in quality of care and health-care options (Barry et al. 2010; Druss et al. 2002).

Table 3.2 Discrimination categories and examples

Avoidance and withdrawal	Employers will not hire
	Landlords will not lease
	Doctors will not treat
	Members of community avoid social interaction
Coercion	Involuntary hospitalization
	Outpatient commitment
	Forced medication
	Guardianship of person or finances
Segregation	State hospitals
	Mental health ghettos
	Jails

Segregation Segregation reflects large-scale, systematic avoidance and paternalism. Although large mental asylums of the past have been replaced by more community-based options, those with psychiatric disabilities may have symptoms that preclude earned income or may experience discrimination in hiring and housing (Corrigan et al. 2006a, b, c; Newman and Goldman 2009). Having few options for housing, people with psychiatric disability may be segregated in nursing homes, group homes, or other residential housing that provides few opportunities for inclusion and social participation with the community. Additionally, people with mental illness disproportionately end up in poor neighborhoods with substandard housing, violence, and limited access to transportation and health care (Draine et al. 2002; Topora et al. 2014). Although this has changed with the advent of supported employment, historically, people with psychiatric disabilities were segregated in sheltered workshops rather than employment in more integrated settings.

Coercion Stereotypes depicting those with mental illness as incompetent, weak, incurable, or violent lead to coercive practices. Involuntary hospital commitments were historically wrought with claims of coercion. While legislation to protect rights has expanded in the past decades, specific practices associated with involuntary hospitalization such as seclusion, restraint, forced medication, and harsh police interactions are still overly controlling (Strauss et al. 2013). In an examination of psychiatric inpatients in one Veteran's Administration hospital, nearly half had been transported to the hospital by law enforcement, 28 % had been physically restrained, and 22 % had been forced to take medications (Strauss et al. 2013). Emotional reactions to involuntary hospitalization, more than the specific coercive practices themselves, are connected to well-being for people with mental illness (Rüsch et al. 2014).

Mandatory treatments outside the hospital setting are common in the USA. Involuntary outpatient commitment or community treatment orders are sometimes applied to those leaving the criminal justice system or inpatient treatment, While court-ordered treatment may have a positive impact on symptoms and social functioning, these consumers may perceive the practice as overly coercive, endorse greater stigma, and enjoy a lower quality of life (Hiday and Ray 2010; Link et al. 2008; Swartz and Swanson 2004). The method by which the mandatory treatment is presented and implemented may also impact the perception of coercion, suggesting the need for peer involvement and development of more accountable and transparent practices (Munetz and Frese 2001).

Subtle forms of coercion occur in the community as well. In the practice of representative payeeship, a designated individual or organization (such as a mental health agency) manages money for the person with mental illness to ensure that basic needs for housing and food are met (Luchins et al. 2003). However, a representative payee can potentially withhold money unless the person engages in treatment or acquiesces to the payees' preferences (Swartz and Swanson 2004). In regard to police interactions, people describe coercive practices in which they are rushed, given little opportunity to explain the situation, or addressed disrespectfully

(Watson et al. 2010). Additionally, when people with mental illness feel discouraged from starting a family (Harangozo et al. 2014), excluded from a parenting role (Jeffery et al. 2013), or given depot medications (Patel et al. 2010), these actions are often perceived as coercive by the diagnosed individual.

Interactional Discrimination

Some of the examples of avoidance, segregation, and coercion involve subtle behavior change that emerges during interactions with a stigmatized person. Link and Phelan (2014) use the term interactional discrimination to describe this phenomenon, a concept which parallels the concept of microaggression as described in the racial discrimination literature (Wong et al. 2014). Microaggressive acts might involve white people locking their door or clutching their purse when a young, black male walks by. During interactional discrimination for someone with a visible mental illness, a store clerk may speak with an air of superiority, disgust, annoyance, or reticence. Over time, interactional discrimination solidifies the differences between stigmatized and "normal," leading to social exclusion or erosion of social status (Link and Phelan 2014). When these subtle behaviors occur on a daily basis, the person with mental illness may avoid contact with the store clerk and others who talk to them in a patronizing way. As a result, the person can become socially isolated, angry, or ashamed. In fact, verbal and nonverbal stigma messages within the context of anonymous social interactions were the most commonly cited by people with schizophrenia as a source of daily stigma (Jenkins and Carpenter-Song 2009).

Interactional discrimination can also be experienced in communications with more proximal social relationships. Over one-third of people with schizophrenia have felt disrespected by mental health workers (Harangozo et al. 2014), which may come in the form of disregard for personal preferences or doubt of decision-making capabilities. In the workplace, people with mental illness report disrespectful language, jokes, and other small interactions that contribute to an uncomfortable work environment (Russinova et al. 2011). Supervisors sometimes doubt the worker's ability to meet work demands, expecting the person with a mental diagnosis to work harder in order to compensate (Russinova et al. 2011).

Types of Stigma

Thus far, we have focused primarily on the type of public stigma. We now examine the effect of public stigma on the stigmatized individual, their family, and society at large. We define and discuss different types of stigma, including self-stigma, label avoidance, structural stigma, courtesy stigma, double stigma, stigma power, and automatic stigma (see Table 3.3).

Table 3.3 Types of stigma

Stigma type	Definition
Public stigma	Public endorsement of prejudice and discrimination toward minority group
Self-stigma	Person in minority group internalizes public stereotypes/ prejudices and applies them to his or her life
Label avoidance	Person with mental illness avoids engaging in activities that reveal his/her diagnosis
Structural stigma	Public and private sector policies that unintentionally restrict opportunities of the minority group
Courtesy stigma	Stigma experience by those who are in close contact with the stigmatized group (mental health workers, friends, family)
Stigma power	A means through which stigmatizers maintain social power through control, exploitation, and exclusion of the stigmatized group
Automatic stigma	Stigmatizing thoughts, feelings, and behaviors that occur automatically with little or no conscious awareness
Double stigma or multiple stigma	Stigma which is compounded by membership in more than one stigmatizing group (LGBT, poor, obese, etc.)

Self-Stigma

When individuals with mental illness are aware of public stereotypes (i.e., public stigma) and incorporate those stereotypes into their self-concept, internalized or self-stigma results (Munoz et al. 2011). Three steps are involved in the development of self-stigma (see Fig. 3.2). The person with mental illness is *aware* of the public stigma ("People with depression are lazy"), must then *agree* with the stigma ("Yes, that's true – depressed people are lazy"), and finally *apply* the stigma to their own lives ("I have depression, so I'm lazy") (Corrigan and Calabrese 2005; Corrigan et al. 2006a, b, c). Internalized stigma can hurt self-esteem ("I'm a lazy slob") (Drapalski et al. 2013; Boyd et al. 2014) or invoke feelings of shame and self-contempt (Rüsch et al. 2014). Self-efficacy suffers ("I can't beat this feeling") (Drapalski et al. 2013), and the person experiences the "why try" effect (Corrigan et al. 2009): "Why should I try to get out of the house and visit friends? They will not want to associate with a person like me" or "Why try to get a job? I'm disabled." Those endorsing higher self-stigma are less empowered to take action and make important life choices (Rüsch et al. 2014; Drapalski et al. 2013). One recent longitudinal study lends support to the process whereby public stigma becomes internalized (Vogel et al. 2013). In a sample of college students, public stigma endorsement at the initial interview predicted self-stigma 3 months later, whereas self-stigma at 3 months was not predictive of initial public stigma levels. Self-stigma appears relatively stable over time (Lysaker et al. 2012) and has been connected to lower quality of life (Rüsch et al. 2014).

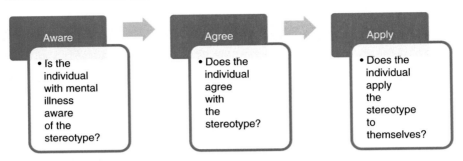

Fig. 3.2 Steps in development of self-stigma

Label Avoidance

When a person with mental illness is conscious of the stigma surrounding the diagnosis, they may engage in label avoidance to evade the stigmatic label. Consequently, psychiatric care is compromised as individuals avoid entering treatment centers, taking psychiatric medications, or asking employers for job accommodations. A majority of people with schizophrenia express some desire to conceal their diagnosis from others (Harangozo et al. 2014). In fact, members of the public who more readily assign labels to those with mental illness are also more likely to believe that people with schizophrenia are dangerous and desire a greater social distance from them (Angermeyer et al. 2004; Pattyn et al. 2013). To elude the label, some refrain from seeking services, do not utilize services fully, or drop out completely (Corrigan et al. 2014; Clemente et al. 2014; Parcesepe and Cabassa 2013; Ben-Zeev et al. 2012). Being seen as someone who takes psychiatric medications is particularly stigmatizing and may lead to discontinuation or sporadic use of medications (Jenkins and Carpenter-Song 2009). In a study exploring posttraumatic stress and depression among US Army members, barriers to care included leaders who discouraged the use of mental health-care services and the fear that mental health assistance would be viewed as a weakness and damaging to participants' military careers (Chapman et al. 2014). A large population study in the Netherlands and Belgium examined relationships between self-stigma and help-seeking (Reynders et al. 2014). Although the two countries have comparable access to quality mental health services, Flemish individuals experience greater shame and self-stigma as well as engage in lower rates of help-seeking behavior than their Dutch counterparts. Accompanying suicide rates in Belgium are significantly higher than those in the Netherlands, pointing to the salience of label avoidance.

Labeling is a function of visibility; those with more apparent symptoms will be readily labeled and will have more extensive supports available in terms of health care, family, and friends. However, these same individuals will be more vulnerable to the pernicious effects of public stigma in the form of social rejection and discrimination from those outside their support network. This is referred to as the labeling paradox (Perry 2011). A person with schizophrenia who is poorly groomed and is responding to auditory hallucinations may have an easier time enrolling in treatment, qualifying for disability benefits, and receiving intensive services than an individual whose disability is less pronounced. However, when this same person rides the subway train or applies for job, he will likely experience negative reactions because of the greater visibility.

While some individuals have little choice in the labels applied to them, others with less visible symptoms must make decisions about whether to talk about a mental health diagnosis. In the employment arena, those who disclose a psychiatric disability are entitled to reasonable accommodations under the Americans with Disabilities Act (ADA) to help them perform the job. This can include time off to attend doctor appointments, job protection in case of hospitalization, or a job coach to provide support. When people with psychiatric disabilities engage in label avoidance, they conceal their condition fearing discrimination but also forego these important benefits (Cummings et al. 2013). Similarly, when people do not talk about their experiences with mental illness, they avoid being labeled but cannot reap the returns of social support. Some individuals use an informal process to evaluate how, and if, they should disclose their diagnosis (Michalak et al. 2011), while formal programs to facilitate disclosure decisions have also been developed (e.g., Corrigan et al. 2013). This judicious process of disclosure can depend on the situation or setting and even the person receiving the information (Michalak et al. 2011).

Structural Stigma

When the policies of governmental and private institutions restrict the opportunities of people with mental illness, either intentionally or unintentionally, this leads to structural stigma (Angermeyer et al. 2014a, b; Corrigan et al. 2004). Jim Crow laws in the USA are an example of intentional structural stigma that prevented African Americans from equal access to employment, education, and public resources. One example of intentional structural stigma in relation to mental illness is statutes that restrict parental rights because of past history of mental illness (Corrigan et al. 2005). In addition, some states restrict those with a mental health diagnosis from voting, serving on juries, or holding public office (Corrigan et al. 2004). These laws stem from public stigmas of incompetency, violence, and treatment resistance of mental illness and become especially problematic when enforced without regard for reinstatement of rights upon recovery or remittance of disability (Corrigan et al. 2004).

Examples of unintentional structural stigma may involve biased media characterizations (Corrigan et al. 2004), diminished quality of care (Thornicroft 2013), access to care (Link and Phelan 2001), or exclusion from community participation (Zubritsky et al. 2006). Those with mental illness and other disabilities sometimes live in institutionalized care such as nursing homes, despite the fact that they can live in more integrated housing in the community if provided the support and opportunity (Cremin 2012). Olmstead v. L.C. (1999) in the USA directed states to offer individuals with disabilities who were living in nursing homes access to community living rather than institution (Zubritsky et al. 2006).

Another example of structural stigma is lack of mental health parity. Historically, mental health coverage through insurance companies has not been on par with that of physical health coverage (Barry et al. 2010). Health insurance systems cap mental health expenditures and yearly visits to lower than those for physical health conditions or fail to provide coverage at all for mental health or substance abuse. Link and Phelan (2001) argue that less money is allocated to research and treatment for mental illness in comparison to other health disorders and mental health professionals opt out of public systems that offer less lucrative employment options. Legislation and court decisions such as the Mental Health Parity Act of 2008 and the Patient Protection and Affordable Care Act have recently challenged structural stigma by expanding insurance coverage and reducing out-of-pocket costs for those with mental illness (Cummings et al. 2013). However, disparities in mental health funding and insurance coverage continue to exist; all individuals with psychiatric disabilities are not uniformly protected (Cummings et al. 2013).

Courtesy Stigma

Goffman (1963) coined the term *courtesy stigma* to describe the negative stereotypes, prejudice, and discrimination experienced by those who are associated with the stigmatized person. Courtesy stigma, also called stigma by association or associative stigma, may apply to friends, family, service providers, employers, or other individuals who appear connected to the stigmatized group (Pryor et al. 2012; Halter 2008; Kulik et al. 2008; van der Sanden et al. 2013). Kulik and colleagues (2008) describe courtesy stigma occurring within the workplace when coworkers associate with the stigmatized person; stigma "spills over" onto them. Excluding and providing social distance between ourselves and stigmatized others may serve to avoid courtesy stigma (Pryor et al. 2012). Mental health providers experience courtesy stigma when they feel shameful about sharing their professional identity with others or avoid being seen with their clients in public situations. A survey of nurses revealed that of ten nursing specialties, psychiatric nursing was perceived as the least preferred, and psychiatric nurses were described as less skilled, less logical, less dynamic, and less respected than those of other specialties (Halter 2008).

Family Stigma Family stigma is a special case of courtesy stigma that applies to parents, siblings, spouses, children, and other relatives of those with mental illness (Corrigan and Miller 2004). Family stigma manifests in the form of ridicule, gossip, or disinterest about the impacted family member. It may also appear in structural ways such as lack of respite services, self-help support groups, and bureaucratic hurdles to obtaining care for family members (Angermeyer et al. 2003). Ethnic minority families may experience stronger family stigma than those of European heritage (Wong et al. 2009).

Stereotypes vary according to family member role (Corrigan et al. 2006a, b, c). For example, parents of children with mental illness experience blame for onset of illness (onset responsibility), whereas spouses and siblings are seen as more responsible for offset. Historically, parental blame for creating a home environment as cause of mental illness was much stronger in the public sentiment than it is today; however, these ideas continue to persist (Mukolo and Heflinger 2011). To some degree, spouses and siblings are perceived as unsupportive or detrimental to their loved one's recovery toward mental illness, whereas children of those with mental illness are seen as contaminated by their parent's illness (Burk and Sher 1990; Corrigan et al. 2006a, b, c). When the public views mental illness as having a genetic basis, they are more likely to believe that a child of someone with schizophrenia or depression will develop the same illness and will thus apply a higher level of courtesy stigma (Koschade and Lynd-Stevenson 2011).

Just as individuals with mental illness internalize public stigma into self-stigma, family members may also feel shame when they blame themselves for contributing to a family member's illness (Moses 2013). Family members who feel greater stigma by association may be at greater risk of distancing themselves from their loved one and experiencing greater psychological distress (van der Sanden et al. 2013). When families fear stigmatizing labels, they may try to keep the diagnosis a secret, avoiding seeking help for their family member and for themselves (Corrigan et al. 2014).

Double Stigma

Those who belong to more than one socially disadvantaged group may have multiple identity statuses and experience double stigma (Gary 2005; Roe et al. 2007; Sanders et al. 2004). About half of people with serious mental illness report discrimination resulting either from mental health status, physical disability, substance abuse problems, ethnic or sexual minority status, or other stigmatizing conditions (Sanders Thompson et al. 2004). Research on the combination of obesity and mental illness concludes that advocacy should address multiple sources of stigma (Mizock 2012). In these cases, the effects of stigmatization could be multiplicative or differentially impact facets of life (Mizock 2012; Glover et al. 2010). Sexual minority status may also impact leisure and social activities, whereas psychiatric disability stigma would be more relevant for employment.

According to minority stress theory, members of ethnic minorities experience stress as a result of low social status (Meyer 2003). The stress of being a minority may in turn lead to psychological distress and impact performance in social situations such as the workplace (Velez et al. 2013). For those with mental illness who are also of minority ethnic status, this additional stress may exacerbate mental health symptoms and increase likelihood of discriminatory treatment. Consistent with this model, USA Marines members who experience racial discrimination during military service are more likely to develop mental health problems (Foynes et al. 2013).

Stigma Power

Link and Phelan (2014) suggest that those in power marginalize others. Stigma power functions to keep people *down*, *in*, and *away*. Stigmatized individuals are kept *down* through denial of resources such as wealth and status, are kept *in* through secrecy of their condition, and are kept *away* to avoid contamination, either physically or socially by the condition (Link and Phelan 2014). Likewise, Kelly (2006) argues that special interest groups supporting mental health have limited power and that people with mental illness have been systematically limited from participation in important life areas. Supporting these assumptions, in a large UK survey, people with mental illness reported fewer social resources (i.e., social capital) than those without a mental diagnosis. Especially when stigma was perpetrated by friends and family and when there was less community participation due to the anticipation of stigma, people with mental illness experienced lower levels of social capital (Webber et al. 2014). Thus, although this idea should be more thoroughly explored empirically, the subtle and systematic processes of stigma power are important to include in the discussion of stigma.

Automatic Stigma

Whereas explicit attitudes are within the realm of conscious control, implicit attitudes are those that occur beyond the individual's conscious awareness (Brener et al. 2013). An example of explicit stigma is the conscious belief that a person with mental illness is helpless or dangerous. In contrast, implicit bias or automatic stigma would be the unconscious tendency to limit a person's autonomy (e.g., control over finances, medications, etc.).

Implicit stigma is manifest in more subtle and concealed forms and requires different measurement techniques than explicit, self-report measures (Stier and Hinshaw 2007). Proponents of implicit attitude measures contend that prejudices are revealed when research participants are unable to consciously mask their socially unacceptable beliefs (Stier and Hinshaw 2007). A key tool designed to measure implicit stigma is the Implicit Association Test (IAT) (Greenwald et al. 1998), consisting of computer-administrated association tasks between opposite targets and attributes (Schnabel et al. 2008). The IAT has been used to measure many types of automatic stigma, including those relating to racial, gender, and socioeconomic differences. The test measures the amount of time that it takes to respond to a stimulus, allowing researchers to quantify the strength of the association. For example, if participants respond more quickly to the key corresponding to blameworthy when seeing a mental illness-related stimulus, then this would indicate a stronger association between people with mental illness and blameworthiness (Teachman et al. 2006).

Although the IAT is a popular method of implicit measurement, very few studies have examined the predictive validity of the test. Greenwald and colleagues (2009) concluded that the IAT performed better on certain socially sensitive topics (e.g., racial bias), while explicit self-report measures predicted attitudes on topics such as consumer preferences and intimate relationships. Oswald and colleagues (2013) conducted a meta-analysis to further determine the IAT's predictive validity on a broader range of domains related to racial discrimination and how these compared to explicit measures. However, this meta-analysis did not reveal a link between IAT scores and verbal or nonverbal behavior. In order to completely trust in the interpretations of the IAT, greater improvement is required in the correlations between implicit and explicit measures of racial discrimination (Oswald et al. 2013). Despite this controversy over the IAT, it is still a common tool used to measure implicit attitudes including those related to mental illness.

Stull and colleagues (2013) applied the IAT to a study examining bias among assertive community treatment (ACT) practitioners and its influence on the endorsement of control treatment mechanisms. ACT is intensive case management, or care coordination for individuals with mental illness that includes extensive monitoring of medications, control over the patient's finances, and outpatient commitment (i.e., involuntary treatment of community members). Research shows implicit bias was found to predict a higher endorsement of the more controlling aspects of ACT treatment (Stull et al. 2013). Additionally, clinical professionals and graduate students with higher implicit bias were more likely to overdiagnose patients (Peris et al. 2008). In another study, Brener and colleagues (2013) found that although mental health-care workers showed positive explicit attitudes, the IAT uncovered implicit bias. Negative implicit attitudes predicted decrease in helping intent among the workers, while explicit attitudes did not (Brener et al. 2013). These findings suggest that implicit attitudes of mental health-care workers may have a stronger influence, relative to explicit bias, on the quality of care that is provided for individuals with mental illness.

Researchers have also examined automatic self-stigma or unconscious negative attitudes toward the self. A study by Rüsch and colleagues (2010) administered implicit measures to people with serious mental illness to examine whether internalized stigma manifests through automatic processes. The results of two brief IATs showed that implicit and explicit self-stigma independently predicted a lower quality of life (Rüsch et al. 2010). Overall, both implicit public stigma (particularly stigma from providers) and implicit self-stigma may prove destructive for those with mental illness; more research on automatic stigma is particularly needed to further evaluate its relationship to outcomes.

Stigma Across Diagnoses

We know that being diagnosed with a mental illness often results in prejudice and discrimination, but differences in stigma exist across diagnoses. In regard to personality disorders, mental health-care professionals often see these patients as uncooperative, hostile, manipulative, and complaining (Fairfax 2011). Alonso and colleagues (2008) noted certain increases in perceived public stigma between individuals with mood and anxiety disorders. Greater stigma was reported among individuals with anxiety disorders in the absence of mood disorders, and the reports increased among individuals with mood disorders in the absence of anxiety disorders. However, even greater stigma was reported among individuals that possessed both a mood and anxiety disorder diagnosis showing that a comorbid diagnosis results in greater discrimination (Alonso et al. 2008). A common misperception of an individual with bipolar disorder (BD) is that he or she is psychotic when, in fact, bipolar I is the only category of BD with prevalence of psychosis. This often leads individuals with BD to be misdiagnosed with a more severe illness. Nevertheless, even if they acquire the correct diagnosis, these individuals often learn to cover up their symptoms and emotions in order to avoid the misconceptions that society places on them (Jasko 2012).

Stigma of Suicide

Many individuals with mental illness have experienced suicidal thoughts or attempted suicide, pointing to the importance of examining public opinions toward suicide and its interaction with mental illness stigma. Using fake obituary vignettes, people who took their own lives were viewed more negatively than those who died from cancer (Sand et al. 2013). Over half of the college students said they would not have a romantic relationship with someone who has attempted suicide in the past year; 20 % would deny a suicide attempter from obtaining US citizenship (Lester and Walker 2006).

Although the stereotypes of people who think about, attempt, or completed suicide may have substantial overlap with those of mental illness, suicide stigma seems to include additional components related to morality, impulsivity, attention seeking, and religious devotion (Witte et al. 2010; Sudak et al. 2008). People who attempt or complete suicide may be seen as refuting religious teachings, selfishly leaving behind loved ones or dependents, or failing to carefully consider all the options. Those who take their own lives are variously identified as irresponsible, cowardly, brave, isolated, and dedicated (Batterham et al. 2013). Thus, stigma of mental illness in general may be compounded by the stigma applied to people who think about or attempt suicide.

Support for those who attempt or consider suicide can be limited by their anticipation of stigma. Just as with mental illness, people who have attempted suicide often conceal or minimize these experiences to avoid labeling and subsequently miss out on opportunities for support or treatment (Czyz et al. 2013). Religious communities and families who endorse stigma of suicide may discourage expression and treatment of suicidal ideation, limiting access to care.

Additionally, courtesy stigma appears to effect the grief process of family survivors. Family members experience negative reactions themselves from extended community upon loss of loved ones to suicide, including tense relations and withdrawal of support (Feigelman et al. 2009). Family members may internalize stigma and blame themselves for the death or for missing any warning signals. when family members of survivors experience more stigma, they also experience greater levels of grief, depression, and suicidal thinking themselves (Feigelman et al. 2009).

Some suggest that life insurance policies that deny payment for suicide deaths reflect intentional structural stigma related to suicide. Others have asserted that funding disparities reflect structural stigma of suicide. For example, the Center for Disease Control (CDC) budget for research on HIV was 50 times higher than that for suicide, despite suicide being the 11th leading cause of death in the USA (Curry et al. 2006). Overall, these findings point to the importance of examining the stigma of suicide as a factor above and beyond the stigma of mental illness.

Summary

The understanding of mental illness stigma has evolved significantly since Goffman's original categorization. Although stereotypes of mental illness vary across diagnoses, three stereotypes are often applied to those with mental illness: (a) people with mental illness are dangerous or unpredictable, (b) people with mental illness are incompetent, and (c) mental illness is chronic and incurable. Prejudice and discrimination occur when people endorse these stereotypes and then act on them. This can mean avoiding the individual in hiring and housing situations, segregating the individual into a special community or institution, or coercing the individual into treatment.

Often times, public stigma can be so influential that the individual also begins to incorporate it into their own self-concept, leading to the construct of self-stigma and causing them to resist the label of mental illness (i.e., label avoidance). The stigma of mental illness can also spill over onto the individual's family and others by association. Mental illness stigma may be further complicated by the fact that people with mental illness may fall into more than one stigmatized group, experiencing prejudice and discrimination based on race, age, ethnicity, physical disability status, or the presence of suicidality. Additionally, stigma power works to socially subjugate those with mental diagnoses, while automatic stigmas operate below the level of consciousness. Although a discussion of erasing stigma is beyond the scope of this chapter, we hope that understanding the types and mechanisms of stigma is useful for starting the discussion of stigma change (Fig. 3.3).

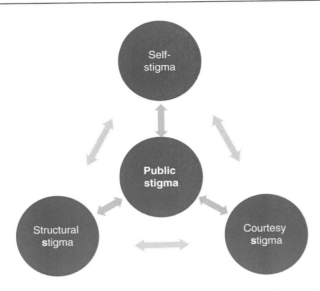

Fig. 3.3 Relationship between types of stigma (Adapted from Pryor and Reeder 2011)

References

Alonso J, Buron A, Bruffaerts R, He Y, Posada-Villa J, Lepine J-P, Angermeyer MC, Levison D, de Girolamo G, Tachimori H, Mneimneh ZN, Medina-Mora ME, Ormel J, Scott KM, Guereje O, Haro JM, Gluzman S, Lee S, Vilagut G, Kessler RC, Von Korff M (2008) Association of perceived stigma and mood and anxiety disorders: results from the world mental health surveys. Acta Psychiatr Scand 118:305–314. doi:10.1111/j.1600-0447.2008.01241

Angermeyer MC, Matschinger H (2005) Labeling-stereotype-discrimination: an investigation of the stigma process. Soc Psychiatry Psychiatr Epidemiol 40:391–395. doi:10.1007/s00127-005-0903-4

Angermeyer MC, Schulze B (2001) Reinforcing stereotypes: how the focus on forensic cases in news reporting may influence public attitudes towards the mentally ill. Int J Law Psychiatry 24(4–5):469–486

Angermeyer MC, Schulze B, Dietrich S (2003) Courtesy stigma: a focus group study of relatives of schizophrenia patients. Soc Psychiatry Psychiatr Epidemiol 38:593–602. doi:10.1007/s00127-003-0680-x

Angermeyer MC, Matschinger H, Corrigan PW (2004) Familiarity with mental illness and social distance from people with schizophrenia and major depression: testing a model using data from a representative population survey. Schizophr Res 69(2–3):175–182. doi:10.1016/S0920-9964(03)00186-5

Angermeyer MC, Matschinger H, Carta MG, Schomerus G (2014a) Changes in the perception of mental illness stigma in Germany over the last two decades. Eur Psychiatry 29(6):390–395. doi:10.1016/j.eurpsy.2013.10.004

Angermeyer MC, Matschinger H, Link BG, Schomerus G (2014b) Public attitudes regarding individual and structural discrimination: two sides of the same coin? Soc Sci Med 103:60–66. doi:10.1016/j.socscimed.2013.11.014

Barry CL, Huskamp HA, Goldman HH (2010) A political history of federal mental health and addiction insurance parity. Milbank Q 88(3):404–433. doi:10.1111/j.1468-0009.2010.00605.x

Batterham PJ, Calear AL, Christensen H (2013) Correlates of suicide stigma and suicide literacy in the community. Suicide Life Threat Behav 43:406–417. doi:10.1111/sltb.12026

Ben-Zeev D, Corrigan PW, Britt TW, Langford L (2012) Stigma of mental illness and service use in the military. J Ment Health 21(3):264–273. doi:10.3109/09638237.2011.621468

Bodenhausen GV, Richeson JA (2010) Prejudice, stereotyping, and discrimination. In: Baumeister RF, Finkel EJ (eds) Advanced social psychology. Oxford University Press, Oxford, pp 341–383

Bos AER, Pryor JB, Reeder GD, Stutterheim SE (2013) Stigma: advances in theory and research. Basic Appl Soc Psychol 35:1–9. doi:10.1080/01973533.2012.746147

Boyd JE, Otilingham PG, DeForge BR (2014) Brief version of the internalized stigma of mental illness (ISMI) scale: psychometric properties and relationship to depression, self-esteem, recovery orientation, empowerment, and perceived devaluation and discrimination. Psychiatr Rehabil J 37:17–23. doi:10.1037/prj0000035l7

Brener L, Grenville R, von Hippel C, Wilson H (2013) Implicit attitudes, emotions, and helping intentions of mental health workers toward their clients. J Nerv Ment Dis 201:460–463. doi:10.1097/NMD.0b013e318294744a

Broussard B, Goulding SM, Talley CL, Compton MT (2012) Social distance and stigma toward individuals with schizophrenia: findings in an urban, African-American community sample. J Nerv Ment Dis 200(11):935–940. doi:10.1097/NMD.0b013e3182718c1b

Chapman PL, Elnitsky C, Thurman RM, Pitts B, Figley C, Unwin B (2014) Posttraumatic stress, depression, stigma and barriers to care among U.S. Army healthcare providers. Traumatol: Int J 20:19–23. doi:10.1037/h009937

Choe JY, Teplin LA, Abram KM (2008) Perpetration of violence, violent victimization, and severe mental illness: balancing public health concerns. Psychiatr Serv 59(2):153–164. doi:10.1176/appi.ps.59.2.153

Clemente S, Schauman O, Graham T, Maggioni F, Evans-Lacko S, Bezborodovs N, Morgan C, Ruschm, N, Brown JS, Thornicroft G (2014) What is the impact of mental health-related stigma on help-seeking? A systematic review of quantitative and qualitative studies. Psychol Med 45(1):11–27. doi:10.1017/S0033291714000129

Corrigan PW, Calabrese JD (2005) Strategies for assessing and diminishing self-stigma. In: Corrigan PW (ed) On the stigma of mental illness: practical strategies for research and social change. American Psychological Association, Washington, DC, pp 239–256. doi:10.1037/10887-011

Corrigan PW, Miller FE (2004) Shame, blame and contamination: a review of the impact of mental illness stigma on family members. J Ment Health 13:537–548. doi:10.1080/09638230400017004

Corrigan PW, Watson AC (2005) Findings from the national comorbidity survey on the frequency of dangerous behavior in individuals with psychiatric disorders. Psychiatry Res 136(2–3):153–162. doi:10.1016/j.psychres.2005.06.005

Corrigan PW, Green A, Lundin R, Kubiak MA, Penn DL (2001) Familiarity with and social distance from people who have serious mental illness. Psychiatr Serv 52(7):953–958

Corrigan PW, Rowan D, Green A, Lundin R, River P, Uphoff-Wasowski K, White K, Kubiak MA (2002) Challenging two mental illness stigmas: personal responsibility and dangerousness. Schizophr Bull 28:293–309

Corrigan PW, Markowitz FE, Watson AC (2004) Structural levels of mental illness stigma and discrimination. Schizophr Bull 30(3):481–491

Corrigan PW, Watson AC, Heyrman M, Warpinski A, Gracia G, Slopen N, Hall LL (2005) Structural stigma in state legislation. Psychiatr Serv 56:557–563. doi:10.1176/appi.ps.56.5.557

Corrigan PW, Larson JE, Watson AC, Boyle M, Barr L (2006a) Solutions to discrimination in work and housing identified by people with mental illness. J Nerv Ment Dis 194:716–718. doi:10.1097/01.nmd.0000235782.18977.de

Corrigan PW, Watson AC, Barr L (2006b) The self-stigma of mental illness: implications for self-esteem and self-efficacy. J Soc Clin Psychol 25:875–884. doi:10.1521/jscp.2006.25.8.875

Corrigan PW, Watson AC, Miller FE (2006c) Blame, shame, and contamination: the impact of mental illness and drug dependence stigma of family members. J Fam Psychol 20:239–246. doi:10.1037/0893-3200.20.2.239

Corrigan PW, Larson JE, Rusch N (2009) Self-stigma and the "why try" effect: impact on life goals and evidence-based practices. World Psychiatry 8:75–81. doi:10.1002/j.2051-5545.2009. tb00218.x

Corrigan PW, Kosyluk KA, Rüsch N (2013) Reducing self-stigma by coming out proud. Am J Public Health 103(5):794–800. doi:10.2105/AJPH.2012.301037

Corrigan PW, Druss BG, Perlick DA (2014) The impact of mental illness stigma on seeking and participating in mental health care. Psychol Sci Public Interes 15(2):37–70. doi:10.1177/1529100614531398

Cremin KM (2012) Challenges to institutionalization: the definition of "institution" and the future of Olmstead litigation. Tex J Civ Liberties Civ Rights 17(2):143–180. doi:10.1177/136345930200600204

Cummings JR, Lucas SM, Druss BG (2013) Addressing public stigma and disparities among persons with mental illness: the role of federal policy. Am J Public Health 103(5):781–785. doi:10.2105/AJPH.2013.301224

Curry CW, De AK, Ikeda RM, Thacker SB (2006) Health burden and funding at the centers for disease control and prevention. Am J Preventative Med 30(3):269–279. doi:10.1016/j.amepre.2005.10.0

Czyz EK, Horwitz AG, Eisenberg D, Kramer A, King CA (2013) Self-reported barriers to professional help seeking among college students at elevated risk for suicide. J Am Coll Health 61(7):398–406. doi:10.1080/07448481.2013.820731

Draine J, Salzer MS, Culhane DP, Hadley TR (2002) Role of social disadvantage in crime, joblessness and homelessness among persons with serious mental illness. Psychiatr Serv. 53(5):565–573. doi:10.1176/appi.ps.53.5.565

Drapalski AL, Lucksted A, Perrin PB, Aakre JM, Brown CH, DeForge BR, Boyd JE (2013) A model of internalized stigma and its effects on people with mental illness. Psychiatr Serv 64:264–269. doi:10.1176/appi.ps.001322012

Druss BG, Rosenheck RA, Desa MM, Perlin JB (2002) Quality of preventative medical care for patients with mental disorders. Med Care 40(2):129–136

Fairfax H (2011) Re-conceiving personality disorders: adaptations on a dimension? Couns Psychol Q 24:313–322. doi:10.1080/09515070.2011.6305

Feigelman W, Gorman BS, Jordan JR (2009) Death Stud 33(7):591–608. doi:10.1080/07481180902979973

Foynes MM, Shipherd JC, Harrington EF (2013) Race and discrimination in the marines. Cult Divers Ethn Minor Psychol 19:111–119. doi:10.1037/a0030567

Gary FA (2005) Stigma: barrier to mental health care among ethnic minorities. Issues Ment Health Nurs 26:979–999. doi:10.1080/01612840500280638

Glover CM, Corrigan P, Wilkniss S (2010) The effects of multiple categorization on perceptions of discrimination, life domains, and stress for individuals with severe mental illness. J Vocat Rehabil 33:113–121. doi:10.3233/JVR-2010-0520

Goffman E (1963) Stigma: notes on the management of spoiled identity. Prentice-Hall, Englewood Cliffs

Greenwald AG, McGhee DE, Schwartz JLK (1998) Measuring individual differences in implicit cognition: the implicit association test. J Pers Soc Psychol 74:1464–1480

Greenwald AG, Poehlman AT, Uhlmann EL, Banaji MR (2009) Understanding and using the implicit association test: III. Meta-analysis of predictive validity. J Pers Soc Psychol 97:17–41. doi:10.1037/a00155

Haller B, Dorries B, Rahn J (2006) Media labeling versus the US disability community identity: a study of shifting cultural language. Disabil Soc 21(1):61–75. doi:10.1080/09687590500375416

Halter MJ (2008) Perceived characteristics of psychiatric nurses: stigma by association. Arch Psychiatr Nurs 22:20–26. doi:10.1016/j.apnu.2007.03.003

Harangozo J, Reneses B, Brohan E, Sebes J, Csukly G, Lopez-Ibor JJ, Sartorius N, Rose D, Thornicroft G (2014) Stigma and discrimination against people with schizophrenia related to medical services. Int J Soc Psychiatry 60(4):359–366. doi:10.1177/0020764013490263

Hayward P, Bright J (1997) Stigma and mental illness: a review and critique. J Ment Health 6:345–354

Hiday VA, Ray B (2010) Arrests two years after exiting a well-established mental health court. Psychiatr Serv 61:463–468. doi:10.1176/appi.ps.61.5.463

Insurance Institute for Highway Safety (2013) Unpublished analysis of data from the U.S. Department of Transportation's Fatality Analysis Reporting System and the National Household Travel Survey. Arlington. Retrieved from http://www.iihs.org/iihs/topics/t/general-statistics/fatalityfacts/gender

Janulis P, Ferrari JR, Fowler P (2013) Understanding public stigma toward substance dependence. J Appl Soc Psychol 43(5):1065–1072. doi:10.1111/jasp.12070

Jasko A (2012) The scarlet letter of mental illness: de-stigmatizing bipolar disorder. Pastor Psychol 61:299–304. doi:10.1007/s11089-012-0436-

Jeffery D, Clement S, Corker E, Howard LM, Murray J, Thornicroft G (2013) Discrimination in relation to parenthood reported by community psychiatric service users in the UK: a framework analysis. BMC Psychiatry 13:120–129. doi:10.1186/1471-244X-13-120

Jenkins JH, Carpenter-Song EA (2009) Awareness of stigma among persons with schizophrenia. J Nerv Ment Dis 197:520–529. doi:10.1097/NMD.0b013e3181aad5e9

Jorm AF, Griffiths KM (2008) The public's stigmatizing attitudes towards people with mental disorders: how important are biomedical conceptualizations? Acta Psychiatr Scand 18:315–321. doi:10.1111/j.1600-0447.2008.01251.x

Kelly BD (2006) The power gap: freedom, power and mental illness. Soc Sci Med 63(8):2118–2128. doi:10.1016/j.socscimed.2006.05.015

Koschade JE, Lynd-Stevenson RM (2011) The stigma of having a parent with mental illness: genetic attributions and associative stigma. Aust J Psychol 63:93–99. doi:10.1111/j.1742-9536.2011.00009.x

Kulik CT, Bainbridge HTJ, Cregan C (2008) Known by the company we keep: stigma-by-association effects in the workplace. Acad Manag Rev 33:216–230. doi:10.2307/20159384

Lester D, Walker RL (2006) The stigma for attempting suicide and the loss to suicide prevention efforts. Crisis J Crisis Interv Suicide Prev 27:147–148. doi:10.1027/0227-5910.27.3.147

Li G, Baker SP, Langlois JA, Kelen GD (1998) Are female drivers safer? An application of the decomposition method. Epidemiology 9:379–384

Link B, Phelan J (2001) Conceptualizing stigma. Annu Rev Sociol 27:363–385

Link BG, Phelan J (2014) Stigma power. Soc Sci Med 103:24–32. doi:10.1016/j.socscimed.2013.07.035

Link BG, Phelan JC, Bresnahan M, Stueve A, Pescosolido BA (1999) Public conceptions of mental illness: labels, causes, dangerousness, and social distance. Am J Public Health 89:1328–1333

Link B, Castille DM, Stuber J (2008) Stigma and coercion in the context of outpatient treatment for people with mental illness. Soc Sci Med 67:409–419. doi:10.1016/j.socscimed.2008.03.015

Luchins DJ, Roberst DL, Hanrahan P (2003) Representative payeeship and mental illness: a review. Adm Policy Ment Health 30(4):341–353. doi:10.1023/A:1024089317630

Lysaker PH, Tunze C, Yanos PT, Roe D, Ringer J, Rand K (2012) Relationships between stereotyped beliefs about mental illness, discrimination experiences, and distressed mood over 1 year among persons with schizophrenia enrolled in rehabilitation. Soc Psychiatry Psychiatr Epidemiol 47:849–855. doi:10.1007/s00127-011-0396-2

Malterud K, Ulriksen K (2011) Obesity, stigma, and responsibility in health care: a synthesis of qualitative studies. Int J Qual Stud Health Well-Being 6(4):1–11. doi:10.3402/qhw.v6i4.8404

Meyer IH (2003) Prejudice, social stress, and mental health in lesbian, gay, and bisexual populations: conceptual issues and research evidence. Psychol Bull 129(5):674–697. doi:10.1037/0033-2909.129.5.674

Michalak E, Livingston JD, Hole R, Suto M, Hale S, Haddock C (2011) 'It's something that I manage but it is not who I am': reflections on internalized stigma in individuals with bipolar disorder. Chronic Illn 7:209–224. doi:10.1177/1742395310395959

Mizock L (2012) The double stigma of obesity and serious mental illnesses: promoting health and recovery. Psychiatry Rehabil J 35:466–469. doi:10.1037/h0094581

Moses T (2013) Stigma & family. In: Corrigan PW (ed) Stigma of disease and disability: understanding causes and overcoming prejudices. American Psychological Association, Washington, DC, pp 247–268. doi:10.1037/14297-013

Mosher CE, Danoff-Burg S (2007) Death anxiety and cancer-related stigma: a terror management analysis. Death Stud 3:885–907. doi:10.1080/07481180701603360

Mukolo A, Heflinger CA (2011) Factors associated with attributions about child health conditions and social distance preference. Community Ment Health J 47(3):286–299. doi:10.1007/s10597-010-9325-1

Munetz MR, Frese FJ III (2001) Getting ready for recovery: reconciling mandatory treatment with the recovery vision. Psychiatry Rehabil J 25(1):35–42

Munoz M, Sanz M, Perez-Santos E, de los Angeles Quiroga M (2011) Proposal of socio-cognitive-behavioral structural equation model of internalized stigma in people with severe and persistent mental illness. Psychiatry Res 186:402–408. doi:10.1016/j.psychres.2010.06.019

Newman S, Goldman H (2009) Housing policy for persons with severe mental illness. Policy Stud J 37(2):299–324. doi:10.1111/j.1541-0072.2009.00315.x

Olmstead VLC (1999) Brief for Amici Curiae American Association on Mental Retardation, et al., http://www.apa.org/about/offices/ogc/amicus/olmstead.pdf. Accessed 15 Apr 2015

Oswald FL, Mitchell G, Blanton H, Jaccard J, Tetlock PE (2013) Predicting ethnic and racial discrimination: a meta-analysis of IAT criterion studies. J Pers Soc Psychol 150:171–192. doi:10.1037/a0032734

Parcesepe AM, Cabassa LJ (2013) Public stigma of mental illness in the United States: a systematic literature review. Adm Policy Ment Health Ment Health Serv Res 40:384–399. doi:10.1007/s10488-012-0430-z

Patel MX, de Zoysa N, Bernadt M, Bindman J, David AS (2010) Are depot antipsychotics more coercive than tablets? The patient's perspective. J Psychopharmacol 24:1483–1489. doi:10.1177/0269881109103133

Pattyn E, Verhaeghe M, Sercu C, Bracke P (2013) Medicalizing versus psychologizing mental illness: what are the implications for help seeking and stigma? A general population study. Soc Psychiatry Psychiatr Epidemiol 48:1637–1645. doi:10.1007/s00127-013-0671-5

Peris TS, Teachman BA, Nosek BA (2008) Implicit and explicit stigma of mental illness: links to clinical care. J Nerv Ment Dis 196:752–760. doi:10.1097/NMD.0b013e3181879dfd

Perry BL (2011) The labeling paradox: stigma, the sick role, and social networks in mental illness. J Health Soc Behav 52:460–477. doi:10.1177/0022146511408913

Pescosolido BA, Olafsdottir S, Martin JK, Long JS (2008) Cross-cultural aspects of the stigma of mental illness. In: Arboleda-Flórez J, Sartorius N (eds) Understanding the stigma of mental illness: theory and interventions. Wiley, Chichester, pp 19–35. doi:10.1002/9780470997642.ch2

Pescosolido BA, Medina TR, Martin JK, Long JS (2013) The "backbone" of stigma: identifying the global core of public prejudice associated with mental illness. Am J Public Health 103(5):853–860. doi:10.2105/AJPH.2012.301147

Pryor JB, Reeder GD (2011) HIV - related stigma. In J.C. Hall, B.J. Hall & C.J. Cockerell (Eds.), HIV/AIDS in the Post - HAART Era: anifestations, treatment, and Epidemiology (pp. 790–806). Shelton, CT: PMP H- USA, Ltd.

Pryor JB, Reeder GD, Monroe AE (2012) The infection of bad company: stigma by association. J Pers Soc Psychol 102:224–241. doi:10.1037/a0026270

Reynders A, Kerkhof AJFM, Molenberghs G, Van Audenhove C (2014) Attitudes and stigma in relation to help-seeking intentions for psychological problems in low and high suicide rate regions. Soc Psychiatry Psychiatr Epidemiol 49(2):231–239. doi:10.1007/s00127-013-0745-4

Roe D, Rudnick A, Gill KJ (2007) The concept of 'being in recovery'. Psychiatry Rehabil J 30:171–173. doi:10.2975/30.3.2007.171.173

Rüsch N, Corrigan PW, Todd AR, Bodenhausen GV (2010) Implicit self-stigma in people with mental illness. J Nerv Ment Dis 198(2):150–153. doi:10.1097/NMD.0b013e3181cc43b5

Rüsch N, Muller M, Lay B, Corrigan PW, Zahn R, Schonenberger T, Bleiker M, Lengler S, Blank C, Rössler W (2014) Emotional reactions to involuntary psychiatric hospitalization and stigma-related stress among people with mental illness. Eur Arch Psychiatry Clin Neurosci 264:35–43. doi:10.1007/s00406-013-0412-5

Russinova Z, Griffin S, Bloch P, Wewiorski NJ, Rosoklija I (2011) Workplace prejudice and discrimination toward individuals with mental illnesses. J Vocat Rehabil 35:227–241. doi:10.3233/JVR-2011-0574

Sand E, Gordon KH, Bresin K (2013) The impact of specifying suicide as the cause of death in an obituary. Crisis J Crisis Interv Suicide Prev 34:63–66. doi:10.1027/0227-5910/a000154

Sanders Thompson VL, Noel JG, Campbell J (2004) Stigmatization, discrimination, and mental health: the impact of multiple identity status. Am J Orthopsychiatry 74:529–544. doi:10.1037/0002-9432.74.4.529

Schnabel K, Asendorpf JB, Greenwald AG (2008) Assessment of individual differences in implicit cognition: a review of IAT measures. Eur J Psychol Assess 24:210–217. doi:10.1027/1015-5759.24.4.210

Schomerus G, Matschinger H, Angermeyer MC (2014) Causal beliefs of the public and social acceptance of persons with mental illness: a comparative analysis of schizophrenia, depression and alcohol dependence. Psychol Med 44:303–314. doi:10.1017/S003329171300072X

Stier A, Hinshaw SP (2007) Explicit and implicit stigma against individuals with mental illness. Aust Psychol 42:106–117. doi:10.1080/00050060701280599

Stout PA, Villegas J, Jennings NA (2004) Images of mental illness in the media: identifying gaps in the research. Schizophr Bull 30(3):543–561

Strauss JL, Zervakis JB, Stechuchak KM, Olsen MK, Swanson J, Swartz MS, Weinberger M, Marx CE, Calhoun PS, Bradford DW, Butterfield MI, Oddone EZ (2013) Adverse impact of coercive treatments on psychiatric inpatients' satisfaction with care. Community Ment Health J 49:457–465. doi:10.1007/s10597-012-9539-5

Stull LG, McGrew JH, Salyers MP, Ashburn-Nardo L (2013) Implicit and explicit stigma of mental illness: attitudes in an evidence-based practice. J Nerv Ment Dis 201:1072–1079. doi:10.1097/NMD.0000000000000056

Sudak H, Maxim K, Carpenter M (2008) Suicide and stigma: a review of the literature and personal reflections. Am Psychiatry 32:136–142. doi:10.1176/appi.ap.32.2.136

Swartz MS, Swanson JW (2004) Involuntary outpatient commitment, community treatment orders and assisted outpatient treatment: what's in the data? Can J Psychiatry 49:585–591

Teachman BA, Wilson JG, Komarkovskayam I (2006) Implicit and explicit stigma of mental illness in diagnosed and healthy samples. J Soc Clin Psychol 25:75–95. doi:10.1521/jscp.2006.25.1.75

Thornicroft G (2013) Premature death among people with mental illness. Br Med J, 346:F2969. doi:10.1080/09540260701278937

Topora A, Anderssonb G, Denhovcd A, Holmqvistc S, Mattssone M, Claes-Göran Stefanssone C, Bülowf P (2014) Psychosis and poverty: coping with poverty and severe mental illness in everyday life. Psychosis Psychol Soc Integr Approaches 6(2):117–127. doi:10.1080/17522439.2013.790070

Vahabzadeh A, Wittenauer C, Erika J (2011) Stigma, schizophrenia and the media: exploring changes in the reporting of schizophrenia in major U.S. newspapers. J Psychiatr Pract 17(6):439–446. doi:10.1097/01.pra.0000407969.65098.35

Van der Sanden RLM, Bos AER, Stutterheim SE, Pryor JB, Kok G (2013) Experiences of stigma by association among family members of people with mental illness. Rehabil Psychol 58:73–80, doi: 0.1037/a0031752

Velez BL, Moradi B, Brewster ME (2013) Testing the tenets of minority stress theory in workplace contexts. J Couns Psychol 60:532–542. doi:10.1037/a0033346

Vogel DL, Bitman RL, Hammer JH, Wade NG (2013) Is stigma internalized? The longitudinal impact of public stigma and self-stigma. J Couns Psychol 60:311–316. doi:10.1037/a0031889

Watson AC, Angell B, Vidalon T, Davis K (2010) Procedural justice and coercion among persons with mental illness in police encounters: the police contact experience scale. J Community Psychol 38(2):206–226. doi:10.1002/jcop.20360

Webber M, Corker E, Hamilton S, Weeks C, Pinfold V, Thornicroft G, Henderson C (2014) Epidemiol Psychiatr Serv 23(2):155–165. doi:10.1017/S2045796013000243

Weiner B (1995) Judgment of responsibility: a foundation for a theory of social conduct. Guilford Press, New York

Witte TK, Smith AR, Joiner TE (2010) Reason for cautious optimism? Two studies suggesting reduced stigma. J Clin Psychol 66(6):611–626. doi:10.1002/jclp

Wong C, Davidson L, Anglin D, Link B, Gerson R, Malaspina D, McGlashan T, Corcoran C (2009) Stigma in families of individuals in early stages of psychotic illness: family stigma and early psychosis. Early Interv Psychiatry 3:108–115. doi:10.1111/j.1751-7893.2009.00116.x

Wong G, Derthick AO, David EJR, Saw A, Okazaki S (2014) The what, the why, and the how: a review of racial microaggressions research in psychology. Race Soc Probl 6(2):181–200. doi:10.1007/s12552-013-9107-9

Zubritsky C, Mullahy M, Allen M, Alfano E (2006) The state of the Olmstead decision and the impact of consumer participation in planning. Am J Psychiatr Rehabil 9(2):131–143. doi:10.1080/15487760600876345

Stigma in Different Cultures

4

Mirja Koschorke, Sara Evans-Lacko, Norman Sartorius, and Graham Thornicroft

Introduction

Most stigma research to date has considered the stigma of mental illness to be a universal occurrence, but one that presents with different manifestations in different contexts. Yang et al., for example, observe that 'stigma appears to be a universal phenomenon, a shared existential experience' (Yang et al. 2007) (p. 1528). In a review of the global evidence on stigma and discrimination, Thornicroft concludes that 'there is no known country, society or culture where people with mental illness (diagnosed or recognised as such by the community) are considered to have the same value or be as acceptable as persons who do not have mental illness'(Thornicroft 2006).

Research has shown that high levels of ignorance and misinformation about mental illness are ubiquitous, and attitude surveys in different countries have generally demonstrated unfavourable views of people with mental disorders (Murthy 2005; Thornicroft 2006). International surveys on discrimination have shown high

M. Koschorke (✉) • S. Evans-Lacko • G. Thornicroft
Department of Health Service and Population Research, Institute of Psychiatry, Psychology and Neuroscience, King's College London, London, UK
e-mail: mirja.koschorke@kcl.ac.uk; Sara.Evans-Lacko@kcl.ac.uk; graham.thornicroft@kcl.ac.uk

N. Sartorius
Association for the Improvement of Mental Health Programmes, Geneva, Switzerland
e-mail: sartorius@normansartorius.com

© Springer International Publishing Switzerland 2017
W. Gaebel et al. (eds.), *The Stigma of Mental Illness - End of the Story?*,
DOI 10.1007/978-3-319-27839-1_4

67

levels of experienced and anticipated discrimination across a range of international sites (Lasalvia et al. 2013; Thornicroft et al. 2009; Ucok et al. 2012).

Yet, while stigma may indeed constitute a universal phenomenon, specific experiences of stigma and discrimination are local and subject to the influence of cultural factors (Murthy 2002). As Yang et al. put it, 'across cultures, the meanings, practices and outcomes of stigma differ, even when we find stigmatisation to be a powerful and often preferred response to illness, disability and difference' (Yang et al. 2007).

In his review of 'psychiatric stigma in non-western societies'[1] published in 1991, Fabrega describes factors bearing on social stigma and concludes that 'there is much variety in the way mental illnesses are labelled and handled with respect to the question of stigmatization' in different settings (Fabrega 1991a, b). Since his seminal work, a number of studies have demonstrated cultural specificities in the understanding of illness and, related to it, public acceptance of illness, pathways of help seeking and manifestations of stigma and discrimination in the lives of people with mental illness (Kohrt and Harper 2008; Quinn and Knifton 2014; Rosen 2003).

This chapter aims to explore how culture shapes the manifestations of stigma through three key domains, (i) notions of 'mental illness' and causal attributions, (ii) cultural meanings of the impairments and manifestations caused by the disorder and (iii) notions of self and personhood, and we then go on to discuss how such stigmatisation and discrimination can be measured and assessed in a cross-cultural context.

Notions of 'Mental Illness' and Causal Attributions

The concept of 'culture', as defined by Pool and Geissler, refers to an 'ideational system: a system of shared ideas, systems of concepts and rules and meanings that underlie and are expressed in the ways that humans live' (Pool and Geissler 2005) (p. 8). In this sense, the concept of 'culture' is inherently connected to the construct of 'stigma', which is often defined to include notions and beliefs about the stigmatised condition as well as its attributions.

A number of studies in different countries have explored the relationship between what is viewed in various contexts as 'mental illness' and the notion of 'stigma' and discussed stigma in relation to the question whether categorisations of mental disorders hold true in all societies (Fabrega 1991b; Kleinman 1987). Fabrega points out that what is called a 'psychiatric condition' in 'Western' systems of medicine (etic perspective) may or may not be judged to be an 'illness' in different local contexts (emic perspective) and that even if it is considered an illness, divisions between psychiatric and nonpsychiatric conditions rarely apply. What, then, do we know

---

[1] The word 'western' is used here because it appears in Fabrega's work. It is a misnomer, usually referring to what happens in the USA and possibly in few European countries. Countries of Europe show vast cultural differences, and there is no justification to making them a group which shares a 'western' culture (Sartorius 2002).

about the relationship between labelling a presentation or behaviour as 'illness' and the social responses it elicits in different contexts?

Several scholars have observed that in settings where people hold notions of mental illness that attribute an external causation to mental illness such as witchcraft or sorcery, there appears to be less associated stigma. Waxler, for example, who observed this phenomenon in Sri Lanka hypothesised that local notions of illness removed responsibility from the person with mental illness, thereby facilitating better outcome and prognosis (Waxler 1976) cited in Littlewood (1998). Sartorius has pointed out that the stigma of mental illness is linked to being recognised as mentally ill, not to extraordinary behaviour per se: for example, shamans and religious healers may go into states of trance or behave in extraordinary ways but are not stigmatised because of this (Stuart et al. 2012). He posits that stigma starts when the person with an extraordinary behaviour is declared ill and when the concept of illness indicates that there is no hope for cure or making the person again a valuable member of the community. Thus, he argues, the stigmatisation of a person with unusual behaviour will depend on whether that behaviour is considered to be due to mental illness (i.e. on what in that culture is considered to be a mental illness). This is illustrated, for example, by the case of a person with schizophrenia who was well looked after by his tribe of Bedouins until they were told that the behaviour of that person was not due to a curse thrown upon him but caused by a mental illness: The tribe promptly rejected the person (Stuart et al. 2013). The hypothesis that propagating a concept of 'mental illness' may enhance stigma would be supported by recent stigma intervention research indicating that providing certain forms of knowledge, particularly information which projects a biomedical model of mental illness, may increase rather than decrease people's desire for social distance from people with mental illness (Corrigan 2007; Schomerus et al. 2012).

Yet, other studies indicate that the relationship between notions of illness and stigma is complex and the evidence somewhat conflicting, not least because people commonly hold several often contradictory explanations for mental illness simultaneously (Littlewood 1998; Saravanan et al. 2008; Srinivasan and Thara 2001). A study among people with schizophrenia and their family members in South India, for example, found that higher stigma was positively associated with the disease model of illness but also with external non-stigmatising beliefs relating to karma and evil spirits (Charles et al. 2007). Qualitative findings of another Indian study on stigma suggest that as long as people with schizophrenia were able to keep up with role expectations in work and marriage, they had little benefit to expect from conceptualising their problems as an 'illness', but that for those too ill to keep up work or another accepted social role, knowledge allowing the attribution of symptoms to an illness rather than to volitional 'misbehaviour' was able to provide some relief from blaming social responses and harsh self-criticism about failure to achieve key markers of social worth (Koschorke et al. 2014).

Stigma research from South Africa suggests that traditional beliefs concerning the causes of mental illness, including the notion that people with mental illness were bewitched or were pretending to be ill, were perpetuating stigma and had negative consequences for people with mental illness through social isolation, neglect and maltreatment, delayed medical help seeking and being ignored by healthcare staff (Su et al. 2013).

Several other studies of mental illness stigma in low- and middle-income (LAMIC) settings have documented the coexistence of supernatural attributions of mental illness and high levels of perceived stigma (Girma et al. 2013; Shibre et al. 2001; Thirthalli and Kumar 2012).

Overall, the importance of considering culture-specific explanatory models and notions of illness in stigma research is now widely acknowledged (Bhui and Bhugra 2007; Evans-Lacko et al. 2012a; Kingdon et al. 2008a, b; Link et al. 1999; Rusch et al. 2010; Shefer et al. 2012; Yang 2007; Yang et al. 2010). The complexities outlined above highlight that it is necessary to assess the role of these factors for each study context separately and seek to avoid regional generalisations.

The Meaning of Stigma and the Impairments Caused by Mental Disorders

Yet, cultural differences in mental illness stigma go beyond differences in illness models and attributions. Link et al. argue that cultural meanings are already relevant in determining which characteristics (e.g. skin colour, body height, particular visible marks or manifestations of illness) reach the social salience required for an attribute to become a potential 'stigma' (Link and Phelan 2001). Similarly, it is worth noting that symptoms of mental illness that are stigmatised in one context may not be associated with social devaluation in another context, particularly when the condition is not considered as an illness. For example, in some cultures, people who hallucinate may be highly respected and seen as privileged because they are able to hear God's voice, as discussed above (Stuart et al. 2012).

In addition to differences in the meaning of symptoms and impairments caused by mental illness, there may be culture-specific differences in the qualitative meaning of specific features and manifestations of stigma: Weiss et al., for example, examined and compared psychiatric stigma in Bangalore and London and found that concerns about the impact of stigma on marital prospects were prominent in both centres but consistent with other indicators of stigma only in India, illustrating the different meaning of marriage in that context. In contrast, study participants in London did not speak about concerns about marriage in a way which suggested they formed part of a coherent concept of stigma (Weiss et al. 2001).

The importance of the social and cultural context in understanding stigma has been further emphasised by Yang and colleagues, who propose that understanding differences in prevalence and severity of experiences of stigma alone does not provide a complete picture of how stigma marginalises individuals and social groups, and that a 'more comprehensive formulation can be reached by understanding how stigma threatens the moral experience of individuals and groups' (Yang et al. 2007) p. 1529. They hypothesise that 'stigma exerts its core effects by threatening the loss or diminution of what is most at stake' and 'what matters most' in a given local context (Yang et al. 2007) p. 1524. Thus, Yang, Kleinman and colleagues advocate for stigma research to investigate the unique cultural and moral processes that undergird stigma in different contexts (Kleinman and Hall-Clifford 2009; Yang et al. 2007). Using examples from schizophrenia and AIDS (Yang et al. 2007; Yang 2007; Yang and Kleinman 2008), the authors describe the processes by which stigma and the stigmatised condition threaten 'what matters most' to ordinary people in China, namely, the 'vital connections that link the person to a social network of support, resources, and life chances' including material opportunities and the chance to get married, have children and perpetuate the family structure and kinship line'. Understanding the meaning of stigma in the context of China therefore demands an acknowledgement that stigma cannot just be considered a matter of the individual affected but that it reaches the significance it has due to its impact on an entire social network and family lineage (Yang et al. 2007). Similarly, qualitative findings of the abovementioned study among people with schizophrenia in India suggest that 'what matters most' to the moral status of people with schizophrenia in India is to be able to meet gender-specific role expectations in work and marriage, and that what is 'at stake' through the stigma of schizophrenia is not only the well-being and status of an individual but that of the whole family for generations to come (Koschorke et al. 2014).

Notions of Personhood and Patterns of Social Cohesion

This leads on to a third aspect of looking at cross-cultural differences with regard to stigma and discrimination: the idea that different cultures hold different notions of personhood and self and that the way the individual relates to its social network differs vastly between different contexts. In her article on 'selfhood and social distance: toward a cultural understanding of psychiatric stigma in Egypt' which reports the results of a qualitative study of psychiatric stigma in Egypt, Coker proposes that 'aspects of self and identity coupled with the specific meanings given to mental illness in Egypt lead to the specific meanings given to the unique form that stigma takes in this context' (Coker 2005) p. 922. She compares conceptualisations of the 'self' in Northern European Protestant culture, where the person is 'experienced as constant, yet alterable through individual effort' and considered separately from its social network, and the Mediterranean culture,[2] where 'the self is constructed and experienced in relation to others in the environment' and 'evaluated by others in relation to the social context as well' (Coker 2005) p. 922. Summarising the findings of her study, she explains that 'strange words or behaviours did not by themselves elicit social distance as long as the person's place in the social fabric was assured' and that, instead, increased social distance was faced by individuals who

[2] As with the word 'western' referring to Fabrega's work, we have kept the words Mediterranean and Northern European being fully aware that the differences among the countries bordering the Mediterranean – ranging from the culture prevailing Albania or Croatia and Italy to Morocco and Israel – are generalisations that are not very meaningful nor useful.

were decontextualised, had become isolated due to the nature and severity of their condition (e.g. psychiatric hospitalisation) and therefore experienced a social death (Coker 2005) p. 928. Coker concludes that 'the ability of a syndrome to (…) lead to stigma is therefore highly dependent on the meanings given to both the person and the illness' (Coker 2005) p. 928.

Differences in patterns of social cohesion and their importance for the local meaning of stigma have been demonstrated for several other low- and middle-income country (LAMIC) contexts, including India, China, Nigeria and South Africa where people with mental illness usually live with their family members and where social networks are usually more cohesive than in Western settings. The observation that there is often higher social cohesion in non-Western than in Western settings has been used to sustain the argument that psychiatric stigma is lower in non-Western settings (Waxler 1976) and also to support the argument that the impact of stigma may be enhanced due to the threat to an entire kinship (Phillips et al. 2002; Yang et al. 2007; Yang 2007; Yang and Kleinman 2008).

'Culture' and the Role of Other Contextual Factors

Finally, it is worth noting that when we seek to compare stigma between different settings, for example, between high-income countries (HIC) and LAMIC settings, more than just 'cultural' differences (i.e. differences relating to beliefs and norms) are at play. Socioeconomic factors, such as poverty and access to health care, have long been found to be associated with outcomes of mental illness (Lund et al. 2011). Similarly, socioeconomic factors determine the context in which stigma is enacted and experienced. While the role of socioeconomic factors in determining stigma is complex and the evidence somewhat inconsistent (Livingston and Boyd 2010; Switaj et al. 2009; Thornicroft et al. 2009), some studies illustrate how the impact and meaning of experiences of stigma can differ according to social circumstances. The findings of a study carried out in 27 European countries to study the mental health consequences of economic recession, for example, suggest that the social exclusion of people with mental health problems may intensify in times of economic hardship (Evans-Lacko et al. 2013a). In India and other LAMIC settings where most people with mental illness do not have access to social welfare benefits, the negative consequences of stigma and discrimination in work may be so severe as to threaten the economic survival of entire families (Koschorke et al. 2014).

A study among Chinese immigrants in the USA by Yang et al., for example, showed that experiences of mental illness stigma were contingent on the degree to which immigrants were able to participate in work to achieve what mattered most in their local context, i.e. the accumulation of financial resources. The authors concluded that the study illustrates how structure, local cultural processes and stigma shape each other, in that stigma is responsive to structural conditions but in turn influences exposure to these structural conditions (Yang et al. 2014a).

Global Patterns of Stigma and Discrimination

There are few studies comparing the frequency of experiences of stigma and discrimination in different contexts, and much of the available information comes from research conducted among ethnic minorities living in high-income countries rather than populations living in their own countries. In addition, findings from studies of stigma in different contexts are often difficult to compare given the heterogeneous methodologies used and differences in the sociocultural meanings of the experiences reported.

To address this gap in the literature and inform international efforts to combat stigma, recent research has sought to investigate the burden of stigma and discrimination across multiple settings using the same research design and a consistent methodology:

An international survey of experienced and anticipated discrimination conducted by the INDIGO Study Group among people with schizophrenia carried out in 27 countries including HIC and LAMIC settings found rates of both outcomes to be consistently high across cultures (Thornicroft et al. 2009; Ucok et al. 2012). Significant between-country variation was found for experienced discrimination but not anticipated discrimination reported by people with schizophrenia using the Discrimination and Stigma Scale (DISC) (Thornicroft et al. 2009). A report on the qualitative data collected as part of the same study, on the other hand, found few transnational differences (Rose et al. 2011). To examine international levels of discrimination associated with major depressive disorders, the same research group conducted a cross-sectional survey in 39 countries using the DISC (Thornicroft et al. 2009) and found that over 79 % of participants had experienced discrimination in at least one domain of their lives (Lasalvia et al. 2013).

Another international study by Alonso et al. analysed population-wide data from 16 countries collected as part of the World Mental Health Survey Initiative, to examine the prevalence of stigma across different settings. Results indicated that, overall, 21.9 % of people with a mental disorder reported stigma (defined as the concurrent experience of embarrassment and unfair discrimination), with higher rates in developing (31.2 %) than in developed (20 %) countries (Alonso et al. 2008).

Given the relative dearth of studies comparing stigma across multiple cultural settings using consistent methodologies, it is also warranted to take a brief look at studies that have compared stigma between two or three different settings. Several studies from LAMIC settings, for example, have reported that rates of experienced discrimination found were lower than those commonly reported from HIC studies: A study of experienced stigma in China (Chung and Wong 2004), for example, found rates of actual discrimination reported by people receiving community mental health services to be considerably lower than the levels of discrimination reported by people affected by a range of mental disorders in the UK (MentalHealthFoundation 2000) – a result which the authors attribute to the high level of functioning of their study participants and low levels of actual disclosure

(Chung and Wong 2004). Similarly, an Indian study found that participants reported levels of negative discrimination much lower than those reported in most HIC settings, but levels of anticipated discrimination and alienation in line with HIC studies (Koschorke et al. 2014).

Does this indicate that stigma and discrimination because of mental illness are less of a problem in LAMIC settings? Since the early days of cross-cultural research on stigma, there have been studies suggesting that the stigma of mental illness may be less marked in nonindustrialised societies due to a more supportive environment with less risk of prolonged rejection, isolation, segregation and institutionalisation (Cooper and Sartorius 1977; Waxler 1979). Some authors have argued that nonindustrialised societies are more cohesive (Waxler 1976) and that the non-Western model of extended families offers more acceptance to individuals with a mental illness (Askenasy 1974; El-Islam 1979) cited in Littlewood (1998). The better prognosis of schizophrenia found in international studies by the World Health Organization (WHO) such as the International Pilot Study of Schizophrenia (WHO 1979), the Determinants of Outcome of Severe Mental Disorder (DOSMeD) (Jablensky et al. 1992) and the International Study of Schizophrenia (ISoS) (Harrison et al. 2001; Hopper et al. 2007) has also sometimes been attributed to less stigmatisation in LAMIC (Rosen 2003).

Contradicting the above, there is now a considerable body of evidence documenting that in many LAMIC settings, experiences of stigma, discrimination and human rights abuses due to mental illness are common and severe (Alonso et al. 2008; Barke et al. 2011; Botha et al. 2006; Drew et al. 2011; Lasalvia et al. 2013; Lauber and Rossler 2007; Lee et al. 2005, 2006; Murthy 2005; Phillips et al. 2002; Sorsdahl et al. 2012; Thara et al. 2003). While there is emerging evidence that certain forms of experiences of stigma and discrimination, i.e. experienced discrimination, may be less commonly reported in some LAMIC settings than in HIC settings (as outlined above), there is also evidence that not all aspects of the experience of stigma and discrimination may be equally subject to cross-cultural variation. For example, even where discrimination rates are found to be low, other aspects and manifestations or stigma may still be very burdensome to people with mental illness (Koschorke et al. 2014). Further, it is possible that the frequency of some forms of stigma experience may influence the frequency of other forms, e.g. higher levels of internalised stigma, avoidance and withdrawal may lead to less exposure to enacted discrimination (Koschorke et al. 2014).

To throw light on the forces that drive intercultural differences in the manifestation of stigma, further research which takes into account a range of forms of stigma and discrimination and their associated, context-specific burden and meanings is needed. Understanding the factors that shape stigma differently in different contexts will serve to inform the development of context-specific anti-stigma interventions and encourage the sharing of successful forms of social integration of people with mental illness between different cultural settings.

Measuring Stigma in Different Cultural Contexts

Challenges Encountered when Measuring Stigma in Different Cultural Contexts

The assessment and validation of instruments to measure stigma and discrimination against people with mental illness have been underway since the 1960s. Although early scales such as the OMI (Opinions About Mental Illness Scale) (Cohen and Struening 1962; Link et al. 2004) and the CAMI (Community Attitudes Towards the Mentally Ill) (Taylor and Dear 1981) are still used in some studies, there have been many developments in both the breadth and quantity of measures to assess stigma, reflecting the growing interest in the field, incorporation of a wider range of perspectives (especially that of service users) (Chatterjee et al. 2014; Lee et al. 2005) and the changing aims and targets of anti-stigma interventions. Nevertheless, studies which include measures developed or validated in low- and middle-income countries (LAMICs) and/or Central or Eastern European cultures are still rare, and only a few include a component focused on stigma developed specifically in a LAMIC country and/or non-Western European cultural setting (Thornicroft et al. 2015). A recent systematic review (Yang et al. 2014b) assessed studies of stigma in non-Western European cultural groups and found that 77 % of identified studies assessed stigma using an adaptation of an existing measure which was developed in some of the European countries. Moreover, only 2 % of studies used stigma measures which were derived within a non-Western European cultural group. Even among identified research studies which used a qualitative research methodology, 82 % applied generic qualitative approaches which tended to be inductive and which did not incorporate a theoretical framework of stigma.

As described earlier, stigma against people with mental illness is an issue which persists across countries and cultures. Variations in the manifestation of stigma and hence the 'cultural validity' of stigma indicators suggest that measurement of stigma-related constructs also requires local adaptation (Weiss et al. 2001). Although applying a proper translation and incorporating appropriate language or relevant idioms are important for comprehensibility and understanding of questions, forward and back translation of an instrument is not sufficient to address the 'cultural validity' of stigma concepts. There may be important differences in the nature of stigma, what is stigmatised and how it is stigmatised (Weiss et al. 2001) according to different population subgroups. Thus, local cultural adaptation of an instrument may require consideration of a variety of factors including, for instance, geographic region, race, ethnicity, nationality, social class or other factors which might influence language, beliefs and experiences. All of these are critical considerations for measurement as they also relate to the consequences of stigma and potential targets of anti-stigma interventions.

Currently, there seem to be two approaches which are mainly used when developing a culture-specific measure (Yang et al. 2014b). In the first instance, an instrument which was developed in the UK or some other European country is translated and then psychometrically validated in a new subpopulation, potentially with some slight adaptations. The second involves the development of a 'composite measure' which incorporates experiences which were assessed across a range of contexts and/ or cultures. As outlined above, Yang et al. have recently proposed a third approach, that is incorporating a 'what matters most' perspective (Yang et al. 2013, 2014a). This approach would require investigating and operationalising everyday activities which are significant in participants' lives and which play a role in shaping stigma and/or have consequences for the stigmatised person.

Developing or Adapting Stigma Interventions for Different Cultural Contexts

Lessons from Adapting Stigma Interventions for Different Cultural Contexts

Efforts towards reducing stigma and discrimination against people with mental illness have been made across a number of countries. In 1996, the World Psychiatric Association initiated several national and regional efforts through the Open the Doors programme (http://www.openthedoors.com/english/index.html) which aimed to reduce public stigma, specifically in relation to people with schizophrenia (Sartorius and Schulze 2005; Warner 2008). More recently, additional national initiatives have been launched alongside evaluations including Like Minds Like Mine New Zealand in 1997 (http://www.likeminds.org.nz/) (Vaughan and Hansen 2004), Beyond Blue Australia in 2000 (http://www.beyondblue.org.au/), See Me Scotland in 2002 (http://www.seemescotland.org.uk/) and Time to Change England in 2009 (http://www.time-to-change.org.uk/), all of which are ongoing and which have published evaluations (Dunion and Gordon 2005; Evans-Lacko et al. 2013b; Jorm et al. 2006; Thornicroft et al. 2014). Overall, interest in large-scale anti-stigma programmes has increased, especially in Europe, and there are now at least 21 anti-stigma campaigns across European countries and regions (Borschmann et al. 2014). A variety of studies have been undertaken in midsized European countries (Beldie et al. 2012). There are also broad international networks which aim to share best practices about what works in terms of reducing stigma and discrimination including INDIGO (International Study of Discrimination Stigma Outcomes) (Lasalvia et al. 2012; Thornicroft, et al. 2009), ASPEN (Anti-Stigma Partnership European Network) (www.antistigma.eu) (Quinn et al. 2013) and the International Anti-Stigma Alliance (see http://www.time-to-change.org.uk/gaas). A main aim of these networks is to find common themes in terms of what works and then to consider how effective strategies can best be translated across countries, cultures and contexts.

Three main anti-stigma strategies in relation to mental illness which are described in the literature include protest, education and contact (Corrigan et al. 2001). Social contact, involving direct contact with people with a psychiatric disorder, has been recognised as one of the most effective ways to fight stigma and discrimination (Corrigan et al. 2012; Evans-Lacko et al. 2012b). Although contact has the strongest level of evidence, multifaceted strategies are encouraged and it is important to target anti-stigma work at the type of stigma we seek to reduce and the type of community in which this is done. Education on its own, for instance, is often not sufficient. Some types of information on description of mental illness or epidemiological data could be perceived by people as reinforcing stigmatising beliefs held by people who are prejudiced.

Discussion

This chapter argues that while the *occurrence* of stigma and discrimination is universal, their *manifestations and implications* are often highly contextually and culturally specific. Further, it appears, against the weight of previous evidence, that having, or having had, experience of *any* mental disorder is more important as a predictor of experiencing stigma and discrimination than being determined by the specific condition (Corker et al. 2013, 2014). Cultural considerations need to be kept in mind not only in seeking to understand the nature of stigma but also in appreciating the role of context in efforts to reduce stigma. The approach drawn from social psychology of 'attribution theory' argues that explanations for mental illness that do not refer to their being a role played or the consequence of action by the person affected by mental illness in its causation will be associated with greater public compassion and support for treatment. According to this theory, explanations for mental illness which are based upon genetic or biochemical causal mechanisms are likely to lead to less stigma. But in fact the evidence is to the contrary with emerging data to show that genetic (Phelan et al. 2006) or biochemical/neurotransmitter models (Pescosolido et al. 2010; Angermeyer et al. 2013) are in fact associated with greater public expressions of social distance to people with mental illness. This suggests that any benefit of the attribution theory may be more than offset by concerns about the indelible stain of stigma upon the person affected and his or her family members, at least in high-income countries where this has been most extensively studied.

In recent years there has been greater research interest in how stigmatisation and discrimination processes occur in low- and middle-income countries, across different population groups (Egbe et al. 2014), in groups such as health-care staff (Li et al. 2014) and among specific patient groups (Han et al. 2014). Recent research is also increasingly focussing not only upon the nature of stigmatisation but also upon its consequences, including profound social exclusion (Fekadu et al. 2014; Fekadu and Thornicroft 2014). Beyond this a new domain of research is being developed, namely, whether stigmatisation is a risk factor for suicide. To take the 'counterfactual' or hypothetical situation: In a world without stigma, would we expect lower suicide rates? Would more people seek help, or seek help sooner, and would fewer experience profound hopelessness? The case for this association is now being discussed at the hypothesis generation stage (Rusch et al. 2014), and we can expect such empirical studies, concerning this issue in the coming years.

References

Alonso J, Buron A, Bruffaerts R, He Y, Posada-Villa J, Lepine JP et al (2008) Association of perceived stigma and mood and anxiety disorders: results from the World Mental Health Surveys. Acta Psychiatr Scand 118(4):305–314

Angermeyer MC, Matschinger H, Schomerus G (2013) Attitudes towards psychiatric treatment and people with mental illness: changes over two decades. Brit J Psychiatry J Ment Sci 203:146–151

Askenasy A (1974) Attitudes towards mental patients: a study across cultures. Mouton, Hague

Barke A, Nyarko S, Klecha D (2011) The stigma of mental illness in Southern Ghana: attitudes of the urban population and patients' views. Soc Psychiatry Psychiatr Epidemiol 46(11): 1191–1202

Beldie A, den Boer JA, Brain C, Constant E, Figueira ML, Filipcic I et al (2012) Fighting stigma of mental illness in midsize European countries. Soc Psychiatry Psychiatr Epidemiol 47(Suppl 1):1–38

Bhui K, Bhugra D (2007) Culture and mental health. Edward Arnold, London

Borschmann R, Greenberg N, Jones N et al (2014) Campaigns to reduce mental illness stigma in Europe: a scoping review. Die Psychiatr 11(1):43–50

Botha UA, Koen L, Niehaus DJ (2006) Perceptions of a South African schizophrenia population with regards to community attitudes towards their illness. Soc Psychiatry Psychiatr Epidemiol 41(8):619–623

Charles H, Manoranjitham S, Jacob K (2007) Stigma and explanatory models among people with schizophrenia and their relatives in Vellore, South India. Int J Soc Psychiatry 53(4):325–332

Chatterjee S, Naik S, John S, Dabholkar H, Balaji M, Koschorke M et al (2014) Effectiveness of a community-based intervention for people with schizophrenia and their caregivers in India (COPSI): a randomised controlled trial. Lancet 383(9926):1385–1394

Chung K, Wong M (2004) Experience of stigma among Chinese mental health patients in Hong Kong [l]. Psychiatr Bull 28(12):451–454

Cohen J, Struening EL (1962) Opinions about mental illness in the personnel of two large mental hospitals. J Abnorm Psychol 64:349–360, 0096–851X (Print)

Coker EM (2005) Selfhood and social distance: toward a cultural understanding of psychiatric stigma in Egypt. Soc Sci Med 61(5):920–930

Cooper J, Sartorius N (1977) Cultural and temporal variations in schizophrenia: a speculation on the importance of industrialization. Br J Psychiatry 130:50–55

Corker E, Hamilton S, Henderson C, Weeks C, Pinfold V, Rose D et al (2013) Experiences of discrimination among people using mental health services in England 2008–2011. Br J Psychiatry Suppl 55:s58–s63

Corker EA, Beldie A, Brain C, Jakovljevic M, Jarema M, Karamustafalioglu O et al (2014) Experience of stigma and discrimination reported by people experiencing the first episode of schizophrenia and those with a first episode of depression: The FEDORA project. Int J Soc Psychiatry 61(5):438–445

Corrigan PW (2007) How clinical diagnosis might exacerbate the stigma of mental illness. Soc Work 52(1):31–39

Corrigan PW, River LP, Lundin RK, Penn DL, Uphoff-Wasowski K, Campion J et al (2001) Three strategies for changing attributions about severe mental illness. Schizophr Bull 27:187–195, 0586-7614 (Print)

Corrigan PW, Morris SB, Michaels PJ, Rafacz JD, Rusch N (2012) Challenging the public stigma of mental illness: a meta-analysis of outcome studies. Psychiatr Serv 63(10):963–973

Drew N, Funk M, Tang S, Lamichhane J, Chavez E, Katontoka S et al (2011) Human rights violations of people with mental and psychosocial disabilities: an unresolved global crisis. Lancet 378(9803):1664–1675 [S0140-6736(11)61458-X pii; 10.1016/S0140-6736(11)61458-X doi]

Dunion L, Gordon L (2005) Tackling the attitude problem. The achievements to date of Scotland's 'see me' anti-stigma campaign. Mental Health Today (Brighton, England), 22–25

Egbe CO, Brooke-Sumner C, Kathree T, Selohilwe O, Thornicroft G, Petersen I (2014) Psychiatric stigma and discrimination in South Africa: perspectives from key stakeholders. BMC Psychiatry 14:191

El-Islam EF (1979) A better outlook for schizophrenics living in extended families. Br J Psychiatry 135:343–347

Evans-Lacko S, Brohan E, Mojtabai R, Thornicroft G (2012a) Association between public views of mental illness and self-stigma among individuals with mental illness in 14 European countries. Psychol Med 42(8):1741–1752

Evans-Lacko S, London J, Japhet S, Rusch N, Flach C, Corker E et al (2012b) Mass social contact interventions and their effect on mental health related stigma and intended discrimination. BMC Public Health 12:489

Evans-Lacko S, Knapp M, McCrone P, Thornicroft G, Mojtabai R (2013a) The mental health consequences of the recession: economic hardship and employment of people with mental health problems in 27 European countries. PLoS One 8(7):e69792

Evans-Lacko S, Malcolm E, West K, Rose D, London J, Rusch N et al (2013b) Influence of Time to Change's social marketing interventions on stigma in England 2009–2011. Br J Psychiatry Suppl 55:s77–s88. doi:10.1192/bjp.bp.113.126672 [202/s55/s77 pii]

Fabrega H Jr (1991a) The culture and history of psychiatric stigma in early modern and modern Western societies: a review of recent literature. Compr Psychiatry 32(2):97–119

Fabrega H Jr (1991b) Psychiatric stigma in non-Western societies. Compr Psychiatry 32(6):534–551

Fekadu A, Thornicroft G (2014) Global mental health: perspectives from Ethiopia. Glob Health Action 7:25447

Fekadu A, Hanlon C, Gebre-Eyesus E, Agedew M, Solomon H, Teferra S et al (2014) Burden of mental disorders and unmet needs among street homeless people in Addis Ababa, Ethiopia. BMC Med 12(1):138

Girma E, Tesfaye M, Froeschl G, Moller-Leimkuhler AM, Muller N, Dehning S (2013) Public stigma against people with mental illness in the Gilgel Gibe Field Research Center (GGFRC) in southwest Ethiopia. PLoS One 8(12):e82116

Han DY, Lin YY, Liao SC, Lee MB, Thornicroft G, Wu CY (2014) Analysis of the barriers of mental distress disclosure in medical inpatients in Taiwan. Int J Soc Psychiatry 61(5):446–455

Harrison G, Hopper K, Craig T, Laska E, Siegel C, Wanderling J et al (2001) Recovery from psychotic illness: a 15- and 25-year international follow-up study. Br J Psychiatry 178:506–517

Hopper K, Harrison G, Wanderling JA (2007) An overview of course and outcome in ISoS. In: Hopper K, Harrison G, Janca A, Sartorius N (eds) Recovery from schizophrenia: an international perspective: a report from the WHO collaborative project, the international study of schizophrenia. Oxford University Press, New York, pp 23–38 [References]

Jablensky A, Sartorius N, Ernberg G et al (1992) Schizophrenia: manifestations, incidence and course in different cultures. A World Health Organization ten-country study. Psychol Med Monogr Suppl 20:1–97

Jorm AF, Christensen H, Griffiths KM (2006) Changes in depression awareness and attitudes in Australia: the impact of beyond blue: the national depression initiative. Aust N Z J Psychiatry 40:42–46, 0004-8674 (Print)

Kingdon D, Gibson A, Kinoshita Y, Turkington D, Rathod S, Morrison A (2008a) Acceptable terminology and subgroups in schizophrenia: an exploratory study. Soc Psychiatry Psychiatr Epidemiol 43(3):239–243

Kingdon D, Vincent S, Vincent S, Kinoshita Y (2008b) Destigmatising schizophrenia: does changing terminology reduce negative attitudes? Psychiatrist 32:419–422

Kleinman A (1987) Anthropology and psychiatry. The role of culture in cross-cultural research on illness. Br J Psychiatry 151:447–454

Kleinman A, Hall-Clifford R (2009) Stigma: a social, cultural and moral process. J Epidemiol Community Health 63(6):418–419

Kohrt BA, Harper I (2008) Navigating diagnoses: understanding mind-body relations, mental health, and stigma in Nepal. Cult Med Psychiatry 32(4):462–491

Koschorke M, Padmavati R, Kumar S, Cohen A, Weiss HA, Chatterjee S et al (2014) Experiences of stigma and discrimination of people with schizophrenia in India. Soc Sci Med 123C:149–159

Lasalvia A, Zoppei S, Van BT, Bonetto C, Cristofalo D, Wahlbeck K et al (2012) Global pattern of experienced and anticipated discrimination reported by people with major depressive disorder: a cross-sectional survey. Lancet (1474-547X (Electronic))

Lasalvia A, Zoppei S, Van Bortel T, Bonetto C, Cristofalo D, Wahlbeck K et al (2013) Global pattern of experienced and anticipated discrimination reported by people with major depressive disorder: a cross-sectional survey. The Lancet 381(9860):55–62

Lauber C, Rossler W (2007) Stigma towards people with mental illness in developing countries in Asia. Int Rev Psychiatry 19(2):157–178

Lee S, Lee MT, Chiu MY, Kleinman A (2005) Experience of social stigma by people with schizophrenia in Hong Kong. Br J Psychiatry 186:153–157

Lee S, Chiu MY, Tsang A, Chui H, Kleinman A (2006) Stigmatizing experience and structural discrimination associated with the treatment of schizophrenia in Hong Kong. Soc Sci Med 62(7):1685–1696

Li J, Thornicroft G, Huang Y (2014) Levels of stigma among community mental health staff in Guangzhou, China. BMC Psychiatry 14(1):231

Link BG, Phelan JC (2001) Conceptualising stigma. Am Sociol Rev 27:363–385

Link BG, Phelan JC, Bresnahan M, Stueve A, Pescosolido BA (1999) Public conceptions of mental illness: labels, causes, dangerousness, and social distance. Am J Public Health 89(9):1328–1333

Link BG, Yang LH, Phelan JC, Collins PY (2004) Measuring mental illness stigma. Schizophr Bull 30:511–541, 0586-7614 (Print

Littlewood R (1998) Cultural variation in the stigmatisation of mental illness. Lancet 352(9133): 1056–1057

Livingston JD, Boyd JE (2010) Correlates and consequences of internalized stigma for people living with mental illness: a systematic review and meta-analysis. Soc Sci Med 71(12):2150–2161

Lund C, De Silva M, Plagerson S, Cooper S, Chisholm D, Das J et al (2011) Poverty and mental disorders: breaking the cycle in low-income and middle-income countries. Lancet 378(9801):1502–1514

Mental Health Foundation (2000) Pull yourself together: a survey of the stigma and discrimination faced by people who experience mental distress. Mental Health Foundation, London

Murthy RS (2002) Stigma is universal but experiences are local. World Psychiatry 1(1):28

Murthy RS (2005) Stigma of mental illness in the third world. In: Okasha A, Stefanis CN (eds) Perspectives on the stigma of mental illness. World Psychiatric Association, Cairo

Pescosolido BA, Martin JK, Long JS, Medina TR, Phelan JC, Link BG (2010) "A disease like any other"? A decade of change in public reactions to schizophrenia, depression, and alcohol dependence. Am J Psychiatr 167(11):1321–1330

Phelan JC, Yang LH, Cruz-Rojas R (2006) Effects of attributing serious mental illnesses to genetic causes on orientations to treatment. Psychiatr Serv 57(3):382–387

Phillips MR, Pearson V, Li F, Xu M, Yang L (2002) Stigma and expressed emotion: a study of people with schizophrenia and their family members in China. Br J Psychiatry 181:488–493

Pool R, Geissler W (2005) Medical anthropology. Open University Press, Maidenhead

Quinn N, Knifton L (2014) Beliefs, stigma and discrimination associated with mental health problems in Uganda: implications for theory and practice. Int J Soc Psychiatry 60(6):554–561

Quinn N, Knifton L, Goldie I, Van Bortel T, Dowds J, Lasalvia A et al (2013) Nature and impact of European anti-stigma depression programmes. Health promotion international, das076

Rose D, Willis R, Brohan E, Sartorius N, Villares C, Wahlbeck K et al (2011) Reported stigma and discrimination by people with a diagnosis of schizophrenia. Epidemiol Psychiatr Sci 20(2): 193–204

Rosen A (2003) What developed countries can learn from developing countries in challenging psychiatric stigma. Australas Psychiatry 11(Suppl1):S89–S95

Rusch N, Todd AR, Bodenhausen GV, Corrigan PW (2010) Do people with mental illness deserve what they get? Links between meritocratic worldviews and implicit versus explicit stigma. Eur Arch Psychiatry Clin Neurosci 260(8):617–625

Rusch N, Zlati A, Black G, Thornicroft G (2014) Does the stigma of mental illness contribute to suicidality? Br J Psychiatry J Ment Sci 205(4):257–259, Editorial

Saravanan B, Jacob K, Deepak M, Prince M, David AS, Bhugra D (2008) Perceptions about psychosis and psychiatric services: a qualitative study from Vellore, India. Soc Psychiatry Psychiatr Epidemiol 43(3):231–238

Sartorius N (2002) Fighting for Mental Health. Cambridge: Cambridge University Press; English. p. 256. (ISBN 0-521-58243-1)

Sartorius N, Schulze H (2005) Reducing the stigma of mental illness. Cambridge University Press, Cambridge

Schomerus G, Schwahn C, Holzinger A, Corrigan PW, Grabe HJ, Carta MG et al (2012) Evolution of public attitudes about mental illness: a systematic review and meta-analysis. Acta Psychiatr Scand 125(6):440–452

Shefer G, Rose D, Nellums L, Thornicroft G, Henderson C, Evans-Lacko S (2012) 'Our community is the worst': the influence of cultural beliefs on stigma, relationships with family and help-seeking in three ethnic communities in London. Int J Soc Psychiatry 59(6):535–544

Shibre T, Negash A, Kullgren G, Kebede D, Alem A, Fekadu A et al (2001) Perception of stigma among family members of individuals with schizophrenia and major affective disorders in rural Ethiopia. Soc Psychiatry Psychiatr Epidemiol 36(6):299–303

Sorsdahl KR, Kakuma R, Wilson Z, Stein DJ (2012) The internalized stigma experienced by members of a mental health advocacy group in South Africa. Int J Soc Psychiatry 58(1):55–61

Srinivasan TN, Thara R (2001) Beliefs about causation of schizophrenia: do Indian families believe in supernatural causes? Soc Psychiatry Psychiatr Epidemiol 36(3):134–140

Stuart H, Arboleda-Florez J, Sartorius N (2012) Paradigms lost – fighting stigma and the lessons learned. Oxford University Press; p. 304. (ISBN 978-0-19-979763-9)

Stuart H, Arboleda Florez J, Sartorius N (2013) Paradigms Lost, Published by Oxford University Press

Su X, Lau JT, Mak WW, Chen L, Choi KC, Song J et al (2013) Perceived discrimination, social support, and perceived stress among people living with HIV/AIDS in China. AIDS Care 25(2):239–248

Switaj P, Wciorka J, Smolarska-Switaj J, Grygiel P (2009) Extent and predictors of stigma experienced by patients with schizophrenia. Eur Psychiatry 24(8):513–520

Taylor SM, Dear MJ (1981) Scaling community attitudes toward the mentally ill. Schizophr Bull 7:225–240, 0586-7614 (Print)

Thara R, Kamath S, Kumar S (2003) Women with schizophrenia and broken marriages – doubly disadvantaged? Part I: patient perspective. Int J Soc Psychiatry 49(3):225–232

Thirthalli J, Kumar CN (2012) Stigma and disability in schizophrenia: developing countries' perspective. Int Rev Psychiatry 24(5):423–440

Thornicroft (2006) Shunned: discrimination against people with mental illness. Oxford University Press, Oxford

Thornicroft G, Brohan E, Rose D, Sartorius N, Leese M, Group, I. S (2009) Global pattern of experienced and anticipated discrimination against people with schizophrenia: a cross-sectional survey. Lancet 373(9661):408–415

Thornicroft C, Wyllie A, Thornicroft G, Mehta N (2014) Impact of the "Like Minds, Like Mine" anti-stigma and discrimination campaign in New Zealand on anticipated and experienced discrimination. Aust N Z J Psychiatry 48(4):360–370

Thornicroft G, Mehta N, Clement S, Evans-Lacko S, Doherty M, Rose D et al (2015) Evidence for effective interventions to reduce mental-health-related stigma and discrimination: narrative review. Lancet

Ucok A, Brohan E, Rose D, Sartorius N, Leese M, Yoon CK et al (2012) Anticipated discrimination among people with schizophrenia. Acta Psychiatr Scand 125(1):77–83

Vaughan G, Hansen C (2004) 'Like Minds, Like Mine': a New Zealand project to counter the stigma and discrimination associated with mental illness. Australas Psychiatry 12(2):113–117

Warner R (2008) Implementing local projects to reduce the stigma of mental illness. Epidemiol Psichiatr Soc 17(1):20–25

Waxler N (1976) Social change and psychiatric illness in Ceylon: traditional and modern conceptions of disease and treatment. In: Lebra W (ed) Culture-bound syndromes, ethnopsychiatry and alternative therapies. University Press of Hawaii, Honolulu

Waxler N (1979) Is outcome of schizophrenia better in non-industrial societies? The case of Sri Lanka. J Nerv Mental Dis 167:144–158

Weiss MG, Jadhav S, Raguram R, Vounatsou P, Littlewood R (2001) Psychiatric stigma across cultures: local validation in Bangalore and London. Anthropol Med 8(7):71–87

WHO (1979) Schizophrenia: an international follow-up study. Wiley, Chichester

Yang LH (2007) Application of mental illness stigma theory to Chinese societies: synthesis and new directions. Singap Med J 48(11):977–985

Yang LH, Kleinman A (2008) 'Face' and the embodiment of stigma in China: the cases of schizophrenia and AIDS. Soc Sci Med 67(3):398–408

Yang, Kleinman A, Link B, Phelan J, Lee S, Good B (2007) Culture and stigma: adding moral experience to stigma theory. Soc Sci Med 64(7):1524–1535

Yang LH, Phillips MR, Lo G, Chou Y, Zhang X, Hopper K (2010) "Excessive thinking" as explanatory model for schizophrenia: impacts on stigma and "moral" status in Mainland China. Schizophr Bull 36(4):836–845

Yang LH, Valencia E, Alvarado R, Link B, Huynh N, Nguyen K et al (2013) A theoretical and empirical framework for constructing culture-specific stigma instruments for Chile. Cad Saúde Coletiva 21(1):71–79

Yang C, Sia L, Lam N et al (2014a) "What matters most:" a cultural mechanism moderating structural vulnerability and moral experience of mental illness stigma. Soc Sci Med 103:84–93

Yang LH, Thornicroft G, Alvarado R, Vega E, Link BG (2014b) Recent advances in cross-cultural measurement in psychiatric epidemiology: utilizing 'what matters most' to identify culture-specific aspects of stigma. Int J Epidemiol 43(2):494–510

Disorder-specific Differences

Claire Henderson

Introduction

Disorder-specific differences in stigma may be most visible on the part of people who are most often aware of what the disorder is during their contact with the potential targets of stigma. As those who make or are informed of the diagnosis as part of their job, health professionals are the most obvious group in which to seek evidence for such differences. However, public education campaigns mean that the general public is increasingly knowledgeable about those disorders included in the content of such campaigns. Therefore, this chapter summarises evidence for mental disorder-specific differences in stigma on the part of both the general public and health professionals. It also considers the evidence for disorder-specific interventions to reduce stigma and discrimination, including those targeted to either or both of health professionals and the general public. In addition to reviewing evidence from surveys and intervention studies with respect to these two groups, I review disorder-specific studies of newspaper coverage, as media depictions of mental illness exert considerable influence on public attitudes.

C. Henderson
Institute of Psychiatry, Psychology and Neuroscience, King's College London,
De Crespigny Park, Box P029, London SE5 8AF, UK
e-mail: claire.1.henderson@kcl.ac.uk

© Springer International Publishing Switzerland 2017
W. Gaebel et al. (eds.), *The Stigma of Mental Illness - End of the Story?*,
DOI 10.1007/978-3-319-27839-1_5

General Public

Public Knowledge, Attitudes and Intended Behaviour

Interpersonal stigma can be considered as consisting of problems of knowledge (ignorance or misinformation), attitudes (prejudice) and behaviour (discrimination, targeted violence and hostility and human rights abuses) (Thornicroft 2006). Attitudes to mental illness have been measured using a variety of instruments which assess emotional reactions to people with mental illness, endorsement of stereotypes (Rogers 1998), opinions about civil rights (Magliano 2004) and social restrictiveness (Nordt 2006) or desire for social distance (Lauber et al. 2004), although the latter is also used to measure behavioural intent.

Surveys of public attitudes to mental disorders have been conducted in a number of countries, and those which also assess knowledge of different mental disorders allow some comparison of attitudes and intended behaviour towards people with these disorders. More accurately, they allow comparison of these aspects of stigma towards people who fit the descriptions of symptoms and behavioural signs provided in the surveys' vignettes; in keeping with the surveys' aim of assessing knowledge through testing recognition, the names of the disorders are not provided. Most often, respondents are asked questions about their desire for social distance from a person such as that described in the vignette. The disorders most commonly included in these surveys are schizophrenia and depression, the former on the basis of its severity and the latter because it is common. Alcohol dependence has also been included in some surveys, as the commonest severe substance misuse disorder (Pescosolido et al. 2010).

Generally, respondents desire greater social distance when responding to vignettes describing a person with schizophrenia compared to someone with depression (Schomerus et al. 2012). For example, among respondents to the 2006 US General Social Survey, 62 % were unwilling to work closely with someone fitting the schizophrenia vignette description, compared to 47 % for the depression vignette. The pattern was similar for unwillingness to have someone as a neighbour (45 % for schizophrenia and 20 % depression), socialise (52 % vs 30 %), make friends (35 % vs 21 %) and have someone marry into the family (69 % vs 53 %). The repetition of this and other surveys suggests that, in addition to there being a greater desire for social distance from people fitting a description of schizophrenia compared to one of depression, responses to the two descriptions show different time trends.

While there has been little change over time in responses to the depression vignette, those to the schizophrenia vignette show an increasing desire for social distance. For example, from the 1996 to the 2006 US General Social Survey, unwillingness to have someone as a neighbour increased from 34 % to 35 % (p-0.01); other changes were not statistically significant but all followed this direction. The same questions have been asked based on vignettes of schizophrenia and depression in repeated surveys in Australia, Germany and Scotland. A meta-regression analysis by Schomerus et al. (2012) estimated that over the 16-year period covered (1900–2006), the accumulated decline for accepting someone with schizophrenia as a neighbour was 15.5 % and 17.8 % for acceptance as a colleague at work.

The reasons for this increased desire for social distance from people fitting the schizophrenia description are not clear. The evidence for change in the common stereotypes for mental disorder, i.e. people with mental disorder are more likely to be violent and are to blame for their illness, is weak; Schomerus et al. (2012) found only a trend for reduced blame, and this applied to both schizophrenia and depression. In the US survey (Pescosolido et al. 2010), there were non-significant increases in the perception of dangerousness to self or others between 1996 and 2006 for the schizophrenia vignette and non-significant declines for the depression vignette. Endorsement of neurobiological attributions increased significantly for both disorders between 1996 and 2006; for both disorders, holding such an attribution was either unrelated to stigmatising responses or positively associated with it, for schizophrenia in the case of desire for social distance in the workplace and for depression perceived dangerousness. Where there was a relationship between neurobiological attributions and stigma, it was stronger in 2006 than in 1996. Considered in isolation, for schizophrenia, this relationship suggests that the rise in neurobiological attribution may have contributed to greater social distance. However, despite a similar rise in neurobiological attributions for depression, and intensification of the association between such attributions and perceived dangerousness among people with depression, stigmatising responses to vignettes fitting a description of depression have not become more frequent. It may be that despite this finding from the USA, neurobiological attribution has less impact on the desire for social distance from people with depression, as has been found in Germany, Russia and Mongolia (Dietrich et al. 2004).

This survey also showed an increase in neurobiological attribution for alcohol dependence, from 38 to 47 % ($p=0.04$) between 1996 and 2006. However, social and moral attributions did not fall over this period, indeed for 'bad character' they increased from 49 to 65 % ($p<0.001$). Desired social distance from someone with alcohol dependence changed little between the two time points. For this disorder, it seems that there is little impact of greater neurobiological attribution on any widely held beliefs and attitudes.

Besides the use of survey questions based upon vignettes which do not include a diagnosis, other surveys comparing attitudes towards different mental illnesses have included questions about a number of disorders. The surveys by Crisp et al. (2005) in 1998 and 2003 asked questions based on common stereotypes rather than the desire for social distance: tendency to be violent, blameworthiness, being hard to talk to, feeling different to others, likelihood of recovery and response to treatment. They show a number of disorder-specific differences which were consistent across time. Drug dependence was viewed unfavourably by the greatest percentage of respondents, with 74 % of respondents recording overall negative opinions and only 5 % recording positive ones in 2003. Alcohol dependence elicited 66 % overall negative opinions and only 6 % positive ones. These disorders were viewed as among the most treatable and people who experience them as the most blameworthy; drug dependence was also the most highly rated as resulting in violence, at 75 % in 2003. Alcohol dependence and schizophrenia were rated slightly less often as being linked to violence, at 64 % and 66 %, respectively. These three disorders were rated similarly and most highly with respect to violence, unpredictability and being hard to talk with, but differed significantly in terms of blameworthiness; over half of respondents blamed people with substance misuse for their disorder, while only 6 % did so for schizophrenia. Due in part to this difference, the substance misuse disorders elicited the fewest overall neutral responses, while schizophrenia elicited the most at 70 %; 21 % were negative and 9 % were positive. Severe depression (16 % negative and 28 % positive), panic attacks (14 % negative and 36 % positive) and eating disorder (13 % negative and 32 % positive) were in an intermediate position. Eating disorders attracted the most blame after substance use disorders, at 33 % in 2003. Dementia, with only 3 % overall negative and 35 % positive opinions, was viewed most favourably despite being rated as the least treatment-responsive disorder.

Mass Media Representation

There is evidence that negative media coverage of people with mental disorders can worsen prejudicial attitudes within the general public (Philo 1996; Borinstein 1992; Thornton 1996; Dietrich 2006), although it should be bone in mind that media representation also reflects public attitudes. The extensive literature on media coverage points to its negative tone and frequent portrayal of people with mental illness as dangerous, incapable or strange (Wahl 1992; Francis 2001; Stout 2004; Klin and Lemish 2008). A study of newspaper coverage of mental illnesses examined whether there had been any change over time and whether this applied equally across diagnoses (Goulden et al. 2011). Samples were created from 1992, 2000 and 2008, from newspapers representing the UK market. A coding frame based on previous studies was developed which took into account both the content and style of reporting. In general, there was an increase over the period covered in the number of articles, reflecting a small increase in the number of 'bad news' articles likely to contribute to stigma, a doubling of 'services and advocacy' articles and more than a threefold increase in 'understanding mental illness' articles. There was thus a proportionate increase in non-stigmatising articles; however, when comparing coverage of different diagnoses, this applied to depression but not to schizophrenia. The treatment of these disorders has become more different over the three time points, such that in 2008 significantly more of the articles only about schizophrenia were negative compared to those about depression. These results are thus to some extent similar to those for public attitudes described above in terms of widening differences between the two disorders: public attitudes regarding depression have stayed the same, while those about schizophrenia have deteriorated; UK newspaper coverage about depression has improved but that about schizophrenia has not.

Regarding other mental disorders, Goulden et al. (2011) found that the reporting of anxiety, bipolar disorder and eating disorders either improved over time or was always largely favourable. In contrast, along with schizophrenia, personality disorders and general references to mental illness appeared mainly in the context of 'bad news' and saw little or no change in their coverage over time. Both schizophrenia and personality disorders rarely appeared in a context not somehow related to violence, tragedy or misfortune.

In Scotland, the See Me anti-stigma campaign included work with media and messaging to reduce the association between schizophrenia and violence. Analysis of Scottish newspapers over the course of the campaign (Knifton and Quinn 2008) showed a proportional reduction in articles about schizophrenia which had violence as a theme; however, coverage of schizophrenia become more negative overall during this time period, due to increases in other forms of negative depiction such as 'lack of capability'.

Experiences of Discrimination

Clinical factors associated with higher levels of reported discrimination include longer time since diagnosis and previous experience of involuntary treatment (Thornicroft et al. 2009; Cechnicki et al. 2011). Severity of psychiatric symptoms has been associated with higher levels of rejection from family and friends (Cechnicki et al. 2011) and higher levels of internalised stigma (Yen et al. 2005; Livingston and Boyd 2010). The effect of specific psychiatric diagnosis has been less researched. Studies examining public attitudes suggest that people have more negative attitudes towards people with schizophrenia compared to depression (Mann and Himelein 2004), and there is some evidence for this from two international surveys of people with each of these two diagnoses (Thornicroft et al. 2009; Lasalvia et al. 2012).

A cross-sectional telephone interview survey was conducted annually between 2008 and 2011 with separate samples of users of specialist mental health services. Full details of the method are reported in Corker et al. (2013). The sample was recruited through National Health Service (NHS) mental health trusts (service provider organisations). A total of 3,579 people using mental health services in England took part in a structured interview between 2008 and 2011. The Discrimination and Stigma Scale (DISC) (Brohan et al. 2013) was used to measure service users' reports of experienced discrimination, anticipated discrimination, social distancing and positive discrimination. Briefly, the scale is interviewer administered and contains 22 items related to negative experiences of mental health-related discrimination in different life areas and three (in 2008) or four (in 2009–2011) items related to anticipated discrimination. All responses are given on a 4-point scale, from 0, not at all, to 3, a lot. A 'not applicable' option is used for items about situations that were not relevant to the participant in the previous 12 months (e.g. items about having children or seeking employment) or to situations in which others could not have known that the respondent had a diagnosis. Discrimination scores were calculated as the number of items in which discrimination was experienced divided by the number of items recorded as applicable and multiplied by 100 to provide a percentage score.

In the univariate analyses, the only diagnosis which was associated with higher levels of discrimination was personality disorder, but even this association dropped out in the regression model. The overall model is statistically significant and accounts for 20.93 % of the variance. In this model, study year, age, employment status, length of time in mental health services, disagreeing with the diagnosis, anticipating discrimination in personal relationships and feeling the need to conceal a diagnosis from others remain significant following Bonferroni adjustment for multiple testing at $p < 0.003$.

The hypothesis that people with schizophrenia would experience higher levels of discrimination than people with other mental health diagnoses was not supported by the data. This finding may indicate that discrimination is a reaction to mental illness in general and not to any specific diagnosis. This is at odds with suggestions from previous studies that people hold more stigmatising attitudes towards people with schizophrenia than people with depression (Mann and Himmelein 2004), but consistent with two other studies comparing the experiences of people with schizophrenia to those affective disorders (Sarkin et al. 2015; Farrelly et al. 2014). It is likely that in some instances, the people identified by participants as sources of discrimination were not aware of the diagnosis itself but were reacting to a more generalised awareness of a mental illness, use of mental health services, symptoms or behaviours. We did not collect additional data concerning the severity of symptoms for participants. As a result, these diagnostic labels may encompass a wide array of illness experiences and symptoms.

Health Professionals

Disorder-specific differences in stigma may be most visible on the part of people who are most often aware of what the disorder is during their contact with the potential targets of stigma. As those who make or are informed of the diagnosis as part of their job, health professionals are the most obvious group in which to seek evidence for such differences. There is ample evidence of stigmatising attitudes among both mental health professionals (Wahl and Aroesty-Cohen 2010; Schulze 2007) and other health professionals (Bell et al. 2006; Bjorkman et al. 2008; Minas et al. 2011; Jorm et al. 1999; Rogers and Kashima 1998), although comparisons with general public samples yield different results depending on the professional group, setting of the study and measures used (Henderson 2014).

Considering stigma again in terms of knowledge, attitudes and behaviour, health professionals generally have more mental illness knowledge than the general public, but may still be affected by specific problems of knowledge related to stigma, for example, lack of knowledge about how to treat specific disorders such as borderline personality disorder (Commons Treloar and Lewis 2008b). Professionals are exposed to the same stereotypes about mental illness as the rest of the general public prior to professional training; thus, their attitudes are likely to reflect those of the general public to some extent in addition to attitudes acquired as a result of professional training and experience.

Using the same measure as Crisp et al. (2005) and Bjorkman et al. (2008) carried out a survey in Sweden of nurses working in general and psychiatric health care. The pattern of responses was similar to that among the general public, in that the most negative attitudes concerning dangerousness and unpredictability were found regarding drug addiction, alcohol addiction and schizophrenia. Compared to psychiatric nurses, nurses working in general health care reported a higher degree of perceived dangerousness regarding people with schizophrenia and unpredictability and found it hard to talk to regarding people with schizophrenia, eating disorders and drug addiction.

Surveys comparing the attitudes of different groups of doctors towards people with specific disorders have also found that people with alcohol and drug addiction were also relatively more stigmatised, whether in London (Mukherjee et al. 2002), Lahore (Naeem et al. 2006) or Colombo (Fernando et al. 2010). However, there was an interesting difference between the UK and Colombo, in that Sri Lankan doctors' attitudes towards people with schizophrenia were less stigmatising than those in the UK (Fernando et al. 2010). A multidisciplinary sample from eight European countries (Gilchrist et al. 2011) found that professionals' regard for working with people with substance use disorders was consistently lower than for working with people with depression or diabetes, especially among primary care professionals as compared to mental health professionals.

In summary, professionals' attitudes to people with different disorders vary in similar ways to the general public, especially among professionals who do not work in mental health care. However, while mental health professionals' attitudes are generally more positive, many aspects of mental health care can be experienced as discriminatory. A qualitative study of people with schizophrenia identified a variety of such experiences (Schulze and Angermeyer 2003). They felt rejected by a focus on diagnostic testing, which they experienced as a lack of interest in their person and being reduced to their symptomatology. They further felt that there was only one standard psychiatric treatment for everyone which mainly revolved around medication, about which they were given insufficient information. Coercive measures and professionals' therapeutic pessimism were also experienced as discriminatory. In addition, undesired effects of psychotropic drugs, such as extrapyramidal symptoms and weight gain, were described as having a negative effect on service users' social relationships by rendering their condition visible to others, thus involuntarily "outing" them.

Self-Harm and Borderline Personality Disorder

The surveys cited above on disorder-specific differences did not include self-harm or borderline personality disorder. However, it is well recognised that professionals find people with these problems difficult to treat and that avoidance and rejection can occur as a result. Within mental health services, the most attention has been paid to people with borderline personality disorder in this respect. The term 'malignant alienation' was coined in 1979 (Morgan 1979) to describe the process whereby therapeutic relationships broke down leading to rejection by professionals, including discharge from care, thus increasing the risk of suicide. This rejection can be understood in psychodynamic terms as acting out a counter transference, i.e. the therapist's emotional reaction to the patient (Watts and Morgan 1994). However, differential treatment such as selective discharge of, and negative interactions (Fraser and Gallop 1993) with, people with borderline personality disorder also constitutes discrimination and is experienced as such by people given this diagnosis, who describe feeling excluded from mental health care on the basis that professionals are unable to or do not wish to help (Schulze 2010; Bonnington 2013). Psychiatric nurses meanwhile describe fear of the consequences of self-harm, frustration at what they feel is manipulative behaviour, lack of support from other colleagues, anger and insufficient knowledge (Deans and Meocevic 2006; Wilstrand et al. 2007).

Stigma Reduction Interventions for Specific Disorders

Some national programmes to reduce stigma have taken a general approach to mental illness (Borschmann 2014), while others have taken a more disorder-specific approach, either targeting a highly stigmatised illness, as in the case of the Open the Doors programme regarding schizophrenia, or a very common disorder, as in the case of depression. We discuss these programmes and the evidence for their impact below.

Schizophrenia

'Open the Doors'

In 1996, the WPA introduced a strategy to reduce stigma and discrimination associated with schizophrenia entitled 'Open the Doors' (www.openthedoors.com). The campaign has gone on to establish over 200 projects in more than 20 countries (including eight in Europe) (Warner 2005). Conducting Open the Doors projects involves:

1. Establishing a local action committee
2. Conducting a survey of local sources of stigma
3. Selecting target groups for the intervention
4. Designing locally relevant messages and media
5. Evaluating the impact of the interventions while continuously refining them

National experts and non-government organisations are involved from the beginning and all materials are tested on local populations and adapted as necessary to the different settings. Professor Norman Sartorius, founder of Open the Doors, has stated that successful anti-stigma programmes can be launched in any country or region irrespective of its size, economic status or level of development (Sartorius 2006). However, published articles of rigorously designed evaluation are limited to Austria and Germany.

Austria

Findings from one Open the Doors programme showed that a combination of education and contact with people with mental illness may improve attitudes towards mental illness (Beldie et al. 2012). Findings from another campaign were less positive; 5 years after it finished, a general population survey showed that 64.1 % agreed with the statement that people with schizophrenia were dangerous; this figure was significantly higher than that reported in a study 5 years earlier (Schöny 1998). Additionally, only 18.7 % of respondents expressed a desire to become better informed about the illness.

Germany

Evaluation findings have mixed (Gaebel et al. 2003). On one hand, there was a decrease in negative stereotypes and social distance towards people with schizophrenia over the course of Open the Doors (Stuart et al. 2005). However, although schoolchildren's stereotypes about people with schizophrenia reduced after the intervention, the positive changes in social distance did not reach statistical significance (Schulze et al. 2003). Worse, evaluation of the film screenings and theatre productions about mental illness revealed that there was an increase in stigmatising beliefs (Stuart et al. 2005).

Depression

Defeat Depression

The 'Defeat Depression' was launched in 1991 (Dillner 1992; Priest 1991). Its target groups were the general public and general practitioners, and its aims were to increase recognition of depression, reduce stigma, promote help seeking and improve evidence-based treatment. Its evaluation showed significant improvements regarding both target groups. Public attitudes towards depression improved (Paykel et al. 1998). Attitudes to treatment were found to be mostly favourable, especially towards counselling and except towards antidepressants, which were viewed by many as addictive (Paykel et al. 1997; Vize and Priest 1993). Two thirds of general practitioners surveyed were aware of the campaign and between 25 and 40 % had changed their practice as a result (Rix et al. 1999; Macaskill et al. 1997).

The Nuremberg Alliance Against Depression

This 2-year community-based educational intervention started at the beginning of 2001. There were three main components: training of primary care professionals on recognition and treatment of depression, a public education campaign and engagement with local media to improve their coverage on mental illness, especially with respect to suicide reporting. The public education campaign used multiple media (posters, a cinema trailer, flyers and a website) to convey three key messages: (1) depression can be treated, (2) depression has many faces and (3) depression can affect everybody (Hegerl et al. 2003, 2006; Dietrich et al. 2010). Evaluation findings showed, while that there was a significant reduction in some aspects of depression-related stigma at follow-up (Dietrich et al. 2010; Hegerl et al. 2003), there was no significant change for statements regarding general attitudes towards depression, beliefs about symptoms or beliefs about side effects of antidepressants. There was a significant reduction in the number of suicidal acts over each of the 2 years of the campaign when compared to a control-comparison region (Hegerl et al. 2006), but no difference was observed in the number of completed suicides between the regions.

beyondblue

'beyondblue: the national depression initiative' was started in Australia in October 2000 as a 5-year programme, whose mission was to 'Provide a national focus and community leadership to increase the capacity of the Australian community to prevent depression and respond effectively to it' (Jorm et al. 2005). It had five priority areas: public awareness and destigmatisation, consumer and carer support, prevention and early intervention, primary care training and support and applied research. Different levels of campaign uptake in different Australian states and territories during the initial stage created a natural experiment, allowing comparisons of public mental health literacy and attitudes between these areas before (1995) and after (2003–2004) its launch. While recognition of depression had improved throughout the country, this was a little more so in participating areas, where there were also more positive attitudes about helpseeking and the potential benefits of counselling and medication. beyondblue has continued and currently addresses anxiety and suicide prevention in addition to depression. There is evidence that among young people, awareness of beyondblue is associated with better recognition of some other psychiatric disorders and with first aid intentions and recommendations for interventions which agree with professionals' (Yap et al. 2012). This is a cross-sectional finding, but is suggestive of a possible positive effect of depression literacy on more general mental health literacy.

Substance Misuse

In the USA, the Substance Abuse and Mental Health Services Administration has promoted Recovery Month http://www.recoverymonth.gov/ since 1989. The stated aim of Recovery Month is to spread 'the positive message that behavioural health is essential to overall health, that prevention works, treatment is effective and people can and do recover'. However, a PubMed search found no articles evaluating whether these messages are now more commonly endorsed.

In summary, as far as public attitudes and primary care professionals' practice are concerned, there is stronger evidence for the effectiveness of depression-specific education campaigns than for those concerning schizophrenia, or indeed those about mental illness in general (Crisp et al. 2005; Evans-Lacko et al. 2013; Corker et al. 2013). This is partly due to stronger evaluation design, through the availability of control areas for the evaluation of beyondblue and the Nuremberg Alliance Against Depression. It is also possible that attitudes towards depression are more amenable to public education, perhaps because it is common, so that once people are able to identify it, they are more likely to experience familiarity with someone with depression; this is associated with

Table 5.1 Disorder-specific public education programmes

Country/region	Campaign	Time period	Website	Formal evaluation completed?
Australia	*beyondblue*	2000–present	http://www.beyondblue.org.au/	Yes (Jorm et al. 2005)
Austria	*Open the Doors*	1998–present	www.openthedoors.com/greek/01_05_01.html	Yes: (Grausgruber et al. 2009; Kohlbauer et al. 2010)
Germany	*Open the Doors*	1999–present	www.openthedoors.com/greek/01_05_05.html	Yes: (Stuart et al. 2005)
	Nuremberg Alliance Against Depression	2001–2003		Yes: (Dietrich et al. 2010; Hegerl et al. 2003, 2006)
United Kingdom	*Defeat Depression*	1991–1996		Yes: (Macaskill et al. 1997; Paykel et al. 1997, 1998; Rix et al. 1999; Vize and Priest 1993)

more positive attitudes (Evans-Lacko et al. 2013). It may also be that stereotypes held regarding depression (such as blameworthiness) are more amenable to change, rather than those which evoke fear, such as unpredictability and dangerousness, which more often help with respect to schizophrenia and substance misuse (Crisp et al. 2005) (Table 5.1).

Other Disorders: Interventions with Health Professionals

Self-Harm and Borderline Personality Disorder

Much of the evidence for stigma reduction in health professionals comes from evaluation of training to improve mental health and general medical professionals' attitudes to people with self-harm and borderline personality disorder, whom they find particularly difficult to treat, as noted above. Commons Treloar and Lewis (Commons Treloar 2008a) point out that this is in part because the medical model does not provide the knowledge and skills professionals need to treat people with these problems. The psychologists in their Australian study had more positive attitudes than doctors and nurses, but their attitudes showed no association with having had specific training, while those of doctors and nurses were more positive if they had received such training. This association was also found among a sample in Belgium (Muehlenkamp 2013) and is consistent with several evaluations of training (Miller and Davenport 1996; Shanks 2011; Krawitz 2008; Commons Treloar 2008b; Samuelsson 2002). One study (Krawitz 2008) included a 6-month follow-up showing little if any reduction in the improvement in attitudes among mental health professionals. However, training may be differentially effective within professional groups; another study found that improvements in attitudes were only seen among female professionals and those with under 15 years' experience (Commons Treloar 2008b). The authors suggest that women's greater empathy, and entrenched attitudes in those with over 15 years' experience, may explain these respective differences.

Substance Misuse

At the structural level, a recent systematic review on stigma among health professionals towards people with substance misuse disorders (van Boekel et al. 2013) found some evidence for the positive impact of supportive organisational factors such as supervision and training policies on professionals' attitudes to working with this group. There have also been a number of intervention studies to improve any or all of knowledge, attitudes and behaviour towards people with substance misuse problems on the part of health professionals. One randomised study of acceptance and commitment therapy in comparison to multicultural training for substance abuse counsellors showed that ACT was more effective at 3-month follow-up for both stigma and burnout (Hayes et al. 2004). Another, of advanced training in drug misuse for general practitioners, showed improved knowledge, attitudes, prescribing confidence and greater involvement in treating drug misusers than those in the waiting list group (Strang 2007). As the authors point out, this was a self-selecting group which wanted training, whose attitudes towards drug misusers were already relatively positive. An older survey (Bander 1987) provides grounds for optimism that stereotypes can change over time. While professionals' attitudes showed considerable room for improvement, they no longer endorsed the view that people with alcohol dependence were easily recognisable as homeless people; this had formerly been the perception, which precluded earlier recognition and treatment (Table 5.2).

The evidence for many studies of education and training for professionals to reduce stigma towards people with self-harm, borderline personality and addictions is limited largely to their effects on knowledge and attitudes rather than behaviour, and follow-up periods tend to be short. Nevertheless, the results of educational interventions should not be ignored, as they suggest that education may also be an effective strategy for health professionals who have had little

Table 5.2 Disorder-specific interventions with health professionals

Citation	Study author, date	Study aim	Study design	Total sample size and sampling strategy	Type(s) of professional, setting	Country	Measure	Intervention	Follow-up	Results	Limitations
86	Commons Treloar (2008)	Assess attitudes of mental health and emergency medicine clinicians towards patients with BPD	Survey	*N* = 140 (response rate: postal 89.4 %, face-to-face 92.3 %). Self-selecting convenience sample	Mental health staff and emergency department staff	Australia New Zealand	ADSHQ. No vignettes	None	None	Mental health clinicians had significantly more positive attitude score towards BPD compared to emergency medicine clinicians. Allied health professionals had significantly higher attitude ratings towards BPD than nursing or medical staff	As self-selected convenience sample may be unable to generalise results

87	Muehlenkamp (2013)	Evaluate association between self-injury training and attitudes across different HCPs	Cross-sectional study	N = 342. Self-selected convenience sampling	Psychologists, social workers, psychiatric and medical nurses from general and psychiatric hospitals	Belgium	Purpose written qu'aire. No vignettes	Educational. Self-injury training	None	Professionals with training had more positive empathy and less negative attitudes. Mental health providers had more positive attitudes than medical professionals	Information on type of training received was not assessed, unclear what type of training is most useful in promoting positive attitudes
88	Miller and Davenport (1996)	Effect of self-instructional programme on nurses' attitudes towards patients with BPD	Controlled follow-up study	N = 32 (unknown). Convenience sample	Registered nurses. Acute adult inpatient psychiatric units, general community hospitals	USA	BPDQ. (Unpublished). No vignettes	Educational. Self-paced programmed module booklet. 3 sections, each taking 30 min to complete	After intervention	Significant differences post-test between groups in knowledge of and attitudes towards patients with BPD	Non-randomised. Low reliability of instrument in measuring behavioural intention

(continued)

Table 5.2 (continued)

Citation	Study author, date	Study aim	Study design	Total sample size and sampling strategy	Type(s) of professional, setting	Country	Measure	Intervention	Follow-up	Results	Limitations
89	Shanks (2011)	Impact of education on attitudes towards patients with BPD	Follow-up study	$N = 271$ (unknown). Convenience sample	Social workers, mental health counsellors, psychologists, psychiatrists, nurses, physician assistants and substance abuse counsellors	USA	Purpose written qu'aire. No vignettes	Educational. One-day workshop. Involved formal didactics, video presentations and case examples	After intervention	Clinicians reported greater empathy towards patients with BPD, greater awareness, feeling of increased competency, improved attitudes towards patients with BPD and their desire to work with them and significantly less likely to express dislike for BPD patients	Participants self-selected. No comparison group. No information as to whether change in attitudes leads to change in outcomes of patients with BPD

90	Krawitz (2008)	Effect of training workshop on clinician attitudes to people with BPD	Follow-up study	N=418 (delivered to 910, 241 excluded, 251 lost to follow-up). Non-convenience sample	Nurses, psychologists, social workers, occupational therapists, drs. Mental health and substance abuse services	Australia	Purpose written qu'aire. No vignettes	Educational. 2-day training workshop	After intervention; 6 months	Post-workshop: statistically significant improvement in all 6 items of questionnaire. 6-month follow-up: score remained the same or showed non-significant decrease	Survey questions not tested for reliability and validity. Selection bias
91	Commons Treloar (2008)	Impact of education on attitudes of HCPs towards working with patients exhibiting DSH behaviour	Controlled follow-up study	N=99 (response rate 13.39–42.42 %). Convenience sample (self-selected)	Nurses, doctors, allied health professionals	Australia New Zealand	ADSHQ. No vignettes	"Educational package" on dealing with BPD. 2 days	After intervention	Statistically significant improvement in clinician attitude ratings towards working with DSH behaviours in patients with BPD	Small sample size. Lack of long-term follow-up

(continued)

Table 5.2 (continued)

Citation	Study author, date	Study aim	Study design	Total sample size and sampling strategy	Type(s) of professional, setting	Country	Measure	Intervention	Follow-up	Results	Limitations
92	Samuelsson (2002)	Impact of training programme on psychiatric nursing personnel attitudes towards patients who attempted suicide	Follow-up study	N=47 (unknown). Convenience sample	Psychiatric nurses	Sweden	Purpose written qu'aire, vignettes	Educational. 12 class sessions (36 h total)	After intervention	Understanding and willingness to care increased; suicide risk of patients in case vignettes estimated more accurately	Limited number of participants. No concurrent control group
95	Strang (2007)	Measure changes in knowledge, attitudes and clinical practice of GPs enrolled to receive training in the management of drug misusers	RCT.	N=112 (original population – 137)	GPs working in primary care practices	England	DDPPQ, DPOPQ, other qu'aires	Educational. Certificate course. The course comprised 5 training days over 6 months	After intervention	Improvements in attitudes and behaviour greatest among intervention group, only 'role security' and 'situational constraint' statistically significant	None stated by study authors

Not cited	Livingston (2012)	Provides a systematic review of existing research that has empirically evaluated interventions designed to reduce stigma related to substance use disorder	Systematic review	Papers identified from 7 databases, reference lists and consulting experts. 13 papers, sample sizes ranged from 28 to 445 (median = 108)	Medical students, drug and alcohol counsellors, psychiatrists	USA, UK, Canada, Australia	Study quality appraisal checklist, Hedges' g effect size. Standardised stigma-related measures were used in 11 (85 %) studies	10 educational based, 2 involved contact education and 1 involved plastic surgery	3 studies (23 %) assessed stigma beyond the immediate post-intervention period	All but one study indicated that their intervention produced positive effect	Adverse events not measured or reported No blinding of assessors or participants Power calculation not performed Small no. of studies Heterogeneity among studies
Not cited	Gerace (1995)	To investigate whether an educational intervention improved practising nurses' recognition of and responses to substance-misusing patients	Follow-up study	N = 32, self-selected. Convenience sample	General health nurses	USA	Substance Abuse Knowledge Survey (SAKS), Substance Abuse Experience Survey (SAES) and Substance Abuse Attitude Scale (SAAS). No vignettes	Educational. 2 full-day workshops, spaced 1 week apart, each year for 3 years	After intervention completion of 5 workshops, 3 years apart	Clinical confidence ratings of the nurses increased significantly in relation to both alcohol- and drug-related clinical skills. Attitude changes were reflected in the responses to only one subscale of the Substance Abuse Attitude Scale: that of treatment optimism	Nurses enrolled had to volunteer to take part Quantitative data only

(continued)

Table 5.2 (continued)

Citation	Study author, date	Study aim	Study design	Total sample size and sampling strategy	Type(s) of professional, setting	Country	Measure	Intervention	Follow-up	Results	Limitations
Not cited	Happell (2001)	To investigate whether access to liaison services from specialist drug and alcohol unit leads to a change in attitudes, confidence and perceived knowledge related to the care of clients with drug and alcohol problems	Cross-sectional study	N = 106, response rate 53 %. Self-selected convenience sampling	General hospital nurses working in a large, private medical-surgical hospital in Melbourne	Australia	Purpose written qu'aire. No vignettes	Access to liaison drug and alcohol service	After intervention	There was little difference between the groups who have used and haven't used the drug and alcohol liaison service with the exception of the perceived knowledge category which indicated a statistically significant difference	Only conducted in one hospital Low sample size Low response rate to some questions

Not cited	Patterson (2007)	Testing the effectiveness of an educational intervention aimed at changing attitudes to self-harm	Controlled follow-up study	Intervention group: $N=69$ Control group: $N=22$. Self-selected convenience sampling	Nurses	UK	Self-Harm Antipathy Scale (SHAS)	Educational. Course titled 'Understanding and Managing Self-Harm and Suicide' over 12 days	After intervention, 18 months to 4 years later	There was evidence of a 20 % reduction in antipathy towards self-harm among course attenders maintained over a period of at least 18 months compared to a reduction of 9 % in the comparison group	Non-randomised Social desirability bias
Not cited	Shirazi (2009)	To assess the impact of an educational intervention on depression in GPs in Iran	RCT	Intervention group: $N=96$ Control group: $N=96$ Randomisation.	GPs	Iran	2 purpose written qu-aires. Vignettes included	Educational. 8 h course.	After intervention	Knowledge and attitude improved in the intervention group compared to the control group	Small sample size Social desirability bias

(continued)

Table 5.2 (continued)

Citation	Study author, date	Study aim	Study design	Total sample size and sampling strategy	Type(s) of professional, setting	Country	Measure	Intervention	Follow-up	Results	Limitations
Not cited	Wang (2012)	To assess whether nonpsychiatric physicians would benefit from a national depression training programme	Follow-up study	N=375, response rate 72 %. Self-selected convenience sampling	Physicians	China	DAQ and adapted intention to change depression management practices. No vignettes	Educational. 2-day course	After intervention	Physicians showed significantly increased knowledge score and willingness to implement new treatment strategies, as well as more positive attitude towards and confidence in treating depression	No control group Social desirability bias

SAKS Substance Abuse Knowledge Survey, *GHQ* General Health Questionnaire, *SAES* Substance Abuse Experience Survey, *SF-36* Short Form 36 Health Survey, *SAAS* Substance Abuse Attitude Scale, *MHL* Mental Health Literacy, *GP* General Practitioner, *SHAS* Self-Harm Antipathy Scale, *BPD* Borderline Personality Disorder, *ADSHQ* Attitude Towards Deliberate Self-Harm Questionnaire, *DAQ* Depression Attitude Questionnaire, *RCT* Randomised Controlled Trial, *BPDQ* Borderline Personality Disorder Questionnaire, *HCP* Health Care Professionals mental health training. In addition, the study on acceptance and commitment therapy (Hayes et al. 2004) suggests that interventions to prevent and reduce burnout should be explored further for their potential to reduce the enactment of stigma in health care.

Conclusions

There is reasonable evidence to delineate disorder-specific stigma with respect to a number of disorders, which is likely to be more differentiated among health professionals then the general public. There is also evidence that disorder-specific stigma is amenable to reduction, but this evidence varies by disorder, being best for depression and weakest for schizophrenia. Although there is no current evidence that people with schizophrenia experience more discrimination overall, there is a risk that this will become the case if current trends continue. Anti-stigma efforts directed at both the general public and specific groups should therefore consider how to avoid the development of this inequality.

References

Bander KW, Goldman DS, Schwartz MA, Rabinowitz E, English J (1987) Survey of attitudes among three specialities in a teaching hospital toward alcoholics. J Med Educ 62:17–24

Beldie A, Den Boer JA, Brain C, Constant E, Figueira ML, Filipcic I, Gillain B, Jakovljevic M, Jarema M, Jelenova D, Karamustafalioglu O, Kores Plesnicar B, Kovacsova A, Latalova K, Marksteiner J, Palha F, Pecenak J, Prasko J, Prelipceanu D, Ringen PA, Sartorius N, Seifritz E, Svestka J, Tyszkowska M, Wancata J (2012) Fighting stigma of mental illness in midsize European countries. Soc Psychiatry Psychiatr Epidemiol 47(Suppl 1):1–38

Bell JS, Johns R, Chen TF (2006) Pharmacy students' and graduates' attitudes towards people with schizophrenia and severe depression. Am J Pharm Educ 70:77

Bjorkman T, Angelman T, Jonsson M (2008) Attitudes towards people with mental illness: a cross-sectional study among nursing staff in psychiatric and somatic care. Scand J Caring Sci 22:170–177

Bonnington O (2013) Experiences of stigma and discrimination amongst people with a diagnosis of bipolar disorder or borderline personality disorder and their informal carers: an exploratory study. Ph D, University of London

Borinstein A (1992) Public attitudes towards persons with mental illness. Health Aff (Millwood) 3:186–196

Borschmann RG, Jones N, Henderson RC (2014) Campaigns to reduce mental illness stigma in Europe: a scoping review. Die Psychiatrie, in press

Brohan E, Slade M, Clement S, Rose D, Sartorius N, Thornicroft G (2013) Development and psychometric validation of the Discrimination and Stigma Scale (DISC). Psychiatry Research. http://dx.doi.org/10.1016/j.psychres.2013.03.007i

Cechnicki A, Angermeyer MC, Bielańska A (2011) Anticipated and experienced stigma among people with schizophrenia: its nature and correlates. Soc Psychiatry Psychiatr Epidemiol 46(7):643–650. doi: 10.1007/s00127-010-0230-2. Epub 2010 May 22

Commons Treloar AJ, Lewis AJ (2008a) Targeted clinical education for staff attitudes towards deliberate self-harm in borderline personality disorder: randomized controlled trial. Aust N Z J Psychiatry 42:981–988

Commons Treloar AJ, Lewis AJ (2008b) Professional attitudes towards deliberate self-harm in patients with borderline personality disorder. Aust N Z J Psychiatry 42:578–584

Corker E, Hamilton S, Henderson C, Weeks C, Pinfold V, Rose D, Williams P, Flach C, Gill V, Lewis-Holmes E (2013) Experiences of discrimination among people using mental health services in England 2008–2011. Br J Psychiatry 202:s58–s63

Crisp A, Gelder MG, Goddard E, Meltzer H (2005) Stigmatization of people with mental illnesses: a follow-up study within the changing minds campaign of the Royal College of Psychiatrists. World Psychiatry 4:106–113

Deans C, Meocevic E (2006) Attitudes of registered psychiatric nurses towards patients diagnosed with borderline personality disorder. Contemp Nurse 21:43–49

Dietrich S, Beck M, Bujantugs B, Kenzine D, Matschinger H, Angermeyer MC (2004) The relationship between public causal beliefs and social distance toward mentally ill people. Aust N Z J Psychiatry 38:348–354

Dietrich S, Heider D, Matschinger H, Angermeyer MC (2006) Influence of newspaper reporting on adolescents' attitudes toward people with mental illness. Soc Psychiatry Psychiatr Epidemiol 41:318–322

Dietrich S, Mergl R, Freudenberg P, Althaus D, Hegerl U (2010) Impact of a campaign on the public's attitudes towards depression. Health Educ Res 25:135–150

Dillner L (1992) Colleges join together to fight depression. BMJ 304:337

Evans-Lacko S, Henderson C, Thornicroft G (2013) Public knowledge, attitudes and behaviour regarding people with mental illness in England 2009–2012. Br J Psychiatry 202:s51–s57

Farrelly S, Clement S, Gabbidon J, Jeffery D, Dockery L, Lassman F, Brohan E, Henderson RC, Williams P, Howard LM, Thornicroft G (2014) Anticipated and experienced discrimination amongst people with schizophrenia, bipolar disorder and major depressive disorder: a cross sectional study. BMC Psychiatry 14:157

Fernando SM, Deane FP, McLeod HJ (2010) Sri Lankan doctors' and medical undergraduates' attitudes towards mental illness. Soc Psychiatry Psychiatr Epidemiol 45:733–739

Francis C, Pirkis J, Dunt D, Blood RW (2001) Mental health and illness in the media. Australian Department of Health and Aged Care, Melbourne

Fraser K, Gallop R (1993) Nurses' confirming/disconfirming responses to patients diagnosed with borderline personality disorder. Arch Psychiatr Nurs 7:336–341

Gaebel W, Baumann AE (2003) Interventions to reduce the stigma associated with severe mental illness: experiences from the open the doors programme in Germany. Can J Psychiatry 48:657–662

Gerace LM, Hughes TL, Spunt J (1995) Improving nurses' responses toward substance-misusing patients: a clinical evaluation project. Arch Psychiatr Nurs 9(5):286–294. PubMed PMID: 1995031825. Language: English. Entry Date: 19951101. Revision Date: 20091218. Publication Type: journal article

Gilchrist G, Moskalewicz J, Slezakova S, Okruhlica L, Torrens M, Vajd R, Baldacchino A (2011) Staff regard towards working with substance users: a European multi-centre study. Addiction 106:1114–1125

Goulden R, Corker E, Evans-Lacko S, Rose D, Thornicroft G, Henderson C (2011) Newspaper coverage of mental illness in the UK, 1992–2008. BMC Public Health 11:796

Grausgruber A, Schöny W, Grausgruber-Berner R, Koren G, Frajo AB, Wancata J, Meise U (2009) "Schizophrenia has many faces" – evaluation of the Austrian anti-stigma-campaign 2000–2002 (German). Psychiatr Prax 36:327–333

Happell BT (2001) Negative attitudes towards clients with drug and alcohol related problems: Finding the elusive solution. Aust N Z J Ment Health Nurs 10:87–96

Hayes SC, Bissett R, Roget N, Padilla I, Kohlenberg BS, Fisher G, Masuda A, Pistoreleo J, Rye AK, Berry K, Niccolls R (2004) The impact of acceptance and commitment training and multicultural training on the stigmatizing attitudes and professional burnout of substance abuse counselors. Behav Ther 35:821–835

Hegerl U, Althaus D, Stefanek J (2003) Public attitudes towards treatment of depression: effects of an information campaign. Pharmacopsychiatry 36:288–291

Hegerl U, Althaus D, Schmidtke A, Niklewski G (2006) The alliance against depression: 2-year evaluation of a community-based intervention to reduce suicidality. Psychol Med 36:1225–1234

Henderson C, Noblett J, Parke H, Clement S, Caffrey A, Gale-Grant O, Schulze B, Druss B, Thornicroft G (2014) Mental health related stigma in health care and mental health care settings. Lancet Psychiatry 1:467–482

Jorm AF, Korten AE, Jacomb PA, Christensen H, Henderson S (1999) Attitudes towards people with a mental disorder: a survey of the Australian public and health professionals. Aust N Z J Psychiatry 33:77–83

Jorm AF, Christensen H, Griffiths KM (2005) The impact of beyondblue: the national depression initiative on the Australian public's recognition of depression and beliefs about treatments. Aust N Z J Psychiatry 39:248–254

Klin A, Lemish D (2008) Mental disorders stigma in the media: review of studies on production, content, and influences. J Health Commun 13:434–449

Knifton L, Quinn N (2008) Media, mental health and discrimination: a Frame of reference for understanding reporting trends. Int J Ment Health Promot 10:23–31

Kohlbauer D, Meise U, Schenner M, Sulzenbacher H, Frajo-Apor B, Meller H, Günther V (2010) Does education focusing on depression change the attitudes towards schizophrenia? A target-group oriented anti-stigma-intervention]. Neuropsychiatrie: Klin Diagn Therapie Rehab: Organ Ges Österreichischer Nervenärzte Psychiater 24:132

Krawitz R (2008) Borderline personality disorder: attitudinal change following training. Aust N Z J Psychiatry 38(7):554–559

Lasalvia A, Zoppei S, Van BT, Bonetto C, Cristofalo D, Wahlbeck K, et al (2012) Global pattern of experienced and anticipated discrimination reported by people with major depressive disorder: a cross-sectional survey. Lancet 381:55–62.

Lauber C, Anthony M, Jdacic-Gross V, Rossler W (2004) What about psychiatrists' attitude to mentally ill people? Eur Psychiatry 19:423–427

Livingston JD, Boyd JE (2010) Correlates and consequences of internalized stigma for people living with mental illness: a systematic review and meta-analysis. Soc Sci Med 71(12):2150–2161. doi: 10.1016/j.socscimed.2010.09.030

Livingston JD, Milne T, Fang ML, Amari E (2012) The effectiveness of interventions for reducing stigma related to substance use disorders: a systematic review. Addiction 107(1):39–50

Macaskill A, Macaskill ND, Nicol A (1997) The defeat depression campaign a mid-point evaluation of its impact on general practitioners. Psychiatr Bull 21:148–150

Magliano L, De Rosa C, Fiorillo A, Malangone C, Guarneri M, Marasco C, Maj M, The Working Group of the Italian National Study on Families of Persons with Schizophrenia (2004) Beliefs of psychiatric nurses about schizophrenia: a comparison with patients' relatives and psychiatrists. Int J Soc Psychiatry 50:319–330

Mann CE, Himelein MJ (2004) Factors associated with stigmatization of persons with mental illness. Psychiatr Serv 55(2):185–187

Miller SA, Davenport NC (1996) Increasing staff knowledge of and improving attitudes toward patients with borderline personality disorder. Psychiatr Serv 47

Minas H, Zamzam R, Midin M, Cohen A (2011) Attitudes of Malaysian general hospital staff towards patients with mental illness and diabetes. BMC Public Health 11:317

Morgan H (1979) Death wishes: the understanding and management of deliberate self harm. Wiley, Chichester

Muehlenkamp JL, Claes L, Quigley K, Prosser E, Claes S, Jan D (2013) Association of training on attitudes towards self-injuring clients across health professionals. Arch Suicide Res 17:462–468

Mukherjee R, Fialho A, Wijetunge A, Checinski K, Surgenor T (2002) The stigmatisation of psychiatric illness: the attitudes of medical students and doctors in a London teaching hospital. Psychiatr Bull 26:178–181

Naeem F, Ayub M, Javed Z, Irfan M, Haral F, Kingdon D (2006) Stigma and psychiatric illness. A survey of attitude of medical students and doctors in Lahore, Pakistan. J Ayub Med Col Abbottabad: JAMC 18:46–49

Nordt C, Rossler W, Lauber C (2006) Attitudes of mental health professionals toward people with schizophrenia and major depression. Schizophr Bull 32:709–714

Patterson P, Whittington R, Bogg J (2007) Measuring nurse attitudes towards deliberate self-harm: the Self-Harm Antipathy Scale (SHAS). J Psychiatr Ment Health Nurs 14(5):438–445

Paykel E, Tylee A, Wright A, Priest R (1997) The defeat depression campaign: psychiatry in the public arena. Am J Psychiatry 154:59–65

Paykel E, Hart D, Priest R (1998) Changes in public attitudes to depression during the defeat depression campaign. Br J Psychiatry 173:519–522

Pescosolido BA, Martin JK, Long JS, Medina TR, Phelan JC, Link BG (2010) "A Disease Like Any Other"? A decade of change in public reactions to schizophrenia, depression, and alcohol dependence. Am J Psychiatry 167:1321–1330

Philo G (1996) The media and public belief. In: Philo G (ed) Media and mental distress. Longman, London

Priest RG (1991) A new initiative on depression. Br J Gen Pract 41:487

Rix S, Paykel E, Lelliott P, Tylee A, Freeling P, Gask L, Hart D (1999) Impact of a national campaign on GP education: an evaluation of the defeat depression campaign. Br J Gen Pract 49:99

Rogers TS, Kashima Y (1998) Nurses' responses to people with schizophrenia. J Adv Nurs 27:195–203

Samuelsson M, Asberg M (2002) Training program in suicide prevention for psychiatric nursing personnel enhance attitudes to attempted suicide patients. Int J Nurs Stud 39:115–121

Sarkin A, Lale R, Sklar M, Center KC, Gilmer T, Fowler C, Heller R, Ojeda VD (2015) Stigma experienced by people using mental health services in San Diego County. Soc Psychiatry Psychiatr Epidemiol 50(5):747–756

Sartorius N (2006) Lessons from a 10-year global programme against stigma and discrimination because of an illness. Psychol Health Med 11:383–388

Schomerus G, Schwahn C, Holzinger A, Corrigan P, Grabe H, Carta M, Angermeyer M (2012) Evolution of public attitudes about mental illness: a systematic review and meta-analysis. Acta Psychiatr Scand 125:440–452

Schöny W (1998) Schizophrenia – an illness and its treatment reflected in public attitude [German]. Wien Med Wochenschrift 148:284

Schulze B (2007) Stigma and mental health professionals: a review of the evidence on an intricate relationship. Int Rev Psychiatry 19:137–155

Schulze B, Angermeyer MC (2003) Subjective experiences of stigma. A focus group study of schizophrenic patients, their relatives and mental health professionals. Soc Sci Med 56:299–312

Schulze B, Richter-Werling M, Matschinger H, Angermeyer M (2003) Crazy? So what! Effects of a school project on students' attitudes towards people with schizophrenia. Acta Psychiatr Scand 107:142–150

Schulze B, Janeiro M, Kiss MH (2010) Das kommt ganz drauf an... Strategien zur Stigmabewältigung von Menschen mit Schizophrenie und Borderline-Persönlichkeitsstörung. [It all depends... Strategies for managing stigma among people with schizophrenia and borderline personality disorder]. Psychiatr Psychol Psychother 58:275–285

Shanks C, Pfohl B, Blum N, Black DW (2011) Can negative attitudes toward patients with borderline personality disorder be changed? The effect of attending a STEPPS workshop. J Pers Disord 25:806–812

Shirazi M, Parikh SV, Alaeddini F, Lonka K, Zeinaloo AA, Sadeghi M, Arbabi M, Nejatisafa AA, Shahrivar Z, Wahlstrom R (2009) Effects on knowledge and Attitudes of Using Stages of Change to Train General Practitioners on Management of Depression: A Randomised Controlled Study. Canadian Journal of Psychiatry - Revue Canadienne de Psychiatrie 54(10):693–700

Stout P, Villegas J, Jennings NA (2004) Images of mental illness in the media: identifying gaps in the research. Schizophr Bull 30:543–561

Strang J, Hunt C, Gerada C, Marsden J (2007) What difference does training make? A randomized trial with waiting-list control of general practitioners seeking advanced training in drug misuse. Addiction 102:1637–1647

Stuart H, Arboleda-Flórez H, Sartorius N (2005) Stigma and mental disorders: international perspectives. World Psychiatry 4:1–62

Thornicroft G (2006) Shunned: discrimination against people with mental illness. Oxford University Press, Oxford

Thornicroft G, Brohan E, Rose D, Sartorius N, Leese M (2009) Global pattern of experienced and anticipated discrimination against people with schizophrenia: a cross-sectional survey. Lancet 373:408–415

Thornton J, Wahl OF (1996) Impact of a newspaper article on attitudes toward mental illness. J Community Psychol 24:17–25

Van Boekel LC, Brouwers EP, Van Weeghel J, Garretsen HF (2013) Stigma among health professionals towards patients with substance use disorders and its consequences for healthcare delivery: systematic review. Drug Alcohol Depend 131:23–35

Vize C, Priest R (1993) Defeat depression campaign: attitudes to depression. Psychiatr Bull 17:573–574

Wahl O (1992) Mass media images of mental illness: a review of the literature. J Community Psychol 20:343–352

Wahl O, Aroesty-Cohen E (2010) Attitudes of mental health professionals about mental illness: a review of the recent literature. J Community Psychol 38:49–62

Wang Y-H, Huang H-C, Liu S-I, Lu R-B (2012) Assessment of changes in confidence, attitude, and knowledge of non-psychiatric physicians undergoing a depression training program in Taiwan. Int J Psychiat Med 43(4):293–308. PubMed PMID: 2012-25679-001

Warner R (2005) Local projects of the World Psychiatric Association programme to reduce stigma and discrimination. Psychiatr Serv 56:570–575

Watts D, Morgan G (1994) Malignant alienation. Dangers for patients who are hard to like. Br J Psychiatry 164:11–15

Wilstrand C, Lindgren BM, Gilje F, Olofsson B (2007) Being burdened and balancing boundaries: a qualitative study of nurses' experiences caring for patients who self-harm. J Psychiatr Ment Health Nurs 14:72–78

Yap MB, Reavley NJ, Jorm AF (2012) Associations between awareness of beyond blue and mental health literacy in Australian youth: results from a national survey. Aust N Z J Psychiatry 46:541–552

Yen CF, Chen CC, Lee Y, Tang TC, Yen JY, Ko CH (2005) Self-stigma and its correlates among outpatients with depressive disorders. Psychiatr Serv 56(5):599–601

Who Is Contributing?

6

Alexandre Andrade Loch and Wulf Rössler

Introduction

In this chapter, we will address the question of who might potentially hold stigmatizing beliefs toward persons with mental illness. While examining these potential contributors, we want to show that, by harboring such beliefs, these groups and individuals perpetuate the stigmatization process now present in popular culture. This process, as we shall see, is inherent to every society and is generalized rather than focused. Therefore, anyone can, hypothetically, add to the stigma of mental illness, including even some healthcare and mental health professionals who might maintain such prejudices. As such, we start with a short introduction that shows how stigmatization does not apply exclusively to mental disorders but, rather, is a natural activity within every society. We then course through the stigmatization process, beginning at the macrolevel, which comprises society as a whole as well as the mass media. We then continue to the intermediate level, comprising healthcare professionals, and finally to the microlevel, which includes the individual with mental illness himself, who also contributes to this process via self-stigmatization.

A.A. Loch (✉)
Laboratory of Neuroscience (LIM-27), Institute of Psychiatry, School of Medicine,
University of São Paulo, R. Dr. Ovidio Pires de Campos, 785, São Paulo, Brazil
e-mail: alexandre.loch@usp.br

W. Rössler
Psychiatric University Hospital, University of Zurich, Zurich, Switzerland
e-mail: wulf.roessler@uzh.ch

© Springer International Publishing Switzerland 2017
W. Gaebel et al. (eds.), *The Stigma of Mental Illness - End of the Story?*,
DOI 10.1007/978-3-319-27839-1_6

Stigma: Potentially Everyone Might Be Contributing

Gerhard Falk, a German sociologist and historian, presented an interesting perspective on stigma: "We and all societies will always stigmatize some conditions and some behaviors because doing so provides for group solidarity by delineating 'outsiders' from 'insiders'" (Falk 2001). That is, in-group love is related to out-group hate (Brewer 1999), such that the latter feeds the former. However, is this relationship necessarily inevitable?

As social assemblies have become increasingly larger, the human species has evolved to depend upon cooperation rather than strength. Moreover, each cooperative system has had to rely upon trust. However, trust that one does not choose for oneself is not viable and, therefore, a person must delimit a group of individuals who are deemed trustworthy and with whom altruism can be exchanged. This mechanism is natural to all societies and is as old as civilization; it is how "insiders" bind one to another. One important and mandatory way to reinforce this trust system and, consequently, further strengthen the in-group is to do the opposite with outsiders. Thus, outsiders are commonly the recipients of negative attributions, mistrust, disdain, and hatred. Sociologists argue that in-group attachment is linked to out-group prejudice, being two sides of the same coin. That is, if no society or group were to gather, then there would be no necessity or utility in excluding outsiders and, ultimately, no discrimination against them.

Taking these ideas into account, one can suppose that there will always be stigma and prejudice toward a certain group of persons, as acknowledged by Falk. Accordingly, Foucault (2006) has related the story of how outsiders' attributions, which had spanned the ages, moved several centuries ago from individuals with leprosy to those with mental illness. Although this transfer occurred long ago, the characteristic of being an outsider is still linked to persons who suffer from these disorders, as demonstrated through various studies in the past two decades.

Nevertheless, among all the various health conditions that exist, why would individuals with mental illness be at special risk for stigmatization? As we know, psychiatric disorders are characterized by changes in behavior and social performance (Fig. 6.1). For example, schizophrenia is the prototypical disorder of psychiatry and is characterized by positive and negative symptoms. Those positive symptoms comprise hallucinations and delusions, perceptions, and beliefs that are incongruent with socially shared observations and ideas. Likewise, negative symptoms encompass social withdrawal, diminished capacity for affective resonation with the surrounding world (affective blunting), apathy, and abulia. These two symptom dimensions are metaphors for a certain degree of dissonance with society and, therefore, place individuals with schizophrenia at greater risk for stigmatization, especially when they find themselves in exacerbated episodes of the disorder. They are then more vulnerable to being labeled an "outsider." Other diagnoses, e.g., depression, anxiety, and substance use disorders, are equally susceptible to stigmatization once they, to a certain extent, fall into the same

Fig. 6.1 Mental illness and the vulnerability to stigma

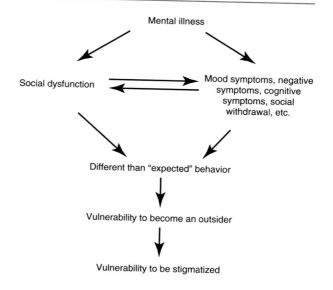

Fig. 6.2 The different levels of stigma

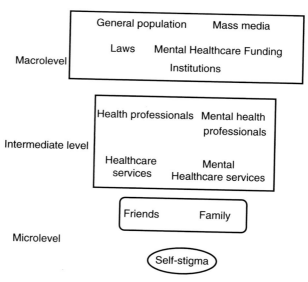

category. That is, all of them are invariably established using the criterion of (social) dysfunctioning.

When all is considered, we acknowledge that stigmatization is a common social mechanism of societies and that individuals with mental disorders are at special risk for being made scapegoats by those attitudes. Therefore, as presented previously, virtually everyone, from the broad macrolevel of the general population to the microlevel of persons with mental illnesses, can contribute to this stigma (Fig. 6.2).

Society: The Macrolevel

Society as a whole exhibits a high degree of stigmatizing beliefs regarding mental illness. These beliefs within the general population are commonly expressed as stereotypes, i.e., units of information that serve to simplify one's understanding about groups. They have an economic function because they collect several subjects with similar characteristics or traits under the same denominational umbrella. Therefore, instead of perceiving individuals according to their singularity and different traits/qualities, the collective group uses stereotypes to simplify that process, depicting a set of individuals with short-word concepts that generalize themselves to all members of the determined group, even to those who do not manifest the specific stereotypical characteristic. Such negative stereotypes are inflexible and tend to become attached to persons with mental illness.

In Germany, a survey of 5,025 participants from the general population indicated that persons with schizophrenia are stereotyped as unpredictable and incompetent (Angermeyer and Matschinger 2004). Moreover, such persons are invariably considered dangerous. A study in Argentina showed that the majority of the 1,254 participants declared that persons with schizophrenia are dangerous and suffer from split personalities (Leiderman et al. 2011). In the USA, 66 % of survey participants reported that, in their opinion, individuals with cocaine dependence are bad characters; for individuals with alcohol dependence, that rate is 51 % (Link et al. 1999). An investigation in Italy revealed that 85 % of the general population sample also characterizes individuals with schizophrenia as dangerous. In the past 15 years, a review of research on population-based attitudes conducted by Angermeyer and Dietrich (2006) has concluded that substance abuse and schizophrenia are the most negatively characterized mental disorder by the general population. Phelan et al. have reinforced this outcome. Phelan et al. (2000) reported that stigmas persist and stereotypes might be inflexible to change. That research group compared two opinion surveys conducted in 1950 and 1996 and found that the concept of mental illness had broadened, such that psychosis did not dominate people's descriptions in 1996 to the same extent as it had in 1950. Nevertheless, the mention of dangerousness had become significantly more frequent in respondents' descriptions of mental illness.

Concerning stereotypes, an important contributor to these false beliefs held by society is the mass media. Over time, their coverage of mental illnesses has been consistently and overwhelmingly negative and imprecise. Thus, media such as television news and entertainment programming, films, and newspapers have a central role in disseminating biased information about mental illness and strengthening negative stereotypes. Sensationalist reports of violence and crimes committed by individuals with these disorders receive much more attention than those committed by mentally healthy persons. This, then, crystallizes a biased image of individuals with mental disorders as dangerous persons who endanger society. Day and Page (1986) have analyzed Canadian newspapers and observed that they generally depict persons with mental illnesses as dangerous, unpredictable, unsociable, unemployed, and transient. An analysis of German newspapers has shown a propensity to associate mental illness with violent crime (Angermeyer and Schulze 2001). In a New

Zealand study, newspaper stories about persons with mental illnesses were found to be negative, placing more emphasis on violent and criminal behavior than the official reports (Nairn et al. 2001). Signorielli (1989) analyzed actors' roles on prime-time television in the USA between 1969 and 1985 and found that 72 % of characters with mental illness were depicted as violent, compared with 42 % of "normal" characters. Another study of television programming showed that characters with mental illnesses are violent nearly ten times more frequently than "normal" characters (Diefenbach 1997). Rose (1998) observed in Great Britain that persons with mental illnesses are portrayed as violent most of the time in television news stories. Another survey demonstrated that approximately 8 % of cartoons contain references to mental illnesses, with most depicting those disorders as a loss of control and portraying characters as devoid of any positive traits (Wilson et al. 2000). Thus, transcultural assessments have further strengthened the evidence that, in countries where media coverage of these incidents is more stigmatizing, negative views of persons with such diagnoses are reinforced (Angermeyer et al. 2004).

With regard to the style of language employed in the mass media, special remarks should be made concerning the term "schizophrenia" because it is often used in a metaphorical way that usually denotes poor attributes. This has been demonstrated by various studies that analyzed the use of this word in newspaper coverage (Clement and Foster 2008). Consequently, the schizophrenia label itself has frequently become associated with negative connotations. Investigations of this issue have revealed that a negative characterization is much more frequent when the diagnostic term used is schizophrenia than when another diagnosis, e.g., "depression," is employed. Angermeyer and Matschinger (2003) have shown in their sampling of the general population that labeling someone with schizophrenia triggers negative reactions such as fear and a desire for social distance. The cognitive process is usually described as follows: labeling evokes well-established negative stereotypes that, in turn, generate discrimination. Studies in Japan identified a significant change in stigma levels after changing the name of the disorder from "mind-split disease" to "integration disorder" (Sato 2006). While the immediate effect was a reduction of stigma, the risk still existed that a stigma would migrate from one name to another in the long term.

While stigma related to mental disorders is fueled by these ideas, they additionally increase discrimination toward persons with the diagnosis. One of the most well-known measures of such discrimination is the desire for social distance from persons with mental disorders, which is usually very strong (Link et al. 1999). Accordingly, an important investigation in Germany observed that this desire for distance intensified the more that persons watched TV (Angermeyer et al. 2005). This confirms the abovementioned hypothesis that the media are a main source of stigma.

Another way to comprehend macrolevel societal discrimination toward individuals with mental illness is through the concept of "structural stigma," or "institutional stigma" (Corrigan et al. 2004), which can be either intentional or unintentional. Intentional applications are manifested by the rules, policies, and procedures of private and public entities in positions of power that consciously and purposefully restrict the rights and opportunities of individuals with mental illness. This includes the abovementioned news media that deliberately denigrate the image of afflicted individuals, as well as laws that limit the rights of those individuals and constrain budgets for public mental healthcare. By contrast, unintentional, or subtle, discrimination means that, despite a commitment to neutrality, a policy or principle may result in less opportunity for a stigmatized group than for the majority. For example, Link and Phelan (2001) have argued that less money is allocated to research on psychiatric treatment than for other conditions that usually dominate the public health agenda (e.g., HIV and cancer). In addition, because of low salaries, many mental health professionals opt out of public systems that serve persons with the most serious psychiatric and substance use disorders.

Healthcare Professionals: The Intermediate Level

Liggins and Hatcher (2005) have observed that, in a general hospital, when there is a suspicion or confirmation that a particular patient suffers from a mental disorder, staff members tend to react negatively toward that person. Moreover, Arvaniti et al. (2009) have demonstrated that an important part of their sample, comprising the staff and medical students of a general university hospital, can hold negative attitudes about patients with mental illness. Such attitudes can lead to social restriction and discrimination in particular. However, an investigation in Istanbul has revealed that medical students in their sixth year of study have better attitudes toward individuals with mental illness when compared with first-year students (Ay et al. 2006). Those researchers hypothesized that this reduction in discrimination might possibly result because the medical school encourages increased contact with such patients. In England, 108 healthcare professionals answered the five-item Attitude to Mental Illness Questionnaire after having been read a vignette about a fictitious patient with an acute psychotic episode, schizophrenia, or no psychiatric disorder (Rao et al. 2009). Schizophrenia received the most negative opinions in comparison with the no-disorder vignette.

Because healthcare and even mental health professionals cultivate stigmatizing beliefs about individuals with mental disorders, two questions must be addressed: (1) what is the degree of stigma displayed by healthcare professionals when compared with the general population and (2) do mental health professionals in particular stigmatize their patients? If these professionals inevitably have more contact with individuals who suffer from psychiatric disorders and it is generally acknowledged that this type of increased contact can decrease such stigma (Couture and Penn 2003) then, accordingly, could these professionals serve as role models for society by demonstrating less-prejudiced beliefs?

Although the latter hypothesis has not been confirmed in the literature, Hori et al. (2011) have examined the opinions toward schizophrenia by 197 individuals from the general population, 100 from the medical staff, 112 general practitioners, and 36 psychiatrists. General practitioners and the general population hold the most negative beliefs. Psychiatrists generally have positive views but express a certain amount of desire for social distance from these patients. Jorm et al. (1999) have investigated 2,031 individuals from the general population plus 1,128 psychiatrists. Persons in both groups consider schizophrenia to be worse than depression. A Swiss evaluation of 90 psychiatrists and 786 individuals from the general population found that members of the former group are more in favor of community psychiatry for persons with severe mental illnesses (Lauber et al. 2006). Interestingly, when the desire for social distance is assessed, the scores are similar for both groups of participants. The researchers explain this response as a "not in my backyard" phenomenon, in which psychiatrists display politically correct opinions as long as they are not affected personally. Nordt et al. (2006) interviewed 1,073 mental health professionals and 1,737 members of the public regarding their attitudes toward a person with or without psychiatric symptoms such as for depression or schizophrenia. Regardless of the interview group, less social distance is desired toward persons with either major depression or no symptoms than toward those with schizophrenia. A study in Brazil indicated that psychiatrists have a stronger prejudice than the general population toward schizophrenia (Loch et al. 2013). In that sampling, groups of participants were divided according to their knowledge about schizophrenia, measured as the recognition of a vignette, and the researchers noted that the more a person recognizes the vignette, the more they stigmatize. Except for social distance, psychiatrists rank highest when scoring the degree of their stigma. The same sample groups also applied a high level of stigma when surveyed about various other psychiatric diagnoses (Hengartner et al. 2013). Caldwell and Jorm (2001) have found that, among general practitioners, psychiatrists, psychologists, and nurses, members of the nursing staff cultivate the worst beliefs about individuals with mental illness. Moreover, a review conducted by Schulze (2007) has revealed that contact with mental health professionals and the quality of mental health services are two of the most stigmatic experiences reported by individuals with mental illness.

In theory, one might expect healthcare professionals and, specifically, mental health professionals, to have the most positive beliefs and attitudes toward individuals with mental illness. However, based on these investigations described above, this is not the case. Results show us that, in this closer social circle of individuals with mental disorder, professionals contribute negatively to the stigma of the disorder. They display at least equal or, in some cases, even stronger negative beliefs and attitudes toward these individuals than do persons in the general population. Consequently, one of the recommendations of the Royal College of Psychiatrists in the UK has been that healthcare professionals, especially psychiatrists, be alerted to this problem (Crisp et al. 2004). As Magliano et al. (2004) stated, mental health professionals should be made aware of their possibly prejudices against individuals with psychiatric disorders because such behavior can influence the perception of nonprofessionals as well as the social acceptance of persons with those diagnoses.

Friends, Family, and Self-Stigma: The Intimate Microlevel

One important issue that stands out in stigma research is family burden, which can arise from a lack of mental health and rehabilitation services, as well as behavior and attitudes expressed toward relatives (Tsang et al. 2003). One common mechanism by which stigma can be transferred from the individual with a mental illness to his/her family is to blame the family for the onset of the disorder and to accuse them of contamination, by which family members are perceived to have the same negative attributes as the mentally ill individual (Corrigan et al. 2006). The usual term for this is "courtesy stigma," or "stigma by association," coined by Erving Goffman to refer to the stigma attached to those merely associated with a stigmatized person.

A common way to deal with this labeling is to reject the stigmatized individual so as to "return" the stigma to its generator, which consequently increases the stigma. A study assessing factors related to rehospitalization of individuals with bipolar disorder or psychosis has found that the most important predictor of readmission is familial stigma (Loch 2012). Despite illness severity and the number of previous hospitalizations, familial rejection of the relative with mental illness can be the main determinant of further hospitalizations. In that case stigma is the primary cause of readmission, but readmission itself also greatly worsens the stigma. As such, a vicious circle is created where readmission strengthens stigma and vice versa. In an examination conducted in Sweden with family members of individuals with mental disorders, an important group of them stated that the ill relative would be better off dead and/or wished that the patient and the relative had never met or that the patient had never been born (Ostman and Kjellin 2002). Hypothetically, another vicious circle can then develop in which relatives fail to provide adequate treatment due to neglect; individuals are undertreated and often symptomatic, thereby increasing their stigma and increasing the level of family rejection, which in turn feeds this loop and worsens the situation. Such a process also incorporates the friends and closer social circle of individuals with mental illnesses, again tending to isolate them in order to avoid association stigma.

Finally, but certainly not the least important, is the contribution of self-stigma, a concept that usually describes a process in which an individual with mental illness internalizes the stigma and then experiences diminished self-esteem and self-efficacy, limiting one's prospects for recovery. Social psychologists argue that this process begins even before that person is afflicted with a mental illness because it is during that period that he/she usually learns and internalizes culturally disseminated stereotypes about such illnesses. Thus, when that individual then faces an outbreak of the first episode, those commonly held knowledge structures become prominent and relevant to the self. Consequently, individuals narrow their social networks in anticipation of stigma-related rejection and then isolate themselves. This in turn causes them to lose jobs and other gainful opportunities and even to refrain from seeking medical help for their symptoms. In doing so, they may go undertreated, their symptoms and prognosis worsen, and they become more disabled and more isolated, ultimately increasing the level of attached stigma.

A suggested model of this process can be simplified as follows: first is stereotype awareness, when an individual becomes familiar with the stereotypes displayed in society by media and the general population. Second, stereotype agreement occurs when the individual endorses those public stereotypes. The third step specifically implies self-stigma, i.e., "self-concurrence," where the individual applies culturally internalized stereotypes to him or herself, yielding the consequences described above (Watson et al. 2007). Thus, self-stigmatization originates from the innermost social layer of the individual with a mental illness.

Conclusion

Stigma toward mental illness is resilient and resistant to intervention. As an example, in a 10-year follow-up investigation conducted in the USA, anti-stigma campaigns directed toward mental illness were successful in increasing the population's acceptance of neurobiological theories and in improving society's support of treatment for persons with mental disorders. However, there was no real change in the level of stigmatization (Pescosolido et al. 2010). Another study evaluating data from 1994 to 2003 in Scotland and England observed that, despite the implementation of anti-stigma efforts, stigma in fact increased during that time frame (Mehta et al. 2009).

Recalling the work by Foucault mentioned earlier in this chapter, although much progress has been made in enhancing one's understanding of various mental illnesses within the past century, and despite anti-stigma campaigns conducted during that time period, stigma still exists toward persons with such diagnoses. Some possible reasons for this are (1) stigmatization is a common mechanism by which societies improve in-group connections, (2) individuals with mental illnesses are especially vulnerable due to the nature of their diagnoses, and (3) the fact that virtually everyone can negatively contribute to stigma, from the macro- to the microlevel. Therefore, this poses an important challenge because, in order to fight stigma, one cannot take a single-target approach but must, instead, present broader interventions aimed at eliminating stigma at all levels.

Information Box 6.1
- Stigmatization is a common mechanism within all societies.
- Individuals with mental illnesses are especially vulnerable to stigma due to the nature of their disorders.
- Virtually every social strata encompassing an individual with mental illness can contribute to stigma.
- Even the individual with mental illness himself can contribute to this problem through self-stigmatization.

References

Angermeyer MC, Dietrich S (2006) Public beliefs about and attitudes towards people with mental illness: a review of population studies. Acta Psychiatr Scand 113(3):163–179

Angermeyer MC, Matschinger H (2003) Public beliefs about schizophrenia and depression: similarities and differences. Soc Psychiatry Psychiatr Epidemiol 38(9):526–534

Angermeyer MC, Matschinger H (2004) The stereotype of schizophrenia and its impact on discrimination against people with schizophrenia: results from a representative survey in Germany. Schizophr Bull 30(4):1049–1061

Angermeyer MC, Schulze B (2001) Reinforcing stereotypes: how the focus on forensic cases in news reporting may influence public attitudes towards the mentally ill. Int J Law Psychiatry 24(4–5):469–486

Angermeyer MC, Buyantugs L, Kenzine DV, Matschinger H (2004) Effects of labelling on public attitudes towards people with schizophrenia: are there cultural differences? Acta Psychiatr Scand 109(6):420–425

Angermeyer MC, Dietrich S, Pott D, Matschinger H (2005) Media consumption and desire for social distance towards people with schizophrenia. Eur Psychiatry 20(3):246–250

Arvaniti A, Samakouri M, Kalamara E, Bochtsou V, Bikos C, Livaditis M (2009) Health service staff's attitudes towards patients with mental illness. Soc Psychiatry Psychiatr Epidemiol 44(8):658–665

Ay P, Save D, Fidanoglu O (2006) Does stigma concerning mental disorders differ through medical education? A survey among medical students in Istanbul. Soc Psychiatry Psychiatr Epidemiol 41(1):63–67

Brewer MB (1999) The psychology of prejudice: ingroup love or outgroup hate? J Soc Issues 55(3):429–444

Caldwell TM, Jorm AF (2001) Mental health nurses' beliefs about likely outcomes for people with schizophrenia or depression: a comparison with the public and other healthcare professionals. Aust N Z J Ment Health Nurs 10(1):42–54

Clement S, Foster N (2008) Newspaper reporting on schizophrenia: a content analysis of five national newspapers at two time points. Schizophr Res 98(1–3):178–183

Corrigan PW, Markowitz FE, Watson AC (2004) Structural levels of mental illness stigma and discrimination. Schizophr Bull 30(3):481–491

Corrigan PW, Watson AC, Miller FE (2006) Blame, shame, and contamination: the impact of mental illness and drug dependence stigma on family members. J Fam Psychol 20(2):239–246

Couture SM, Penn DL (2003) Interpersonal contact and the stigma of mental illness: a review of the literature. J Ment Health 12(3):291–305

Crisp A, Cowan L, Hart D (2004) The college's anti-stigma campaign, 1998–2003. Psychiatr Bull 28:133–136

Day DM, Page S (1986) Portrayal of mental illness in Canadian newspapers. Can J Psychiatry 31(9):813–817

Diefenbach DL (1997) The portrayal of mental illness on prime-time television. J Community Psychol 25(3):289–302

Falk G (2001) Stigma: how we treat outsiders. Prometheus Books, Amherst

Foucault M (2006) History of madness. Routledge, London

Hengartner MP, Loch AA, Lawson FL et al (2013) Public stigmatization of different mental disorders: a comprehensive attitude survey. Epidemiol Psychiatr Sci 22(3):269–274

Hori H, Richards M, Kawamoto Y, Kunugi H (2011) Attitudes toward schizophrenia in the general population, psychiatric staff, physicians, and psychiatrists: a web-based survey in Japan. Psychiatry Res 186(2–3):183–189

Jorm AF, Korten AE, Jacomb PA, Christensen H, Henderson S (1999) Attitudes towards people with a mental disorder: a survey of the Australian public and health professionals. Aust N Z J Psychiatry 33(1):77–83

Lauber C, Nordt C, Braunschweig C, Rossler W (2006) Do mental health professionals stigmatize their patients? Acta Psychiatr Scand Suppl 429:51–59

Leiderman EA, Vazquez G, Berizzo C et al (2011) Public knowledge, beliefs and attitudes towards patients with schizophrenia: Buenos Aires. Soc Psychiatry Psychiatr Epidemiol 46(4):281–290

Liggins J, Hatcher S (2005) Stigma toward the mentally ill in the general hospital: a qualitative study. Gen Hosp Psychiatry 27(5):359–364

Link BG, Phelan JC (2001) Conceptualizing stigma. Annu Rev Sociol 27:363–385

Link BG, Phelan JC, Bresnahan M, Stueve A, Pescosolido BA (1999) Public conceptions of mental illness: labels, causes, dangerousness, and social distance. Am J Public Health 89(9):1328–1333

Loch AA (2012) Stigma and higher rates of psychiatric re-hospitalization: Sao Paulo public mental health system. Rev Bras Psiquiatr 34(2):185–192

Loch AA, Hengartner MP, Guarniero FB et al (2013) The more information, the more negative stigma towards schizophrenia: Brazilian general population and psychiatrists compared. Psychiatry Res 205(3):185–191

Magliano L, Fiorillo A, De Rosa C, Malangone C, Maj M (2004) Beliefs about schizophrenia in Italy: a comparative nationwide survey of the general public, mental health professionals, and patients' relatives. Can J Psychiatry 49(5):322–330

Mehta N, Kassam A, Leese M, Butler G, Thornicroft G (2009) Public attitudes towards people with mental illness in England and Scotland, 1994–2003. Br J Psychiatry 194(3):278–284

Nairn R, Coverdale J, Claasen D (2001) From source material to news story in New Zealand print media: a prospective study of the stigmatizing processes in depicting mental illness. Aust N Z J Psychiatry 35(5):654–659

Nordt C, Rossler W, Lauber C (2006) Attitudes of mental health professionals toward people with schizophrenia and major depression. Schizophr Bull 32(4):709–714

Ostman M, Kjellin L (2002) Stigma by association: psychological factors in relatives of people with mental illness. Br J Psychiatry 181:494–498

Pescosolido BA, Martin JK, Long JS, Medina TR, Phelan JC, Link BG (2010) "A disease like any other"? A decade of change in public reactions to schizophrenia, depression, and alcohol dependence. Am J Psychiatry 167(11):1321–1330

Phelan JC, Link BG, Stueve A, Pescosolido BA (2000) Public conceptions of mental illness in 1950 and 1996: what is mental illness and is it to be feared? J Health Soc Behav 41(2):188–207

Rao H, Mahadevappa H, Pillay P, Sessay M, Abraham A, Luty J (2009) A study of stigmatized attitudes towards people with mental health problems among health professionals. J Psychiatr Ment Health Nurs 16(3):279–284

Rose D (1998) Television, madness and community care. J Community Appl Soc Psychol 8(3):213–228

Sato M (2006) Renaming schizophrenia: a Japanese perspective. World Psychiatry 5(1):53–55

Schulze B (2007) Stigma and mental health professionals: a review of the evidence on an intricate relationship. Int Rev Psychiatry 19(2):137–155

Signorielli N (1989) The stigma of mental-illness on television. J Broadcast Elec Media 33(3):325–331

Tsang HW, Tam PK, Chan F, Cheung WM (2003) Sources of burdens on families of individuals with mental illness. Int J Rehabil Res 26(2):123–130

Watson AC, Corrigan P, Larson JE, Sells M (2007) Self-stigma in people with mental illness. Schizophr Bull 33(6):1312–1318

Wilson C, Nairn R, Coverdale J, Panapa A (2000) How mental illness is portrayed in children's television – a prospective study. Br J Psychiatry 176:440–443

Discrimination and Stigma

7

Dzmitry Krupchanka and Graham Thornicroft

Introduction and Terminology

Since Goffman's seminal work on stigma (Goffman 1963), research in this field has steadily grown (Abelev et al. 2006). Until recently, most stigma research in relation to mental illness consisted of surveys among the general public of attitudes towards people with mental illness (Sartorius and Schulze 2005; Rabkin 1974; Link et al. 1999; Thornicroft 2006a). Much less is known about the subjective experiences of stigma and discrimination faced by people with mental illness (Thornicroft 2006a) or about the effective interventions to reduce stigma (Thornicroft 2006a).

The various approaches used in stigma research have evolved from a focus on the 'mark of shame' itself, to address the ways in which relationships are affected by such stigmatisation, describing both the sociological processes of labelling and stereotyping and the internal psychological aspects of coping with stigma. More recent work has also considered social factors (in particular the implications of power relationships for stigma (Yang et al. 2007, 2010; Link and Phelan 2001; Hatzenbuehler et al. 2013) and anthropological perspectives on stigma (e.g. work carried out in China (Yang 2007; Yang and Kleinman 2008), India (Raguram et al.

D. Krupchanka (✉) • G. Thornicroft
Institute of Psychiatry, Psychology and Neuroscience, King's College London, London SE5 8AF, UK
e-mail: dmitry.krupchenko@gmail.com; graham.thornicroft@kcl.ac.uk

© Springer International Publishing Switzerland 2017
W. Gaebel et al. (eds.), *The Stigma of Mental Illness - End of the Story?*,
DOI 10.1007/978-3-319-27839-1_7

2004; Weiss et al. 2001) and Nepal (Yang et al. 2007, 2010; Kohrt and Harper 2008; Kohrt and Hruschka 2010)).

Several theoretical approaches have been developed. The social cognitive model of stigma (Corrigan 2000; Cooper et al. 2003; Corrigan and Kleinlein 2005) focuses on three core features of stigma, namely, stereotypes (negative beliefs about a group), prejudice (agreement with stereotyped beliefs and/or negative emotional reactions such as fear or anger) and discrimination (a behavioural consequence of prejudice, such as exclusion from social and economic opportunities) (Rusch et al. 2005). They define self-stigma as occurring when people with mental illness, or another stigmatised attribute, accept the discrediting beliefs (stereotypes) held against them, agree with these beliefs (i.e. prejudice themselves) and lose self-esteem and self-efficacy. This may then lead to adverse behavioural consequences (discrimination) (Corrigan and Kleinlein 2005; Corrigan and Larson 2008; Corrigan et al. 2009).

In contrast, sociological approaches consider stigma as a societal force which affects both the targeted individual or group and the society as a whole. Sociological models use labelling theory to describe the processes through which stigma is created and are based on the idea that the meaning of interpersonal interactions is socially constructed (Yang et al. 2010). In this tradition, Link and Phelan have conceptualised stigma as a broader concept that occurs 'when elements of labelling, stereotyping, separation, status loss and discrimination co-occur in a power situation that allows the components of stigma to unfold' (Link and Phelan 2001).

The conceptualisation we adopt for the purpose of this chapter incorporates elements of these models and describes stigma as an overarching construct which consists of three major domains: problems of knowledge (ignorance), problems of attitudes (prejudice) and problems of behaviour (discrimination) (Thornicroft 2006a; Thornicroft et al. 2007; Clement et al. 2011). These three elements represent the cognitive, affective and behavioural elements referred to in social psychological research on stigma (Corrigan and Kleinlein 2005; Dovidio et al. 2000). This knowledge-attitude-behaviour approach to stigma has also been adopted by the National Institute for Health and Care Excellence (NICE) in relation to public health interventions (Excellence NIfHaC 2007).

It may be helpful to distinguish two different broad types of discrimination: individual discrimination and structural discrimination (Link et al. 2001, 2004; Thornicroft 2006a; Corrigan et al. 2004, 2005a). Until recently, it was felt that practically nothing was known about how attitudes regarding individual and structural discrimination relate to each other (Matschinger and Angermeyer 2004). Angermeyer has reported that 'In fact the attitudes of the German public towards structural discrimination in the area of health care of people with depression have substantially improved during the first decade of this century' (Schomerus et al. 2015). At the same time, further studies in Germany suggest that specific strategies may be necessary to counteract specific forms of stigma and discrimination. Interventions successfully employed with one form of discrimination may not necessarily work with another form (Schomerus et al. 2007).

Several studies have reported naturalistic trends in recent years in public opinions about people with mental illness and have shown that without specific national anti-stigma programmes, social distance towards people with common mental disorders does not seem to have changed, whilst attitudes towards people with mental illness have deteriorated in the USA and Germany (Pescosolido et al. 2010; Angermeyer et al. 2013). Where national anti-stigma programmes have been rigorously assessed, the results to date have shown moderate-sized improvements in aspects of social distance, stigma and discrimination (Thornicroft et al. 2014; Henderson and Thornicroft 2009; Henderson et al. 2012).

Processes and Levels of Discrimination

Discrimination is usually defined as a behavioural component of stigma, and it is deemed to be one of the core elements through which people with mental disorders are exposed to status loss and unfair distribution of life chances after being labelled, set apart and associated with negative stereotypes (Thornicroft 2006a; Link et al. 2001).

The exact mechanisms of transformation of cognitive and attitudinal components of stigma into actions, resulting in a lower position of those being stigmatised in social hierarchy, are not clearly understood. But it has been suggested that these mechanisms are complex, pervasive and interchangeable, with direct and indirect or conscious and unconscious ways of implementation. It is offered that even after fixing or blockage of one of the mechanisms of discrimination, the pre-existing labelling, stereotypes and prejudices from a group in power can easily be implemented in another way (Link and Phelan 2001). Some authors argue that this process of hidden and complicated discrimination may play a role of power retention of stigmatisers by keeping people with mental illnesses 'in concerns, away or down' (Link and Phelan 2014).

However, although the exact way through which stigma is transformed into negative behavioural actions towards people diagnosed with mental disorders is often difficult to apprehend, actual discrimination is experienced in almost every domain of everyday life. The broad scope of discrimination may be systematised and grouped into 3 main levels:

1. Macro-social level: structural discrimination
2. Micro-social level: interpersonal discrimination
3. Intrapersonal level: anticipated discrimination and self-discrimination

Macro-social Level: Structural Discrimination

One of the important extensions of the sociological approach to stigma and discrimination offered by Link and Phelan is the idea of unequal distribution of power, which unfolds and strengthens the underlying and pre-existing ignorance, prejudices and separation of a stigmatised group, who are limited in power (Link and Phelan 2001, 2014). In such a perspective, it is important to understand the power distribution in the society and the role of a major group, as well as the contribution of the state and governmental institutions that represent them.

A concept of 'institutional racism' was offered to describe practices of discrimination and a failure to meet the demands of racial minority groups by institutional practices (Mehta and Thornicroft 2010). The very broad governmental and societal structures, practices and functioning may be created in a way that limits life chances of stigmatised groups. Superposition of the concept into discrimination associated with mental illness leads to the formulation of 'structural' or 'institutional' discrimination of them (Corrigan 2004a). It is defined as a type of stigma 'formed by sociopolitical forces and represents policies of private and government institutions that restrict the opportunities of the groups that are stigmatised' (Corrigan and Kleinlein 2005).

One of the main problems of structural stigma and discrimination is that on a macro level, it is very difficult to detect the exact stigmatiser or stigmatising group, as power may be distributed among a very broad group within the whole society. This is the reason why institutional stigma is often covert and indirectly occurring through the everyday operations of institutions, buried beneath layers of rules and regulations and sustained by traditions. For example, in the US study, conducted with a purpose to examine the experience of stigma from a family members' perspective, it was revealed that institutional stigma was viewed as the most problematic, although the way of its implementation and exact discriminatory practices were very subtle (Muhlbauer 2002).

But structural discrimination exists so widely that may be related to the whole structure and functioning of the society, which creates a 'disabling environment' for some of its members even in the absence of individual discrimination (Angermeyer et al. 2004, 2014; Gee 2008). It is implemented both through intended (policies that intentionally restrict the rights and opportunities of a stigmatised group) and unintended (practices that unintentionally hinder life chances) discrimination (Corrigan 2004b). In relation to mental illness, the manifestation of structural stigma has been found in an array of different dimensions, including resource allocation, policy and legislation, statements of development priorities, health care, economic and social inclusion and media coverage.

Discrimination in Resource Allocation

The importance of appropriate resource allocation to support mental health services is obvious and has been multiply emphasised (Saxena et al. 2007). The significant burden of mental disorders (WHO|The global burden of disease 2004), huge economic and social impact have been abundantly shown in the existing literature and repeatedly accompanied by calls for actions to increase attention to mental health care (Prince et al. 2007).

Nevertheless, the gap between the existing burden and the resources allocated remains significant (Saxena et al. 2007). Data from the WHO's Atlas project showed that among countries which have a separate mental health budget, one forth spend <1 % of the total health budget on mental health. In general the results of the project demonstrate that the resources that the world spends on mental health are grossly inadequate in comparison to the needs (Saxena et al. 2006a). It is especially relevant for LMIC as the poorer the country, a lower percentage of their overall health budget is spent on mental health (Chisholm et al. 2007).

Furthermore the inequality of resources appears not only in its insufficient allocation to mental health care but also within their distribution inside of services, nearly three quarters of mental health expenditure is spent inside of institutional care. Globally, 67 % of financial resources are directed towards mental hospitals, continuing to support the institutional nature of mental health services. It is also obvious that there is a shortage in the number of mental health professionals (Saxena et al. 2006b), one of the reasons for which is an additional stigma and discrimination experienced when working in mental health care (Gaebel et al. 2014). In general, the infrastructural, financial and human resources available for mental health are a small fraction of what are needed, even to provide basic care to the population (Saxena et al. 2006b; Schomerus et al. 2006).

A partial explanation to such a disparity could be found in research on public preferences of resource allocation (Beck et al. 2003). Several studies have investigated the area with the results reaffirming that mental health stigma has an adverse effect on public desire to allocate resources to mental health care (Corrigan 2004c; Corrigan et al. 2004; Sharac et al. 2010): people are far less willing to allocate financial resources to the care of people with psychiatric disorders compared to other medical diseases (Matschinger and Angermeyer 2004). It has been suggested that although structural and individual discrimination are different aspects of stigma, the possible connections between them sometimes might be followed. For instance, policymakers involved in decision-making and responsibility for resource allocations may be sharing stigmatising public beliefs, which inevitably influence their professional vision and activity.

Discrimination in Legislation, Policies and Priorities

Both intended and unintended structural discrimination might be represented in legislation, policies and stated priorities for societal development. One clear example of such an unreasonable lack of priority of mental health is the fact it was not included in the Millennium Development Goals, despite the strong evidence of a huge burden and importance (Eaton et al. 2014).

The issue of stigma is very closely connected to the problem of human rights violations of people with mental illnesses, and almost every aspect of discrimination may be considered and interpreted from the perspective of human rights and vice versa (Drew et al. 2011). Article 1 of the Universal Declaration of Human Rights states that 'all human beings are born free and equal in dignity and rights' that very much remains the necessity of non-discrimination and equal distribution of life chances (The Universal Declaration of Human Rights n.d.). At the same time, legislation and policies may play the opposite role. Sometimes they directly create barriers for people with mental illnesses, for example, through limiting legal capacity, prohibiting employment and access to different social goods. In other cases mental health policy and legislation may indirectly contribute and facilitate discrimination and human rights violations through its faultiness, for example, through hampering access to care by supporting hospital-based services and underfunding community-based treatment, through allowing arbitrary involuntary admission and the absence of independent review bodies (WHO Resource Book on Mental Health, Human Rights & Legislation: World Health Organization n.d.).

Development of new mental health policies and legislation must play a leading role in prevention of human rights violations and discrimination of people with mental illnesses. Some substantial progress has been achieved through the development and promotion of the Convention on the Rights of Persons with Disabilities (CRPD) (Convention on the rights of persons with disabilities n.d.). The convention presents the important paradigm shift from a medical and biological vision of disability to a social model, which removes responsibility from overloaded people, and to a society that discriminates and fails to accept them. The emphasis on social rights and civic participation in turn creates a background for inclusion, better legal defence and advocacy for people with disabilities and promotes subsequent important amendments and improvements, such as the creation of the Institutional Treatment, Human Rights and Care Assessment (ITHACA) (Randall et al. 2013).

On the other hand, even the best and most profound mental health policy and legislation can't insure success in overcoming discrimination. Discrimination is implemented through an array of complex and interchangeable mechanisms, which partially explain why stigma is such a persistent predicament, so difficult to overcome. The existence of a gap between law, policy and real practice may represent a further barrier for the lives of people with mental disorders even if the legal framework is felicitous (Lockwood et al. 2014; Callard et al. 2012).

Discrimination in Health Care and Treatment

The right to the 'highest attainable standard of health conducive to living a life in dignity' is stated as a fundamental human right in Article 12 and the General Comment 14 on the International Covenant on Economic, Social, and Cultural Rights (ICESCR). This right is extended to all human beings regardless their race, culture, age, presence of disability or mental disorder. However, some elements of health-care provision for people with mental illness are, unfortunately, far beyond these principles, as people with mental illness very often receive both second-class physical health care and are confronted with insensitive, disrespectful or even disabling treatment within psychiatric care (Thornicroft et al. 2010; Skosireva et al. 2014).

At the same time, access to appropriate mental care is one of the indispensable preconditions of healthy life, and it is very often limited for people with mental disorders (Thornicroft 2008; Amaddeo and Jones 2007). Inequity of resource allocation, support of institutional instead of community-based service, low quality of treatment, insufficiency of competent human resources, medications, psychological support and rehabilitation altogether constitute a situation in which proper care is hampered by financial, geographical, lingual, informational, cultural and other barriers (Thornicroft 2006a). Mental health care in many countries of the world is delivered through huge centralised psychiatric hospitals, which are very often situated in a separated location on the city outskirts, and it has been argued that such a model of care is known to strengthen the existing stigma of mental illness, violate the rights to liberty and security of persons (Drew et al. 2011), lead to fear of psychiatric diagnosis and treatment (Thornicroft et al. 2009).

Moreover, it has been shown that within such institutions, inhuman and degrading treatment and conditions can become the norm. In a study by Lee et al. in Hong Kong, it was found that adverse experiences during hospitalisation (such as negative staff attitudes, excessive physical/chemical restraints, inadequate information/complaint systems and limited rights) were reported by 44 % of patients with schizophrenia (Lee et al. 2006). As a result of imperfect and disrepute psychiatric treatment together with stigma towards mental illnesses and their treatment in general, many people choose not to seek care until their need is critical; this will increase costs to the patient, the patient's family and to society (Cooper et al. 2003; Compton et al. 2004; Schomerus et al. 2008).

It has also often been shown that the presence of mental disorder reduces the chance to get sufficient attention within a physical health-care system (De Hert et al. 2011; Thornicroft 2011) with reduced access to primary health care (Levinson et al. 2003), worse treatment for diabetes (Desai et al. 2002), cardiovascular diseases (Druss et al. 2000), improper attention in emergency departments and a higher level of infectious complications after surgical interventions.

Among the implications of such discrimination is an increased mortality rate of people with mental illness (Reininghaus et al. 2015). There is evidence that the life expectancy of people with severe mental illnesses is 10–15 years lower than that of the general population (Lawrence et al. 2013) with an increased risk of death from coronary heart disease and stroke that is not wholly explained by smoking, social deprivation scores (Osborn et al. 2007), antipsychotic medication or clinical variables. The mortality risk of people with first-contact psychosis is nearly double that of the general population (Dutta et al. 2012).

As a partial explanation of the neglect within physical health care, the 'diagnostic and treatment overshadowing' concept has been offered to describe a 'physician bias' when medical practitioners misattribute physical illness signs and symptoms to concurrent mental disorders, leading to underdiagnosis and mistreatment of the physical conditions (Jones et al. 2008; Thornicroft et al. 2007).

Discrimination in Education, Employment and Economic Exclusion

It is well known that the chance to have a good job position is substantially reduced when a person has a history of mental illness (Boardman et al. 2003; Stuart 2006a, b). The problem is very broad as work-related discrimination outspreads to all stages of participation in the labour market, starting much before the immediate employment procedure and continuing long after getting a job position. In general the problem may be called an 'economic exclusion' of a whole part of society who has been shown to have a high willingness to work (Bond et al. 2001). Data from the UK National Labour Force Survey in 2014 shows that the level of employment rate among people with mental illnesses is 36.1 %, much less than among people with other long-term medical conditions (58.8 %) and half of rates in general population (72.7 %) (http://www.ons.gov.uk/). It appeared that adults with long-term mental health problems are one of the most excluded groups in society with high efforts and low rewards (Social Exclusion U 2004).

The situation might be partially explained by the problems of knowledge and prejudices of employers who often express reluctance about employing people with a psychiatric history (Manning and White 1995); there is an issue of underestimation of the capacities and skills of patients and an overestimation of risks to employers by mental health professionals (Thornicroft 2006b), but it is only a part of the whole picture.

Structural barriers for employment may be created by governmental regulations and legislation, for example, in some countries for person having mental disorder, it is forbidden by law to occupy several positions, drive a car, work with money, etc. Some professions may be unreachable by people with mental illnesses because of barriers within the education system, and the occupational skill level in general has been shown to be less. These numerous and overall barriers inevitably contribute to poor self-perception and professional confidence of people with mental disorders resulting in strengthening their self-stigma and social withdrawal (see out at work: http://www.mentalhealth.org.uk/publications/out-at-work/).

There is a necessity for mental health-care restructuring and deinstitutionalisation, not in doubt from the point of view of existing evidence, but this shift has to be accompanied with employment and education assistance programmes (Grove 1999). If it is not, the existing practices of job and education-related discrimination of people with mental illnesses will remain the huge hidden pitfall that even the most sophisticated medical and psychological interventions directed to improve social inclusion will not be able to cover.

Discrimination in the Media and Among the Public

The way in which people both perceive reality and behaviour very much depends on currently existing social norms and practices. The appearance and distribution of these norms is a very complex process depending on many interrelated factors, but the substantial role of the media is more clear. Knowledge about mental illnesses, acceptable attitudes, emotional reactions and understanding of socially acceptable behaviours are very much constructed and transmitted through the media (Thornicroft 2006a). At the same time, one of the main intentions of mass media is 'entertainment' with the principle of 'acceptability to audience'. Such a perspective of mental illness in the mass media represents another important aspect of structural stigma as a reflexion of views, attitudes and behaviour of the lay public (Corrigan 2005a).

The topic of mental illnesses has been associated by the media with violence and aggression or blame and helplessness. In the study analysing newspaper coverage by Corrigan et al., it was found that themes of dangerousness and criminal activity appear in the most stories (near 39 %) covering mental disorders (Corrigan et al. 2005b).

On the other hand, some positive tendencies of media coverage of mental illness have been shown (Thornicroft et al. 2013) and the importance of messages of the mass media, for the education of society, has been emphasised. If used in a correct way, it will play a huge role in overcoming the stigma surrounding mental illness. The evidence of an effect on discrimination, however, is insufficient at the moment and further research is required (Clement et al. 2013).

Micro-social Level of Discrimination: Interpersonal Discrimination

Along with structural stigma, people with mental illness experience interpersonal or 'individual' discrimination in their everyday communications. Individual discrimination is defined as a process taking place in the direct interaction between the stigmatising and the stigmatised person (Angermeyer et al. 2014). The knowledge and attitudes of the stigmatiser transformed into behaviour resulting in discriminatory actions towards stigmatised one. Thus, individual discrimination happens in the living environment of people with mental disorders: in their families, neighbourhoods, communities in general, during contact with policemen and doctors and other everyday communications.

There are a number of papers on public attitude towards people with mental disorders showing a background for the discrimination. It was demonstrated that social rejection, distancing and dehumanisation are a common and stable phenomenon of the public attitude towards people with a history of mental illness (Angermeyer et al. 2014). It may be described in terms of the 'not in my backyard' (NIMBY) principle (Cowan 2003). This is when people refuse to have contact with or live near a person with serious mental illness as they perceive them as dangerous and unpredictable (Cowan 2003). It was shown that people report more comfort with individuals who are deaf or have facial disfigurement than people with mental disorders. In a recent Australian study, it was also shown that GPs expressed an even more pronounced stigmatising attitude than the general population (Reavley et al. 2014).

This data on attitudes towards people with mental disorders indirectly speak about discrimination that appears in the contacts they experience. At the same time, there is relatively fewer studies investigating discrimination experienced by those stigmatised directly. A big international study, conducted in 27 countries, showed that negative discrimination was experienced by 49 % of participants. The most frequent areas of discrimination were mentioned in making or keeping friends (47 %), discrimination within families (43 %), in finding or keeping a job (27 %) and in intimate or sexual relationships (23 %) with rare experience of positive discrimination (Thornicroft et al. 2009). In another study in 35 countries, 79 % of people with depression reported experiencing discrimination in at least one life domain (Lasalvia et al. 2013).

The discrimination within a family context appears in different domains. The concept of 'courtesy' stigma is the stigmatisation experience of family members of people diagnosed with mental disorder (Angermeyer et al. 2003). This can affect children, parents, siblings and spouses (Corrigan 2004a). It has been shown that stigmatisation of families is widespread and occurs in different cultures and continents, regardless of nationality or social status (Girma et al. 2014; Kadri et al. 2004; Shibre et al. 2001; Wahl and Harman 1989). The burden of stigma in families leads to practices of hiding their ill relative, concealing diagnosis, refusing help and avoiding contact with the external world. This in turn may lead to delays in treatment and increase emotional burnout (Ostman 2004). Some family members may decide to distance themselves from their relatives, which contribute to an increased number of divorces and decreased number of years of marriage (Kessler et al. 1998). People with mental illness are then left to live in a 'broken family' (Thara et al. 2003) either with some social contacts or in loneliness.

Intrapersonal Level of Discrimination: Anticipated Discrimination and Self-Discrimination

Experience of both structural and individual discrimination, repeatedly throughout the life of a person with diagnosis of mental disorders, contributes to internalisation of 'spoiled identity', self-stigma and self-discrimination. Results of the INDIGO study showed that 64 % of respondents anticipated discrimination in applying for work, training or education, 55 % in looking for a close relationship and 72 % felt the need to conceal their diagnosis. Over a third of participants anticipated discrimination for job seeking and close personal relationships when even no discrimination was experienced (Thornicroft et al. 2009). Results of the study also showed that anticipated discrimination was reported more frequently than experienced acts of discrimination and not necessarily associated with it.

On the other hand, in another recent study by Lasalvia et al., the experienced discrimination and greater illness awareness have been associated with more anticipated discrimination (Lasalvia et al. 2013).

Although the exact mechanisms of internalisation of stigma are not clear at the moment, several explanations have been suggested. Yang et al. offered the concept of 'moral experience' (or "what is most at stake for actors in a local social world") to explain pervasion of stigma inside the personal world of an individual (Yang et al. 2007). It has also been shown that automatic shame-related reactions to mental illness may increase the vulnerability to mental illness stigma (Rusch et al. 2010). Thus, previous knowledge, self-prejudice and attitude as well as agreement with stereotypes by persons with mental illness may play a role in its internalisation (Rüsch et al. 2005), decreasing self-esteem and self-efficacy (Wright et al. 2000). The decreased self-esteem in turn contributes to self-discriminatory behaviour, when persons do not put effort into applying a job or independent living, which will altogether reduce their chances of getting better position and support existing stereotypes. As a result, self-stigma undermining self-esteem and self-efficacy strengthens the exclusion of person from social interactions (Rusch et al. 2010). This can be even more devastating than the real experience of discrimination (Hansson et al. 2014) and disorder symptoms (Corrigan et al. 2002).

It has also been shown that in countries with less stigmatising attitudes, better access to information, where the public felt more comfortable to talk to people with mental illness, the self-stigma is reduced and people with mental illnesses are more empowered, creating promising directions for future interventions (Evans-Lacko et al. 2012).

Consequences of Stigma

The behavioural consequences of stigma (i.e. discrimination) can compound the disability of people with mental illness and may lead to disadvantages in many aspects of life, including personal relationships, education and work (Thornicroft 2006a; Corrigan 2005b). Such discrimination limits the life opportunities of those affected, through loss of income, unemployment, reduced access to housing or health care, and other important means of recovery (Yang et al. 2010). In addition to experiences of direct discrimination from others, people with mental illness may be disadvantaged through structural discrimination, for example, as manifested in the lesser investment of health-care resources allocated to the care of people with mental disorders, compared with those with physical illnesses. Further, people with mental disorders also often experience unequal treatment for physical health conditions, which may contribute to excess morbidity and premature mortality (Wahlbeck et al. 2011; Thornicroft 2013).

In parallel with external stigmatisation, a process of internalised or self-stigma is also common among people with mental illness. This is manifested in feelings of shame, a loss of emotional well-being and poor self-efficacy. The internal consequences of stigma and discrimination can also be associated with hopelessness and depression, social withdrawal and reduced participation in treatment programmes. Coping responses to the experience or anticipation of discrimination, such as non-disclosure of the condition, and avoidance of others can further feed into the cycle of loss of social and economic opportunities and alienation.

Within health-care settings, stigma may be manifested as human rights violations, for example, as a consequence of poor staff training standards or ineffective care quality inspection systems. Poor quality of care can in turn act as an important barrier to help seeking by people with mental illness and their family members. For example, people with mental disorders may delay seeking treatment or terminate treatment prematurely for fear of labelling and discrimination, or because of perceptions that treatments are not effective or respectful. In societies where services are scarce and support systems are inadequate, families may feel forced to resort to physical measures such as chaining to restrain relatives with mental illness in the absence of any locally available or acceptable alternative.

Stigma and discrimination also affect family members and carers. The effect of negative attitudes towards the family members of people with mental illness has been described as 'stigma by association', 'affiliate stigma' or 'courtesy stigma'. This may lead to direct discrimination, feelings of shame and self-blame, much like the internal consequences of mental illness stigma faced by people with mental disorders. In societies where the cohesion of family networks is high, the impact of stigma by association may be more severe and can include economic consequences as well as impact on work or marital prospects (Thara et al. 2003). In one study from China, for example, stigma was found to exert significant effects on the lives of healthy family members in more than a quarter of the families. Across cultures, it seems clear that vicious cycles of stigma and discrimination seem to operate, in which labelling is related to the generation of stereotypes, leading to social distance, discrimination and status loss. The evidence to date is that these phenomena are common, and in one recent study in England, '93 % of the sample anticipated discrimination and 87% of participants had experienced discrimination in at least one area of life in the previous year'(Farrelly et al. 2014).

Conclusions

This chapter has considered the distinction between stigma and discrimination, the processes and levels at which they operate and their implications for people with experience of mental illness. From the evidence presented here, several issues become clear: (i) Stigma and discrimination remain entrenched worldwide. (ii) Whilst there are some cultural and contextual differences in the manifestations of stigma, the larger picture is that the features and impact are remarkably similar across the world. (iii) Secular trends do not show that stigma related to mental illness reduces over time of its own accord. (iv) Evidence both from local and national level interventions show that stigma and discrimination can be reduced if well-organised interventions, primarily based upon social contact with people with mental illness, are delivered and sustained over time. The key issue is therefore disclosure, to allow social contact to take place, and this is the turnkey for future progress towards the elimination of stigma and discrimination in the future.

References

Abelev BI, Aggarwal MM, Ahammed Z, Amonett J, Anderson BD, Anderson M et al (2006) Longitudinal double-spin asymmetry and cross section for inclusive jet production in polarized proton collisions at square root of s = 200 GeV. Phys Rev Lett 97(25):252001

Amaddeo F, Jones J (2007) What is the impact of socio-economic inequalities on the use of mental health services? Epidemiol Psichiatr Soc 16(1):16–19

Angermeyer MC, Beck M, Matschinger H (2003) Determinants of the public's preference for social distance from people with schizophrenia. Can J Psychiatry 48(10):663–668

Angermeyer MC, Buyantugs L, Kenzine DV, Matschinger H (2004) Effects of labelling on public attitudes towards people with schizophrenia: are there cultural differences? Acta Psychiatr Scand 109(6):420–425

Angermeyer MC, Matschinger H, Schomerus G (2013) Attitudes towards psychiatric treatment and people with mental illness: changes over two decades. Br J Psychiatry 203:146–151

Angermeyer MC, Matschinger H, Link BG, Schomerus G (2014) Public attitudes regarding individual and structural discrimination: two sides of the same coin? Soc Sci Med (1982) 103:60–66

Beck M, Matschinger H, Angermeyer MC (2003) Social representations of major depression in West and East Germany – do differences still persist 11 years after reunification? Soc Psychiatry Psychiatr Epidemiol 38(9):520–525

Boardman J, Grove B, Perkins R, Shepherd G (2003) Work and employment for people with psychiatric disabilities. Br J Psychiatry 182:467–468

Bond GR, Becker DR, Drake RE, Rapp CA, Meisler N, Lehman AF et al (2001) Implementing supported employment as an evidence-based practice. Psychiatr Serv 52(3):313–322

Callard F, Sartorius N, Arboleda-Florez J, Bartlett P, Helmchen H, Stuart H et al (2012) Mental illness, discrimination and the law: fighting for social justice. Wiley Blackwell, London

Chisholm D, Flisher AJ, Lund C, Patel V, Saxena S, Thornicroft G et al (2007) Scale up services for mental disorders: a call for action. Lancet 370(9594):1241–1252

Clement S, Brohan E, Sayce L, Pool J, Thornicroft G (2011) Disability hate crime and targeted violence and hostility: a mental health and discrimination perspective. J Ment Health 20(3):219–225

Clement S, Lassman F, Barley E, Evans-Lacko S, Williams P, Yamaguchi S, Slade M, Rüsch N, Thornicroft G. Mass media interventions for reducing mental health-related stigma. Cochrane Database of Systematic Reviews 2013, Issue 7. Art. No.: CD009453. doi:10.1002/14651858. CD009453.pub2

Compton MT, Kaslow NJ, Walker EF (2004) Observations on parent/family factors that may influence the duration of untreated psychosis among African American first-episode schizophrenia-spectrum patients. Schizophr Res 68(2–3):373–385

Cooper AE, Corrigan PW, Watson AC (2003) Mental illness stigma and care seeking. J Nerv Ment Dis 191(5):339–341

Corrigan P (2000) Mental health stigma as social attribution: Implications for research methods and attitude change. Clin Psychol Sci Pract 7:48–67

Corrigan P (2004a) How stigma interferes with mental health care. Am Psychol 59(7):614–625

Corrigan PW (2004b) Don't call me nuts: an international perspective on the stigma of mental illness. Acta Psychiatr Scand 109(6):403–404

Corrigan PW (2004c) On the stigma of mental illness: practical strategies for research and social change. American Psychological Association, Washington, DC

Corrigan PW (2005a) Dealing with stigma through personal disclosure. In: Corrigan PW (ed) On the stigma of mental illness practical strategies for research and social change. American Psychological Press, Washington, DC, pp 257–280

Corrigan P (2005b) On the stigma of mental illness. American Psychological Association, Washington, DC

Corrigan P, Kleinlein P (2005) The impact of mental illness stigma. In: Corrigan P (ed) On the stigma of mental illness: practical strategies for research and social change. American Psychological Assocation, Washington, DC

Corrigan PW, Larson JE (2008) Stigma. Guilford Press, New York, (2008). Clinical handbook of schizophrenia. (pp. 533–540). xxi, 650 p

Corrigan PW, Rowan D, Green A, Lundin R, River P, Uphoff-Wasowski K et al (2002) Challenging two mental illness stigmas: personal responsibility and dangerousness. Schizophr Bull 28(2):293–309

Corrigan PW, Markowitz FE, Watson AC (2004) Structural levels of mental illness stigma and discrimination. Schizophr Bull 30(3):481–491

Corrigan PW, Watson AC, Heyrman ML, Warpinski A, Gracia G, Slopen N et al (2005a) Structural stigma in state legislation. Psychiatr Serv 56(5):557–563

Corrigan P, Watson A, Gracia G, Slopen N, Rasinski K, Hall L (2005b) Newspaper stories as a measure of structural stigma. Psychiatr Serv 56(5):551–556

Corrigan PW, Larson JE, Rusch N (2009) Self-stigma and the "why try" effect: impact on life goals and evidence-based practices. World Psychiatry 8(2):75–81

Cowan S (2003) NIMBY syndrome and public consultation policy: the implications of a discourse analysis of local responses to the establishment of a community mental health facility. Health Soc Care Community 11(5):379–386

De Hert M, Correll CU, Bobes J, Cetkovich-Bakmas M, Cohen D, Asai I et al (2011) Physical illness in patients with severe mental disorders. I. Prevalence, impact of medications and disparities in health care. World Psychiatry Off J World Psychiatr Assoc (WPA) 10:52–77

Desai MM, Rosenheck RA, Druss BG, Perlin JB (2002) Mental disorders and quality of diabetes care in the veterans health administration. Am J Psychiatr 159(9):1584–1590

Dovidio JF, Major B, Crocker J (2000) Stigma: introduction and overview. In: Heatherton TF, Kleck RE, Hebl MR, Hull JG (eds) The social psychology of stigma. Guildford Press, New York, pp 1–28

Drew N, Funk M, Tang S, Lamichhane J, Chavez E, Katontoka S et al (2011) Human rights violations of people with mental and psychosocial disabilities: an unresolved global crisis. Lancet 378(9803):1664–1675

Druss BG, Bradford DW, Rosenheck RA, Radford MJ, Krumholz HM (2000) Mental disorders and use of cardiovascular procedures after myocardial infarction. JAMA 283(4):506–511

Dutta R, Murray RM, Allardyce J, Jones PB, Boydell JE (2012) Mortality in first-contact psychosis patients in the U.K.: a cohort study. Psychol Med 42:1649–1661

Eaton J, DeSilva M, Regan M, Lamichhane J, Thornicroft G (2014) There is no wealth without mental health. Lancet Psychiatry 1:252–253

Evans-Lacko S, Brohan E, Mojtabai R, Thornicroft G (2012) Association between public views of mental illness and self-stigma among individuals with mental illness in 14 European countries. Psychol Med 42(8):1741–1752

Excellence NIfHaC (2007) Behaviour change at population, community and individual levels. Available from: http://www.nice.org.uk/PH006

Farrelly S, Clement S, Gabbidon J, Jeffery D, Dockery L, Lassman F et al (2014) Anticipated and experienced discrimination amongst people with schizophrenia, bipolar disorder and major depressive disorder: a cross sectional study. BMC Psychiatry 14:157

Freeman, Melvyn, and Soumitra Pathare. (2005) WHO resource book on mental health, human rights and legislation. Geneva: World Health Organization.

Gaebel W, Zäske H, Zielasek J, Cleveland H-R, Samjeske K, Stuart H, et al (2014) Stigmatization of psychiatrists and general practitioners: results of an international survey. Eur Arch Psychiatry Clin Neurosci 265(3):189–197

Gee GC (2008) A multilevel analysis of the relationship between institutional and individual racial discrimination and health status. Am J Public Health 98:S48–S56

Girma E, Moller-Leimkuhler AM, Muller N, Dehning S, Froeschl G, Tesfaye M (2014) Public stigma against family members of people with mental illness: findings from the Gilgel Gibe Field Research Center (GGFRC), Southwest Ethiopia. BMC Int Health Hum Rights 14:2

Goffmann E (1963) Stigma: notes on the management of spoiled identity. Prentice Hall, Englewood Cliffs

Grove B (1999) Mental health and employment. Shaping a new agenda. J Ment Health 8:131–140

Hansson L, Stjernswärd S, Svensson B (2014) Perceived and anticipated discrimination in people with mental illness – an interview study. Nord J Psychiatry 68:100–106

Hatzenbuehler ML, Phelan JC, Link BG (2013) Stigma as a fundamental cause of population health inequalities. Am J Public Health 103(5):813–821

Henderson C, Thornicroft G (2009) Stigma and discrimination in mental illness: time to change. Lancet 373(9679):1928–1930

Henderson C, Corker E, Lewis-Holmes E, Hamilton S, Flach C, Rose D et al (2012) England's time to change antistigma campaign: one-year outcomes of service user-rated experiences of discrimination. Psychiatr Serv 63(5):451–457

Jones S, Howard L, Thornicroft G (2008) 'Diagnostic overshadowing': worse physical health care for people with mental illness. Acta Psychiatr Scand 118(3):169–171

Kadri N, Manoudi F, Berrada S, Moussaoui D (2004) Stigma impact on Moroccan families of patients with schizophrenia. Can J Psychiatry 49(9):625–629

Kessler RC, Walters EE, Forthofer MS (1998) The social consequences of psychiatric disorders, III: probability of marital stability. Am J Psychiatr 155(8):1092–1096

Kohrt BA, Harper I (2008) Navigating diagnoses: understanding mind-body relations, mental health, and stigma in Nepal. Cult Med Psychiatry 32(4):462–491

Kohrt BA, Hruschka DJ (2010) Nepali concepts of psychological trauma: the role of idioms of distress, ethnopsychology and ethnophysiology in alleviating suffering and preventing stigma. Cult Med Psychiatry 34(2):322–352

Lasalvia A, Zoppei S, Van Bortel T, Bonetto C, Cristofalo D, Wahlbeck K et al (2013) Global pattern of experienced and anticipated discrimination reported by people with major depressive disorder: a cross-sectional survey. Lancet 381(9860):55–62

Lawrence D, Hancock KJ, Kisely S (2013) The gap in life expectancy from preventable physical illness in psychiatric patients in Western Australia: retrospective analysis of population based registers. BMJ (Clin Res Ed) 346:f2539

Lee S, Chiu MY, Tsang A, Chui H, Kleinman A (2006) Stigmatizing experience and structural discrimination associated with the treatment of schizophrenia in Hong Kong. Soc Sci Med 62(7):1685–1696

Levinson MC, Druss BG, Dombrowski EA, Rosenheck RA (2003) Barriers to primary medical care among patients at a community mental health center. Psychiatr Serv 54(8):1158–1160

Link BG, Phelan JC (2001) Conceptualizing stigma. Annu Rev Sociol 27:363–385

Link BG, Phelan J (2014) Stigma power. Soc Sci Med 103:24–32

Link BG, Phelan JC, Bresnahan M, Stueve A, Pescosolido BA (1999) Public conceptions of mental illness: labels, causes, dangerousness, and social distance. Am J Public Health 89(9): 1328–1333

Link BG, Struening EL, Neese-Todd S, Asmussen S, Phelan JC (2001) Stigma as a barrier to recovery: the consequences of stigma for the self-esteem of people with mental illness. Psychiatr Serv 52(12):1621–1626

Link BG, Yang LH, Phelan JC, Collins PY (2004) Measuring mental illness stigma. Schizophr Bull 30(3):511–541

Lockwood G, Henderson C, Thornicroft G (2014) Mental health disability discrimination: law, policy and practice. Int J Discrimination Law 14:168–182

Manning C, White P (1995) Attitudes of employers to the mentally ill. Psychiatr Bull 19:541–543

Matschinger H, Angermeyer MC (2004) The public's preferences concerning the allocation of financial resources to health care: results from a representative population survey in Germany. Eur Psychiatry 19(8):478–482

Mehta N, Thornicroft G (2010) Stigmatisation of people with mental illness and of psychiatric institutions. Int Libr Eth Law New 45:11–32

Muhlbauer SK (2002) Experience of stigma by families with mentally ill members. J Am Psychiatry Nurses Assoc 8:76–83

Osborn DP, Levy G, Nazareth I, Petersen I, Islam A, King MB (2007) Relative risk of cardiovascular and cancer mortality in people with severe mental illness from the United Kingdom's General Practice Research Database. Arch Gen Psychiatry 64(2):242–249

Ostman M (2004) Family burden and participation in care: differences between relatives of patients admitted to psychiatric care for the first time and relatives of re-admitted patients. J Psychiatr Ment Health Nurs 11(5):608–613

Pescosolido BA, Martin JK, Long JS, Medina TR, Phelan JC, Link BG (2010) "A disease like any other"? A decade of change in public reactions to schizophrenia, depression, and alcohol dependence. Am J Psychiatr 167(11):1321–1330

Prince M, Patel V, Saxena S, Maj M, Maselko J, Phillips MR et al (2007) No health without mental health. Lancet 370(9590):859–877

Rabkin J (1974) Public attitudes toward mental illness: a review of the literature. Schizophr Bull 10:9–33

Raguram R, Raghu TM, Vounatsou P, Weiss MG (2004) Schizophrenia and the cultural epidemiology of stigma in Bangalore, India. J Nerv Ment Dis 192(11):734–744

Randall J, Thornicroft G, Burti L, Katschnig H, Lewis O, Russo J et al (2013) Development of the ITHACA toolkit for monitoring human rights and general health care in psychiatric and social care institutions. Epidemiol Psychiatry Sci 22(3):241–254

Reavley NJ, Mackinnon AJ, Morgan AJ, Jorm AF (2014) Stigmatising attitudes towards people with mental disorders: a comparison of Australian health professionals with the general community. Aust N Z J Psychiatry 48(5):433–441

Reininghaus U, Dutta R, Dazzan P, Doody GA, Fearon P, Lappin J et al (2015) Mortality in schizophrenia and other psychoses: a 10-year follow-up of the ÆSOP first-episode cohort. Schizophr Bull 41(3): 664–673 first published online 2014 doi:10.1093/schbul/sbu138

Rusch N, Angermeyer MC, Corrigan PW (2005) Mental illness stigma: concepts, consequences, and initiatives to reduce stigma. Eur Psychiatry 20(8):529–539

Rüsch N, Angermeyer MC, Corrigan PW (2005) The stigma of mental illness: concepts, forms, and consequences. Psychiatr Prax 32:221–232

Rusch N, Todd AR, Bodenhausen GV, Corrigan PW (2010) Do people with mental illness deserve what they get? Links between meritocratic worldviews and implicit versus explicit stigma. Eur Arch Psychiatry Clin Neurosci 260(8):617–625

Sartorius N, Schulze H (2005) Reducing the stigma of mental illness. Cambridge University Press, Cambridge

Saxena S, Paraje G, Sharan P, Karam G, Sadana R (2006a) The 10/90 divide in mental health research: trends over a 10-year period. Br J Psychiatry 188:81–82

Saxena S, Van OM, Lora A, Saraceno B (2006b) Monitoring of mental health systems and services: comparison of four existing indicator schemes. Soc Psychiatry Psychiatr Epidemiol 41(6):488–497

Saxena S, Thornicroft G, Knapp M, Whiteford H (2007) Resources for mental health: scarcity, inequity, and inefficiency. Lancet 370(9590):878–889

Schomerus G, Borsche J, Matschinger H, Angermeyer MC (2006) Public knowledge about causes and treatment for schizophrenia: a representative population study. J Nerv Ment Dis 194(8):622–624

Schomerus G, Heider D, Angermeyer MC, Bebbington PE, Azorin JM, Brugha T et al (2007) Residential area and social contacts in schizophrenia. Results from the European Schizophrenia Cohort (EuroSC). Soc Psychiatry Psychiatr Epidemiol 42(8):617–622

Schomerus G, Angermeyer MC, Matschinger H, Riedel-Heller SG (2008) Public attitudes towards prevention of depression. J Affect Disord 106(3):257–263

Schomerus G, Evans-Lacko S, Rusch N, Mojtabai R, Angermeyer MC, Thornicroft G (2015) Collective levels of stigma and national suicide rates in 25 European countries. Epidemiol Psychiatr Epidemiology and Psychiatric Sciences 24(02):166–171 doi:10.1017/S2045796014000109

Sharac J, McCrone P, Clement S, Thornicroft G (2010) The economic impact of mental health stigma and discrimination: A systematic review. Epidemiologia e Psichiatria Sociale,19(3):223–232 doi:10.1017/S1121189X00001159

Shibre T, Negash A, Kullgren G, Kebede D, Alem A, Fekadu A et al (2001) Perception of stigma among family members of individuals with schizophrenia and major affective disorders in rural Ethiopia. Soc Psychiatry Psychiatr Epidemiol 36(6):299–303

Skosireva A, O'Campo P, Zerger S, Chambers C, Gapka S, Stergiopoulos V (2014) Different faces of discrimination: perceived discrimination among homeless adults with mental illness in healthcare settings. BMC Health Serv Res 14:376

Social Exclusion U (ed) (2004) Mental health and social exclusion: social exclusion unit report summary. Office of the Deputy Prime Minister ODPM, London http://www.nfao.org/Useful_Websites/MH_Social_Exclusion_report_summary.pdf

Stuart H (2006a) Mental illness and employment discrimination. Curr Opin Psychiatry 19(5):522–526

Stuart H (2006b) Media portrayal of mental illness and its treatments: what effect does it have on people with mental illness? CNS Drugs 20(2):99–106

Thara R, Kamath S, Kumar S (2003) Women with schizophrenia and broken marriages – doubly disadvantaged? Part II: family perspective. IntJ Soc Psychiatry 49(3):233–240

Thornicroft G (2006) Tackling discrimination. Ment Health Today 2006;26–9. http://www.ncbi.nlm.nih.gov/pubmed/16821392

Thornicroft G (2006a) Shunned: discrimination against people with mental illness. Oxford University Press, Oxford

Thornicroft G (2008) Stigma and discrimination limit access to mental health care. Epidemiol Psichiatr Soc 17(1):14–19

Thornicroft G (2011) Physical health disparities and mental illness: the scandal of premature mortality. Br J Psychiatry 199:441–442

Thornicroft G (2013) Premature death among people with mental illness. BMJ 346:f2969

Thornicroft G, Rose D, Kassam A (2007) Stigma: ignorance, prejudice or discrimination. Br J Psychiatry 190:192–193

Thornicroft G, Brohan E, Rose D, Sartorius N, Leese M, The ISG (2009) Global pattern of experienced and anticipated discrimination against people with schizophrenia: a cross-sectional survey. Lancet 373(9661):408–415

Thornicroft G, Alem A, Dos Santos RA, Barley E, Drake RE, Gregorio G et al (2010) WPA guidance on steps, obstacles and mistakes to avoid in the implementation of community mental health care. World Psychiatry 9(2):67–77

Thornicroft A, Goulden R, Shefer G, Rhydderch D, Rose D, Williams P et al (2013) Newspaper coverage of mental illness in England 2008–2011. Br J Psychiatry Suppl 55:s64–s69

Thornicroft C, Wyllie A, Thornicroft G, Mehta N (2014) Impact of the "Like Minds, Like Mine" anti-stigma and discrimination campaign in New Zealand on anticipated and experienced discrimination. Aust N Z J Psychiatry 48(4):360–370

United Nations. (2007) Universal Declaration of Human Rights 60th anniversary special edition, United Nations Dept. of Public Information. New York 1948–2008.

UN. Ad Hoc Committee on a Comprehensive and Integral International Convention on Protection and Promotion of the Rights and Dignity of Persons with Disabilities (8th sess., resumed: 2006: New York). 2006. Convention on the Rights of Persons with Disabilities. [New York]: UN.

Wahl OF, Harman CR (1989) Family views of stigma. Schizophr Bull 15(1):131–139

Wahlbeck K, Westman J, Nordentoft M, Gissler M, Laursen TM (2011) Outcomes of Nordic mental health systems: life expectancy of patients with mental disorders. Br J Psychiatry 199(6):453–458

Weiss MG, Jadhav S, Raguram R, Vounatsou P, Littlewood R (2001) Psychiatric stigma across cultures: local validation in Bangalore and London. Anthropol Med 8(7):71–87

WHO | The global burden of disease: 2004 update

Wright ER, Gronfein WP, Owens TJ (2000) Deinstitutionalization, social rejection, and the self-esteem of former mental patients. J Health Soc Behav 41(1):68–90

Yang LH (2007) Application of mental illness stigma theory to Chinese societies: synthesis and new directions. Singap Med J 48(11):977–985

Yang LH, Kleinman A (2008) 'Face' and the embodiment of stigma in China: the cases of schizophrenia and AIDS. Soc Sci Med 67(3):398–408

Yang L, Kleinman A, Link BG, Phelan J, Lee S, Good B (2007) Culture and stigma: adding moral experience to stigma theory. Soc Sci Med 64:1524–1535

Yang L, Cho SH, Kleinman A (2010) Stigma of mental illness. In: Patel V (ed) Mental and neurological public health: a global perspective. San Diego, CA : Academic Press/Elsevier, London http://www.worldcat.org/title/mental-and-neurological-public-health-a-global-perspective/oclc/665844048

The Influence of Stigma on the Course of Illness

8

Harald Zäske

Introduction

This chapter deals with the stigma of mental illnesses and its effects on the course of illness. Basically, the course of a psychiatric illness is influenced by a multitude of factors, e.g. treatment, personal and external factors. From a methodological point of view, an examination of these factors would require experimental approaches or long-term panel studies. Yet after more than 20 years of growing research history, the stigma of mental illness is still a dynamic research field with evolving concepts but a limited number of longitudinal and experimental studies. Furthermore, the focus of many experimental studies lies on the development of social distance towards people with mental illness (e.g. Penn et al. 2000; Graves et al. 2005) or on basic mechanisms as the development of self-esteem in stigmatized individuals in general (e.g. Crocker 1999). Other strategies to describe the relationships between stigma and mental illness course are to examine the effects of stigma at specific stages of a mental illness and to consider the duration of illness (cf. Mueller et al. 2006); nevertheless, studies following these approaches are also few in number (cf. Gerlinger et al. 2013).

Examining the association of mental illness stigma and the illness course is also sophisticated due to the diversity of stigma concepts which underlie a continuous development. Aspects of stigma concerning people with a mental illness are commonly summarized with the term *personal stigma* (cf. Brohan et al. 2010). *Personal stigma* comprises consequences of the mental illness stigma on the individuals' level (including the concepts of perceived or anticipated stigma, stigma experiences and self-stigma or internalized stigma) and serves as orientation for this chapter.

Complementary to *personal stigma*, *structural discrimination* undoubtedly aggravates social exclusion and lowers the chances of participation for people with mental illness (cf. Corrigan et al. 2004). According to the definition provided by

H. Zäske
Department of Psychiatry and Psychotherapy, Medical Faculty, Heinrich-Heine-University, LVR-Klinikum Düsseldorf, Bergische Landstrasse 2, 40629 Duesseldorf, Germany
e-mail: harald.zaeske@lvr.de

© Springer International Publishing Switzerland 2017
W. Gaebel et al. (eds.), *The Stigma of Mental Illness - End of the Story?*,
DOI 10.1007/978-3-319-27839-1_8

Corrigan et al. (2004), *structural discrimination* refers to policies of institutions that result in restricted opportunities of people with mental illness. Its relation to the illness course will not be discussed in further detail in this chapter due to the lack of empirical evidence. As the World Health Organization (WHO) summarizes, structural determinants of mental health are "social, cultural, economic, political and environmental factors such as national policies, social protection, living standards, working conditions, and community social supports" (WHO 2013). It can be assumed that effects of *structural discrimination* are associated with an increased risk for mental ill health, in particular due to reduced coping resources and limited access to care, as it is already described for the effects of poverty on health and mental health (Patel and Kleinman 2003; Funk et al. 2012).

Several questions concerning the relationship between the stigma of mental illness and the illness course shall be discussed in this chapter with regard to their empirical foundation. The chapter is divided into three parts: In the first part, the role of stigma during onset of illness and treatment initiation will be examined. Studies will be discussed addressing the personal stigma during the onset of mental health conditions such as schizophrenia, suicidal ideation and obsessive compulsive disorder. In particular, reasons for a prolonged duration of untreated illness (DUI) have been assessed retrospectively. A main conclusion of these studies is that due to the fear of stigmatization, people avoid seeking professional help and treatment.

Next, studies about the burden of stigma at illness onset will be discussed. Some cross-sectional descriptive studies with first-episode psychosis and depression patients have been published. In comparison to the subsequent illness course, experiences of stigma and discrimination seem to be less frequent during the first episode of illness. As Corker et al. (2014) conclude, patients with a longer illness history had more time to experience discrimination in their lives.

The third part of this chapter is dedicated to stigma process models making assertions about the origin of personal stigma and its consequences. Here, the models proposed by Link (modified labelling approach) and Corrigan (progressive model of self-stigma) seem to be the most influencing models in the field of psychiatric stigma research, since a number of longitudinal studies examining the association between personal stigma and illness parameters have been published.

Information Box 8.1
- Generally, long-term panel studies are scarce.
- Best evidence is given for the long-term course of illness with several studies referring to Link's modified labelling approach.
- Personal stigma (comprising perceived, experienced and self-stigma) is associated in the long run with impaired quality of life, decreased self-esteem and higher burden due to depression and further illness symptoms.
- Even though personal stigma is related to the course of illness, it is not simply part of it: illness burden and symptoms usually improve over time while the burden due to stigma remains high.

Effects of Stigma During the Course of Illness: Onset of Illness and Treatment Initiation

It is a complex question whether the duration between illness onset and treatment initiation (duration of untreated illness DUI) has an impact on courses and prognoses of mental illnesses. It is undoubted that the stigma of mental illness contributes to prolonging this duration. However, the contributing factors cannot easily be identified. Corrigan (2004) mentions two relevant mechanisms: persons in need of mental health care actually may be reluctant to seek professional help because they want to avoid the public stigma of mental illness, and they might try to avoid self-stigma just at the point when they are in need of professional help. In line with this, a further examination of stigma effects on treatment initiation has to consider the peculiar mechanisms of illness onset and treatment initiation specifically for different mental illnesses.

In the case of schizophrenia, the duration of untreated psychosis (DUP) characterizes the time period from the beginning of psychotic symptoms until treatment initiation, which is associated with a poorer prognosis (Marshall et al. 2005), even though underlying mechanisms are not yet fully understood. Evidence has been provided that a shorter DUP (achieved through early recognition and treatment services) is associated with better long-term outcome and recovery (Hegelstad et al. 2012). Yet further research is needed to clarify which factors contribute to these improved prognoses. Regardless of these uncertainties, it is important to know whether and how the stigma of mental illness contributes to the prolonging of the time until people with mental health problems seek professional care and treatment. In the following section, selected studies will be discussed examining the factors contributing to the DUP (or DUI, respectively) and the willingness to seek professional help in schizophrenia and other mental health states as suicidality and obsessive compulsive disorder (OCD).

Stigma as a Barrier to Help Seeking: Reports from Patients with First-Episode Psychosis and Their Relatives

The duration of untreated psychosis (DUP) describes the time between the onset of psychotic symptoms and the beginning of criteria treatment (e.g. neuroleptic treatment). Until such criteria treatment can be initiated, the patient must have come to the decision to seek help; and provided that he then has been diagnosed correctly, he needs a referral to a mental health service where the criteria treatment can finally begin. All these steps together account to the total DUP, as shown in a systematic field study in a defined rural catchment area by Brunet et al. (2007). In this study, all referrals to mental health services in the eastern inner-city area of Birmingham (a catchment area without early intervention service) were analysed over 1 year. $N = 80$ persons were identified with a first-episode psychosis, and 55 of them participated in the study reporting a mean DUP of 53.1 weeks. The help-seeking delay accounted for 29.8 weeks, the referral delay for 4.7 weeks, and the delay in mental health services for 18.8 weeks. Thus, the time the patients needed from the onset of psychotic symptoms until they sought help accounted for more than 50 % of the total DUP.

Retrospective interview studies with patients and relatives identify factors affecting help-seeking behaviour. Relatives and close friends are persons, who are long and well acquainted with the person with FEP, and they are often involved into the decision process of help-seeking (Arria et al. 2011; Anderson et al. 2013). E.g., Ienciu et al. (2010) interviewed $N=28$ Rumanian first-episode schizophrenia patients and their relatives ($N=25$), summarizing two major reasons for a delayed seeking of treatment: First, a common uncertainty about the interpretation of behavioural changes both in patients and relatives. Both groups recognized behavioural changes in the patient, but did not attribute them to a mental illness. Second, the fear of stigma and negative labelling was also reported by both relatives and patients.

Semi-structured interviews were also conducted in a study with $N=21$ service users and $N=9$ carers in an early interventions service (Tanskanen et al. 2011). The interviewees addressed several obstacles for seeking professional help. As in the mentioned study of Ienciu and colleagues (2010), the problem of interpreting the symptoms as part of a mental illness was reported by the majority of both users and carers. Furthermore, about half of the users thought that these symptoms were transient and might cease without further intervention. In response to these symptoms, the majority of the interviewees reported withdrawal from social networks and hiding the symptoms from others. Again, most users reported that the stigma of mental illness was a barrier preventing them of seeking help. Patients' fears were related to anticipated negative reactions from other persons, the mental health services itself and the social consequences of mental health service involvement. Most carers were also concerned about possible negative social and psychological effects on their relatives if they utilized mental health services. In addition, some of the users and relatives expressed their lack of knowledge about pathways in the mental health-care system and their difficulties in identifying an appropriate service for their problems.

Help Seeking and Stigma in Other Mental Health Conditions

Suicidal ideation is a rather common phenomenon in youth and adolescence (e.g. Kisch et al. 2005: 9.5 % of students report serious suicidal ideation within the last school year). However, the rate of persons with suicidal ideation or attempts receiving adequate treatment is quite low (Kisch et al. 2005: 20 %). Obstacles of help-seeking in young suicidal adults were examined in a study by Arria et al. (2011) who interviewed $N=158$ American college students with a lifetime history of suicidal ideation. Additionally, the students were asked to name sources of help they utilized in case of psychological distress, which were categorized into informal

Table 8.1 Informal and formal sources of help in case of psychological distress (Arria et al. 2011)

Informal help	Formal help
Family (65 %)	Private psychiatrists (38 %)
Friends (54 %)	Private psychologists (33 %)
Significant other (23 %)	Medical doctor (11 %)
Trusted adult (13 %)	Private social worker (10 %)
Internet research (9 %)	Hospital (9 %)
Self-help books (6 %)	Other private professionals (9 %)

and formal sources of help. Ninety-six percent of the interviewees (who were suicidal at least once in their lifetime) reported episodes of psychological distress when they thought they were in need of any type of help or treatment. The sources of help are summarized in Table 8.1. The family (65 %) and friends (54 %) were most frequently named sources of help, followed by psychiatrists (38 %) and psychologists (33 %).

The reasons not to seek help are similar to those already mentioned by patients with schizophrenia (Arria et al. 2011): First is the uncertainty about the need for help, treatment effectiveness or importance of treatment (e.g. 58 % thought they could handle the problem without treatment; 36 % did not think treatment would help). Second is stigma-related concerns (39 % were afraid that getting treatment might cause people to have a negative opinion of you). Furthermore, the students referred to logistical barriers (24 % did not know where to get treatment) and financial barriers (33%).

In a further study, Poyraz et al. (2015) assessed potential barriers to treatment in obsessive compulsive disorder (OCD) in $N=96$ OCD patients using a checklist with 16 potential barriers. The duration of untreated illness (DUI) in OCD is considerably long with about 6–8 years. However, until now there is no clear evidence whether a longer DUI is associated with a poorer long-term course of illness. The answers of the interviewed OCD patients resemble the answers of the suicidal students in so far that the most often agreed reasons not to seek treatment reflect a lack of perceived need for help, whether due to the lesser severity of symptoms, the belief to handle the symptoms by oneself or the missing association of the symptoms to an illness. The rate of agreement to items related to public or self-stigma is somewhat lower in OCD patients compared to the rate in suicidal students. Nevertheless, 21.9 % of the OCD patients agreed to the statement that they did not seek help because they were ashamed of symptoms and needing help (self-stigma), and 12.5 % were afraid to have a diagnosis of mental illness (public stigma).

The following list presents all barriers to treatment for patients with obsessive compulsive disorder with their relative frequencies, as reported by Poyraz et al. (2015):

- Spontaneous fluctuation of symptoms (61.5 %)
- Belief that OC symptoms are not associated with an illness (60.4 %)
- Belief that one could manage or handle symptoms on his/her own (55.2 %)
- Not being considerably disturbed by OC symptoms (33.3 %)
- Possibility of using medication (24.0 %)
- Ashamed of symptoms and needing help (21.9 %)
- Thinking that symptoms are necessary in order to be tidy/orderly (17.7 %)
- Feeling depressed/hopeless (15.6 %)
- Preferring to go to a neurologist/psychologist or spiritual healer (15.6 %)
- Thinking that symptoms are related to religious problems/being a sinner (15.6 %)
- Perception that treatment will be ineffective (14.6 %)
- Afraid to have a diagnosis of mental illness (12.5 %)
- Family support for overcoming symptoms (12.5 %)
- Logistic or financial factors (12.5 %)
- Not comfortable discussing OCD-related symptoms with the psychiatrist (8.3 %)
- Not starting treatment even after seeing a psychiatrist (6.3 %)

Conclusions

In summary, the reported studies allow the following conclusions:

- A large time gap exists between the onset of illness and treatment initiation in many mental health conditions (duration of untreated illness DUI/duration of untreated psychosis DUP).
- Quality of evidence whether a prolonged DUI/DUP worsens the long-term course of illness varies for different mental illnesses. For schizophrenia, such a relationship is widely accepted.
- The DUI/DUP consists of the components help-seeking delay, referral delay and delay in mental health services.
- Persons with mental health problems seek help in various sources, both informal as family and friends and formal (psychiatrists, psychologists).
- The most often named reasons to abstain from seeking help are related to the uncertainty about the need for help and effectiveness of treatment and to the stigma of mental illness (both perceived and self-stigma).
- Most studies about help-seeking behaviour and stigma are of retrospective and descriptive nature. Long-term studies in high-risk groups examining the relation between stigma and DUI/DUP are lacking.
- Anti-stigma interventions are appropriate means to reduce the DUI/DUP in addition to improving the mental health-care system and early detection services (cf. Lloyd-Evans et al. 2011).

The Burden of Stigma at Illness Onset: First-Episode Psychosis and Discrimination Experiences

Suffering a first-episode psychosis (FEP) is a decisive turning point in a person's life. In an interview study with $N=35$ patients with first-episode psychosis, Tarrier and colleagues (2007) assessed reactions and experiences due to the FEP. Thus, a majority of the interviewed patients experienced persistent loss, pessimistic views about their personal future and being stigmatized. Furthermore, more than 40 % of the interviewees stated being suicidal at that time. The results of the study by Tarrier et al. (2007) are summarized in the following list:

Consequences of psychosis for their lives:
- Persistent loss, change or disruption (84 %)
- Hopes and aspirations no longer achievable (69 %)
- Felt stigmatized (53 %)
- Social exclusion (50 %)
- Suffered physical harassment (38 %)

Suicidal behaviour:
- Suicidal due to psychosis (44 %)

A more detailed view on the frequency and quality of discrimination experiences during the first episode of schizophrenia is provided by a multinational interview study with patients with first-episode schizophrenia ($N=150$) and patients with first-episode major depressive disorder ($N=176$; the FEDORA project; Corker et al. 2014). Discrimination experiences were assessed with the Discrimination and Stigma Scale (DISC-12), a comprehensive interview schedule assessing discrimination experiences in 21 different areas of life. Patients with first-episode major depression episodes reported discrimination experiences in at average 3.0 areas of their life, while patients with first-episode schizophrenia did so in at average 2.3 areas; this difference was statistically significant (t-Test $p=0.03$). Examples for discrimination experiences in selected areas of life and their occurrence in relative frequencies are presented in Table 8.2. Discrimination experiences concerning interactions with the police were the only area of life where people with first-episode schizophrenia had reported significantly more frequently discrimination experiences than people with first-episode depression (t-Test, $p=0.045$).

Table 8.2 Discrimination experiences in selected areas of life (Corker et al. 2014)

Area of life	Schizophrenia (%)	Depression (%)
Neighbours	12.8	25.0
Marriage	10.7	20.5
Dating and intimate relationships	6.7	19.4
Education	6.0	14.8
Physical health	2.0	14.3
Police	8.1	2.9

A further study reports the subjective burden due to stigma experienced by patients with first-episode psychosis (Zäske et al. 2016). $N=48$ patients with first-episode schizophrenia were assessed with a five-item self-rating questionnaire. The quartile of these patients which experienced the most severe burden due to stigma showed also reduced quality of life and self-esteem in comparison to the less burdened patients.

Only few studies exist which address patients and their experiences of being stigmatized due to their first-episode mental illness. According to their cross-sectional nature, only limited conclusions can be drawn about the relationship between the stigma of mental illness during the first episode of illness and the further illness course. Corker et al. (2014) indicate that experiences of discrimination are less frequent during first episode of illness than at later stages of the illness. A simple explanation would be that patients with a longer illness history had more time to experience discriminating situations. It seems that despite the traumatizing character of going through the first episode of a mental illness, a long-term perspective on the illness and the effects of stigma might be more promising for the analysis of the relationship between stigma and course of illness. Two models providing corresponding theoretical frameworks will be discussed in the next section.

Effects of Stigma During the Course of Illness: Stigma Process Models

Perceived Stigma and Coping Strategies: The Modified Labelling Approach

The modified labelling approach has been introduced by Bruce G. Link in the late 1980s (Link et al. 1989). Historically, this work can be seen as one of the most important contributions to modern stigma research in psychiatry since the groundbreaking work of Goffman (1963), as it inspired a large number of empirical studies in this field. Accordingly, from the 1990s onwards, the body of psychiatric stigma research has continuously increased.

The main assertions of the model can be summarized by five steps (Link et al. 1989): First, members of a society share conceptions of what it means to be a mental patient, i.e. perceptions of devaluation and discrimination. Second, in the case that someone is being denoted (labelled) as mentally ill, these societal conceptions become relevant to him or her. Third, the labelled individuals respond with different coping strategies, e.g. secrecy, withdrawal and education. Fourth, labelled persons suffer negative consequences for their self-esteem, earning power or societal network ties. And finally, they are increasingly vulnerable for a more severe and chronic course of illness.

B. G. Link developed several instruments assessing the different facets of stigma rejection experiences, perceived (anticipated) stigma and coping strategies. A series of panel studies was then published by Link's workgroup (Link et al. 1997, 2001; Perlick et al. 2001). Furthermore, long-term studies based on Link's methodology were published by Markowitz (1998, 2001) and Wright et al. (2000). Table 8.3 gives an overview about methodology and main results of these studies.

Table 8.3 Panel studies examining perceived stigma and rejection experiences according to Link's modified labelling approach

Study	Sample	Instruments	Follow-up	Main results
Link et al. (1997)	N=84 male patients with a dual diagnose of mental illness and substance abuse	Perceived stigma (PDDQ) Rejection experiences (proprietary scale from Link) Depressive symptoms (CES-D)	1 year	Experienced stigma has enduring effects on depressive symptoms even in the context of effective mental health and substance abuse interventions and controlled for baseline depression. The long-term effect of perceived stigma on depression is larger (10.9 % explained variance) than the effect of baseline psychopathology (9 %)
Link et al. (2001)	N=88 clubhouse members (mixed diagnoses)	Perceived stigma (PDDQ) Withdrawal as a coping strategy (proprietary scale from Link) Self-esteem (Rosenberg SES) Depressive symptoms (CES-D)	6/24 months	Prediction of self-esteem by PDDQ and withdrawal (combined): explained variance after 6 months, 12.6 %; after 24 months, 18.8 % (regression analysis with controlled baseline self-esteem and depressive symptoms). Both perceived stigma and social withdrawal have a negative effect on self-esteem in the long run
Perlick et al. (2001)	N=264 consecutive bipolar in- and outpatients (university)	Brief Psychiatric Rating Scale (BPRS) Concerns about stigma: aggregation of withdrawal (Link) and PDDQ Social adjustment scale (SAS) subscales extended family and social leisure	7 months	Regression analysis controlling symptom severity, baseline social adaptation and sociodemographic characteristics: Stigma total score at baseline was a significant predictor for SAS-social leisure subscales psychological isolation and behavioural avoidance after 7 months

(continued)

Table 8.3 (continued)

Study	Sample	Instruments	Follow-up	Main results
Markowitz (1998, 2001)	$N = 610$ consumer-run self-help groups and outpatient settings (mixed diagnoses)	Anticipated stigma (adapted from PDDQ) Stigma experiences (proprietary item) Colorado symptom index Rosenberg self-esteem Self-efficacy (derived from the mental health confidence scale) Life satisfaction (interpersonal, economic, proprietary items)	18 months	Experienced stigma is a significant predictor for symptoms and life satisfaction in the follow-up. Effects of anticipated stigma depend on whether stigma experiences are controlled. If stigma experiences are not controlled, effects of anticipated stigma may be overestimated. In general, stigma experiences have a small adverse effect on change in symptoms and life satisfaction across the 18-month interval
Wright et al. (2000)	$N = 88$ inpatients at discharge, mixed diagnoses	Semi-structured interviews; Rosenberg self-esteem Sense of personal control (Pearlin and schooler) Stigma: composed from Link rejection experiences and Link defensive strategies (secrecy and withdrawal)	Three-wave panel survey (at discharge, 1/2 years)	Path models (LISREL): experiences of rejection increase and crystallize patients' self-deprecating feelings. The impact of these rejection experiences appears to persist over time and, indirectly, contributes to a decrease in feelings of mastery and control a year later

Altogether, these studies support the view that personal stigma in terms of perceived stigma, stigma experiences and defensive stigma coping strategies has negative long-term effects on the course of illness. It is associated with increased depressive and further illness symptoms over time and with reduced self-esteem and social adjustment. Link et al. (1997) emphasize that though the stigma is related to the course of illness, it is not merely part of the symptoms or psychopathology, respectively: As they have shown in their long-term studies, illness severity usually decreases over time, while (anticipated) stigma does not show such changes but remains on a (high) level. A further important finding is that some studies suggest that these negative effects of perceived stigma are moderated by stigma experiences (Markowitz 1998; Link et al. 1997).

However, from a critical perspective, validity of these studies is limited. Samples of some of the studies include a mix of diagnoses, with prevailing diagnoses depression and schizophrenia, and, more important, assessments of stigma were partly realized with unvalidated instruments and ad hoc scales or items. Corrigan and colleagues (2006) proposed a progressive model of self-stigma as further development and enhancement of Link's approach which will be discussed in the next section.

The Progressive Model of Self-Stigma

Corrigan argues that the modified labelling approach's focus on perceived stigma is only the first of several steps how the stigma affects persons with mental illness. He calls it *stereotype awareness*, i.e. that people are aware that persons with a mental illness are being discriminated in their society. In his model, Corrigan summarizes effects of stigma concerning the affected person's self (reduced self-worth, reduced self-efficacy and reduced pursue of individuals' life goals) as self-stigma. Self-stigma develops in four stages that build on one another (cf. Corrigan et al. 2006):

- *Stereotype awareness*: the person is aware of the fact that people with mental illness are devaluated in his society.
- *Stereotype agreement*: the person endorses "the same stereotypes perceived to be common in the public".
- *Self-concurrence*: the belief that these stereotype beliefs "in fact apply to them".
- *Self-esteem decrement*: as a consequence, the person's self-esteem "is diminished due to concurrence with the negative belief".

In its essence, the progressive model of self-stigma elaborates the second step of Link's modified labelling approach (asserting that negative beliefs about persons with mental illness become relevant to oneself). To verify the progressive model of self-stigma, Corrigan developed the Self-Stigma of Mental Illness Scale (SSMIS, Corrigan et al. 2006) with four subscales assessing the proposed four stages of self-stigma.

The model was tested in a series of multiple regression analysis using a repeated measurement design (follow-up after 6 months). $N = 85$ patients with mixed psychiatric diagnoses were assessed with the SSMIS, hopelessness (assessed with the Beck hopelessness scale) and self-esteem (assessed with the Rosenberg self-esteem scale). Hence, hopelessness at follow-up was significantly predicted by the SSMIS subscale assessing the stage *self-concurrence* at baseline, even if controlled for baseline depression (assessed with the CES-D). Self-esteem at follow-up was predicted by the SSMIS subscale assessing *self-esteem decrement* at baseline. However, if controlled for depression, the effect was not significant anymore. In sum, the effects were weak. A revised SSMIS scale has been published in the mean time (Corrigan et al. 2012), but long-term studies using the revised SSMIS have not been published so far.

Discussion and Conclusions

This chapter provides an overview about the impact of mental illness stigma on the course of illness. Three different stages of the illness were discussed: the time at illness onset and before treatment initiation, the first illness episode and, third, the long-term course.

For the time from illness onset and in advance of treatment initiation, evidence relies on retrospective interview studies. Nevertheless the results are quite clear and base on studies addressing different mental illnesses: Perceived stigma and the fear of being stigmatized is one of several factors abstaining people from seeking professional help. The deriving question, whether a prolongation of the duration of untreated illness (DUI) contributes to a worsening of the long-term illness course, cannot be answered without regarding each mental illness separately. For schizophrenia it must be assumed that the prolonged duration of psychosis (DUP) contributes to a worsening of the illness course. For other mental illnesses, evidence is less clear. Yet what can be concluded with certainty is that the stigma prolongs the suffering of many persons with mental illness due to their hesitation to seek professional help.

In this context, a new study has been published just in time while finishing this manuscript (Rüsch et al. 2015). It reports new evidence for young people at high risk of psychosis: Perceiving the stigma of mental illness as harmful (as stressor) seems to be predictive for the transition to schizophrenia after 1 year (controlled for psychosis symptoms and antipsychotic medication). However, an interpretation of these results is complicated. Is the higher risk for transition to psychosis caused by the presumed stress due to the perception of being stigmatized in the long run? Or is the higher transition rate due to a more sensitive self-perception of the own mental health state, of probably already being or becoming mentally ill, might be associated with the reported feeling of being threatened and stressed by the stigma? In any case a replication of the study would be informative.

Given the few existing studies about personal stigma before mental illness onset, the situation of research literature about personal stigma at illness onset is even worse. Only few cross-sectional descriptive studies exist reporting the extent and nature of personal stigma at illness onset. In fact, being diagnosed as mentally ill and starting a psychiatric treatment is a far-reaching life event on its own, where experiences of stigma and discrimination are reported presumably less frequently than during the later course of illness.

Several long-term studies have been conducted addressing the long-term illness course and its relation to the stigma. In line with Link's modified labelling approach, personal stigma negatively affects psychosocial factors as quality of life, self-esteem and social adjustment, as well as illness symptoms and depression over time. As Corrigan concludes, the stigma impairs people with mental illness in seeking professional help and pursuing their personal life goals (Corrigan et al. 2009), what he called the "why try effect". In other words, stigma acts as "disempowerment" to people with mental illness.

At this point it is important to note that people react differently to the stigma. Some patients with mental illness react with righteous anger and develop offensive strategies (e.g. with self-disclosure) to cope with the stigma (Bos et al. 2009; Corrigan et al. 2010). Hence, stigma can also be seen as acting point for personal empowerment. This leads to the strategies how to overcome the stigma of mental illness. Two major strategies emerge: fighting against the public stigma on the one hand and supporting patients to cope with stigma and reducing negative consequences of personal stigma on the other hand. Both strategies are equally important; and both have advantages and flaws.

The fight against the public stigma is not a challenge that can be done within a couple of years. Stakeholders (both mental health professionals as organized service users) must adopt this fight as an essential part of their professional acting. But even then, full equality for people with mental illness seems as a somehow utopian idea today. Societies are based on diversity, and thinking (in particular, social judgements) and acting of human beings are influenced by fundamental processes which are well described in social psychology and which sow the seeds for stigma and discrimination. Hence, to overcome the willingness to stigmatize people who deviate from the expectations of the majority (as it is the case for many people with mental illness) is a cultural achievement that has to be reached again and again in every new generation. Public anti-stigma campaigns should therefore formulate realistic goals and take on a continuous long-term perspective.

The second major strategy is supporting people with mental illness, their relatives and caregivers in their struggle with the stigma. From the perspective of the mental health service provider, it requires mental health staff that is aware of the stigma and informed about at least two things: first, preventing discriminating behaviour within their own professional field (Zäske et al. 2014) and, second, supporting patients, relatives and caregivers in coping the stigma on their own (Sibitz et al. 2013; Zäske et al. 2013). Research has just begun to develop and evaluate such interventions (Mittal et al. 2012).

Finally, the combat against the stigma of mental illness does not only happen within professional institutions. Initiatives on grassroots level, local self-help and mutual help groups are of equal importance, because they provide support on a tangible individual level and therefore build the foundation of any large-scale anti-stigma initiative.

References

Anderson KK, Fuhrer R, Malla AK (2013) "There are too many steps before you get to where you need to be": help-seeking by patients with first-episode psychosis. J Ment Health 22:384–395

Arria AM, Winick ER, Garnier-Dykstra LM et al (2011) Help seeking and mental health service utilization among college students with a history of suicide ideation. Psychiatr Serv 62:1510–1513

Bos AE, Kanner D, Muris P et al (2009) Mental illness stigma and disclosure: consequences of coming out of the closet. Issues Ment Health Nurs 30:509–513

Brohan E, Slade M, Clement S, Thornicroft G (2010) Experiences of mental illness stigma, prejudice and discrimination: a review of measures. BMC Health Serv Res 10:80. doi:10.1186/1472-6963-10-80

Brunet K, Birchwood M, Lester H, Thornhill K (2007) Delays in mental health services and duration of untreated psychosis. Psychiatr Bull 31:408–410

Corker EA, Beldie A, Brain C et al (2014) Experience of stigma and discrimination reported by people experiencing the first episode of schizophrenia and those with a first episode of depression: the FEDORA project. Int J Soc Psychiatry. doi:10.1177/0020764014551941

Corrigan PW (2004) How stigma interferes with mental health care. Am Psychol 59:614–625

Corrigan PW, Markowitz FE, Watson AC (2004) Structural levels of mental illness stigma and discrimination. Schizophr Bull 30:481–491

Corrigan PW, Watson AC, Barr L (2006) The self-stigma of mental illness: implications for self-esteem and self-efficacy. J Soc Clin Psychol 25:875–884

Corrigan PW, Larson JE, Rüsch N (2009) Self-stigma and the "why try" effect: impact on life goals and evidence-based practices. World Psychiatry 8:75–81

Corrigan PW, Morris S, Larson J et al (2010) Self-stigma and coming out about one's mental illness. J Community Psychol 38:259–275

Corrigan PW, Michaels PJ, Vega E et al (2012) Self-stigma of mental illness scale – short form: reliability and validity. Psychiatry Res 199:65–69

Crocker J (1999) Social stigma and self-esteem: situational construction of self-worth. J Exp Soc Psychol 35:89–107

Funk M, Drew N, Knapp M (2012) Mental health, poverty and development. J Pub Ment Health 11:166–185

Gerlinger G, Hauser M, De Hert M et al (2013) Personal stigma in schizophrenia spectrum disorders: a systematic review of prevalence rates, correlates, impact and interventions. World Psychiatry 12:155–164

Goffman E (1963) Stigma. Notes on the management of spoiled identity. Prentice-Hall, Englewood-Cliffs

Graves RE, Cassisi JE, Penn DL (2005) Psychophysiological evaluation of stigma towards schizophrenia. Schizophr Res 76:317–327

Hegelstad WT, Larsen TK, Auestad B et al (2012) Long-term follow-up of the TIPS early detection in psychosis study: effects on 10-year outcome. Am J Psychiatry 169:374–380

Ienciu M, Romoşan F, Bredicean C, Romoşan R (2010) First episode psychosis and treatment delay – causes and consequences. Psychiatr Danub 22:540–543

Kisch J, Leino EV, Silverman MM (2005) Aspects of suicidal behavior, depression, and treatment in college students: results from the spring 2000 national college health assessment survey. Suicide Life Threat Behav 35:3–13

Link BG, Cullen FT, Struening E et al (1989) A modified labeling theory approach to mental disorders: an empirical assessment. Am Sociol Rev 54:400–423

Link BG, Struening EL, Rahav M et al (1997) On stigma and its consequences: evidence from a longitudinal study of men with dual diagnoses of mental illness and substance abuse. J Health Soc Behav 38:177–190

Link BG, Struening EL, Neese-Todd S et al (2001) Stigma as a barrier to recovery: the consequences of stigma for the self-esteem of people with mental illnesses. Psychiatr Serv 52:1621–1626

Lloyd-Evans B, Crosby M, Stockton S et al (2011) Initiatives to shorten duration of untreated psychosis: systematic review. Br J Psychiatry 198:256–263

Markowitz FE (1998) The effects of stigma on the psychological well-being and life satisfaction of persons with mental illness. J Health Soc Behav 39:335–347

Markowitz FE (2001) Modeling processes in recovery from mental illness: relationships between symptoms, life satisfaction, and self-concept. J Health Soc Behav 42:64–79

Marshall M, Lewis S, Lockwood A et al (2005) Association between duration of untreated psychosis and outcome in cohorts of first-episode patients: a systematic review. Arch Gen Psychiatry 62:975–983

Mittal D, Sullivan G, Chekuri L et al (2012) Empirical studies of self-stigma reduction strategies: a critical review of the literature. Psychiatr Serv 63:974–981

Mueller B, Nordt C, Lauber C et al (2006) Social support modifies perceived stigmatization in the first years of mental illness: a longitudinal approach. Soc Sci Med 62:39–49

Patel V, Kleinman A (2003) Poverty and common mental disorders in developing countries. Bull World Health Organ 81:609–615

Penn DL, Kohlmaier JR, Corrigan PW (2000) Interpersonal factors contributing to the stigma of schizophrenia: social skills, perceived attractiveness, and symptoms. Schizophr Res 45:37–45

Perlick DA, Rosenheck RA, Clarkin JF et al (2001) Stigma as a barrier to recovery: adverse effects of perceived stigma on social adaptation of persons diagnosed with bipolar affective disorder. Psychiatr Serv 52:1627–1632

Poyraz CA, Turan Ş, Sağlam NG et al (2015) Factors associated with the duration of untreated illness among patients with obsessive compulsive disorder. Compr Psychiatry 58:88–93

Rüsch N, Heekeren K, Theodoridou A et al (2015) Stigma as a stressor and transition to schizophrenia after one year among young people at risk of psychosis. Schizophr Res. doi:10.1016/j.schres.2015.05.027 [Epub ahead of print]

Sibitz I, Provaznikova K, Lipp M et al (2013) The impact of recovery-oriented day clinic treatment on internalized stigma: preliminary report. Psychiatry Res 209:326–332

Tanskanen S, Morant N, Hinton M et al (2011) Service user and carer experiences of seeking help for a first episode of psychosis: a UK qualitative study. BMC Psychiatry 11:157

Tarrier N, Khan S, Cater J, Picken A (2007) The subjective consequences of suffering a first episode psychosis: trauma and suicide behaviour. Soc Psychiatry Psychiatr Epidemiol 42:29–35

World Health Organization (2013) Mental health action plan 2013–2020. WHO, Geneva

Wright ER, Gronfein WP, Owens TJ (2000) Deinstitutionalization, social rejection, and the self-esteem of former mental patients. J Health Soc Behav 41:68–90

Zäske H, Sauter S, Ohmann C, Icks A, Gaebel W (2013) Improving empowerment and stigma coping in people with mental illness [Poster in German]. Poster presented at the 12th German Conference for Healthcare Research, Berlin, 23–25 Oct 2013

Zäske H, Freimüller L, Wölwer W, Gaebel W (2014) Anti-stigma competence for mental health professionals: results of a pilot study of a further education programme for people working in psychiatric and psychosocial settings [Article in German]. Fortschr Neurol Psychiatr 82:586–592

Zäske H, Degner D, Jockers-Scherübl M et al (2016) Experiences of stigma and discrimination in patients with first-episode schizophrenia [Article in German]. Nervenarzt 87:82–87.

Changes of Stigma over Time

9

Georg Schomerus and Matthias C. Angermeyer

Introduction

Stigma is not static. As a cultural phenomenon, it changes over time, just as public values, attitudes, and preferences in many areas of life change. Changes of stigma are particularly relevant: They indicate whether the discrimination experienced by persons with mental illness has diminished, or whether it has grown. Time trends of stigma may reveal areas of successful anti-stigma work and thus endorse certain anti-stigma strategies, or they may point out areas where more work is necessary, where novel approaches are needed. Looking at the changes of stigma may reveal something about the nature of stigma. Which attitudes develop in parallel, which attitudes seem independent from each other? Which aspects of stigma are most amenable to changes, which are the most persistent?

To capture changes of stigma on population level over time, repeated cross-sectional surveys among the general population are necessary. Fortunately, the last 25 years have seen tremendous efforts to examine and understand public attitudes toward persons with mental illness, and numerous surveys in many countries have yielded a wealth of data. However, for a valid assessment of time trends, an identical methodology employed among the same population in repeated surveys is needed. Items have to be worded identically and use similar answer scales, and identical

G. Schomerus (✉)
Department of Psychiatry, University of Greifswald, Greifswald, Germany
e-mail: georg.schomerus@uni-greifswald.de

M.C. Angermeyer
Department of Public Health, University of Cagliari, Cagliari, Italy
e-mail: angermeyer@aon.at

© Springer International Publishing Switzerland 2017
W. Gaebel et al. (eds.), *The Stigma of Mental Illness - End of the Story?*,
DOI 10.1007/978-3-319-27839-1_9

stimuli like case vignettes need to be used. Sampling should follow the same procedure, so that differences between surveys are not due to different biases inherent in every sampling method. Finally, the same interview method should be used (face to face, telephone, postal survey, online survey, etc.), because each method has its specific strengths and weaknesses. A personal interview, for example, is probably hampered by social desirability bias, but provides the reliability of a thorough interview, while an online survey has the advantage of anonymity, but may be impeded by superficial, hasty answers by some respondents.

In this chapter, we summarize the findings of time-trend studies that largely meet these methodological requirements. They are mostly from Western industrialized countries and provide a fairly consistent picture of time trends of mental health-related attitudes. However, since attitude research in other cultures and less-developed countries has mostly started later and is still developing, the evolution of stigma in many parts of the world remains unknown. We will look at how causal beliefs regarding mental illness have changed and how the image of psychiatry and psychiatric treatment has evolved. Then we will evaluate how the public stigma and the perceived stigma of mental illness have changed over the last 30 years and whether there are indications for changes in structural stigma.

Changes of Illness Models Among the General Population

Studies that have looked at public conceptions of mental illness within the last 25 years have found a fairly consistent pattern: Biological illness models have become more and more popular. Agreement with the statement that schizophrenia is genetically caused did increase, for example, from 61 to 71 % in the USA between 1996 and 2006 (Pescosolido et al. 2010) and from 59 to 75 % in Australia between 1995 and 2011 (Reavley and Jorm 2014). A meta-regression analysis of national time-trend studies found a common linear trend of increasing biological illness beliefs for both schizophrenia and, from a lower baseline, depression between 1990 and 2006 (Schomerus et al. 2012) (Fig. 9.1). However, the rising popularity of biological illness models does not imply that psychosocial causes are seen as less important: Consistently, an even greater proportion of the public endorses psychosocial causes compared to biological causes. For example, while 75 % of Australians considered schizophrenia an inherited condition, 91 % saw day-to-day problems as a possible cause (Reavley and Jorm 2014).

The similar direction of changes in illness beliefs seen in the meta-analysis indicates broad trends of attitude change occurring across countries, illustrating the connectedness of the countries on a cultural level. There seems to be some common zeitgeist of how mental illness is seen by the general public in quite different countries.

Recent surveys indicate that the trend toward greater endorsement of biological causes might have peaked: Biological illness explanations of depression are not further increasing in Australia (Pilkington et al. 2013) or even declining in Germany (Angermeyer et al. 2013b). In Germany, a survey in 2011 still showed increasing endorsement of "brain disease" as a cause for schizophrenia compared to 1990, but

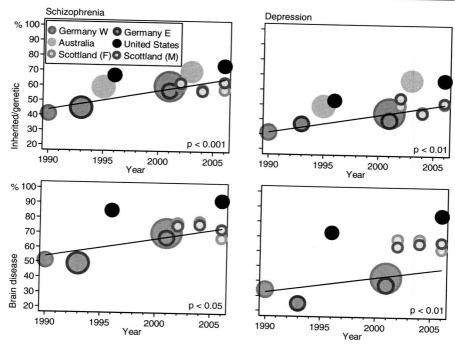

Fig. 9.1 Evolution of causal explanations for schizophrenia and depression. Results from representative, national trend studies using unlabelled case vignettes. Agreement to a specific cause, meta-regression analysis controlled for study site, reference category: West Germany. The position of each *circle* represents the result (*y*-axis) and year (*x*-axis) of one national survey, and circle size is proportional to sample size. Surveys from different countries/trend analyses are distinguished by different *shades of gray*. *Germany W* West Germany (old FRG), *Germany E* East Germany (former GDR), *F* Female vignette, *M* Male vignette (From: Schomerus et al. 2012. © 2012 John Wiley & Sons A/S)

the strong increase of genetic illness beliefs visible between 1990 and 2001 (Angermeyer and Matschinger 2005a) was no longer visible in 2011 (Angermeyer et al. 2013b). In depression, particularly work related, stress had become more popular in recent years (Angermeyer et al. 2013b), which could be attributed to changing working conditions in a globalized economy that suffered a severe crisis in 2008.

Causal Beliefs and Stigma

Causal beliefs have been shown to interact with the stigma of mental illness. While attribution of mental illness to stressful circumstances increases feelings of anger toward the affected, it reduces notions of differentness and dangerousness. Conversely, biological illness beliefs have been shown to be associated with stronger notions of differentness, dangerousness, and fear, reactions that increase the desire for social distance toward a person with mental illness (Kvaale et al. 2013; Schomerus et al. 2014a).

Most studies group childhood causes into "psychosocial causal explanations," but they differ in important ways from causal beliefs like day-to-day problems or work-related stress: Different to these present stressful conditions, childhood-related causes are in the past and cannot be changed. A correlational study among the general public found childhood-related causes associated with stronger stigmatizing attitudes in depression (Schomerus et al. 2014a). For this group of causal explanations, time trends are inconsistent between different countries. In Australia, "childhood problems" became a more popular cause for both depression and schizophrenia between 1996 and 2011 (Pilkington et al. 2013; Reavley and Jorm 2014), being endorsed by more than 90 % in 2011. Contrarily, childhood-related causes seem to lose popularity in Germany and the USA (Angermeyer et al. 2013b; Pescosolido et al. 2010). For example, a broken home was considered a possible cause for depression and schizophrenia in Germany by more than 50 % in 1990, while in 2011, only 31 % (schizophrenia) and 26 % (depression) considered this a possible cause (Angermeyer et al. 2013b).

> **Information Box 9.1: Changes of Illness Models Among the General Population**
> There has been a broad trend toward more biological illness explanations over the last 25 years, but psychosocial explanations, particularly current stress, continue to enjoy high popularity. There is evidence linking biological causal models to increased stigma.

Changes of the Image of Psychiatry and Psychiatric Treatment

Over the last decades, psychiatric reform has triggered fundamental changes in psychiatric services in many countries (McDaid and Thornicroft 2005). This ongoing process of deinstitutionalization, the development of community mental health services, and the integration of mental health care with general health services certainly has had profound impact on the way psychiatric services are provided (Priebe 2012). Departing from a psychiatry that had been described as a "total institution" (Goffman 1961), it was hoped that psychiatric reform would improve the public image of psychiatric services and make it an accepted medical specialty among other specialties (Bundestag 1975). But there are concerns that the old, negative image of psychiatry prevails, that psychiatry even carries a stigma on its own (Sartorius et al. 2010). A recent campaign by the World Psychiatric Association explicitly targeted the stigma of psychiatry and psychiatrists, not the least because it was perceived as a barrier to taking up a psychiatric career among junior doctors (Gaebel et al. 2015).

Hospital-Based Psychiatry

Only few studies examine time trends of attitudes toward psychiatric institutions, but they show that the image particularly of the psychiatric hospital has improved over the last decades. A study from Germany compared agreement with negative stereotypes about the psychiatric hospital in 1990 and in 2011 (Angermeyer et al. 2013c). It shows that most fears have diminished, while expectations regarding adequate help and protection have increased. For example, agreement with the statement that psychiatric hospitals are more like prisons than like hospitals decreased by half from 32 to 16 %, while agreement with the statement that they offer necessary protection during a personal crisis increased from 44 to 66 %. Agreement with the statement that psychiatric hospitals are making you ill instead of offering treatment dropped from 26 to 16 %, while now 62 % (compared to 55 % in 1990) agreed that psychiatric hospitals are hospitals just like other hospitals. This development was especially pronounced in persons that stated that they had some personal experience of psychiatric treatment. The psychiatric hospital, once seen as prisonlike and far from offering effective treatment, is now more frequently seen as a place where adequate treatment is provided to persons who are in need (Angermeyer et al. 2013c). However, the same study also showed that more people in 2011 compared to 1990 consider psychiatric hospitals necessary to protect society from persons with mental illness (49 % vs. 39 %), indicating developments like increased fear from persons with mental illness, or reduced tolerance of nonconforming behavior.

Community Psychiatry

A somewhat different development has been observed with regard to community psychiatry. Again the only time-trend study on this topic was conducted in Germany (Angermeyer et al. 2013a). It enquired how many people preferred patients with mental illness being treated in the same hospital as other patients and how many would welcome a group home for persons with mental illness in their neighborhood. A small but stable proportion of respondents firmly opposed both aspects of community psychiatry. However, the share of persons welcoming these developments clearly dropped: The proportion of respondents explicitly welcoming a psychiatric ward at a general hospital decreased from 41 to 26 %, and the percentages of respondents welcoming a group home lessened from 34 to 25 % between 1990 and 2011. Thus communities seem to show less enthusiasm welcoming community psychiatric services than earlier during psychiatric reform.

Apart from this, one broad and stable trend regarding psychiatric treatment has been observed almost universally: Medication is enjoying growing popularity and is more and more seen as an adequate treatment for both depression and schizophrenia. Psychiatrists are more readily seen as an appropriate source of help, and psychotherapy remains popular at high levels (Angermeyer et al. 2013b; Schomerus et al. 2012). Thus, academic-, hospital-, or office-based psychiatric care has improved its image considerably over the last decades, and probably this is indeed a success of a more open, patient-centered, and human right-informed psychiatry that has evolved in many countries. However, the limited existing evidence suggests that community psychiatric services have not fully participated in this image gain, are seen with more indifference than 20 years ago, and have thus not yet arrived at the heart of the community.

> **Information Box 9.2: Changes of the Image of Psychiatry and Psychiatric Treatment**
> Hospital- and office-based psychiatric treatment is clearly more accepted now than it was 25 years ago. Few studies examine acceptance of community psychiatric services, showing more indifference and less enthusiasm today than in the 1990s.

Changes of Public Stigma

Stigma has been conceptualized as a process of interrelated cognitive and emotional steps (Corrigan 2000; Link and Phelan 2001; Rüsch et al. 2005). At the end of this process, discrimination and status loss are inflicted on those with mental disorders. Looking at time trends of stigma, we will distinguish between public stigma, stigma experience or self-stigma, and structural stigma. With regard to public stigma, we will look at both measures of individual discrimination like the desire for social distance and measures of common stereotypes like dangerousness, unpredictability, or blame.

Many studies have provided evidence that stigmatizing attitudes of the general public differ between different mental disorders. Consistently, substance-related disorders and schizophrenia are stigmatized most, whereas other disorders like depression, anxiety disorders, and eating disorders are stigmatized to a lesser extent (Crisp et al. 2005; Schomerus et al. 2011). Looking at time trends of attitude change, these differences between mental disorders appear even more profound.

Social Distance and Emotional Reactions

Figure 9.2 shows more results from the meta-regression analysis of international time-trend studies (Schomerus et al. 2012). It summarizes time rends of social distance, depicted as willingness to engage in two hypothetical situations with a person with either schizophrenia or depression: Respondents were asked to indicate whether they would be willing to accept someone with depression or schizophrenia as a neighbor or as a colleague at work. Overall, willingness to get close to someone with depression did not change between 1990 and 2006, while willingness to engage in personal contact with a person with schizophrenia declined.

Here, the obvious differences in time trends between the two disorders greatly increase the validity of the findings: If reluctance to get closer to another person would have been a general phenomenon not specific to mental illness, trends for both disorders would have been similar, even more so since studies in Germany, the USA, and Scotland used identical methodology not only across surveys but also between the two disorders. Instead, persons suffering from schizophrenia clearly fare worse than those suffering from depression – even though there is no significant improvement in depression, either. The same disorder-specific trend was corroborated in another German study comparing attitudes elicited in 2011 with those

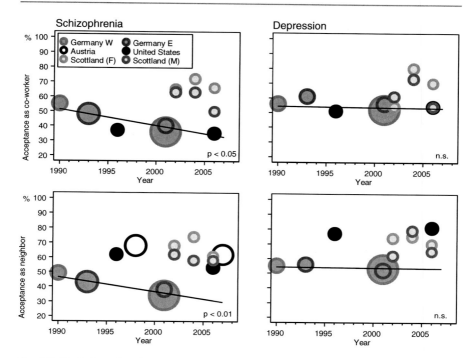

Fig. 9.2 Evolution of social acceptance of persons with schizophrenia or depression. Results from representative, national trend studies using unlabelled case vignettes. Willingness to engage in specific forms of social contact, meta-regression analysis controlled for study site, reference category: West Germany. The position of each *circle* represents the result (*y*-axis) and year (*x*-axis) of one national survey, and *circle* size is proportional to sample size. Surveys from different countries/trend analyses are distinguished by different *shades of gray*. *Germany W* West Germany (old FRG), *Germany E*, East Germany (former GDR), *F* female vignette, *M* male vignette (From: Schomerus et al. 2012. © 2012 John Wiley & Sons A/S)

in 1990. In all seven hypothetical situations elicited with a social distance scale, respondents were less willing to interact with a person suffering from schizophrenia (predicted probability change for rejection 5–18 % across all social distance items), while willingness to interact with a person with depression or with alcohol dependence hardly changed (Angermeyer et al. 2013b).

In the same study, social distance toward a person with depression increased in only one situation: Respondents were more unwilling to recommend a person with depression for a job in 2011 than they had been in 1990. Looking at this trend in more detail, the authors examined social distance toward a male person with depression in 1990, 2001, and 2011. In fact, reluctance to recommend someone with depression for a job remained stable from 1990 to 2001, but increased between 2001 and 2011 from 41 to 49 % (Angermeyer et al. 2013d). This trend was even more pronounced among those respondents who were currently employed. These findings likely reflect the economic crisis: In times of uncertainty, people might be more likely to restrict the opportunities of persons with mental illness on a competitive field – or, alternatively, they might be more skeptical whether a person with depression is fit for the job market.

Inconsistent with these findings, a study from Australia based on surveys from 2003/2004 and 2011 showed more persons willing to let someone with either schizophrenia or depression marry into their family, but no significant changes in more distant social relationships like living next door or making friends (Reavley and Jorm 2012). Since sampling and interviewing methodology varied from a personal face-to-face interview in 2003/2004 to a telephone interview in 2011, the contribution of methodological biases to these findings remains unknown.

Not all studies examine illness-specific attitudes, and certainly the cultural climate surrounding mental illness in general is also important. Studies from other countries examining social distance toward a person with "mental illness" did, however, also fail to find improvements. In the Netherlands, growing social acceptance between 1976 and 1987 was followed by declining social acceptance until 1997 (Kwekkeboom 2000). Surveys in Scotland and England, conducted between 1994 and 2003, showed very little changes in the Community Attitudes toward Mental Illness (CAMI) scale until 1997 but some interesting differences between both countries between 2000 and 2003: While during that time, 17 of 25 items of the scale deteriorated in England, this effect was markedly less in Scotland, where, accompanied by the national anti-stigma campaign *see me*, only 4/25 items deteriorated (Mehta et al. 2009). Conversely, a series of population surveys conducted in England between 2009 and 2012 during the nationwide Time to Change anti-stigma campaign showed a trend toward more positive attitudes in the CAMI and slight decreases in social distance toward a person with "mental health problems" as measured with the Reported and Intended Behavior Scale (Evans-Lacko et al. 2013). Although not disorder specific, these findings might indicate that nationwide anti-stigma campaigns can to some extent counterbalance negative general time trends and improve attitudes toward persons with mental health problems in general.

Another way to find out about pending individual discrimination is to ask respondents about their emotional reactions toward a person with mental illness described in a case vignette. The stigma model of Link and Phelan sees negative emotional reactions as precedents of separation, status loss and discrimination (Link and Phelan 2001; Link et al. 2004). A German study following this approach found increasing fear between 1990 and 2011 solely in reaction to a person with schizophrenia, and not depression (Angermeyer et al. 2013b). Similarly, the percentage of respondents feeling the need to help a person with depression increased between 1990 and 2011, while it decreased with regard to a person with schizophrenia. More persons felt uncomfortable around a person with schizophrenia in 2011 compared to 1990, while less did so around a person with depression (Angermeyer et al. 2013b). Annoyance or anger did not change in depression and schizophrenia, the latter being expressed by less than 10 %. Only in alcohol dependence, more persons stated being annoyed and feeling anger in 2011 (22/24 %) compared to 1990 (15 %).

Overall, there is a clear trend separating schizophrenia from other mental disorders like depression and alcohol dependence. While in depression and alcohol dependence, the desire for social distance remained stable, social distance toward persons with schizophrenia deteriorated. It is a pressing question in stigma research to understand the reasons for this development.

Fear, Dangerousness, and Guilt

Individual discrimination as measured with various adoptions of the social distance scale is the most widely used outcome in psychiatric attitude research, but negative stereotypes are probably not less relevant, because they have been shown to be closely related to social distance (Angermeyer and Matschinger 2005b) – stigma models see them as a driving force for stigma (Corrigan 2000; Link and Phelan 2001). To a different degree, persons with different mental disorders are seen as dangerous and unpredictable, as self-responsible for their condition, or as both dangerous and self-responsible. For example, while persons with schizophrenia are rarely blamed for their condition, many people regard them as dangerous and unpredictable. Persons with eating disorders, in contrast, are seen as self-responsible, but not dangerous. Persons with substance use conditions finally are seen as both dangerous/unpredictable and guilty for their condition, making their stigma particularly severe (Crisp et al. 2005; Schomerus et al. 2011). Some studies have examined time trends of these stereotypes.

A study in England accompanying the Changing Minds campaign of the Royal College of Psychiatrists found decreasing notions of dangerousness and unpredictability between 1998 and 2005 for schizophrenia and, to a lesser extent, depression, while notions of blame remained unchanged at very low levels (Crisp et al. 2005). The comparison of results from the General Social Survey in 1996 and 2006 in the USA revealed no changes with regard to unpredictability, dangerousness, and blame with regard to schizophrenia, slightly less blame with regard to depression, but significantly more blame toward a person with alcohol dependence (Pescosolido et al. 2010). A study from New Zealand (1999–2002), in contrast, showed a growing notion that people with mental illness are more likely to be dangerous than other people (Vaughan and Hansen 2004). Similarly, surveys from Australia found increasing notions of dangerousness and unpredictability for both depression and schizophrenia between 2003/2004 and 2011 (Reavley and Jorm 2012).

Overall, time trends related to stereotypes are more inconsistent than those related to social distance or emotional reactions. Accordingly, the meta-analysis of time trends found no consistent trend for studies on stereotypes, although there was an insignificant trend toward less blame in depression and schizophrenia (Schomerus et al. 2012). So results on the prevalence of negative stereotypes add little to explain the differential development of social distance toward persons with different mental disorders.

Age and Cohort Effects

To identify net changes of attitudes regardless of demographic changes between survey years, time-trend studies usually control their results for age. However, it is a frequent finding in cross-sectional studies of mental illness stigma that stigmatizing attitudes increase with the age the respondents. This could reflect a cohort effect if younger cohorts develop more tolerant attitudes toward persons with mental illness, or it could be a true age effect if attitudes do in fact worsen over the life-span (Jorm and Oh 2009). A study from Germany, based on population surveys in 1990, 2001, and 2011, calculated age-period-cohort models to disentangle the different contributions of age, birth cohort, and time period to changes in social distance (Schomerus et al. 2015). Based on reactions to case vignettes of either schizophrenia or depression, this study found that while younger cohorts tend to be more open toward a person with depression, no such cohort effect could be observed for schizophrenia. The authors speculate that reactions to symptoms of depression could be subject to cultural change that is reflected in changing socialization experiences of younger cohorts. In contrast, symptoms of schizophrenia, being outside of most people's everyday experiences, could be perceived equally strange and frightening regardless of subtle cultural changes across different birth cohorts.

The same study found a consistent linear age effect across both disorders: Over the life-span, the respondents' willingness to interact with persons with mental illness declined significantly, irrespective of birth cohort or time period (Schomerus et al. 2015). Given the demographic change in most Western societies, this development alone will lead to increases of population-level stigma for both schizophrenia and depression. This study illustrates the need to target anti-stigma activities not only to younger individuals, as has frequently been done so far (Griffiths et al. 2014), but also to elderly persons.

Information Box 9.3: Changes in Public Stigma
There is little indication that individual attitudes toward persons with mental illness among the general population improve. With regard to schizophrenia, there are consistent findings from many countries that stigmatizing attitudes have even become worse, particularly during the 1990s and early 2000s, and that negative stereotypes like dangerousness or unpredictability prevail.

Changes in Perceived Stigma and Discrimination Experiences

How do population attitudes affect those who develop a mental illness? Looking at discrimination experiences of persons with schizophrenia and depression worldwide, Thornicroft and co-workers found high prevalence of both experienced and anticipated discrimination (Thornicroft et al. 2009). The important role of anticipated discrimination is noteworthy, because it shows that stigma experience is not limited to situations where overt discrimination occurs, but might be experienced even absent of discriminatory behavior. It would be shortsighted to discard anticipated discrimination as less real or relevant than actual discrimination. Many persons with mental illness chose not to disclose their illness or even withdraw from certain situations because of anticipated discrimination, so perceived stigma has profound effect on their life and well-being even absent of any overt discriminatory behavior.

Trends in Discrimination Experience

Measuring time trends in stigma experience is challenging, because it requires repeated large representative surveys among service users. In England, anticipated and experienced discriminations among service users were monitored in annual surveys during the Time to Change anti-stigma campaign from 2008 to 2011 (Corker et al. 2013), using random samples of users from different mental health trusts across England. Although this study was hampered by unexpected low response rates, which made the introduction of incentives and foreign language questionnaires during follow-up surveys necessary, it is the largest and most comprehensive attempt to establish time trends of stigma experiences. It showed a significant reduction of experienced discrimination in 4 out of 21 domains and a nonsignificant trend toward less anticipated discrimination. The median of discrimination ratings fell by 11 % (Corker et al. 2013). This study covered a time period of 3 years in close context to a national anti-stigma campaign. So far, long-term developments of stigma experiences have not been examined.

Trends in Perceived Stigma

Other studies have measured perceptions of stigma among the general population. These perceptions are relevant, because they indicate the level of stigma a person anticipates if he or she develops a mental illness. A large study from Germany analyzed data from three repeated surveys in 1990, 2001, and 2011 (Angermeyer et al. 2014a) using Link's Perceived Devaluation and Discrimination Scale (PDDS) (Link et al. 1989), covering a time period of 21 years. The PDDS is a 12-item scale asking respondents to rate how likely it is, in their opinion, that most people will discriminate or devalue a person with a history of psychiatric treatment. Compared to the measure of social distance employed in the same German study, this scale is different in two respects. First, it asks what the respondents believe most other persons think – thereby stopping short from eliciting the respondent's own personal attitudes and thus circumventing social desirability bias, but rather enquiring about the perceived attitudes of others. Studies employing parallel measures of personal and perceived attitudes showed only low correlations between both aspects of stigma (Griffiths et al. 2004), demonstrating that perceived stigma and personal stigma are not the same.

The second difference is that the scale elicits reactions to a person that is described as having received psychiatric treatment. Different to the case histories used as stimulus for the social distance scale, the person is not described as showing symptoms of any acute mental disorder. This approach was originally chosen by Link and co-workers to focus on reactions associated with the label mental illness, not with symptoms of a specific mental disorder (Link et al. 1989).

Perceived stigma as measured with the PDDS decreased significantly in Germany between 1990 and 2011. While in 1990 more respondents disagreed than agreed with the statement that "most people believe that a former mental patient is just as trust-worthy as the average person," 21 years later the opposite was true. In 1990, more than half of the respondents disagreed with the statement that "most people in my community would treat a former mental patient just as they would treat anyone"; in 2011, only one third disagreed with that statement. While almost half of the respondents in 1990 shared the view that once a person had been in a psychiatric hospital, most people would not take his or her opinion seriously, 21 years later the percentage has dropped by half. Overall, the reduction of perceived stigma cumulated to 0.77 standard deviations (SD) between 1990 and 2011 (Angermeyer et al. 2014a).

In a similar study comparing the perceived stigma of alcohol dependence, representative samples in Germany in 1990 and 2011 were presented with an adapted version of the PDDS referring to a person that had been treated for alcoholism. Here, too, perceptions of discrimination and devaluation diminished considerably between 1990 and 2011, showing an overall reduction of 0.44 SD (Schomerus et al. 2014b).

Among many discouraging findings on stable negative personal attitudes among the general public, the improvement of perceived stigma clearly is good news. It suggests that a person experiencing a mental illness might today anticipate less discrimination than in the early 1990s. It is, however, also puzzling. Why should perceptions of attitudes of other people improve so markedly, while personal attitudes remained unchanged or even worsened?

One reason could be that media reports on anti-stigma campaigns, although not changing personal attitudes, could have nourished the impression that "something is being done," so people expect that most other persons' attitudes should have improved. Along similar lines, the predominance of biogenetic illness models in media reports on mental illness (Lewison et al. 2012) could have led individuals to conclude that an increasing biomedical understanding of mental illness should have reduced its stigma – although there is ample evidence that biological illness models do not reduce stigma, but carry a danger of increasing notions of dangerousness and differentness (Angermeyer et al. 2011; Kvaale et al. 2013; Schomerus et al. 2014a).

Another reason could be the focus of the PDDS on treated persons with mental illness without any reference to mental illness symptoms. While actually having a mental illness is clearly as stigmatizing as it was more than 20 years ago, having a history of treated mental illness seems more acceptable nowadays. This would be in line with findings on the growing public acceptance of professional mental health treatment that were outlined at the beginning of this chapter. It would also imply, however, that mental illness is only acceptable when under control, when it is treated, when it is something of the person's past, and not if it presents as a current, yet unsolved problem.

The surveys from Germany provide several indications that unpredictable, nonconformist behavior is seen as less acceptable today than it was 21 years ago: Respondents showed more fear and felt more uncomfortable when confronted with a person with schizophrenia (Angermeyer et al. 2013b), they stated greater willingness to admit a person with mental illness to a hospital against his/her will if she provoked public nuisance (Angermeyer et al. 2014c), and they agreed more frequently with the statement that psychiatric hospitals are important to protect society from persons with mental illness (Angermeyer et al. 2013c). A reduction in perceived stigma does carry some hope for those who experience mental illness, who might feel less stigmatized and more comfortable disclosing their mental illness, which in fact could contribute to a substantial de-stigmatization because it would create more situations of overt contact with mental illness. However, there seems to be a real danger that a de-stigmatization of those who have a past treated mental illness comes at the expense of growing social exclusion of those who presently suffer from mental illness.

> **Information Box 9.4: Changes in Perceived Stigma**
> Perceived stigma of someone with a history of mental illness clearly diminished in Germany between 1990 and 2011. This stands in contrast to unchanged or worsening personal attitudes toward persons with mental illness. It is unclear whether this is due to a discrepancy between personal and perceived attitudes or whether there is a widening gap between attitudes toward persons with past as opposed to persons with present mental illness.

Changes in Structural Stigma

Structural discrimination is defined as institutional practices and policies that work to the disadvantage of a stigmatized group even in the absence of individual discrimination. This facet of stigma is drawing increasing scientific attention (Hatzenbuehler and Link 2014), since structural stigma has severe consequences for persons with mental disorders, but at the same time might well be amenable to change. So far, there are no studies measuring changes in structural stigma over time. However, the German study on time trends of attitudes included a question on resource allocation preferences of the public within the health-care sector. Respondents were instructed that, since funds for health care were increasingly scarce, resources for the treatment of certain disorders need to be cut, and they should name those three conditions out of a list of nine diseases that should be saved from such cuts (Angermeyer et al. 2014b). In 2001, when the question was first employed, most respondents chose "cancer" (chosen by more than 80 %), followed by "AIDS" and "diabetes" – the same three disorders being chosen most frequently in 2011. The lowest priority for funding was given to the three mental disorders included in the list: "schizophrenia," "depression," and "alcoholism," all chosen by less than 10 % of respondents in 2001. Ten years later, there was only one difference: "Depression" was now chosen to be excluded from funding cuts by about 20 %, while "schizophrenia" and "alcoholism" remained below 10 % (Angermeyer et al. 2014b). The same study showed that in both surveys, attitudes indicating individual discrimination did correlate only weakly with attitudes regarding structural discrimination. Although not measuring structural discrimination directly, the study shows that public preferences regarding a crucial structural aspect of health care, its funding, are biased against mental disorders.

Information Box 9.5: Changes in Structural Stigma
Studies on changes in structural stigma are warranted. Studies on public attitudes toward resource allocation in health care show particularly schizophrenia and alcohol use disorder persistently at risk for structural discrimination.

Conclusion

Time-trend analyses of mental health-related public attitudes provide us with a complex picture of attitude change over the last 25 years. Due to their high methodological demands, these analyses are rare, and hence our picture is imbalanced: We know a lot about attitude changes in relatively few countries. Although reviews and meta-analyses indicate that broad trends of attitude change are not confined within national boundaries, developments in other cultural contexts or in specific national/political circumstances likely remained unnoticed.

From what we know, it appears that there are different trends. Overall, only perceived stigma, but not personal attitudes among the general population, has improved. There is growing rejection of persons with severe mental illness. Biological causal beliefs have been shown to be associated with more stigmatizing attitudes, based on stronger notions of differentness and dangerousness. The growing popularity of biological illness models over the last 25 years could contribute to the growing rejection of persons with schizophrenia. Psychiatric treatment has lost much of its negative image, but simultaneously community psychiatry has lost outspoken support and enthusiasm in the community. Stigma increases with growing age, and younger cohorts are just as intolerant toward a person with schizophrenia as older cohorts. While treatment of depression enjoys a somewhat higher esteem now, treatment of alcohol dependence and schizophrenia has very low priority with the public. The stigma of mental illness remains a troublesome, complex phenomenon aggravating the burden of mental illness. Future research will show whether the divide between less stigmatized and more stigmatized mental disorders as it has been observed for depression and schizophrenia widens further.

Acknowledgment We wish to thank Herbert Matschinger, whose methodological excellence has enabled many of the studies cited in this chapter.

References

Angermeyer MC, Matschinger H (2005a) Causal beliefs and attitudes to people with schizophrenia – trend analysis based on data from two population surveys in Germany. Br J Psychiatry 186:331–334
Angermeyer MC, Matschinger H (2005b) Labeling – stereotype – discrimination – an investigation of the stigma process. Soc Psychiatry Psychiatr Epidemiol 40:391–395

Angermeyer MC, Holzinger A, Carta MG, Schomerus G (2011) Biogenetic explanations and public acceptance of mental illness: systematic review of population studies. Br J Psychiatry 199:367–372

Angermeyer MC, Matschinger H, Holzinger A, Carta MG, Schomerus G (2013a) Psychiatric services in the community? The German public's opinion in 1990 and 2011. Epidemiol Psychiatr Sci 22:339–344

Angermeyer MC, Matschinger H, Schomerus G (2013b) Attitudes towards psychiatric treatment and people with mental illness: changes over two decades. Br J Psychiatry 203:146–151

Angermeyer MC, Matschinger H, Schomerus G (2013c) Has the public taken notice of psychiatric reform? The image of psychiatric hospitals in Germany 1990–2011. Soc Psychiatry Psychiatr Epidemiol 48:1629–1635

Angermeyer MC, Matschinger H, Schomerus G (2013d) Public attitudes towards people with depression in times of uncertainty: results from three population surveys in Germany. Soc Psychiatry Psychiatr Epidemiol 48:1513–1518

Angermeyer MC, Matschinger H, Carta MG, Schomerus G (2014a) Changes in the perception of mental illness stigma in Germany over the last two decades. Eur Psychiatry 29:390–395

Angermeyer MC, Matschinger H, Link BG, Schomerus G (2014b) Public attitudes regarding individual and structural discrimination: two sides of the same coin? Soc Sci Med 103: 60–66

Angermeyer MC, Matschinger H, Schomerus G (2014c) Attitudes of the German public to restrictions on persons with mental illness in 1993 and 2011. Epidemiol Psychiatr Sci 23:263–270

Bundestag D (1975) Bericht über die Lage der Psychiatrie in der Bundesrepublik Deutschland – Zur psychiatrischen und psychotherapeutischen/psychosomatischen Versorgung der Bevölkerung. Hans Herger, Bonn

Corker E, Hamilton S, Henderson C, Weeks C, Pinfold V, Rose D, Williams P, Flach C, Gill V, Lewis-Holmes E (2013) Experiences of discrimination among people using mental health services in England 2008–2011. Br J Psychiatry 202:s58–s63, %@ 0007-1250

Corrigan PW (2000) Mental health stigma as social attribution: implications for research methods and attitude change. Clin Psychol-Sci Pract 7:48–67

Crisp AH, Gelder MG, Goddard E, Meltzer HI (2005) Stigmatization of people with mental illnesses: a follow-up study within the Changing Minds campaign of the Royal College of Psychiatrists. World Psychiatry 4:106–113

Evans-Lacko S, Henderson C, Thornicroft G (2013) Public knowledge, attitudes and behaviour regarding people with mental illness in England 2009–2012. Br J Psychiatry 202:s51–s57, %@ 0007-1250

Gaebel W, Zäske H, Zielasek J, Cleveland H-R, Samjeske K, Stuart H, Arboleda-Florez J, Akiyama T, Baumann AE, Gureje O (2015) Stigmatization of psychiatrists and general practitioners: results of an international survey. Eur Arch Psychiatry Clin Neurosci 265:189–197, %@ 0940-1334

Goffmann E (1961) On the Characteristics of Total Institutions. In: E. Goffmann: Asylums. Essays on the Social Situation of Mental Patients and Other Inmates. Anchor Books: Garden City, New York, pp 1–124

Griffiths KM, Christensen H, Jorm AF, Evans K, Groves C (2004) Effect of web-based depression literacy and cognitive-behavioural therapy interventions on stigmatising attitudes to depression – randomised controlled trial. Br J Psychiatry 185:342–349

Griffiths KM, Carron-Arthur B, Parsons A, Reid R (2014) Effectiveness of programs for reducing the stigma associated with mental disorders. A meta-analysis of randomized controlled trials. World Psychiatry 13:161–175

Hatzenbuehler ML, Link BG (2014) Introduction to the special issue on structural stigma and health. Soc Sci Med 103:1–6

Jorm AF, Oh E (2009) Desire for social distance from people with mental disorders. Aust N Z J Psychiatry 43:183–200

Kvaale EP, Gottdiener WH, Haslam N (2013) Biogenetic explanations and stigma: a meta-analytic review of associations among laypeople. Soc Sci Med 96:95–103

Kwekkeboom MH (2000) Sociaal draagvlak voor de vermaatschappelijking in de geestelijke Gezondheidswetenschappen. Ontwikkelingen tussen 1976 en 1997. Tijdschr Gezondheidswetenschappen 78:165–171

Lewison G, Roe P, Wentworth A, Szmukler G (2012) The reporting of mental disorders research in British media. Psychol Med 42:435–441

Link BG, Phelan JC (2001) Conceptualizing stigma. Annu Rev Sociol 27:363–385

Link BG, Cullen FT, Struening E, Shrout PE, Dohrenwend BP (1989) A modified labeling theory approach to mental disorders: an empirical assessment. Am Sociol Rev 54:400–423

Link BG, Yang LH, Phelan JC, Collins PY (2004) Measuring mental illness stigma. Schizophr Bull 30:511–541

McDaid D, Thornicroft G (2005) Policy brief mental health II. Balancing institutional and community based care. WHO Regional Office for Europe, Copenhagen

Mehta N, Kassam A, Leese M, Butler G, Thornicroft G (2009) Public attitudes towards people with mental illness in England and Scotland, 1994–2003. Br J Psychiatry 194:278–284

Pescosolido BA, Martin JK, Long JS, Medina TR, Phelan JC, Link BG (2010) "A disease like any other"? A decade of change in public reactions to schizophrenia, depression, and alcohol dependence. Am J Psychiatry 167:1321–1330

Pilkington PD, Reavley NJ, Jorm AF (2013) The Australian public's beliefs about the causes of depression: associated factors and changes over 16 years. J Affect Disord 150:356–362

Priebe S (2012) Where is the progress? Psychiatr Prax 39:55–56

Reavley NJ, Jorm AF (2012) Stigmatising attitudes towards people with mental disorders: changes in Australia over 8 years. Psychiatry Res 197:302–306

Reavley NJ, Jorm AF (2014) The Australian public's beliefs about the causes of schizophrenia: associated factors and change over 16 years. Psychiatry Res 220:609–614

Rüsch N, Angermeyer MC, Corrigan PW (2005) Mental illness stigma: concepts, consequences, and initiatives to reduce stigma. Eur Psychiatry 20:529–539

Sartorius N, Gaebel W, Cleveland HR, Stuart H, Akiyama T, Arboleda-Flórez J, Baumann AE, Gureje O, Jorge MR, Kastrup M (2010) WPA guidance on how to combat stigmatization of psychiatry and psychiatrists. World Psychiatry 9:131

Schomerus G, Lucht M, Holzinger A, Matschinger H, Carta MG, Angermeyer MC (2011) The stigma of alcohol dependence compared with other mental disorders: a review of population studies. Alcohol Alcohol 46:105–112

Schomerus G, Schwahn C, Holzinger A, Corrigan PW, Grabe HJ, Carta MG, Angermeyer MC (2012) Evolution of public attitudes about mental illness: a systematic review and meta-analysis. Acta Psychiatr Scand 125:440–452

Schomerus G, Matschinger H, Angermeyer MC (2014a) Causal beliefs of the public and social acceptance of persons with mental illness: a comparative analysis of schizophrenia, depression and alcohol dependence. Psychol Med 44:303–314

Schomerus G, Matschinger H, Lucht MJ, Angermeyer MC (2014b) Changes in the perception of alcohol-related stigma in Germany over the last two decades. Drug Alcohol Depend 143:225–231

Schomerus G, Van der Auwera S, Matschinger H, Baumeister SE, Angermeyer MC (2015) Do attitudes towards persons with mental illness worsen over the life span? An age-period-cohort analysis. Acta Psychiatr Scand 132:357–364

Thornicroft G, Brohan E, Rose D, Sartorius N, Leese M (2009) Global pattern of experienced and anticipated discrimination against people with schizophrenia: a cross-sectional survey. Lancet 373:408–415

Vaughan G, Hansen C (2004) 'Like Minds, Like Mine': a New Zealand project to counter the stigma and discrimination associated with mental illness. Australas Psychiatr 12:113–117

The Viewpoint of GAMIAN*-Europe

10

Pedro Manuel Ortiz de Montellano[†]

Introduction

Every society categorises its members according to a set of attributes of many different types and results in the association of each member with the various groups that exist, according to the combination of those attributes. This process will lead to the placement of each individual in that society.

Having a mental illness is one of the attributes that can be used to make that categorisation, by marking, differentiating and including the affected individuals in a specific group within society. This process is similar to the one the Greeks used when they made marks on the body of certain people to mark their moral status, to which they called stigmas.

Unfortunately, in all societies, a mental illness has always been considered a very negative attribute, a stigma that causes a high level of social devaluation and leading people with a mental health disorder to experience prejudice, social discrimination and exclusion.

Stigma represents a heavy burden that affects people with a mental health disorder, constituting a severe obstacle to their recovery and inclusion in society as equals.

In this chapter, we are going to consider two types of stigma, one from the interaction with the members and institutions of society (family, friends, other individuals,

*GAMIAN-Europe (Global Alliance of Mental Illness Advocacy Networks-Europe) is a patient-driven, pan-European organisation that represents the interests of people affected by mental illness and advocates their rights (www.gamian.eu).

[†]Deceased on October 2nd, 2015

P.M.O. de Montellano
GAMIAN-Europe, Washingtonstreet 40, Brussels 1050, Belgium

© Springer International Publishing Switzerland 2017
W. Gaebel et al. (eds.), *The Stigma of Mental Illness - End of the Story?*,
DOI 10.1007/978-3-319-27839-1_10

workplaces, schools, hospital, church), the social stigma; and the other related to the self-reflexive analysis made by the person with mental illness about his condition as a result of its social experiences, the self-stigma.

Both these stigmas have a tremendous impact in several domains of the lives of the people with mental illness: on social relations, access to care, access to work, access to education and equality of rights among other things that have a very relevant role in the full integration of any individual in any society.

In this chapter, we will see, from the perspective of the people with a mental disorder, some of the impacts social stigma and self-stigma has in their lives.

Self-Stigma

The stigma associated to mental illness is not an intrinsic characteristic of the individual; it implies the existence of symptoms and a diagnosis, something that only arises at a certain point in the life of a person with mental health problem.

Thus, two very distinct periods have to be considered in the lifetime of a person with a mental health problem: before the diagnosis and after the diagnosis.

The first period, before diagnosis, although is not relevant where stigma is concerned, as the mental illness has not been disclosed yet, is a very important period for someone that will develop a mental illness in the future. During this period, as a consequence of the interactions and experiences with the other members of society (individuals, groups and institutions), a perception about the way that people are categorised by others and also by themselves is established. This will be relevant to the stigma that will come in the second period.

The second period starts when the mental illness appears and, besides having to deal with the effects of the symptoms, the person with a mental health problem also has to face the effects of stigma. The effects caused by stigma will have implications in a social dimension, related to social stigma, and an individual dimension, related to self-stigma.

Before the diagnosis, as the great majority of the members of the society, the person with mental health problems most likely had the same prejudice that resulted from misconceptions about mental illness, considering people with a mental disorder as members of a devalued group.

Thus, the acceptance of the diagnosis is emotionally very difficult for any person because besides representing a breakthrough into an unknown and frightening disease, it also implicates the assumption that from that moment he/she belongs to a group that is segregated and devalued by the other members of society.

They say I have a mental illness, bipolar disorder, the psychiatrist says he has no doubts. How could this happen to me? Now how is it going to be? How will I face everybody, my family and my friends? How is it going to be at the university? How is it going to be at the rugby club? Will they think I'm crazy? Will I be able to have a normal life? (Pedro, 28 December 2014)

The perception of a downgrade of the self-condition, the self-image, the self-esteem and even self-respect, eventually, can lead to situations where the individual feels ashamed of himself and uncomfortable about this new 'identity'.

> There is so much I used to enjoy and so much I felt like I wanted to achieve but this part of me seems to have disappeared and is nowhere to be found at present. People ask me why? It is so difficult to explain to those that have not suffered with depression themselves as they think there must be a reason, something must have happened to make you feel this way but the truth of the matter is that I cannot explain it myself.
>
> The only way I can attempt to is to ask you to imagine a haze that clouds your mind and consequently your judgment and that leaves you constantly in a state of confusion and despair. Unfortunately, I reacted as many do, and for a while blamed only me. Why am I like this? What's wrong with me that I can't just snap out of it? Feeling ashamed and considering depression as a sign of weakness, I put on a pretence. Once I grew tired of this pretence I excluded myself from social situations as much as possible but in doing so, only ended up hurting those I care most about (Amber, November 1, 2013). (Time to Change 2013a)

The effect of this self-stigma in the self-perceptions has a very strong impact in psychological terms and can be a great obstacle to normal functioning, namely, by the impact on the motivation to perform the normal activities or to seek help.

This internalisation of stigma is very damaging because it results in people believing that they do indeed have undesirable attributes and they are of less value than a 'normal' person.

> When I was first diagnosed seven years ago, I didn't share my story with anyone. I was so ashamed at what I had been through. I always considered myself such a strong, capable person but that seemed to no longer be the case – I mean, hell, I could barely function or take care of myself. And I certainly didn't want to face the fact that I had actually tried to end my life at one point. Only a little over two years later did I finally share it with a few close friends.
>
> I guess I felt like a life loser. I couldn't really hold a job. I used to be super successful and was given every opportunity in the world to succeed. I went to private school and to a College from which I graduated with honours. Once the bipolar hit and I was diagnosed, I started to isolate. I avoided social situations because I never wanted to answer the impending questions: "How are you?" and "What are you doing these days?" I always deflected and turned the questions back around onto the person asking them.
>
> I guess the real honest truth is that I'm still somewhat ashamed of my illness and don't want to be completely honest with the world or myself about it. I did, however, choose to come clean with some people because I was tired of hiding (Hilary, 32 years). (Healthyplace 2012)

Very often mental health diseases are chronic conditions, they last for all life-time, with periods where the symptoms are present that alternate with other periods that there are no symptoms.

Because very often it is very hard to cope with these symptoms, people realise that they prevent them from having total control over their lives during those periods. This can be very frightening and lead to a self-perception of vulnerability and incapacity to have a normal functioning in society.

Things started to spiral whilst I was on holiday. Everything should have been perfect. I'd got into a top uni[versity], we were staying in a beautiful place. But for me, nothing much seemed beautiful. I had this terrible feeling that something very awful was going to happen. I knew then that it wasn't logical, but that didn't help to ease the intensity. I cried hysterically and told my boyfriend that I knew I was going to fail, and that I was a disappointment to everybody. I was terrified to be alone with my thoughts.

I spent a lot of my time alone at uni[versity], and things only got worse. I was convinced that I wasn't good enough to be on my course and that I wasn't like anybody else. It was like my mind was in overdrive, and it was a voice in my head was just saying over and over 'you can't do it'. I could literally hear myself saying it, and once I even said it out loud without realising. I really felt as if I was losing my mind, I felt so unexplainably out of control. I thought that if I couldn't even control what I was thinking or saying, what was I capable of? I worried that because I thought I was 'going crazy', I wouldn't know what I was doing and I would hurt myself (Emily, May 15, 2014). (Time to Change 2014a)

The Global Alliance of Mental Illness Advocacy Networks-Europe (GAMIAN-Europe), a patient-driven pan-European organisation that represents the interests of people affected by mental illness and advocates their rights made a study in 2010 to measure:

1. The levels of stigma that people with a mental illness feel towards themselves, across Europe (internalised or self-stigma)
2. The degree to which people with a mental illness believe that the general public hold negative attitudes towards the mentally ill (perceived devaluation/discrimination)
3. To measure the levels of self-esteem and feelings of power/control that people with a mental illness report (empowerment)

Surveys were sent out through the GAMIAN-Europe network of members in 21 European countries.

Some of the results obtained for the Internalised Stigma of Mental Illness (ISMI) – 29 items (Ritsher et al. 2003) – are presented in Table 10.1.

Table 10.1 GAMIAN-Europe stigma study 2010

Internalised stigma of mental illness (ISMI) – 29 items (Ritsher et al. 2003)	%
Living with mental illness has made me a tough survivor	58.46
People with a mental illness make important contributions to society	57.73
People discriminate against me because I have a mental illness	52.25
I am disappointed in myself for having a mental illness	49.14
I don't talk about myself much because I don't want to burden others with my mental illness	48.32
Being around people who do not have a mental illness makes me feel out of place or inadequate	32.05
Because I have a mental illness, I need others to make most decisions for me	31.64
I cannot contribute anything to society because I have a mental illness	31.23
People can tell that I have a mental illness by the way I look	30.17
Nobody would be interested in getting close to me because I have a mental illness	27.56

Table 10.2 GAMIAN-Europe stigma study 2010

Perceived devaluation and discrimination scale 12 items (Link 1987) (PPD %)	%
Most people would not hire a mental health patient to take care of their children, even if she or he had been well for some time	69.34
Most employers will pass over the application of a former mental patient in favour of another applicant	68.11
Most people think less of a person who has been in a mental hospital	67.38
Most people believe that a person who has been in a mental hospital is just as intelligent as the average person	45.54
Most people would accept a fully recovered former mental patient as a teacher of young children in a public school	43.99
Most people believe that a former mental patient is just as trustworthy as the average citizen	43.58

Social Stigma

When someone is diagnosed with a mental health problem, he knows by his previous social interactions that this disease has a very negative stigma attached, which will contribute to the devaluation and discrimination in his social relations, both with individuals and institutions.

As it can be seen in Table 10.2, people with a mental illness believe that the general public hold negative attitudes towards the mentally ill in several relevant domains.

Stigma and Family

In this item of this chapter, stigma and the family are addressed from the patient's perspective, more related to self-stigma, because the perspective of the other members of the family (husband, wife, parents, sibling and others) is going to be addressed in a specific chapter of this book.

The self-stigma that the person acquires, as a result of the diagnosis of a mental illness, has a significant effect on the relationships inside the family.

The perception of self-devaluation the person has might cause them to feel that they are no longer so valid or doesn't have the same role in the family as they used to have.

The first person I talked to about my diagnosis was my mum. I was nervous about how she'd react and even more nervous about how I was going to tell her. We don't have the closest of relationships. It's not bad but being one of 4 sisters I am possibly the least close to her out of my siblings. The only way I felt comfortable enough to tell her was by text. I felt weak and pathetic doing so but it stimulated a reasonably open conversation face to face. She was sympathetic and most of all caring. She asked no questions and just simply accepted it. This was exactly what I needed but not what I expected. I thought my Mum would try and understand or find out why I was the way I was but she didn't and it was perfect. From time to time we will have these open conversations just so she is aware of what state I am in, other than that is not something we talk about. It's too uncomfortable but just knowing she is accepting and sympathetic of the condition is plenty (Harriet Marie, May 24, 2013). (Time to Change 2013b)

The person might feel less confident to participate in the conversations than before, not having the same ease to express his/her opinions.

He might also think that he hasn't got the same rights as before, being afraid or ashamed that his condition might cause some embarrassment to the other members of the family.

All these perceptions and behaviours can lead him to be more isolated keeping his emotions and thoughts to himself. This can also contribute to his not asking for help due to this stigma.

> The hardest issue I had to face was to tell my parents I was ill. They were worried, understandably, and wondered why I hadn't come to them earlier. They didn't understand what was going on and had no idea what it was that I was facing.
>
> I was a mess. Only certain friends knew that I was unwell, I felt that I couldn't tell the others something was wrong. I self-stigmatised myself, ashamed at how I could be so stupid and unable to do something. Here was a Cambridge graduate that could no longer cook pasta! (Natalie Anne Read, June 18, 2013). (Time to Change 2013c)

In all the families, there are balances in the relationships that are established among its members according to their living experiences. When mental illness arises in the family, it can cause very disturbing damages in these balances.

Some families, despite the difficulties, manage to get through, providing a support that is extremely important to the mentally ill person.

> My teenage life has been one hell of a ride. The up-down ride that is bipolar. My family were by my side throughout.
>
> When I first became ill, it was difficult for them to support me. We were unaware of mental health problems and none of us knew what was to come – it all came as rather a shock. They didn't know what to do.
>
> It was scary for them, just as it was scary for me.
>
> My family love me and they were desperate to support me. They did everything they could to understand what I was going through.
>
> As time went on they gained a much better understanding and were better equipped to support me. I spent two years in hospital – 2 hours away from home. Despite the distance, my parents would visit most weekends. My brother would often drive down to see me. Seeing him always made me smile. As time went on we became more able to talk about mental health (Emma P., November 12, 2014). (Time to Change 2014b)

Unfortunately, there are others that would not resist to the pressure of all the implications of the illness, stigma being one of the more relevant ones, and fall apart.

> I was first diagnosed with a mental health disorder five years ago after the birth of my youngest daughter. The stigma I faced within my family was crushing: talking about me whilst I was sat in the same room and generally treating me in a way that was about my illness and not me.
>
> I became a walking label. Social services became automatically involved with my family. No one was very interested in what I was actually doing, just the risks associated with the label. I was no longer an individual, a person, I was what was written about me; the doctors' opinions and the old fashioned ideas that my family held about mental illness.
>
> I have found the journey through discrimination and stigma to be the biggest fight for survival. I had all my children removed from my care. I lost my career as a police officer. Finally I began to lose the will to fight. However, I slowly but surely began to rebuild my life.

I took work in a local shop where my colleagues were just really supportive. I took up a new hobby – modern jiving and made new friends. The constant stigma I faced from my daughters' fathers was completely devastating. Frighteningly I was called names in the street like 'nutter' and 'mental case'. And, as for court proceedings involving my children, I was treated like a social outcast. The humiliation of being judged as an 'unfit' mother and facing the constant verbal and sometimes physical attacks from 'suitable' parents left scars that although have healed will always be there.

As the years passed by I met and fell in love with a man who I am marrying. My life has changed in so many ways and I avoided all those people that saw me as nothing but a label. My eldest daughters returned to live back at home of their own accord. I have finally been blessed with being surrounded by people to whom I am just Lisa (mum). My labels are irrelevant. Life is about living and being happy and moving forward.

The stigma, however, from social workers and family court social workers, is still alive and kicking. There I am a label, a disorder and a subject to be discussed. I still attend court to see my youngest daughter. Still I am discussed like I wasn't in the room.

There is hope however and it is really time to change! (Lisa, October 15, 2013). (Time to Change 2013d)

In many cases the stigma prevents families from getting information and help on how to deal with the illness and how to help their relatives.

An eating disorder affects the whole family, not just the sufferer. If I could control it, I would stop this right now and decide to get better to put my family at rest but it is not as simple as that. To my family, I am the one who is "crazy" because I have mental health issues. I know they care and they do not understand the reasons behind why things are so hard for me. If they did, they would not think like they do. Support is what I need. They do not like to admit that I am suffering. It is very much like I am a different person to them, whom they wish was not abnormal. I seem to have become such a burden to my family and that makes me feel incredibly guilty.

This stigma has left me feeling rather lost and alone and like I have no one to turn to. Family is an important part in recovery and when you feel like you cannot talk to the people who you live with, your world seems even darker than it already is (Habiba, October 22, 2013). (Time to Change 2013e)

Stigma and Friends

In the early stages of the disease, very often friends don't know very well how they should behave towards the person with mental illness.

My friends were very sympathetic when I told them about my diagnosis, especially when I talked about the awful side effects of the medication I'd been put on. But they couldn't really relate to my condition – schizophrenia was almost like something mystical to them (Yvonne Stewart-Williams, 52). (Rethink 2013)

Most of the times they want to help, to show their sympathy and friendship despite the disease, but they don't know how to do it and without noticing end up talking in a way different from the usual, which causes a discomfort to the person with mental illness who doesn't feel happy with this change and becomes afraid that the relationship has changed.

I am excellent at pretending. Pretending I am interested in whatever the current topic of conversation may be; when, in fact, I am entirely, momentarily (hopefully), hollowed out, numb, incapable of communication on anything other than a basic level: "Yes. No. Okay"; when all I want is the conversation to end, as soon as possible, as painlessly as possible, but for it to do so would involve me being able to talk, to explain – a dark irony not lost on me as I stare at the table top (Gregory, December 20, 2012). (Time to Change 2012a)

The person with mental illness tends to feel shame in relation to friends, namely, after being admitted in a psychiatric hospital, or because he has no job, and that causes changes in relationships, namely, by avoiding social contacts and talking about him.

It's hard, really hard. The one thing I'm finding harder than anything though is the stigma, ignorance and frustration being lobbed at me from certain people who are supposed to be my friends (Lana S, December 19, 2013). (Time to Change 2013f)

The support of friends is very important to the recovery of the person affected by mental illness. It contributes to increased self-esteem and the sense of inclusion.

I have some incredible friends who have literally saved my life on several occasions; not all of them have first-hand experience of mental illness, which proves that the ability to be supportive or empathetic isn't only a consequence of going through it (Rachael, January 14, 2015). (Time to Change 2015)

Stigma, Dating and Relationships

Self-stigma impacts on self-esteem and self-confidence and can affect the capacity to cope with romantic situations. To engage in a relationship or to keep it can be a very challenging task.

It's our first date…I am excellent at pretending. Pretending I'm happily joining in, laughing along, when, in fact, I am grossly irritated and impatient, overwhelmed by the noise in the restaurant, ready to explode at the slightest imagined slight. I am unpredictable. It's our first date and I'm wondering if she has noticed these things. Should I tell her that often I'm not myself. It doesn't define me but I worry she'll think I'm making excuses for myself, so I sit there, silently, stupidly collapsing before this beautiful girl.
I so desperately want to tell her I'm not always this way. I want to tell her that my brain often fizzes like the drink she's sipping, that the world vibrates with infinite possibilities, endless beauty, a thousand profound connections a second. Much of this can contribute to my mania but, just like the negative stuff, some of it is me, too. I want to tell her how I don't feel pity for myself, quite the opposite, I am often proud. Mostly, I just want to tell her (Gregory, December 20, 2012). (Time to Change 2012a)

Stigma and Professionals

Sometimes the professionals that work with mental health patients don't have the personal skills or the right education to take care of them in a suitable way. This might have a very damaging impact in the recovery and access to care of those patients. All the efforts should be done to increase the use of the best practices that will contribute to stop this situation.

My experience of mental health services started 10 years ago, when I first started being treated under CAMHS services for depression and an eating disorder. I also developed OCD and after two years under the care of community services, I spent a few months as an inpatient. I continued to be treated in the community after this, until being discharged at 18.

Particularly whilst as an inpatient, I felt valued and respected, and as though it was ok for me to be unwell but that it was possible to recover. This, along with the experiences I had whilst I was ill, encouraged me to base my career in mental health. I was inspired to be as caring as the people who had looked after me, and wanted to be able to support people – particularly young people – to recover. I started my career in mental health services in 2009, and began studying to train as a mental health nurse.

I initially didn't hide my past involvement in services, as I had never felt that I needed to. However, I soon found the attitudes and prejudices of those working in services were different to anything I had ever experienced before. Although through school I dealt with a lot of stigma and discrimination, I had assumed that this was through a lack of knowledge rather than genuine prejudice. However, here I was, surrounded by professionals whose idea of how to talk about, and manage, eating disorders was shocking (Cara, April 2, 2014). (Time to Change 2014c)

When my self-harm got bad and when my low mood got bad and I was going to hospital for stitches or treatment for overdoses, I sometimes got a bad reaction from the staff.

Mostly, they were good with me and supportive but a few times they were the complete opposite. I remember having stitches once and the nurse telling me that it was all my fault and that I was going to get an infection and I was to blame for it. I know that it was self-inflicted, but it felt a little harsh to be so full on.

Experiences like that make it even harder to reach out for help when you need it and that's vital. Doctors and nurses should have enough training to know how to manage a situation like the ones I was in. There is nothing better than seeing a really lovely nurse or doctor at A&E after you spent all day plucking up the courage to go there, and getting the support and care you need.

Yes, I may be harming myself, but I'm not doing it because I enjoy it or because that is how I want to live my life. I do it because I feel so bad inside and need a way to cope. So to all those doctors and nurses, imagine how it would feel, to hurt so badly inside that you felt the need to physically hurt yourself.

Sometimes I have to ask myself, are these people really working in mental health? (Jessica, October 24, 2013). (Time to Change 2013g)

When I was young I started to self-harm. This is an issue that I still battle with to this day. I have attempted suicide several times and ended up in hospital as a result of this and self-harm. I have received so many judgemental comments from professionals when in these vulnerable situations such as being told that I must be mad for hurting myself and that personality disorders are not real mental health problems. I was once told by a mental health practitioner, whilst being treated by a crisis resolution and home treatment team, that there was nothing wrong with me because personality disorders don't really exist, and that I was lazy for not challenging my negative thoughts. These types of comments are so hurtful and need to be challenged. It is wrong that so many people out there are being forced to suffer in silence because of stigma and discrimination (Vikki, November 28, 2014). (Time to Change 2014d)

Stigma and School

The children at school can be very cruel, stigmatising and bullying peers that show different behaviours or exhibit any fragility. Children and adolescents with mental illness are victims of this situation, which is mostly a consequence of the lack of awareness and information about mental illnesses. The bullying can also lead to mental illness.

I was bullied during my entire school life. Sometimes I think back about my bullies and feel myself seething with rage, other times I completely understand why they did it. I was always an odd one at school, either bursting into tears at the tiniest thing and not speaking to anyone for days on end, or being so hyper that I'd get sent out of lessons and given detentions every other day.

When I was diagnosed with Borderline Personality Disorder, just before I turned nineteen, everything suddenly made sense. The extreme mood swings, the extreme highs and depressive lows, the feelings of numbness for weeks on end, the suicidal thoughts and self-harm. But after doing some research on my illness and other mental health conditions, I was furious once again; I realized just how badly I'd been discriminated against since I first started showing symptoms as young as ten or eleven years old. I thought back to how teachers had said that I "wasn't REALLY sick" and how I was "just attention seeking" when I had to stay off school because I'd tried to take my own life. I thought about how many doctors had turned away, or told me that my daily self-harming was because of "hormones" (Zoe, August 14, 2014). (Time to Change 2014e)

It is the lack of awareness and information about mental illnesses that leads to prejudice and stigma existing among students as well as among teachers and staff.

When I returned to work I informed the head-teacher that I had been diagnosed bipolar. There was much squirming and gnashing of teeth but mostly there were words of understanding. I can totally understand that people still find the idea of talking about mental illness uncomfortable and that sometimes people feel avoidance is the best way of 'dealing' with the situation. This is why the Time to Change campaign is such an important vehicle to help people.

I began notice a tangible sense of quiet hostility towards me from the management team. An emerging strategy from their meetings was becoming clear: suddenly the pressure was piled on with several random observations of lessons a week, weekly spot checks on books and constant comments about whether I was fit enough for work… I was offered settlement money and had to agree to silence. I took it. I had no choice. I have children to support (Minuteman, December 20, 2011). (Time to Change 2011)

Stigma and Work

Work is much more than a salary; it gives to anyone a sense of inclusion, of responsibility, of capacity, of pride, of productivity and, among many other things, a sense of 'normality' and belonging to society.

For a person with a mental illness as well as for any 'normal' person being employed is something very important to be integrated in society and the absence of employment causes many problems.

Stigma at workplaces is responsible for several barriers that people who have a mental illness have on access to work, job retention and returning to work after a period of sick leave.

As it is shown in Table 10.3 below, the study done by GAMIAN-Europe suggests that there is still a considerable way to go to give people with a mental illness a more fair chance to have a fulfilled working life.

The need that people with mental illness have to hide their condition in the workplace is something that is very stressful, causes anxiety and doesn't contribute, in any way, to good mental health. It is very disturbing that someone needs to hide behind a lie in order to be accepted.

Table 10.3 GAMIAN-Europe stigma study 2010

You work?	%
I work full time	12.92
I work part time	16.76
I work as a volunteer (not paid)	4.82
I'm looking for a job	11.45
I'd like to work but am afraid of losing my benefits	3.03
I'm not able to work (disabled)	31.23
Student	3.11
Retired	16.68

Although there should be no need to keep one's mental health condition a secret, I can totally understand why many people decide to keep it so as I have firsthand knowledge of the stigma that results from work colleagues finding out about it. Unfortunately, I did not have the luxury of hiding my condition as I was spectacularly and publically 'outed' as psychologically damaged when 19 years of undiagnosed, and therefore untreated, depression and stress caused me to have a breakdown at work.

I was seen as less than the man I once was. I had suddenly been given the nickname 'psycho' and people were reluctant to approach me. The little respect I once had amongst my fellow workers diminished visibly and I was seen as less than the man I once was. Oh, there was sympathy shown towards me by some but there was also a distance that I had to fight against and some took liberties with my personal belongings that they would never have taken before. I had to fight twice as hard to gain half the respect that seemed to be lavished on the others.

Every time the nickname 'psycho' was used it felt like a rapier (sword) being thrust deep into my heart and it simply added to the self-hatred I had been feeling on the 19-year journey along the dark path of depression I had endured alone. Every fearful glance in my direction and every cautious approach made me feel damaged, alone, isolated. Every disrespectful use of my personal belongings made me feel less human than the people I was surrounded by on a daily basis because it did not seem to matter to them that the belongings were mine; they seemed to be of the opinion that I no longer deserved the respect of being asked because I was somehow broken (Valen, April 28, 2014). (Time to Change 2014f)

Sometimes it would only be necessary that employers and employees make small adjustments in order to get a mutual benefit solution, increasing job retention and assuring that skilled and experienced employees can continue to work.

When stigma prevails, both parties lose.

Although work knew about my mental health condition, they seemed to refuse to accept it. In my review meetings I was told that I needed to be more consistent and looking back this just demonstrated their lack of understanding about mental health problems. Basically they wanted me to perform in my normal/hypomanic phases all the time. It's not like I had any control over it!

Redundancies were being made at work and I just knew it would be me. They applied a selection criteria which was totally unfair and discriminated against me for my disability. I have 100 % support for this from my union, which is absolutely fantastic to have. It demonstrates to me that I haven't been going crazy all this time, I was right. They had no understanding for my needs, they made no adjustments to help me. I will fight them to show that nobody should be allowed to get away with discriminating against those with disabilities (Marie, September, 7, 2012). (Time to Change 2012b)

The stigma that exists on mental illness leads many people to devaluate the ones with such illnesses, assuming they don't have certain skills and thinking that they're weak. This can cause leadership problems in workplaces when there is a mental disorder in the middle.

> My job was managing a small team, many of which I had known for over 10 years. I am lucky in the fact that I have a very supportive HR manager and line manager and we agreed that it would be good for me to make short visits to the office which would help with my return.
>
> During the first visit, the majority of my team snubbed me, some even getting up from their desk and walking away. I was upset and surprised but thought that maybe I had come in at a busy time but this happened again on my second and last visit. Further investigation by senior management revealed that my team were of the opinion that if I was well enough to be out and about and able to visit then I should be at work. This attitude continued throughout my absence and unsurprisingly delayed my return.
>
> I have now returned to work, after a very long phased return I decided I could not continue to manage these people, who I still have to sit with and who continue to make my life uncomfortable daily with whispering and comments about my health. So, after 25 years of hard work and finally understanding why I'm different, I still find myself 'on the outside' (Louise Copson, October 15, 2013). (Time to Change 2013h)

Stigma and the Media

The media hold a very important place in our society. They have the capacity of creating or destroying myths and have a decisive role in influencing people.

Several times the media associate mental health with violence and crime in an inappropriate way. This is wrong, considering that mentally ill people are much more likely to be victims of violence than aggressors.

> But for me the biggest and toughest battle of all about having schizophrenia is living with the stigma attached to it.
>
> Most of us who have schizophrenia are not violent or dangerous and yet this is the only thing the public seem to be constantly told about the condition by the media. Take The Sun's recent front page for example: "1,200 Killed By Mental Patients" (Jonny Benjamin, October 23, 2013). (Time to Change 2013i)

New media platforms such as social media could allow the appearance of initiatives coming from the community to raise awareness on mental health and fight stigma.

> Like many others with mental health issues, I was most afraid that the people around me would no longer think of me in the same way. I felt like I'd let everyone down, like it was my fault that I had come to think and feel the way I did. I also didn't want to feel like a burden to anyone. "These are the best years of your life" I was told. I didn't want to show anyone that I was in fact really suffering. My friend dealt with it brilliantly though and he took me to see my GP.
>
> I struggled to get the care I required for some time, and this wasn't helped by the fact I kept what was happening to me a secret from the rest of my loved ones. The first they knew of my mental illness was when I was admitted to a psychiatric unit and diagnosed with schizoaffective disorder aged 20. Finally, I started to talk to the people around me; doctors, family and friends. I then began to learn how to take control and manage my condition.

Talking to them about my mental health was the best thing I have ever done. They may not have understood what was going on in my head, but the love and support they gave me got me through that very difficult time.

This was exactly why I decided to talk publicly about my mental illness; making YouTube vlogs, speaking at events, and now presenting this BBC Three documentary as part of their mental health season. Within the programme you will see me meet six inspiring young people with various mental health problems who talk incredibly openly about their conditions.

Unfortunately they also didn't get the help they needed when they asked for it. Throughout the documentary I try to uncover why many young people with mental health problems just don't get the support and care they should.

Everyone I interviewed wanted to break down mental health stigma

Everyone that I interviewed within the programme told me they had taken part in it for exactly that reason. We all want to challenge misconceptions that the public may have about mental illness, to help those that may be struggling with their mental health to have the confidence to ask for help.

Please do seek help if this all sounds familiar. There are so many places and people who can support you. Just talking to someone you trust; a friend, family member or teacher, can get you the help you need. (Jonny Benjamin, October 23, 2013). (Time to Change 2013j)

Stigma in Physical and Mental Health

Mental illnesses are the invisible diseases, and when you mix this with ignorance and prejudice, it is expected that people react differently than they do to physical diseases.

If you have a physical health problem, people can see you need help and you can get reasonable adjustment, e.g. a ramp for a person in a wheelchair. But if you have a mental health problem, which is not so obvious to people, they will treat you as a normal person. No reasonable adjustment will be offered, unless you disclose you have mental health problems. This often prevents many people from disclosing their problems as they fear being judged unfavourable (Jeffy, March 15, 2014). (Time to Change 2014g)

For the sake of contrast, I am also a type 1 diabetic. My family all know this, my friends all know this, and many colleagues and acquaintances do too. I am very open with my diabetes and happy to talk about it. I don't fear judgement for my diabetes.

So, why the difference? These are both long term, chronic conditions that affect my everyday life. The fact is that I don't fear judgement for my diabetes. When I tell people I am depressed, I worry that they are thinking I am weak or pathetic. That I am using it as an excuse. Even that I am a danger to myself.

I worry that people will look at me and treat me differently. That blossoming friendships or relationships may flounder because I have too much emotional baggage. And the saddest part is that these are not just paranoid concerns. These are real reactions that I have had from real people (Maggie, November 22, 2013). (Time to Change 2013k)

I broke my arm last year and was bowled over by people's reactions. Nearly everyone I came across asked me if I was ok, what had happened and if there was anything they could do to help.

I could hardly believe I was receiving such attention when I actually felt better than I had done in years! In stark contrast, when I was very ill with bipolar disorder and infinitely more disabled, people didn't know and I didn't think I should say.

Most comments I received when I broke my arm were superficial, but I didn't need anything more. Likewise with my mood, I didn't need support; I had that in abundance from professionals and people close to me. What I needed was acknowledgement that I was disabled and for people to adjust their expectations accordingly. My experience with my broken arm showed me the vast majority of people are compassionate. Mental illnesses and many physical ones are harder to talk about and understand; but that need not stop us from being compassionate! (Fay Walter, June 8, 2012). (Time to Change 2012c)

Stigma and Religion

All the aspects that are part of the cultural/social environment should be considered when we are addressing the way of dealing with mental illness, and religion is a very important subject for the way it determines some behaviour of individuals.

Recently a friend came to visit me, the topic of conversation centred on a young lady living in sheltered accommodation who had been admitted to the psychiatric ward. During the conversation my friend mentioned to me "it's so sad because she comes from such a normal family"! This statement sums up an attitude towards mental illness that I have come across very often within the close-knit Jewish community in which I live (Sara, October 11, 2012). (Time to Change 2012d)

Religion can be an obstacle to the understanding, support and care of the person with mental illness.

In my experience, mental illness is a very taboo subject in Islam. You could argue that it is a taboo subject in general but, specifically in Islam, I have found that it can be incredibly difficult for family members to understand.

For me, this has always been the case. I did not open up to family members about this issue for a long time because I was ashamed to even admit it to them. I was afraid of their reaction and thought they would neglect me. So, after speaking to my eating disorder treatment team about being afraid to speak to my family, they offered to sit down with my family and explain to them about why I have this condition and what they are doing to help me, which has helped my family understand a little bit and reassured them that I can get better. I was surprised by their reaction. It was not as bad as I thought it would be. Now, it is easier for me to talk to my family about it but they still find it hard to understand fully.

I think some Muslim families neglect the issue of mental illness because of a feeling that it brings shame on them and the reputation of the family. In Islam, we rely on God to heal us. If we are depressed or ill, we pray to God to make us better. We do our five prayers every day and make du'aa (invocation) whenever possible. If you are a spiritual and faithful person and rely on God to make you better, then there is nothing wrong with that at all. I think that believing in a higher power when feeling down is the most amazing thing to have in you. However, combining proper treatment to get to the root of the illness will make the sufferer see things in a new light. God will always be there to turn to but, sometimes, we need to talk openly about our problems to someone who can help us practically as well as emotionally and create a support network of friends and family.

There is nothing wrong in asking for help. There is nothing wrong in going to your GP and admitting that you are experiencing a mental health problem and that you need psychological help.

I live within a big Muslim community and there is hardly any talk about mental illness. It is as if the problem does not exist. In fact, it seems like it should not exist because people are so ashamed of it and that makes me feel ashamed to even have an illness. We need to start talking (Habiba, October 22, 2013). (Time to Change 2013l)

Final Considerations

Self-Stigma

Self-stigma results from the self-reflexive analysis made by the person with mental illness about his condition, as a result of its social experiences. It is essential to address this dimension of stigma, as it is the only one that totally relies on the sphere of the mentally ill person. The improvement on this dimension will lead to a better capacity to deal with the disease as well as cope with social stigma.

It is vital that interventions such as psychoeducation, psychotherapy, peer support groups, cognitive behaviour therapy and others, which can contribute to solve this problem, are made widely accessible (physical and financial) by the mental health services.

On the other hand, more research should be developed on how to tackle self-stigma with the direct involvement of patients.

The patients' organisations, with all their experience, can have an important role in providing reliable information and a stigma-free environment to share experiences and other interventions, which can help to increase self-awareness, self-esteem and self-confidence.

Social Stigma

Social stigma is unfortunately a broad reality that, in most cases, is a consequence of the misconceptions about mental illness. This results from the lack of information and prejudice of social stereotypes.

We live in a world that fights racism or intolerance that leads to extremism and in the other hand stands for human rights and freedom (of choice, of religion, of press…).

It's time to put the fight against stigma on the agenda of the causes of mankind.

A very important role has to be played by the media in promoting awareness campaigns on mental health, contributing to the clarification of several taboos that create barriers on the integration of people with mental health problems.

For example, most of the people don't know that, in mental illnesses, there are periods where the symptoms are present which alternate with other periods that there are no symptoms where the person can have a totally functional life. The interval between the appearances of the symptoms can vary from weeks to many years, depending on biological factors as well as social environment factors such as stigma that generate stress and anxiety.

The families have a very important role in the recovery of people affected by a mental illness. They should be helped on the best way to cope with the disease of their relatives as well as in the impact it has in their own lives.

The world needs all kinds of minds. Some of the greatest minds of humanity had mental health problems (Dickens, Tolstoy, Hemingway, Lord Byron, Friedrich

Nietzsche, Ted Turner, Robin Williams, Virginia Woolf, Agatha Christie, Winston Churchill, Bob Dylan, John Nash and many others).

Diversity should always be seen as an opportunity, an additional resource and an alternative option.

The inclusion of difference will lead to diversity, but it poses a challenge and will always face some kind of opposition. Nonetheless, a society that has no capacity to include diversity will become more and more limited in its ability to respond, eventually becoming stagnated and falling.

References

Time to Change (2011) School fails mental health test. Available at: http://www.time-to-change.org.uk/blog/school-fails-mental-health-test/. Accessed 15 Jan 2015

Time to Change (2012a) Bipolar disorder, dating and relationships. Available at: http://www.time-to-change.org.uk/blog/bipolar-disorder-relationships-dating/. Accessed 15 Jan 2015

Time to Change (2012b) Bipolar at work: I was told I needed to be more consistent. Available at: http://www.time-to-change.org.uk/blog/bipolar-type-3-at-work-told-to-be-more-consistent/. Accessed 15 Jan 2015

Time to Change (2012c) Broken arm vs. broken mind. Available at: http://www.time-to-change.org.uk/blog/broken-arm-broken-mind-bipolar-disorder/. Accessed 15 Jan 2015

Time to Change (2012d) Talking about mental illness in my Jewish community. Available at: http://www.time-to-change.org.uk/blog/talking-mental-illness-jewish-community/. Accessed 15 Jan 2015

Time to Change (2013a) I felt ashamed and saw depression as a sign of weakness. Available at: http://www.time-to-change.org.uk/blog/i-felt-ashamed-saw-depression-as-a-sign-of-weakness/. Accessed 15 Jan 2015

Time to Change (2013b) Why should I feel guilty or ashamed about depression? Available at: http://www.time-to-change.org.uk/blog/depression-why-should-i-feel-guilty-ashamed/. Accessed 15 Jan 2015

Time to Change (2013c) Telling my parents I have a mental illness was the hardest part. Available at: http://www.time-to-change.org.uk/blog/telling-my-parents-about-my-mental-illness/. Accessed 15 Jan 2015

Time to Change (2013d) Mental illness: people thought about the label rather than about me. Available at: http://www.time-to-change.org.uk/blog/mental-illness-people-thought-about-label-rather-than-me/. Accessed 15 Jan 2015

Time to Change (2013e) My experience of talking about mental health in a Muslim community. Available at: http://www.time-to-change.org.uk/blog/talking-about-mental-health-in-a-muslim-community/. Accessed 15 Jan 2015

Time to Change (2013f) Depression, stigma and needing people to be by your side. Available at: http://www.time-to-change.org.uk/blog/depression-stigma-and-needing-people-be-your-side/. Accessed 15 Jan 2015

Time to Change (2013g) Some of my friends just didn't seem to understand why I was low. Available at: http://www.time-to-change.org.uk/blog/some-of-my-friends-didnt-understand-why-i-was-low/. Accessed 15 Jan 2015

Time to Change (2013h) I returned to work with the support of my line manager. Available at: http://www.time-to-change.org.uk/blog/returned-to-work-with-full-support-of-my-manager/. Accessed 15 Jan 2015

Time to Change (2013i) What it's like to live with schizoaffective disorder. Available at: http://www.time-to-change.org.uk/blog/living-with-schizoaffective-disorder/. Accessed 15 Jan 2015

Time to Change (2013j) Why I took part in BBC Three's mental health season. Available at: http://www.time-to-change.org.uk/blog/jonny-benjamin-presenting-bbc-three-mental-health-documentary/. Accessed 15 Jan 2015

Time to Change (2013k) When I tell people I am depressed, I worry that they will think I am weak. Available at: http://www.time-to-change.org.uk/blog/when-i-tell-people-i-am-depressed-i-worry-they-will-think-i-am-weak/. Accessed 15 Jan 2015

Time to Change (2013l) My experience of talking about mental health in a Muslim community. Available at: http://www.time-to-change.org.uk/blog/talking-about-mental-health-in-a-muslim-community/. Accessed 15 Jan 2015

Time to Change (2014a) Admitting to myself that I had depression and anxiety was hard, but now I'm in a much better place. Available at: http://www.time-to-change.org.uk/blog/admitting-myself-i-had-depression-and-anxiety-was-hard-now-im-much-better-place/. Accessed 15 Jan 2015

Time to Change (2014b) Living with bipolar disorder and having support from family and friends. Available at: http://www.time-to-change.org.uk/blog/living-with-bipolar-disorder-and-having-support-from-family-and-friends/. Accessed 15 Jan 2015

Time to Change (2014c) Discrimination from within: hoping see a change in mental health professionals' perspectives on eating disorders. Available at: http://www.time-to-change.org.uk/blog/discrimination-within-hoping-see-change-mental-health-professionals-perspectives-eating/. Accessed 15 Jan 2015

Time to Change (2014d) Mental health stigma means people often cope in silence. Available at: http://www.time-to-change.org.uk/blog/mental-health-stigma-means-people-often-cope-in-silence/. Accessed 15 Jan 2015

Time to Change (2014e) It's time to change the stigma associated with mental health. Available at: http://www.time-to-change.org.uk/blog/its-time-change-stigma-associated-mental-health/. Accessed 15 Jan 2015

Time to Change (2014f) I now use my experiences to inform people of the damage caused by negative attitudes towards mental health problems. Available at: http://www.time-to-change.org.uk/blog/i-now-use-my-experiences-inform-people-damage-caused-negative-attitudes-towards-mental-health/. Accessed 15 Jan 2015

Time to Change (2014g) Public speaking: it's rewarding to help other people. Available at: http://www.time-to-change.org.uk/blog/public-speaking-its-rewarding-help-other-people/. Accessed 15 Jan 2015

Time to Change (2015) Why I believe that supporting people with mental illness is important. Available at: https://www.time-to-change.org.uk/blog/why-i-believe-supporting-people-mental-illness-important/. Accessed 15 Jan 2015

Healthyplace (2012) Mental illness ans self-stigma: a personal story. Available at: http://healthyplace.com/stigma/stories/mental-illness-and-self-stigma-a-personal-story/. Accessed 15 Jan 2015

Link B (1987) Understanding labeling effects in the area of mental disorders: an assessment of the effect of expectations of rejection. Am J Comm Psychol 11:261–273

Rethink (2013) I get nasty comments, but I don't let them drag me down. Available at: https://www.rethink.org/news-views/2013/11/i-dont-let-nasty-comments-drag-me-down/. Accessed 15 Jan 2015

Ritsher JB, Otilingam PG, Grajales M (2003) Internalized stigma of mental illness: psychometric properties of a new measure. Psych Res 121(1):31–49

The Role of Family Caregivers: A EUFAMI Viewpoint

11

Bert Johnson

The experience of stigma and discrimination against people with mental illness is by no means confined to them but extends to their families who take responsibility for their care. That responsibility is growing, yet the needs of family carers and the burdens of care they assume are neither sufficiently recognised nor understood and therefore not adequately provided for.

This chapter sees stigma and its consequences as one important aspect among the many which arise out of the role and activities of family carers and their experiences. This role has always been difficult but has been made harder still by the profound changes in policy for providing care which have swept across the world in recent decades and still continue.

Carers' problems start from the huge scale of closure of mental hospitals – so-called nineteenth century "lunatic asylums" – and their replacement by so-called "care in the community". This policy has been in pursuit of apparently laudable and enlightened clinical and social aims. It has though had two major and difficult consequences: one, the money saved from closures has not been transferred to community settings and two, on inspection the community turns out usually to be none other than the family of the person discharged from hospital, often prematurely, who work voluntarily to provide care not otherwise available.

In most cases, community care becomes in reality unfunded family care. Quite by chance, families who are affected have little option but to assume enormously challenging obligations for which they have no training and often little support from the professionals looking after their loved ones. Too much can be expected of the skill and resilience of family carers without the support of corresponding policies and practices to acknowledge and provide for their due place at the heart of the whole network of care and treatment relationships.

B. Johnson
EUFAMI (European Federation of Associations of Families of People with Mental Illness),
Diestsevest 100, Leuven 3000, Belgium
e-mail: bert.johnson@btinternet.com

© Springer International Publishing Switzerland 2017
W. Gaebel et al. (eds.), *The Stigma of Mental Illness - End of the Story?*,
DOI 10.1007/978-3-319-27839-1_11

The Life of a Family Caregiver

Let us then first consider the general role of the family in caring for the mentally ill of which dealing with stigma and discrimination so often forms part. The first step is to understand the daily reality of family caregivers, the uncertainties they face, the overwhelming nature of the difficulties they encounter and the myriad questions they have to resolve which often remain unanswered since too few professionals are said to take the trouble to explain matters in a patient and understandable way.

To begin with, a diagnosis of mental illness in a family member can usually mark a major life crisis which will make a significant impact on the family dynamics. The lives of the other family members change in many ways, sometimes permanently and often long term. They can feel afraid, kept in the dark, misunderstood, judged, isolated, shunned and in other ways stigmatised. The family struggles to deal with its collective sense of helplessness, shame and social exclusion that can go with neighbours' and colleagues' awareness of their situation, while at the same time struggling with the actual tasks of providing care itself.

Against that sombre background, families are there to supply practical, social and emotional support. They provide a lifeline, sometimes lasting a lifetime, which does at least something to make the quality of life of their ill relative as good as it can be. That can include help with basic routines which go under the heading of "life skills" such as personal care, cooking, washing, handling money and recreational and social activities. Incidentally all this saves the public authorities billions, and a cost-benefit analysis shows beyond doubt that family carers are quite indispensible to any efficient and affordable publicly funded provision of mental health services. Family support thus becomes a key factor for successful outcomes in the treatment of mental health problems generally.

A sense of bereavement, sorrow, fear and even guilt are some of the emotions that distress family members, alongside the distress felt by their mentally ill member him- or herself. Many will suffer in silence, not knowing what they should be doing to deal with the turmoil created by aggressive behaviour, delusions, confusions, lack of self-care, apathy and extreme reclusiveness – all of which can be exhausting emotionally and physically. The impact of endless caring can tax the caregiver's patience to the limit. Families ignore or downplay their own physical health problems. They have to struggle to adjust patterns of family and working life. Mutual recriminations, effects on siblings and even the breakdown of marriages are not uncommon. Relations with others outside the family and at work become similarly undermined and that is where stigma and discrimination are most likely to be manifest.

So constant care giving is emotionally demanding work and physically draining too. As well as grappling with feelings of anxiety and grief, caregivers come to recognise their own limitations in dealing with such strong emotions as resentment and anger at the ill loved one or absent relations who refuse to share the burden of care. Constant care giving leads to frustration, stress and burnout. Emotional upheaval unsettles family life and whereas previously there was the security of routines, there is now the insecurity of constant and nerve-racking unpredictability. Planning is abandoned. Family outings and holidays become a thing of the past.

Life as a primary caregiver becomes a lonely place which only magnifies the stress of providing care itself. Some carers naturally express their frustration and fear of becoming unable to cope with the unpredictable behaviour of their ill son or daughter.

And then on top of these emotional distress signals, we have the repercussions on the rest of the family if the main carer falls physically ill or their own mental health is threatened. These consequences can be severe. In fact the health of family caregivers is not sufficiently taken into account by policy makers and health and social care practitioners.

Financial implications also cannot be ignored. Everyone knows that governments are over-reliant on family care giving and the inestimable costs incurred by families in shouldering much of the burden of care. The well-intentioned political discourse on the desirability of "work-life balance" often leaves out of account the reality of family care giving. In times of unstable relationships, the primary caregiver may have to decide to change jobs or quit work altogether to cope with their new responsibilities. No wonder that some families which were never poor start sliding into poverty and others sink further.

And after all that, and even in this day and age, we find ourselves still grappling with the effects of stigma. Stigma makes it that much harder for caregivers to seek help for themselves. They may put on a brave mask for friends, colleagues and acquaintances. But such reactions to stigma only lead to isolation. Caregivers need support to overcome their fear of embarrassment in a number of situations. Fear of being judged, shunned, ridiculed and rejected robs them of self-esteem and confidence and of the opportunity to tackle the situation head on with assurance and hope. Such fear hinders them from seeking support and moving on through another path.

It would however be a mistake to conclude that the role and effects of care giving are wholly negative. The normal loving relationship often pushes family members to assume roles that result in positive outcomes. Some of those roles are of a practical nature. Others, such as sustained emotional support, provide the bedrock on which recovery can be built.

Positive care giving has the potential to enable those cared for to continue to achieve personal growth and development despite the many new challenges they face. It enables them to continue to be an integral part of their cultural surroundings. Affirmation and praise enable the cared for to gain a sense of achievement from developing such personal attributes as patience, gratitude and motivation to embark on a different pathway than was mapped out before the onset of their illness. Positive caring may also enable the mentally ill family member to become empowered through personal experience to help someone they love to improve their own quality of life. And it can strengthen the relationship between caregiver and cared for.

The positive caring relationship can nurture resilience and boost the ability of the cared for to come back to some degree of recovery. It also has the potential to trigger deeper insights into the true meaning of love, friendship, acceptance and duty to care for the loved one whose strength has weakened. When this positive care giving bolsters recovery, the caregiver derives a deep sense of satisfaction and well-being which further renews their commitment to move forward.

So family caregivers become experts in their own right and should be recognised as essential partners with the professionals and their ill member. Supported involvement of families enhances the quality of life of persons with severe mental illness. A well-planned and supported family involvement can even lead to family take up of the key role of case manager: the family learns to assess, monitor and deal with daily problems and crises. The family is thus empowered to make a better job of what it is already doing. In this scenario the role of case manager can be assigned to the stakeholder who is best placed to assume it which in appropriate conditions could actually be the family.

Some Initial Conclusions

There is **no substitute for families** who live with and care for the mentally ill member 24 hours a day every day. Nobody else can provide such care full time. This basic fact should never be forgotten or overlooked by professionals, government policy makers, officials and opinion formers in the media.

Families are an **irreplaceable yet fragile** gift to society. The fragility can be overcome through acknowledgement and appreciation of the role the family plays in caring for its loved ones.

Families have **much to give**. They can no longer be ignored in the framework of policy making and therapeutic partnerships if these are to achieve their full-intended results. The principle of patient/doctor confidentiality should be respected but not used as a pretext for excluding family carers.

It is the family that **provides accommodation** and **prevents homelessness**.

It is the family relatives who **make sure that medication is taken regularly** according to a prescribed regime to avoid relapse.

It is the family relatives who **advocate on behalf of the ill person** when they are unable to speak effectively for themselves.

It is the family relatives who can **provide vital and useful information** to the professionals that the ill person is unwilling or unable to communicate, drawn from firsthand knowledge and observation.

It is the family relatives who **nurture and support the mentally ill member** to sustain some degree of self-reliance.

Families have a **life beyond caring**. They have their own needs which must be recognised. Practitioners take leave but family caregivers often sacrifice their own personal needs to the detriment of society. Caring for caregivers essentially means investing to prevent mental health problems increasing in scale and in severity.

The Role of EUFAMI

It was because of this crucial role played by family carers coupled with their need for support that many began to come together to form self-help groups. These are organised at local, national and regional levels to lobby for the rights of people with mental illness and their care giving relatives to be acknowledged. This movement naturally led on to the idea of a pan European body united in a common crusade to strengthen their voice and influence on a broader stage. Thus it was that the European Federation of Associations of Families of People with Mental Illness – EUFAMI – was established in 1992 to highlight the collective concerns of family caregivers' organisations across the continent.

Today, EUFAMI is the umbrella body for 40 national and regional family associations from 25 countries. It is the only organisation in Europe that seeks to empower families of mentally ill persons to combat the stigma and discrimination they suffer. EUFAMI works to promote best practice in every European country, particularly to help reduce discrepancies in services between Eastern and Western Europe, and campaigns for positive changes to improve the quality of care.

Its stated mission is to represent all family members of persons affected by severe mental illness at the European level so that their rights and interests are protected and promoted. As a means to achieving these goals, EUFAMI strongly advocates and promotes the ideas of partnership and collaboration between these interests for example by identifying and addressing key barriers to partnership. EUFAMI also acts as a conduit to enable EU member states to act jointly at the European level to achieve common aims.

In its campaigns to combat stigma, EUFAMI addresses issues that affect both the mentally ill themselves and their families and also the mental health professionals. One successful method of this broad approach characterised its zero stigma campaign some years ago which was also targeted at policy makers and the media. It was based upon three clear objectives which have stood the test of time and remain as valid as ever today:

To **reduce stigma** against people with severe mental illness
To replace people's **prejudice, ignorance and fear**
To create **acceptance, knowledge and understanding**

Currently EUFAMI has been engaged with LUCAS, the research arm of the Catholic University of Leuven, in conducting a major international family carer survey designed to understand the needs and challenges of carers. This starts from the general recognition that carers' needs and experiences are closely linked with those of the person they care for. The aim is to expand knowledge of carers' role and experience so as to see them recognised as a true and important partner in that whole care process. The findings should be for consideration by professionals and their organisations, including EUFAMI's own member associations and of course to policy makers and opinion formers as well. They should particularly help to inform priorities being set for future policies and programmes to support family carers.

The full report of the survey was published in late 2015, and the analysis provides a valuable extension of our knowledge. To give a flavour, it confirms the way in which the care giving burden encompasses several life domains – emotional, social, physical financial and relational. It reports too on the main worries reported by the caregivers, their positive care giving experiences, which can serve as a counterweight to the negative aspects of caring, and their degree of satisfaction with the support they receive from the various professional groups – doctors, nurses, social care workers and pharmaceutical companies.

Stigma has its own place among the questions asked. What did the caregivers perceive as stigma after contact with professional help? We learn that not all caregivers feel empowered. For example, 18 % of carers began doubting themselves, 16 % began feeling less capable than before, 15 % sometimes began to feel useless, and 13 % began to feel inferior. More than one in 7 sometimes felt ashamed because of their contact with professionals. These responses can be related to the findings that less than four out of ten caregivers were satisfied with their relationships with the key staff and less than four felt that professional staff took seriously what they say.

These are serious revelations for the future of effective caring. The challenge thrown up must be to strengthen the link and the level of understanding between professionals and family caregivers and not just between the professionals and their patients. That argument is reinforced by the concluding finding that more than 90 % of caregivers said they would like additional support in their role and nearly half wanted significantly more help. Following through the conclusions of the survey is an important project for EUFAMI itself.

Experience of Stigma and Discrimination

Let us now continue by illustrating the ways in which these two monsters threaten the lives of family caregivers, quite separately from and in addition to the actual responsibilities of caring themselves. They compound the problems of living with mental illness, already severe enough and sometimes intolerably so, by encouraging attitudes and actions that cause still more distress, where instead sympathy and understanding should be the rule.

First some definitions. Stigma is held to mean a mark or sign of shame, disgrace, reproach or disapproval of being shunned or rejected by others but which is not deserved. Discrimination follows and refers to the practice of making distinctions or treating differently because of one's feelings or prejudices about a person. Both have their origins in a series of myths, especially about people with schizophrenia, that can readily be dispelled.

The first myth is that they are violent and dangerous. However there exists any amount of research findings and statistical evidence to show that they are no more likely to commit such acts than any other group in society, provided they follow their prescribed treatment including medication.

Secondly they are thought to be poor and unintelligent. But in fact mental illness knows no boundaries and appears across all social strata.

Thirdly they have personal weaknesses of some sort, for which there is no evidence whatever.

And fourthly their illness cannot be treated. But a diagnosis of schizophrenia does not necessarily indicate that a lifelong illness is inevitable. Many people do recover with early treatment interventions and many others can improve to a situation where they can make a meaningful and fulfilling quality of life for themselves.

In one phrase the roots of stigma and its partner discrimination lie with those three major enemies: prejudice, ignorance and fear. They can be overcome by our friends' acceptance, knowledge and understanding.

From the family viewpoint, the key to understanding is that stigma affects not only those with the illness but the family members as well. And critically, this effect is most marked in the case of mental illness. One relevant study estimated the degree to which a family member might feel embarrassed when a close relative is suffering from an alcohol, drug or mental health condition versus a general medical condition. The results showed that both mental and physical conditions impose a burden on family members. However what was most notable was that relatives of patients with mental illnesses felt greater stigma than those with physical conditions compare and contrast for example instinctive responses to the sight of a wheelchair case or a blind person using white sticks with the appearance of someone clearly showing signs of abnormal behaviour. A large-scale study to assess the feelings of family members would test and confirm this broader hypothesis and should support the suggestion that anti-stigma campaigns must include relatives within their target audience.

Even when all members of the family have the knowledge to deal with mental illness, which is rarely the case, the family is often reluctant to discuss their family member with others because they do not know how people will react. After all, myths and misconceptions surround mental illness. For many, even their closest friends may not understand. For example, the sister of a young man with schizophrenia pointed out that when a friend's brother had cancer, all his friends were supportive and understanding. But when she told a few close friends that her brother had paranoid schizophrenia, they said little and implied that something must be very wrong in her family to cause this illness.

Family members may become reluctant to invite anyone to the home because the ill person can be unpredictable or is unable to handle the disruption and heightened stimulation of having a number of people in the house. Furthermore, family members may be anxious about leaving the ill person at home alone. They are concerned about what might happen. So they go out separately or not at all.

The result of stigma in so many areas of daily life is that the family becomes more and more withdrawn. When others do not accept the reality of mental illness, families have little choice but to withdraw from existing or previous relationships to protect both themselves and their loved one. They are unwilling to take any more risks of being hurt or rejected. Not surprisingly, all this can lead to withdrawal from actively participating in the life of the community. In such a situation, a trusted friend or companion can be tremendously helpful by reaching out to the family and by working to create an atmosphere of acceptance and hospitality within the community for both the family and the person who is ill.

Some Illustrative Cases

A talk given by a mother who has three sons, all in their twenties and all diagnosed with schizophrenia, provides a live illustration of the experience of stigma. Of her second son, she said:

- "He was able to complete his studies and had been in employment for some time. He was a valued member of a work team and nobody knew about his problem. If they had ever found out, he would have lost his job. But he did lose his job after the disclosure of his illness. It destroyed his dignity. For a long time we had to nurture him to rebuild some self-esteem."
- Of her third son, she said: "Then 23, he had the benefit of effective medicine and nurturing support right from the start. He has been in full remission for several years. After 8 months of TLC (tender loving care) and total rest he was able to return to his studies. He obtained his degree with distinction, being the top student in one of the majors, for which he received a prize last year when he completed a year-long course and won the top student trophy, gaining an average of 93 %. Very occasionally, when stressed, he thinks he hears voices, suffers some paranoia or feels deep guilt about unimportant things. Then likewise I or one of us nurture him through. He has recently found a job which he will start soon. His biggest fear is exposure of his illness". He writes "I cannot disclose my true story. I sit convicted of the heinous crime of mental illness. Maybe, one day, you will all understand. For now I must simply hide but with the hope that I will be found, trying to pass as a human being who can make a valuable contribution. At least I know that life can and does continue after schizophrenia".

Here is another quote from a mother of a son with schizophrenia.

- It has been a living hell. The pain of losing a child to mental illness is bad enough. But now my whole life is a mess. Our marriage has ended. Why? Constant arguing. My husband would come home and it would start. I could not understand why the sudden change. Until during one episode I realised that he was experiencing grief and abuse from his work mates. Telling him that our son was just a lazy good for nothing. It got to him and he began believing it. If only I could have met them and really tell it like it is.

And one from another mother:

- "I now feel it is all my fault that my daughter is the way she is. I could see the neighbours treating me differently. Turning their heads, becoming occupied when I approached. It has got so bad that I now only go out at nights when there is no one around. Sometimes I could kill myself but then I think – who will there be for my daughter?"

That is stigma. People with mental illness also find themselves discriminated against in fundamentally important areas of their lives from finding employment or accommodation to simply making friends. As a result their families and carers suffer too with anxiety and depression which may turn into a mental illness itself. More quotes will illustrate.

- "I have had to take early retirement to support my son who suffers from mental illness. I had no other option, as my employer could only see black and white. The stress of mental illness in a family can have widespread and deep effects, stretching also into the workforce. Although my boss was aware of my circumstances, no allowances were made. Not that I wanted favours. Just some flexibility. I wasn't on any production line. I worked in the office, so there was a reasonable case for some flexibility in shifting working hours. But it began to get worse, with jibes taking over. Eventually I decided for the sanity of all our family to retire. At least I now only have the worry of my son I don't have to live with a continuous strain of feeling worthless in work."

- "Recently our daughter, who suffers with severe mental illness, was judged as being capable of adopting an "independent life style", in other words to live in her own apartment. Both my husband and I were absolutely delighted, as for so long we had been living with what I would call the hell of mental illness. But our joy was short lived after we started to help our daughter in the search for an apartment. Time and time again we got to the stage of locating the ideal one. And then came the question – does your daughter work? Although we were there to assure the landlords that the rent was guaranteed, they all came up with excuses, none truthful bar one who admitted that if others in the block found out about our daughter he would have a lot of trouble. So every night for almost 2 weeks we went home and honestly I cried myself to sleep. Whatever about us – and it was bad – can you imagine what our daughter must have felt? Thankfully we did eventually find an owner of an apartment who agreed to rent. While we were negotiating it emerged that he had had personal experience of mental illness."

- "When our son became ill, our friends and neighbours were there to support us. At that time he was not diagnosed. But after it became known that our son was suffering from mental illness, we noticed a change with our friends, not all thankfully but the majority. You see we had been very active in our community. But it took a while to fully understand what was happening. Excuses were beginning to appear as to why Mr X or Mrs X could not make it to a meeting or some other function where we were involved. When something like this happens you begin to blame yourself for everything. It was our fault that our son was mentally ill. You begin to feel worthless and full of shame. My wife is now reluctant to go out during normal hours. It takes a great toll. If only people could understand."

- "Our son, once considered the brightest of our children, started behaving oddly in his teens. He twice failed his first year university and went to tour India, getting into the expatriate drug culture and arriving home emaciated and dishevelled. Now in his 40s he has never worked since. After a crisis he was admitted to a mental hospital for observation, not speaking to visitors and feigning sleep. After discharge he returned home and lurked in his bedroom all day. He was hearing voices – "the people inside my head" whom he said had made him wrench the telephone off the wall, breaking the cable. A local Consultant Psychiatrist diagnosed schizophrenia. With his help our son was admitted to hospital and initially seemed greatly improved. Subsequently however he began a long decline. He invariably rejects any suggestion of help and will not face the future. Although we are not aware of his ever suffering stigma from others, he himself thinks he is discriminated against. He had no apparent self-esteem or social skills and hides resentfully from any approach. He told the community mental health team that he wanted no contact with his parents and will not speak to them and has never answered a letter or e-mail. Asked by a care home manager what he wanted he replied 'I want to be left alone.' We his parents felt trapped, unable to invite friends to visit still less to stay while this strange figure was haunting the house, lurking in his room but liable to appear without warning to complain or throw away rubbish. Occasionally he would be seen venturing out to buy food or to see his psychiatrist (though he would frequently miss appointments). It was embarrassing to answers neighbours asking after him for fear that any stigma might rub off on the entire household – what is known as self-stigma. The conclusion is that public ignorance about mental illness increases the stress on carers. We need high profile sponsorship and publicity on the same level as that given for example to cancer charities."

- "James was the child of two very successful professional parents. He was always a difficult child. He was physically clumsy, slightly dyslexic and delayed in some of his childhood milestones, although he was very bright and gifted in mathematics. He had never had many friends. As he became adolescent, his behaviour worsened and he took to staying up all night and sleeping during the day. He stopped washing, became withdrawn, irritable and negative towards the family. He was taken to see a psychiatrist privately. The psychiatrist found James to be psychotic and thought he was developing schizophrenia but did not tell the family and instead reassured them that this was probably a case of adolescent behaviour. The psychiatrist later said he was 'reluctant to label James because schizophrenia is such a terrible diagnosis'. He recognised the need for early intervention and prescribed medication but James found the side effects so unpleasant that he stopped taking it. Because his parents had been reassured they did not insist on the medication. Sadly James' illness progressively worsened and 18 months later he was found by the police wandering down the hard shoulder of a motorway and was admitted to hospital with a florid psychotic illness. A chance for early treatment had been missed because the psychiatrist had a stigmatised view of schizophrenia."

- "K's father, Mr Ma, a man of Pakistani origin, worked at an airport in retail. Mrs MA, his wife and his five adult children lived in two adjoining houses. The family generally kept themselves to themselves and were traditional in their approach to life, believing in arranged marriage and being quite strict in the way the children were brought up. Mr MA's youngest daughter, K, was very gifted at school and she decided with the support of her father to go into medicine. She did well but her studies brought her into increasing contact with the wider society in Britain and she found the conflict between her family's traditional values and her own wishes to be quite hard to cope with. K became depressed but soldiered on at medical school without seeking help. Eventually, and sadly, K made a serious suicide attempt and was admitted to hospital. There the story emerged of K's childhood. Her mother had always been withdrawn and aloof, she spoke little did little during the day and never interacted with the children as they were growing up. Mrs MA seldom left the house. K was brought up by her father, who worked long hours, and her older sister. The team supporting K strongly suspected that her mother had a serious mental illness, probably schizophrenia and discussed the matter with Mr MA when he came to visit K. Mr MA was very upset and spoke in confidence to the doctor. He told the team that his wife had indeed been diagnosed with schizophrenia many years previously. He said that he did not want anyone in the community or even his own children to know about this because he believed that if they did the marriage prospects of his children would be ruined. He therefore took the decision to keep his wife at home out of the public eye and he did not want mental health or social services involved. Mrs MA had had no treatment. She had gradually become more and more inward-looking and withdrawn and was able to contribute nothing to family life. Mr MA remained adamant that his wife's diagnosis should remain secret and asked K to keep her depression secret also. K left medical school and was lost to psychiatric follow-up."

- "While caring for our son, Steve, who has schizophrenia, we have found stigma and discrimination to be a major factor to contend with ourselves and one which in our view slowed his recovery considerably. They have also frustrated our attempts to help him.

  Steve was diagnosed with paranoid schizophrenia in the autumn of 1999 at a time when my wife and I were looking forward to our two children 'flying the nest'; when we hoping to rediscover our loving relationship and enjoy spending some of our hard earned savings. Unfortunately this was not to be. By the end of that summer our happiness and optimism had been replaced by fear and despair. Severe mental illness had stuck our beautiful son.

  When Steve was first diagnosed with schizophrenia I wrestled with a sense of shame that somehow I was partially responsible for his illness. I had not given him the time I should have done. I was plagued with the guilt that had I done so, perhaps his illness might have been avoided. Self-doubt and guilt is a burden many carers live with all their lives. The belief that they could have done more. This made worse by misguided academics who proclaim that families are to blame for mental illness. As a carer when you first read such statements tour self-esteem and self-worth are diminished even more and you sense of shame is heightened. Thankfully, as the years have passed I have come to understand that this stigmatising of families is simplistic nonsense and belongs in the university bins. But at the time this nonsense is highly damaging, specifically when you are trying to understand things at such a traumatic period in your life.

The stigmatising of carers by a minority of academics I learnt to ignore but the blatant discrimination we experiences by some health care professionals was and still is much harder to deal with. While the majority of professionals have been kind and have shown genuine empathy, others have displayed outright discrimination against us, refusing to talk to us, cancelling meetings at the last moment, not answering correspondence, not telling us our rights. Often we have been made to feel invisible especially when important decisions have been made about Steve without proper consultation.

Over time my wife and I were able to deal with the stigma and discrimination directed at us but when directed at Steve that was another matter. For the first 3 years of his illness he was a virtual recluse. We spent many months trying to encourage him to walk down to the local shop to get his own cigarettes. Finally he agreed but as he was walking back from the shop a 'white van man' shouted out of his window 'f … nutter'. It took another 2 years to get his confidence back – 10 years on he still worries about seeing a white van man. This was one of a number of incidents, including taunts from local teenagers all of which have damaged his confidence. Some of the media do not help with insensitive headlines which serve to confirm his own feelings of being different. He sees himself a 'nutter'. Not as a person who is cognitively impaired, a person with some chemical imbalance in his brain, above all a good human being.

Lastly the group whose actions put the severely mental ill at greatest risk, in my view, are those who have in fact failed to discriminate positively in favour of the mentally ill. They include some professionals who have failed to understand the complex and problematic nature of conditions such as schizophrenia which are profoundly disabling and require a far more subtle approach than other conditions such as depression. This failure has in my view led to the deprivations of tens of thousands of society's most vulnerable citizens. Many are left to fend for themselves in lonely bedsits, often without any proper support which is cruel, inhuman and an utter disgrace.

How can we expect the general public to adopt a more reasonable approach to the severely mentally ill when many professionals and politicians appear to lack sympathetic understanding of these highly vulnerable people. Until policy makers really grip the situation I see a bleak future for them. Nevertheless I live in hope that one day their needs will be fully understood and met."

Elements of a Remedial Strategy

These quotations drawn from life illustrate vividly the kind of pain and heartache that is the normal experience of countless thousands of family carers. We owe it to them to seek ways of at least ameliorating their situation. From the broadest perspective, this implies raising the whole status of family carers to see them as full members of a three-way care and treatment team on the same level as the mentally ill persons themselves and the responsible clinical and social work professionals.

To this end, part 2 of this chapter offers a condensed version of a carers charter produced by the author some years ago setting out principles which should guide acceptance of their role and thus achieve that broad status-raising aim. More directly we can identify a number of actions to reduce stigma and at least eliminate public expressions of prejudice as is being achieved with regard to other personal characteristics. Deeper internalised changes in attitude do of course rely on the evolution of societies more generally. Here is what we can address right away.

Education Educating society on mental illness both at school and in wider community settings is an effective way of increasing awareness and changing negative attitudes. The object is to help people learn to think about mental illness in the same way as they think about other physical illnesses or conditions.

Talking openly This too is an important goal. It is surprising how many people are affected by mental illness or have a family member or friend who is and are too afraid of rejection or rebuff to discuss it openly. The problem should not be swept under the carpet.

Quality support and treatment To enable people with severe mental illness to participate fully in all areas of community life, they need to be provided with high-quality support and treatment services. Advocacy and support groups need to be proactive in their fight against the stigma surrounding mental illness, both for people with the diagnosis and their families.

Personal role People with mental illness should themselves play an active role in challenging stigma and accordingly develop the skills and strategies to cope with their own stigmatising experiences.

Language The use of particular words often portrays the idea that people with schizophrenia are somehow undesirable. Labelling someone as "schizophrenic" suggests that their illness defines who they are. It puts the illness before the person. It may also suggest that the illness is lifelong and that the symptoms evident in a psychotic episode will always be present. To reduce stigma, a person with schizophrenia should always be referred to as just that – a person who happens to have schizophrenia.

The media The media plays a pervasive role in influencing public opinion. When used effectively mass media can inform and educate people as to the facts about mental illness. Unfortunately, in many cases the media tends to portray people with a mental illness as unpredictable and often violent. As such, it is important to keep a check on the media's representation of mental illness and to confront those involved if poor practice is observed.

Acknowledgements Connie Magro, EUFAMI Vice President contributing her invaluable experience and understanding as a mental health carer

Guiding Principles for Family Support

Bert Johnson

This chapter sets out six principles as guidance to enable the crucial role of family caregivers to be acknowledged and their own needs to be met.

Principle 1

Carers' essential role and expertise should be recognised and respected.

- They should be listened to without bias or prejudice and be taken seriously.
- They should be recognised as someone who is providing support to the person for whom you care.
- They should be treated as someone who has relevant and important knowledge about the person for whom they care.
- All staff should be aware of the distress and anxiety that caring can cause and help carers cope with this.
- They should be asked to give their opinion – this should be respected and valued and where necessary kept confidential.
- Their views should be taken into account in the decisions about the person they care for.
- They should be told how the information they provide will be used.
- They should be able to choose whether they wish to take on, or continue with, the role of carer.

Principle 2

Carers should be given the information that they need to help them provide care.

- They should be helped to obtain, within a reasonable time, the information that they need to get help and support for themselves and the person for whom they care.
- The information should be clear and accurate.
- The information should be provided in a way which is helpful to them – for example orally, in writing or on tape, in their own language, through an interpreting service or in discussion with a qualified professional.

Principle 3

Carers should be involved in planning and agreeing the care plan for the person they care for.

- Their views about the needs of the person for whom they care should be sought and taken into account.

- They should be involved in the decisions made about themselves and (with his or her consent) the person for whom they care, including the preparation of a care plan.
- Even if the person they care for is unwilling for them to be involved in planning and agreeing his or her care, they should be told who to contact in an emergency or in a crisis.
- They should be told of their rights regarding a carer's assessment.
- They should be given a copy of the care plan of the person for whom they care (with his or her consent). This should state the responsibilities of all the people who are involved in providing care.
- If they feel that the care plan is not working or is being improperly implemented, they should be given the opportunity to state their views and to be listened to and be involved in the discussions on the action to be taken to address the problems they have identified.
- When the person they care for is receiving care and treatment in hospital, they should be involved in planning and agreeing the discharge plan, including the date of discharge.
- So far as possible, meetings should be held at a time that suits them and the person they care for.

Principle 4

Carers' needs as carers should be recognised, responded to and reflected in the care plan.

- All staff should recognise that they may have additional commitments to that of their caring role, such as looking after their children or going to work.
- Their ethnicity and culture, religion, gender, sexual preference, age and other characteristics should be respected and taken into account but without general assumptions being made about them.
- If they require assistance in communicating their views, they should be given the appropriate assistance, for example if English is not their first language, they should be assisted by a qualified interpreter.
- If they are told that they are not entitled to a carer's assessment, they should be told why.
- If they have a carer's assessment, this should:
  - If they so wish, be carried out separately from the assessment of the needs of the person for whom they provide care
  - Allow them to have someone to support them while the assessment is taking place
  - Give them the opportunity to assess their own needs
  - Assess their needs without the assumption being made that they are willing or able to take on a caring role or to continue to provide the same level of care
  - Consider how their caring role affects their relationship with other family members and friends and their ability to hold down a job

- Address their own health and wellbeing, their need for emotional and other support and how they would like to be helped in providing care
- Consider whether they would like to take a break from caring and if so, look at what type of support they think would enable them to do this
- When they have a carer's assessment, they should be given a copy of their assessment and care plan.
- They should have their needs regularly reviewed, as circumstances require, but at least annually and, if they so wish, this should be carried out separately from the review of the needs of the person for whom they care.

Principle 5

Carers should be provided with appropriate help and support when they need it.

- They should be told of their rights regarding a carer's assessment.
- They should be told who to contact if they need help and to know that their request will be responded to within a reasonable time.
- Their contribution should be valued and incorporated into the planning, development and evaluation of services.
- Where plans such as hospital admission are being considered, they and the person they care for should be given the opportunity to consider alternative care.
- They should be given information about what to do and whom to contact in times of crisis.
- They should be told about opportunities to take a break from caring.
- They should be given details of local support groups and advocacy services.
- They should be helped to get advice about housing and employment issues and financial matters, including entitlement to benefits and training for carers.
- They should be given a copy of their own care plan in a form which they find useful.
- The services that they receive should be of good quality, appropriate to their needs and provided within an agreed time.
- They should be advised on what action to take if they are not happy with the assessment or the decisions made as a result of the assessment or if they think that the care plan is not being implemented properly.

Principle 6

Carers should be actively involved in the planning, development and evaluation of services.

- They should be given the opportunity to state their views on the quality of services provided and on the range of services which need to be developed.
- They should be told how their views will be taken into account as part of an ongoing evaluation process.

- Their contribution should be valued and incorporated into the planning, development and evaluation of services.
- Where they are invited to meetings, they should be offered help in arranging alternative care for the person they care for and receive payment for travel and alternative care costs.
- They should be given adequate notice of meetings, consultation periods and other relevant events.
- They should be told how the particular consultation process will work.
- They should be told how the information they provide will be used.
- They should receive feedback on the outcome of the consultation within 6 months of completing the consultation.

Stigma, Human Rights and the UN Convention on the Rights of Persons with Disabilities

12

Peter Bartlett

Introduction

> For 650 million persons around the world living with disabilities, today promises to be the dawn of a new era – an era in which disabled people will no longer have to endure the discriminatory practices and attitudes that have been permitted to prevail for all too long.[1]

With these words, Secretary General Kofi Annan celebrated the passage of the United Nations Convention on the Rights of Persons with Disabilities (CRPD)[2] in 2006. The CRPD represents a new high point in the human rights of people with disabilities, including people with mental disabilities.[3] Unlike the previous disability-specific international law, it is a full convention rather than a set of principles or a declaration and as such has the full force of international law. It is not a regional treaty, but is at the UN level, now signed and ratified by 151 countries across the world[4] – 78 % of the 193 members of the United Nations. This means that the considerable bulk of the world's population is covered by the Convention. Of the 12 countries with more than 100 million populations, only the United States of America and the Republic of the Congo have failed to ratify it. Of the additional

---

[1] Statement of Kofi Annan, United Nations Secretary-General (2006).

[2] United Nations A/Res/61/106 (general assembly, 24 January 2007).

[3] In this chapter, 'mental disabilities' is taken to include disabilities related to development such as learning disabilities, psychosocial disabilities (disabilities traditionally associated with mental ill health), disabilities flowing from injury to the brain and mental disabilities associated with later life such as dementia.

[4] A list of signatories and ratifications may be found at http://www.un.org/disabilities/. Accessed 24 November 2014. An additional eight countries have signed but not yet ratified the CRPD – so more than 82 % of UN member states have signed the Convention.

P. Bartlett
Department of Law and Social Sciences, Faculty of Social Sciences,
University of Nottingham, University Park, Nottingham NG7 2RD, UK
e-mail: peter.bartlett@nottingham.ac.uk

© Springer International Publishing Switzerland 2017
W. Gaebel et al. (eds.), *The Stigma of Mental Illness - End of the Story?*,
DOI 10.1007/978-3-319-27839-1_12

34 countries with populations greater than 30 million, only Vietnam, Uzbekistan, Burma and Tanzania have not yet ratified. The vast bulk of the world's population is therefore covered by the Convention.

The Convention contains much that will warm the hearts of those concerned with combating stigma against people with mental disabilities. The Convention's express purpose is 'to promote, protect and ensure the full and equal enjoyment of all human rights and fundamental freedoms by all persons with disabilities, and to promote respect for their inherent dignity.'[5] Its principles include non-discrimination, the full and effective participation and inclusion in society of people with disabilities, respect for difference and acceptance of persons with disabilities as part of human diversity, equality of opportunity and respect for inherent dignity, individual auton-omy including the freedom to make one's own choices – principles that are at the heart of anti-stigma campaigns.[6] People with disabilities are defined to include those with impairments 'which in interaction with various barriers may hinder their full and effective participation in society on an equal basis with others'[7] – a social model of disability which again resounds sympathetically with the understanding of anti-stigma campaigners. The definition expressly includes both 'mental' and 'intel-lectual' disabilities, so both people with learning disabilities and mental health problems are within the scope of the Convention.

The CRPD further has teeth. Its implementation is overseen by a specific UN body, the Committee on the Rights of Persons with Disabilities (the 'CRPD Committee'). Countries that have ratified the Convention are required to establish 'focal points' and 'coordination mechanisms' to oversee implementation and moni-toring of the Convention at the domestic level, and these bodies are specifically required to involve people with disabilities and their representative bodies in the monitoring process.[8] National governments are required to collect evidence, includ-ing statistical evidence, as part of policy formation in implementing the Convention and as part of the process of demonstrating compliance.[9] Upon ratification and every four years thereafter, they are required to report to the CRPD Committee on their progress at implementing the Convention.[10] These reports are public, and the public (either as individuals or civil society organisations) are permitted to file 'shadow reports' commenting on the completeness and accuracy of the government reports. The concluding observations of the Committee are also public.[11] While the

---

[5] CRPD, Article 1.

[6] CRPD, Article 3 (a) to (e). Additional principles contained in Article 3 include accessibility (rel-evant primarily for people with physical disabilities rather than mental disabilities), equality between men and women, acknowledgment of the evolving capacities of children and respecting the right of children with disabilities to preserve their identities.

[7] CRPD, Article 1.

[8] CRPD, Article 33.

[9] CRPD, Article 31.

[10] CRPD, Article 35.

[11] See http://www.ohchr.org/EN/HRBodies/CRPD/Pages/CRPDIndex.aspx, accessed 25 November 2014. At the time of writing, concluding comments had been written for New Zealand, Denmark, the Republic of Korea, Belgium, Ecuador, Mexico, El Savador, Azerbaijan, Costa Rica, Sweden, Australia, Austria, Paraguay, China, Hungary, Argentina, Spain, Tunisia and Peru.

Committee cannot force governments to implement specific measures and it remains for individual national governments to implement the CRPD, these reports do have a political impact: countries cannot assume that failure to implement the Convention will not go unnoticed.

For the 85 countries that have currently signed and ratified the optional protocol to the Convention, the CRPD Committee can also consider complaints from individuals.[12] The process here operates much like a court, with evidence presented and the Committee expressing a view as to whether the CRPD has been violated. Once again, while the Committee cannot formally enforce its judgments, they are public and do create political pressure on governments.

The CRPD is the first significant human rights convention of the twenty-first century. As will be clear, anti-stigma campaigners will laud much of its basis and fundamental direction. It is a human rights treaty, however, and along with the synergies with the anti-stigma movement, there will be tensions. The remainder of this article explores these aspects.

A Convention for the Anti-stigma Movement?

As will be clear from the introduction, there is much in the CRPD that the anti-stigma movement will celebrate. It is not merely the overall direction of the Convention that is consistent with that movement, but a good deal of the detail creates requirements that will work to the de-stigmatisation of people with mental disabilities. For this reason, because the CRPD is likely to be new to many of the readers of this article, it is appropriate to take some time to go into what it actually says.

Article 8: Public Awareness

While the word 'stigma' never appears in the Convention, anti-stigma programmes seem in effect to be required by Article 8:

1. States Parties undertake to adopt immediate, effective and appropriate measures:
   (a) To raise awareness throughout society, including at the family level, regarding persons with disabilities, and to foster respect for the rights and dignity of persons with disabilities.
   (b) To combat stereotypes, prejudices and harmful practices relating to persons with disabilities, including those based on sex and age, in all areas of life.
   (c) To promote awareness of the capabilities and contributions of persons with disabilities.

---

[12] A copy of the first protocol, along with a list of countries ratifying it, may be found at http://www.un.org/disabilities/, accessed 25 November 2014.

2. Measures to this end include:
   (a) Initiating and maintaining effective public awareness campaigns designed
       (i)   To nurture receptiveness to the rights of persons with disabilities.
       (ii) To promote positive perceptions and greater social awareness towards persons with disabilities.
       (iii) To promote recognition of the skills, merits and abilities of persons with disabilities, and of their contributions to the workplace and the labour market.
   (b) Fostering at all levels of the education system, including in all children from an early age, an attitude of respect for the rights of persons with disabilities.
   (c) Encouraging all organs of the media to portray persons with disabilities in a manner consistent with the purpose of the present Convention.
   (d) Promoting awareness-training programmes regarding persons with disabilities and the rights of persons with disabilities.

This article, coupled with the requirements on states to develop statistical evidence as to the implementation of the Convention, provides a powerful political tool for the anti-stigma movement. While the precise form of the awareness-raising programmes are a matter for individual states, they are required to include public awareness campaigns, development of suitable educational curricula at all levels of the education system, and campaigns directed to families (including, presumably, families of people with disabilities), to media awareness and to the labour market. The statistical evidence requirements in Article 31 when applied to Article 8 would suggest that states must also take reasonable steps to determine and record whether the programmes are working. That is a powerful tool for the anti-stigma movement.

Other Articles

While Article 8 is the provision most clearly aligned to the anti-stigma movement per se, the world envisaged by much of the CRPD is one in which people with mental disabilities will be de-stigmatised. Space does not allow a detailed analysis of all the relevant articles, and readers are encouraged to peruse the full text of the Convention. Nonetheless, an overview of some of the pertinent articles may give an indication of the ways in which the CRPD may work towards de-stigmatisation of people with mental disabilities.

The CRPD is at its core a convention to protect people with disabilities from discrimination. Discrimination is taken to mean 'any distinction, exclusion or restriction on the basis of disability which has the purpose or effect of impairing or nullifying the recognition, enjoyment or exercise, on an equal basis with others, of all human rights and fundamental freedoms in the political, economic, social, cultural, civil or any other field.'[13] It thus includes both direct and indirect (adverse effect) discrimination. It further includes a failure to provide 'reasonable accommodation', which is in turn defined as making 'necessary and appropriate modification and adjustments not imposing a disproportionate or undue burden, where needed in a particular case, to ensure to persons with disabilities the enjoyment or exercise on an equal basis with others of all human rights and fundamental freedoms'.[14] This objective of non-discrimination overlaps considerably with the objectives of anti-stigma campaigns, insofar as both are intended to allow people with disabilities to participate fully in the broader community and to normalise the participation of people with disabilities within that community. Particular articles protect in particular the rights of women and children with disabilities, thus acknowledging the particular difficulties arising from intersectional discrimination (and, by extension, intersectional stigmatisation).[15]

That theme of social integration is reflected in many of the CRPD's subsequent substantive articles, and many of these will be of particular relevance to removing stigma from people with mental disability. For example,

- Article 12 provides the right to recognition as persons before the law: people with mental disabilities are thus required to exist in law – a prerequisite for enjoying even the most basic civil rights and the benefits flowing from citizenship.
- Article 19 provides a right to live independently and to be included in the community, including the right to appropriate support services.
- The right to freedom of expression in Article 21 requires states to provide information for the general public in appropriate formats, suggesting people with learning disabilities should have access to easy-read versions of this information. States are also to encourage the use of such formats in the private sector.
- Article 23 protects rights to home and the family, including the right to marry and found a family, expressly protecting the right of persons with disabilities to decide the number and spacing of their children.

---

[13] CRPD, Article 2.

[14] CRPD, Article 2. Note that 'accommodation' is not in this context a term referring to physical accommodation or housing. That is covered in Article 28 (as part of the right to an adequate standard of living and social protection) and by implication in a number of other articles. 'Reasonable accommodation' requires modifications and adjustments in *all* of the areas governed by the CRPD. While 'reasonable accommodation' reflects a long legal usage in anti-discrimination law, 'reasonable adjustments' or 'reasonable adaptations' may be more useful to non-lawyers in understanding the concept.

[15] CRPD, Articles 6 and 7. Perhaps surprisingly, and unfortunately, there is no express article protecting the specific needs of people based on race or other demographic criteria. While this is acknowledged in the recitals at the beginning (see recital (p), located prior to Article 1), it is not reflected in specific articles in the Convention.

- Article 24 provides the right to inclusive education, in an environment that respects the dignity of persons with disabilities. While this article will no doubt be particularly useful for children with disabilities (including those with mental disabilities), it is not restricted to children; adults also have these rights.
- Article 25 provides the right to health, including the requirement that health professionals provide the same quality of care to people with disabilities as to people without disabilities.
- Article 27 provides the right to work and employment, including involvement in the labour market, non-discriminatory work practices, equality of remuneration, trade union membership, favourable conditions of work and healthy workplaces.
- Participation in public and political life is protected by Article 29, including rights to full participation in the selection of government (most notably, the right to vote) and full rights to participate in non-governmental organisations.
- Article 30 provides the right to participate in cultural life, recreation, leisure and sport, both as audience and as participants.

These articles are noted in particular because of their direct relevance to anti-stigma movements. The CRPD does go beyond this, covering matters of more general human rights law, including rights to life (Article 10); access to justice (Article 13); liberty (Article 14); freedom from torture and cruel, inhuman or degrading treatment or punishment (Article 15); freedom from exploitation, violence and abuse (Article 16); the right to integrity of the person (Article 17); the right to liberty of movement and nationality (Article 18); the right to privacy (Article 22) and the right to habilitation and rehabilitation (Article 26). These are less obviously relevant to an anti-stigma agenda. The CRPD is thus not *just* an anti-stigma convention.

A limitation of almost all the CRPD rights should be noted. The CRPD is to protect individuals with disabilities from discrimination, and most of its provisions provide rights to people with disabilities 'on an equal basis with others'. This may be a significant limitation. The right to 'the same range, quality and standard of free or affordable health care and programmes as provided to other persons', contained in Article 25 (a), for example, may be of little assistance in countries where standards of health care are generally poor, particularly for people with limited financial means. It provides only the right to the same poor services that the rest of that society get – perhaps a rather hollow victory. This serves as a reminder that issues of justice for people with disabilities are often inextricably intertwined with issues of justice for the population more broadly.

Nonetheless, there is much that those with an anti-stigma agenda may find of assistance in the CRPD. Does that mean we should understand it as an anti-stigma convention? The previous comments would suggest that this is not far from the truth, but the Convention also highlights how human rights and anti-stigma, at least as it is practised, may be subject to their tensions as well. It is to these that this chapter now turns.

Systemic Issues in the Interface Between Human Rights Law and Stigma

Labelling Disability

The CRPD is designed to protect people with disabilities from discrimination, but in order to do that, it is necessary to define who is within the scope of the anti-discrimination protection. The drafters of the Convention were aware of this problem, and long discussions occurred as to whether a definition was desirable at all, and if so, how it should be phrased. [16] The primary concern of the opponents of an express definition was that people should not be excluded from the protection of the Convention arbitrarily or based on overly technocratic readings of a definition by state courts and bureaucrats. Proponents of a definition, including the disabled peoples' organisations involved in the drafting process, wanted a definition to ensure that the Convention was not read unduly narrowly. The result was a non-exhaustive definition, which allows unanticipated groups to be included in the future as a matter of interpretation.

All that is fine, but it does not change the fact that people with disabilities have to be identified as such for the rights in the Convention to bite. The rights in the CRPD apply only to people with disabilities. For many of the rights, this matters little: the CRPD rights mirror rights in other human rights conventions. Indeed, it is sometimes said that the CRPD does not add any new rights, but merely creates mechanisms by which people with disabilities can enjoy their pre-existing and universal human rights.[17] In some situations, however, identifying a person as having a disability will be pivotal to the implementation of the Convention. Most importantly, the right to reasonable accommodation attaches only to people with disabilities. This is a fundamental mechanism for the realisation of the rights in the CRPD, and it is difficult to see how the objectives of the CRPD could be realised without it. At the same time, it does involve the identification of people with disabilities, and identification of people as having a disability has stigmatising effects. The result is that to access the non-discrimination benefits of the CRPD, an individual must be identified as belonging to a category which, in practice, is likely to involve the stigmatisation of that individual.

This problem does not necessarily fall on all people with disabilities equally. In some cases it is arguable that accommodations should be made as a matter of routine, without waiting for an individual case to arise. This is what we do in architecture for people in wheelchairs, for example: we (at least should) design buildings to have good wheelchair access at the time of construction; we do not wait for a person

---

[16] On the drafting history, see Lawson (2006).

[17] See, e.g., MacKay (2006). While this is generally a fair reading of the CRPD, there has been some debate as to whether the new right to integrity of the person (Article 17) is merely a restatement of an existing right or is instead an extension of previous conventions. Certainly, it does not appear expressly in other conventions. On this point, see Quinn (2009), Weller (2008), Kayess and French (2008), Mégret (2008).

in a wheelchair to ask to enter the building. Similarly, it is reasonable to expect that easy-read versions of documents should be made increasingly available, for the benefit of people with learning disabilities. No stigma would seem to attach in this circumstance. For many people with mental disabilities, however, the disability is much more specific to the individual, and reasonable accommodations must be tailored to the individual's own specific needs: there is no 'one size fits all' equivalent to the wheelchair ramp. For these people, identifying themselves (or being identified) as having a disability seems a prerequisite to enjoying the Convention rights, as it is of enjoying the rights contained in domestic non-discrimination legislation. And at least until stigma is a thing of the past, that will have stigmatising effects.

This serves as a useful reminder of the difference and the interrelations between systems of non-discrimination and anti-stigma movements. For people with mental disabilities (as for so many other minority groups), non-discrimination is not enough. Also required are changes in social attitudes, and that is where the eradication of stigma is vital.

The Scope of Human Rights

As the discussion above shows, there is much in human rights law that is in sympathy with the objectives of anti-stigma movements. The objectives of non-discrimination as well as many of the economic and social rights related to ensuring adequate standards of life and provision of services are obvious examples of intersection between human rights and anti-stigma movements.

Human rights are not restricted to these social and economic rights, however. They also include civil and political rights, and these often concern the protection of individual freedom and choice. The values of these rights are not measured with reference to reduction in stigma. To pick an obvious example, the right to refuse or consent to medical treatment is an important civil right, protected in Article 25 of the CRPD and in other human rights legislation. Refusal of such treatment (whether that treatment is for mental or other disorder) may result in worse therapeutic outcomes, but the right is still broadly accepted because of the importance of the right itself in a democratic society. The CRPD makes it clear that this right extends to people with disabilities, including people with mental disabilities. Such a person may similarly achieve worse therapeutic outcomes than if they had accepted treatment, and that may in turn make the person more visible and sometimes engage in behaviours which re-enforce stereotypes and stigma. Even if that were demonstrably the case, the reinforcement of stigma would not be a convincing human rights argument to override the individual's choices regarding treatment. Civil rights do not work that way. They are based in broadly liberal political philosophies relating to what it is to live in democracy. If the result is increased stigma, so be it: that is to be challenged through other means, not through removal of the individual's civil rights.[18]

---

[18]There are of course a wide array of other reasons why rights may be curtailed. The point here is not that fundamental human rights may never be curtailed, but rather that the effects on stigmatisation is not a reason for doing so.

As the catalogue of rights noted earlier in this paper makes clear, the CRPD is replete with provisions protecting the choice of persons with disability. Indeed, the right to exercise legal capacity contained in Article 12 comes close to providing a free-standing right to make choices. We do not know what the political effects of the exercise of this freedom will be, but their effect on stigma is not in human rights terms relevant to whether the right should be curtailed.

There is a tension that results. For the person with mental disabilities, is the abolition of stigma the objective? Surely the answer is ambiguous. He or she almost certainly wants social respect and social inclusion, but wants that to be consistent with his or her exercise of freedom and autonomy, quite possibly in ways that mark them out from much of the rest of society. The anti-stigma equivalent question is whether the abolition of stigma is to be achieved through developing a society that celebrates social difference and diversity and thus includes people with disabilities as they are or instead through assimilation of people with disabilities into broader society by helping people with disabilities to adapt to the expectations of broader society. Is the message that people with mental disabilities are really a lot like us (an assimilationist message), or that they are different from us but that's fine (a diversity message)? Anti-stigma campaigns often contain elements of both; in a human rights framework, however, individuality and the acceptance of social diversity play the more pivotal role.

It is clear, therefore, that while there is much that human rights law and the CRPD share with anti-stigma movements, there are also systematic tensions. In the sections that follow, these tensions will be examined in a variety of more specific contexts.

Issues of Implementation

Stigma, Medical Models, Social Models and the CRPD

The anti-stigma movement has been spearheaded by concerned medical professionals. The preponderance of medics among the contributors to this book is a reminder of the continuing leadership and influence of the medical profession in the anti-stigma project. This is not meant as a criticism – if anything quite the reverse. At a time when few other people with sufficient social standing to make a difference were prepared to force progress in this area, medics stepped up to the plate.

There has been real progress in recent years in involving people with disabilities as part of the teams that conceptualise, manage and run anti-stigma campaigns. In one sense, the desirability of that involvement seems almost tautological: if part of the point of anti-stigma is to increase the visibility and involvement of people with mental disabilities in society, involving them in the anti-stigma movement seems required by the logic of the project. In that sense, it seems little more than leading by example, but the fact that it is happening is important symbolically for the anti-stigma movement. Nonetheless, in much of the world, political and practical factors (ironically and perhaps most significantly the continued stigmatisation of service users and their organisations) mean that medics will be significant in developing, designing, conceptualising and implementing anti-stigma programmes for some time to come.

These medical roots have of course affected the conceptualisation of the movement. While medics may be acutely aware of the social aspects of disability in their anti-stigma activities, their day job is likely to be treating the impairments associated with the disability. In this conception, 'impairments' are of profound relevance to understanding disability and the legal, social and policy responses to it. These impairments, in the context of mental disability, often phrased in terms of ICD or DSM taxonomies, are located in the individual. While they are not to be viewed in moral terms, they are matters which are to be ameliorated or, if possible, fixed, and they are central to the understanding of disability.

The CRPD is not entirely at odds with this. The definition of disability does require the presence of impairment.[19] The right to health includes the right to 'early identification and intervention as appropriate, and services designed to minimize and prevent further disabilities',[20] suggesting that the right to health includes the right to treatment that will minimise future impairments (based, of course, on the patient's free and informed consent).

Nonetheless, the CRPD is focused on the social model of disability, rather than its biological or medical causes. Its focus is changing social practice to allow the full integration of people with disability. As noted in previous sections, much of this involves standards of service provision and will be familiar to anti-stigma campaigners. Where previous approaches to mental disability law have included a considerable degree of flexibility in the provision of these rights, however, the CRPD is uncompromising. Thus where the United Nations Mental Illness Principles of 1991 had provided a right to live and work in the community 'to the extent possible',[21] the comparable provision in the CRPD contains no such qualifier.[22] Where much of the 1991 Mental Illness Principles had included extensive detail on the nature of procedural and substantive safeguards that were required prior to detention based on mental disability or medical treatment under compulsion, the most authoritative views of the CRPD are that any such compulsory interventions are in violation of the Convention, if disability (including mental illness, learning disability or other mental disability) is even one aspect of the criteria for that compulsion.[23] There is no express acknowledgement that there may be circumstances where the nature of

---

[19] CRPD Article 1.

[20] CRPD, Article 25 (b).

[21] United Nations Mental Illness Principles, adopted by General Assembly resolution 46/119 (17 December 1991), principle 3.

[22] CRPD, Article 19.

[23] Regarding compulsory admission, see UN High Commissioner for Human Rights (2009). This is further consistent with a number of the Committee's concluding observations on individual countries. Regarding compulsory treatment, see Report of the Special Rapporteur on torture and other cruel, inhuman or degrading treatment or punishment, Juan E. Méndez to the United Nations General Assembly, A/HRC/22/53 (1 February 2013). A volume of papers reflecting on this report has been published as *Torture in Healthcare Settings: Reflections on the Special Rapporteur on Torture's 2013 Thematic Report* (Washington: Centre for Human Rights and Humanitarian Law,

the impairment precludes the provision of the right, through suitable reasonable accommodation.[24] All this suggests that it will be necessary to develop new legal and professional models of practice that are currently quite foreign to the ways in which medicine for people with mental disabilities is currently practised. Such structural re-design has barely begun to be considered.

If it is possible to get beyond the initial shock, it is at least arguable that even the most radical of the CRPD provisions may contain much that medics will recognise. Consider Article 12, which would appear to disallow any use of capacity as a concept, when the determination of capacity flows directly or indirectly from an individual's disability.[25] Rather than a binary articulation of capacity, where an individual is capable or not either in general or for a specific decision, Article 12 has been interpreted as requiring a move towards supported decision-making: the individual never entirely loses capacity in law, but instead is to be provided with supports to decision-making that may be tailored as required to the nature and severity of the individual's condition (presumably including the degree of their impairment, their social context and the decisions that need to be taken). This is in a sense a radical move: capacity has been pivotal to determination of rights in most legal systems for centuries, and in some countries has been argued to be a particularly non-stigmatising and non-discriminatory criterion because it applies not merely to people with specific mental disabilities, but to society as a whole.[26] These views are already problematic, given the oppressive and highly stigmatising use of capacity and guardianship in some parts of the world.[27]

Even if the systems of capacity and guardianship are working well, however, it is not obvious that they are desirable. Existing law creates a bright line between capacity and incapacity. A person who just has capacity can make the decision without legal interference of any sort and without any requirement that meaningful support or assistance be provided to that person, whatever the ramifications of the decisions are and whatever the understanding of the individual is (so long as they at least just have capacity). For people who barely do not have capacity, intensive legal regimes come into play which take the decision away from the individual entirely, even

American University Washington College of Law, 2014). It is available at http://antitorture.org/torture-in-healthcare-publication/. Accessed 29 November 2014.

[24] To put it another way, while reasonable accommodations are limited to responses that do not impose a disproportionate or undue burden [CRPD Article 2], the CRPD says nothing about how to understand situations where reasonable accommodation cannot realise the right in question. It would be unthinkable, given the ethos of the Convention, that people with disabilities in this circumstance do not acquire rights under the Convention, but the Convention does not articulate how those rights are to be understood.

[25] CRPD Committee, General Comment on Article 12, CRPD/C/GC/1 (19 May 2014). For a discussion of this article in an English context, see Bartlett (2012).

[26] Dawson and Szmukler (2006), Rees (2010), and the papers in the Horne and Richardson (2010).

[27] For discussions of capacity and guardianship that raise some of these issues, see the country reports of the Mental Disability Advocacy Center (MDAC) relating to Serbia, Russia, the Czech Republic, Bulgaria, Hungary and Kyrgystan from 2006 to 2007 available at http://www.mdac.info/en/resources?goal=137&format=144&page=1. Accessed 17 November 2014.

where the individual may well continue to have a good deal to say about what he or she wants and may have good reasons for this. The bright line does not however correspond to the experience of people working with people with mental disabilities (or, perhaps, without disabilities). Many people require support to develop their views and make decisions regarding, for example, serious medical treatment, even if they have legal capacity. And many people who currently are held not to have legal capacity have views that warrant considerable respect and should not simply be rendered marginal to the decision. To a considerable degree, that is what Article 12 is attempting to do, and once we get used to the idea, there is likely to be much common ground between medics and the Convention in this area.

Admittedly, there will be cases which may prove problematic (as there are in the existing system). Profound disabilities are often used as an example here: what support can be provided to allow a person with profound disabilities (or, in the extreme case, a person in a coma) to reach a meaningful decision? Those situations are indeed problematic, since the required support may perhaps involve a person other than the individual with disability effectively making the decision (albeit, perhaps, according to criteria that focus on the individual's values when in more robust health, if these are known). Such decision-making by others is what Article 12 is meant to be guarding against, so such a solution would be problematic. In any event, the relatively small number of problematic cases should not detract from the overall strength of Article 12, which removes the legal fiction of a bright line between capacity and incapacity.

Can similar arguments be made regarding the other clearest collisions between the CRPD and previous forms of treatment of people with mental disabilities? It is probably too early to tell. We are still at the stage where the CRPD provisions are largely unknown in medical circles and, when known, are still creating shock waves. It is fair to say that much of the compulsion now used may be difficult to justify on evidential grounds, quite apart from the CRPD. Community treatment orders seem never quite able to show that they improve outcomes following discharge,[28] and the limited evidence available suggests that it is similarly doubtful how much good comes from involuntary psychiatric admission.[29] While these techniques have been used for many years, it may be the case that they are not as essential as seems to be assumed.

From all this, it will be clear that there will be tensions between the direction of human rights law and some of the key players in the anti-stigma movement. That is a slightly different question from what the stronger focus on the social model of disability will mean for stigma more generally. If the CRPD is broadly implemented, it is likely to mean that people with mental disabilities will be more visible in the community and making more of their own choices. Some of those choices will be perceived sympathetically by the community; some will not. It is difficult to guess in advance the relative effects and thus the effect on stigma.

---

[28] Churchill et al. (2007); Kisely et al. (2005).
[29] Priebe et al. (2011).

Reasonable Accommodation

It is worth drawing together some of the strands noted above relating to reasonable accommodation, since in combination they raise issues of potential interest to anti-stigma activists. As noted above, some matters of reasonable accommodation may be implemented at a systemic level and ought to become a matter of routine. An obvious example is the provision of easy-read versions of documents, including government policy documents and guidance. Legislation can be introduced to make similar versions available for significant documents in the private sector, such as leases and standard form contracts. Such routine reasonable accommodations can allow people with disabilities to take greater control of their lives and be much more active in the community. This sort of measure is consistent with the objectives of the anti-stigma movement and should be widely embraced by it.

In many cases, however, reasonable accommodations will be much less general and may indeed be person-specific. The accommodations that will be necessary to allow persons with mental disabilities to hold down a specific job, for example, may well depend on the specific nature of the individual's personal situation and the job in question. These may further vary over time and sometimes over a relatively short space of time. The accommodations reached may clash with the needs of the remainder of the relevant group (e.g. the rest of the employees) or indeed with other people with disabilities. Thus a student with autistic spectrum disorder or a similar mental disability may require a relaxed atmosphere in the classroom, without bright lights and distracting images. That may or may not be consistent with best practice for the remainder of the class. It may directly conflict with the needs of a person with a disability related to vision, who may require bright and contrasting colours to see what is in the classroom.

This raises a variety of questions. First, how can reasonable accommodations be made in individual circumstances, when those circumstances may not be static over time? Related to this is the question of how far the accommodations are to be made to allow the individual to mould himself or herself to the job, and how much it is appropriate to require job descriptions to be changed to meet the individual circumstances of people with disabilities? Insofar as the latter is involved – and it is difficult to see that we will see meaningful success if it is not, at least to some degree – numerous practical problems arise. As a legal question, how are those expectations to be identified? Phrases such as 'not imposing a disproportionate or undue burden' may be fine for international conventions, but it does not really provide much concrete guidance to an employer. Even when the expectations are agreed with the person with disabilities, they may nonetheless affect the interests of other employees, whose job descriptions may have to change to incorporate the aspects of the job that have been removed from the person with disabilities. These other employees may or may not be sympathetic to this. Such changes are not impossible. They have occurred, for example, relating to pregnancy and maternity leave, where in many countries and many workplaces, mechanisms to ensure that the work gets done have been successfully implemented, and the remainder of the workforce has accepted these measures (with or without good grace). There is a stigma question that arises, however, as to how this process is managed without the individual with disabilities being stigmatised, and, once again, whether the objective of the anti-stigma movement favours assimilating people with disabilities based on the traits they share with the broader public or developing a society that can accommodate their differences.

Conclusion: Human Rights, Stigma and Greater Forces

In the end, so many of the questions of implementation of human rights and viability of anti-stigma campaigns flow from greater factors related to politics and economics. In much of the world, where there is a long history of long-term institutionalisation of people with mental disabilities, established orthodoxies, often supported by large professional and bureaucratic systems and significant infrastructures, need to be challenged, and these can be remarkably resistant to change. The image is of turning a supertanker. In other parts of the world, there is no such institutional history. Often, these are economically poorer parts of the world, however, where there is little express tradition of providing systematic services for people with disabilities at all. Here, the image is of building services from the ground up, but in an environment where there is little by way of services for any segment of the population and where within the extremely limited provision available, services for people with disability always seem to be a priority for some vague time in the future. These issues apply to both human rights implementation and the furthering of the anti-stigma agenda: the working environment and the impediments to progress are remarkably similar.

The CRPD, like the anti-stigma movement, requires us to ask some fundamental questions about how society works, not just for people with disabilities, but for us all. At the core of this is the relationship between the person with disability and society. When is it that disability makes a real difference that must be provided for? What benefits should be limited to people with disabilities, and what should be available as a matter of right to all citizens, including those with disabilities? Should our societies welcome the diversity of people with disabilities, or expect people with disabilities to fit in? And who do we implement relevant policies without stigmatizing the person we are trying to help?

These are complex questions, with political, legal, economic, social policy and other aspects. The CRPD imports a particular gravitas to its terms: as international law, it is meant to be followed by the nations that have signed and ratified it. Nonetheless, there is much to do in figuring out how to implement it even at an intellectual level. Bringing about meaningful change on the ground will be a long slog – there is no point in pretending the contrary.

References

Bartlett P (2012) The United Nations Convention on the rights of persons with disabilities and mental health law. Mod Law Rev 75(5):752–778

Churchill R, Owen G, Singh S. Hothopf M (2007) International experiences of using community treatment orders. King's College London, London

Dawson J, Szmukler G (2006) Fusion of mental health and incapacity legislation. Br Med J 188:504

Horne J, Richardon G (eds) (2010) A model law fusing incapacity and mental health legislation – is it viable; is it advisable? J Mental Health Law (Being a special issue 20)

Kayess R, French P (2008) Out of darkness into light? Introducing the convention on the rights of persons with disabilities. HRLRev 8:1 at 29

Kisely S, Campbell LA, Preston N (2005) Compulsory community and involuntary outpatient treatment for people with severe mental disorders (Review). Cochrane Library (3)

Lawson A (2006–2007) The United Nations Convention on the rights of persons with disabilities: new era or false dawn? Syracuse J Int'l Law Com 34:563 at 593–595

MacKay D (2006–2007) The United Nations Convention on the rights of persons with disabilities. Syracuse. J Int'l Law Com 34:323–331

Mégret F. (2008) The disabilities convention: human rights of persons with disabilities or disability rights? Hum Rights Q 30:494 at 507

Priebe S et al (2011) Predictors of clinical and social outcomes following involuntary hospital admissions. Eur Arch Psychiatry Clin Neurosci 261:377

Quinn G (2009) Brining the UN Convention on rights for persons with disabilities to live in Ireland. Br J Learn Disab 37:245 at 247

Rees N (2010) The fusion proposal: a next step?. In: McSherry B, Weller P (eds). Rethinking rights-based mental health laws. Hart, Oxford

Statement of Kofi Annan, United Nations Secretary-General, on the occasion of the passage of the UN Convention on the Rights of Persons with Disabilities, 13 December 2006. Full text available at http://www.un.org/News/Press/docs//2006/sgsm10797.doc.htm. Accessed 25 Nov 2014

UN High Commissioner for Human Rights, Annual Report, A/HRC/10/48 (2009) at [48], CRPD Committee, CRPD Committee, Statement on article 14 of the Convention on the Rights of Persons with Disabilities, September 2014. Available at: http://www.ohchr.org/EN/NewsEvents/Pages/DisplayNews.aspx?NewsID=15183&LangID=E. Accessed 17 Nov 2014

United Nations A/Res/61/106 (general assembly, 24 January 2007). The full text of the CRPD may be found at http://www.un.org/disabilities/default.asp?id=199. Accessed 25 Nov 2014

Weller P (2008) Supported decision-making and the achievement of non-discrimination: the promise and paradox of the disabilities convention. In: McSherry B (ed), International trends in mental health law. Federation Press, Sydney, pp 85 at 89

Part II

"Fighting" Stigma and Discrimination:
Programs in Different Parts of the World

Opening Doors: The Global Programme to Fight Stigma and Discrimination Because of Schizophrenia

13

Heather Stuart and Norman Sartorius

Prior to the 1990s, anti-stigma interventions did not receive much research attention. While there was considerable theoretical literature, dating back to the mid-1950s, little in the way of evidence-based anti-stigma practice had emerged (Sartorius and Stuart 2009). At a time when the majority of people with serious mental illnesses were segregated in large mental hospitals, and when social psychiatry was in its infancy, community-based stigmatization may not have seemed like a priority for researchers or funders. In addition, early failed efforts to reduce stigma (Cumming and Cumming 1957) may have inadvertently left a legacy of negativism. Comprehensive stigma-reduction strategies may have seemed beyond the abilities of many health professionals to undertake, or perhaps the social consequences of mental illnesses were outside of the field of vision of mental health providers and systems. The belief that developments in neurosciences would ultimately eliminate mental illnesses meant there would be little need to provide robust funding for the social determinants and consequences of mental illnesses. Indeed, it was not until the 1960s and 1970s that we had the first comprehensive international study to examine the cultural effects on the appearance and course of schizophrenia (Sartorius et al. 1972).

In 1996, the World Psychiatric Association, under the leadership of one of us (Norman Sartorius, then president of WPA), initiated an international programme to fight stigma caused by schizophrenia. It was subsequently implemented in over 20 countries resulting in over 200 interventions. While not all of these interventions

H. Stuart (✉)
Centre for Health Services and Policy Research, Queen's University, 21 Arch Street, Room 324B, Abramsky Hall, Kingston, ON K7L 3 N6, Canada

Department of Public Health Sciences, Mental Health Commission of Canada, Ottawa, ON, Canada
e-mail: heather.stuart@queensu.ca

N. Sartorius
Association for the Improvement of Mental Health Programmes, Geneva, Switzerland
e-mail: sartorius@normansartorius.com

© Springer International Publishing Switzerland 2017
W. Gaebel et al. (eds.), *The Stigma of Mental Illness - End of the Story?*,
DOI 10.1007/978-3-319-27839-1_13

were formally evaluated, many were. This chapter describes the 'Open the Doors' programme and reviews the lessons learned from these various activities in the countries participating in the programme and others that were stimulated by them for improving practices in the field of stigma reduction (see supplement for a description of additional programmes that were developed in small and midsize countries in Europe (Beldie et al. 2012)).

Unless otherwise referenced, material in this chapter is based on Sartorius and Schulze (2005). Additional materials may be found in Arboleda-Flórez and Sartorius (2008) and Stuart et al. (2012).

First Steps

In preparation for a large international anti-stigma programme, a large group of experts from some 20 countries met in Geneva to discuss stigma and how best to address it. The goals of the programme were (i) to examine the nature of stigma and its consequences in different sociocultural settings and (ii) to develop methods that could be used to reduce or prevent it. A strategic consideration was based on the recognition that there was insufficient data describing the scope and magnitude of stigma from the perspective of those who are stigmatized—patients and their families. Therefore, the programme placed high priority on surveying individuals living with mental illnesses and their family members about their experiences of prejudice and discrimination and where possible, encouraged their active participation. The experts planning the programme also recognized that stigma was pervasive and socially derived and that it was therefore necessary to encourage broad participation of experts and other stakeholders in the programme. Stigma reduction was not to be the purview of a single group but would include members of healthcare organizations, governments, private enterprises and those who had experienced stigma first hand. Finally, the group recognized that stigma reduction would be a long haul effort, perhaps taking generations of interventions. Therefore, stigma reduction was conceptualized as an effort to create the basis and the motivation to initiate long-term programmes in participating countries and in others that might wish to benefit from the evidence and the methods developed by the Open the Doors programme.

Three subcommittees were established to develop tools and manuals that could be used to (a) identify best practices in the treatment of schizophrenia, (b) undertake action that would help to integrate individuals in society and (c) start national or local programmes to prevent or reduce stigma and/or its consequences. Members of the expert group produced a volume on schizophrenia, written in the form of a single easily readable and widely accessible review of knowledge that could serve all the participating countries and could be easily translated step-by-step guide for implementing an anti-stigma programme. The manual stressed the need to facilitate the work of the local action groups, to set measurable goals and objectives and to identify opportunities to start local programmes.

Funding to help in the coordination of the programme came from an unrestricted educational grant from Eli Lilly Foundation. Local programmes were funded with local grants and in kind resources from existing services, though considerable work was completed by volunteers.

Several features of the Open the Doors programme made it different from all other programmes developed to deal with stigma. These included (a) the collaboration of a large number of developed and developing countries, (b) the emphasis on the promotion of local action and the creation of a structure for further work against stigma, and (c) the involvement of a variety of community and national partners. The involvement of scientists and world leading experts in the field of stigma reduction helped the exchange of knowledge across the centres and the better resolution of problems arising locally. International meetings and academic congresses were spawned to provide a more formal forum for knowledge exchange. The academic conferences continue to this day. The inaugural *Together Against Stigma International Conference* was held by the members of that programme in Leipzig (Germany) in 2001 with the aim of fostering multidisciplinary interest in anti-stigma programmes—breaking down the silos between disciplines and driving efforts from theory into practice. Open the Doors members then organized a second conference in Kingston (Canada) in 2003. In 2005, the World Psychiatric Association's General Assembly ratified the creation of a scientific section devoted to the prevention and reduction of stigma related to mental illness. Since that time, the section has coordinated international work related to the fight against stigma and organized, in collaboration with local associations and institutions, *Together Against Stigma International Conferences* in Istanbul (Turkey) in 2006, in London (United Kingdom) in 2009, in Ottawa (Canada) in 2012, in Tokyo (Japan) in 2013 and in San Francisco in 2015. The *Together Against Stigma* conferences bring together researchers, mental health professionals, policymakers, members of the media and persons with lived experience to present results of effective interventions aimed at the reduction of stigma of mental illnesses and to develop collaboration between all concerned for further work in this field.

Conceptual Framework

Many of the conceptual models available in the literature that could inform the programme were highly theoretical and a poor guide for public health action. For the Open the Doors programme, the elements of these models were synthesized into a series of interrelated cycles that described the progression of stigma for the individual, the family and mental health programmes. Figure 13.1 illustrates the cycle of stigmatization for the individual (Sartorius and Schulze 2005). It shows a marker (in this case a mental illness) that sets the individual apart from the group. The marker becomes socially salient and emotionally loaded, resulting in stigmatizing attitudes and discriminatory behaviour by those surrounding the person with the marker. This leads to social disadvantage and marginalization, which negatively affects the individual's self-esteem, causing greater disability and diminished stigma resistance.

Similar cycles occur for the family and for mental health programmes (Sartorius and Schulze 2005). The cycle of stigmatization experienced by the family begins with their experiencing shame, guilt and worry. This reduces family reserves and

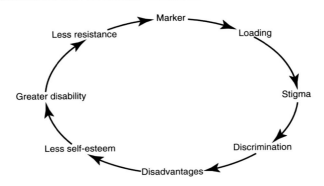

Fig. 13.1 Cycle of stigmatization for the individual

lessens the social support that can be provided to the ill family member. With fewer social supports, there is less possibility for recovery and greater social disadvantage. This increases stress and the possibility of family burnout, increasing the chances that the illness will re-emerge or be prolonged. At the programmatic level, mental health programmes and patients are stigmatized, resulting in a poor reputation (compared to other services), lack of or reduced funding, resulting in deteriorating services, poorer quality of staff, lack of productivity and poor overall quality of care. These cycles reinforce stereotypes, increase cynicism among the public and diminish the hopes of those living with a mental illness that they can improve and recover.

The models described proved to be of pragmatic value and helped to highlight the important and disabling effect of stigma. More importantly, however, they indicated points around which an anti-stigma programme might take as a target for its work and thus interrupt the process. The use of the model made it clear that it is possible to fight stigma at several access points and that therefore there is no one that could not contribute to fighting stigma and its consequences.

Programme Approach

The programme targeted the stigma associated with schizophrenia, rather than mental illnesses in general. The stigma attached to schizophrenia was considered to be greater than other more prevalent disorders such as depression or anxiety. Moreover, when the public thinks of 'mental illness', they often describe symptoms and behaviours that are indicative of schizophrenia. The selection of a well-defined target made it easier to design and implement programmes. In addition, the WPA expert steering group considered that any gains made in reducing the stigma of schizophrenia could be usefully applied to fight stigma related to other mental disorders or indeed stigma related to characteristics of population subgroups (e.g. those of a different race, religion). Targeting the programme to a specific disorder group also made the programme activities simpler to conduct and explain and made the evaluation more focused and easier to implement. The focus on schizophrenia also made it possible to work with community advocacy groups and non-governmental organizations that focused on schizophrenia.

Open the Doors was built on the recognition that the commitment of a small group of people working at the local level would be the key to success. The support of institutions and governments would be helpful but not sufficient to create sustainable change. Thus, the programme recruited countries where a small group of individuals were willing to lead an anti-stigma programme and maintain activities over years. These 'action groups' were expected to be small and based on volunteer labour. They were to meet often and discuss how best to develop a programme. It was also recommended that they have a larger advisory committee that would include individuals of influence who could assist the programme but who would not be involved in the day-to-day activities.

Originally, the International Expert Group that met in 1996 thought that it would be useful to develop a set of specific plans that could then be offered to local action groups—a smorgasbord of potential activities along with timelines. However, it soon became obvious that it would be easier and more effective if local action groups were invited to develop activities based on their own local needs. This became one of the most successful hallmarks of the programme and allowed for a much broader range of activities than originally envisioned.

To assess local needs, action groups were encouraged to canvass people with schizophrenia and their family members to identify their priorities. This exploration typically resulted in a long list of problems, some of which were related to stigma and some of which were not. Then, groups targeted programme interventions to those problems that could be resolved relatively quickly—success of such actions being recognized as a powerful incentive for further work. More difficult to resolve problems were reserved for later in the life of the programme, as the programme's momentum and successes began to build.

Because programmes were encouraged to address local needs, interventions were not standardized across sites. This proved to be an advantage as it allowed programme participants to learn about the success of a wider array of interventions than originally envisioned. In addition, local programmes targeting local priorities were much more likely to gain local support. This enhanced sustainability and effectiveness of local efforts. People who were working with the programmes knew that they were addressing important local needs.

Pilot Testing

Beginning in 1977, three locations in Alberta, Canada (Edmonton, Calgary and Drumheller), started work serving as pilot sites for the global programme. The Canadian action group included 28 members who worked in smaller task groups over an 18-month period. Members came from a broad range of organizations, including hospitals, universities, community treatment programmes, community advocacy groups, governments, the media, local service experts, people with schizophrenia and family members. Many of these groups had not previously worked together and some had worked at cross purposes. The local anti-stigma programme gave them an important common ground and helped them coordinate activities in more cost-effective ways.

In order to provide the best possible evidence to other countries joining the global initiative, the goal of the Canadian programme was to undertake as many different activities as possible, evaluate their effects and understand what worked and what did not.

Based on the combined experience of the local action group, several target groups were identified: healthcare professionals in a variety of settings (including emergency rooms and universities), youth (grades 9–11) and community change agents (such as journalists, clergy and business leaders). In addition, the group planned an education campaign that targeted anti-stigma messages through mass media to the general public. Group members were less convinced that a mass media campaign would be useful but considered it would be important to test and evaluate this approach to empirically assess its usefulness.

Scaling Up

The programme was scaled up to other countries in two phases (see Table 13.1). Australia and New Zealand had existing active programmes so they were not included in the Open the Doors sites but were considered to be collaborating centres. In addition, China and Russia who were originally included among target countries could not be included for local reasons.

Table 13.1 Countries with Open-the-Door sites

Phase	Country
Phase I—pilot programme	Canada
Phase II	Spain
	Austria
Phase III	Germany
	Italy
	Greece
	United States
	Poland
	Japan
Phase IV	Slovakia
	Turkey
	Brazil
	Egypt
	Morocco
	United Kingdom
	Chile
	India
	Romania

Table 13.2 Target groups across 18 countries

Target group	Total
General practitioners and other healthcare professionals	15
Primary or secondary school students	13
Journalists and the media	13
Psychiatrists and mental health providers	12
People with schizophrenia	11
Family members and friends	11
General public	11
Religious communities and clergy	6
Government workers and non-governmental agencies	5
Businesses and employers	5
Medical students	3
Judicial and law enforcement officials and lawyers	2

The approach taken in Spain was particularly instructive for countries where the general public had little knowledge of schizophrenia, where self-reported discrimination was low and where a large public education campaign might increase stigma. The Spanish local action committee targeted the people closest to those with the illness—family members and health providers. Subsequently, nine of the countries with the lowest gross domestic product and the fewest psychiatrists per capita used this model to target family members for intervention and support.

Seven countries used focus groups to identify the priorities of people with schizophrenia and family members so that they could identify relevant target groups and/or define key messages. Four dimensions of stigma were elucidated: interpersonal interaction, structural discrimination, public images of mental illness and access to social roles. Of note is the fact that only one dimension (interpersonal interaction) refers to the stigma experienced during day-to-day social interactions. The remaining dimensions all pertained to structural barriers that are built into social organizations. Thus, for example, people living with schizophrenia often identified access to social roles (such as employment) as the most significant dimension of stigma, whereas mental health professionals identified negative public imagery as most important. Family members were most concerned about structural discrimination. Thus, for example, one of the early activities of the programme was the effort to change the behaviour or general healthcare staff dealing with physical illness of people with schizophrenia. The selection of this activity as a first target (instead of others originally envisaged by the action group) did not only achieve a significant change in the life of people with schizophrenia and their carers but also enhanced the willingness of users and family groups to take an active role in the programme. These results highlighted the importance of identifying anti-stigma priorities from the perspective of the target group chosen, as well as the importance of allowing people with schizophrenia to set priorities that are important to them. An example of results of a focus group study (conducted in Leipzig, Germany) can be found in Schulze and Angermeyer (2003).

Table 13.3 Interventions and activities (as of 2003; 18 countries)

Intervention/activity	Total
Survey of knowledge/attitudes	14
Publications in newspapers/magazines	14
Publications in scientific journals	13
Speaker bureau	12
Education for other health professionals	12
Education for journalists	11
Radio programmes	10
Television programmes	10
Primary/secondary education	9
Education for psychiatrists	9
Education for families	8
Education for general practitioners	7
Stigma watch/stigma busting	6
Art presentations/competitions	6
Education for clergy	5
Anti-stigma awards	5
Theatre/dramatic presentations	4
Story workshops	3
Other	10

Table 13.3 shows the interventions and activities that were undertaken across the 18 countries. Nearly half of the interventions involved education programmes targeting students, healthcare providers, media or other professionals. Also, most local action groups were able to generate press coverage and contribute results of surveys and focus groups to the scientific literature. Almost half of the countries also generated some form of cultural event, such as a play, poetry reading, film project or concert. In some countries, such as Spain and Greece, cultural events were given added profile by high-ranking public or religious officials who also attended. Having a member of the targeted group participate in the local action group facilitated success.

Lessons Learned from Opening the Doors

Formal evaluation and critical reflection on the Open the Doors global programme resulted in a number of lessons learned that can be offered as recommendations for programme development:

1. The programme has to be long lasting. Campaigns, reflecting short bursts of activity, will not unseat deeply held misconceptions and prejudices. To be long lasting, anti-stigma programmes must become part of existing systems; a routine part of health and social service responses to the dilemmas caused by mental illnesses.
2. Programme goals must have local relevance in order to retain interested people and local support.

3. To be effective, the programme must deal with the problems experienced by those who have a mental illness and their family members. Focus groups and surveys were invaluable tools in identifying the needs and priorities of target groups, which differed considerably in their perspectives. Programme developers should not assume that they know what should be done.

4. Because many of the barriers faced by people with a mental illness and their family members are structural, anti-stigma programmes must reach beyond the mental healthcare systems to enlist the participation of a broader community.

5. Anti-stigma programmes should employ people who have had first-hand experience with mental illnesses and their associated stigma.

6. Programmes must rest on a theory of change that links the activities to the outcomes in some logical way. The model used by the WPA showed vicious cycles of stigma occurring at various levels. It has the advantage of offering multiple entry points and supports a broad base of partners.

7. Programmes should plan for sustainability and actively work towards reducing burnout of leaders and volunteers. Giving recognition of achievements and celebrating even small successes is important.

8. In addition to electronic communications, programmes need to invest in face-to-face encounters and knowledge translation through attendance at scientific meetings.

9. The programme has to develop tools to facilitate new members joining the programme and also to facilitate the replication of successful interventions.

The most important finding of the Open the Doors programme was (a) that it had demonstrated that anti-stigma activities can be launched in any country, including those which can only invest minimal resources, and (b) that a devoted small group of people—often composed of community volunteers—is central to the progress in anti-stigma work.

References

Arboleda-Florez J, Sartorius N (eds) (2008) Understanding the stigma of mental illness: theory and interventions. Wiley, Chichester

Beldie A, den Boer J, Brain C, Constant E, Figueira M, Filipcic I et al (2012) Fighting stigma of mental illness in midsize European countries. Soc Psychiatry Psychiatr Epidemiol 47(Suppl 1):1–38

Cumming E, Cumming J (1957) Closed ranks: an experiment in mental health education. Harvard University Press, Cambridge, MA

Sartorius N, Schulze H (2005) Reducing the stigma of mental illness: a report from the global programme of the World Psychiatric Association. Cambridge University Press, Cambridge, UK

Sartorius N, Stuart H (2009) Stigma of mental disorders and consequent discrimination. Kor J Schizophr Res 12(1):5–9

Sartorius N, Shapiro R, Kimura M, Barrett K (1972) WHO international pilot study of schizophrenia. Psychol Med 2(4):422–425

Schulze B, Angermeyer MC (2003) Subjective experiences of stigma. A focus group study of schizophrenic patients, their relatives and mental health professionals. Soc Sci Med 56:299–312

Stuart H, Arboleda-Florez J, Sartorius N (2012) Paradigms lost: fighting stigma and the lessons learned. Oxford University Press, Oxford

Fighting Stigma in Canada: Opening Minds Anti-Stigma Initiative

14

Shu-Ping Chen, Keith Dobson, Bonnie Kirsh,
Stephanie Knaak, Michelle Koller, Terry Krupa,
Bianca Lauria-Horner, Dorothy Luong, Geeta Modgill,
Scott Patten, Michael Pietrus, Heather Stuart, Rob Whitley,
and Andrew Szeto

S.-P. Chen
Centre of Health Services and Policy Research, Mental Health Commission of Canada,
Ottawa, ON, Canada

K. Dobson
Department of Psychology, University of Calgary, Calgary, AB, Canada

B. Kirsh
Department of Occupational Science and Occupational Therapy,
University of Toronto, Toronto, ON, Canada

S. Knaak
Department of Community Health and Epidemiology, Mental Health Commission of Canada,
Ottawa, ON, Canada

M. Koller
Centre for Health Services and Policy Research, Queen's University, Kingston, ON, Canada
Department of Community Health and Epidemiology, Mental Health Commission of Canada,
Ottawa, ON, Canada

T. Krupa
School of Rehabilitation Therapy, Queen's University, Kingston, ON, Canada

B. Lauria-Horner
Department of Psychiatry, Dalhousie University, Halifax, NS, Canada

D. Luong
Department of Occupational Therapy, University of Toronto, Toronto, ON, Canada

G. Modgill • M. Pietrus (✉)
Mental Health Commission of Canada, Ottawa, ON, Canada
e-mail: mpietrus@mentalhealthcommission.ca

S. Patten
Departments of Community Health Sciences and Psychiatry, Mental Health Commission of
Canada, Ottawa, ON, Canada

© Springer International Publishing Switzerland 2017
W. Gaebel et al. (eds.), *The Stigma of Mental Illness - End of the Story?*,
DOI 10.1007/978-3-319-27839-1_14

237

H. Stuart
Department of Public Health Sciences, Mental Health Commission of Canada, Ottawa, ON, Canada

Centre for Health Services and Policy Research, Queen's University, Kingston, ON, Canada

R. Whitley
Department of Psychiatry, McGill University, Montréal, QC, Canada

A. Szeto
Department of Psychology, University of Calgary, Calgary, AB, Canada

The Opening Minds Anti-Stigma Initiative

Mental illnesses continue to gain awareness as a global health problem. Within this international context, Canada has also paid closer attention to mental illnesses and their related stigma. The Mental Health Commission of Canada was formed in 2007 as a federal government initiative to be a catalyst for improving the mental health system. Since then, the Commission has examined the many ways in which people living with mental illnesses are viewed in society and devised a series of initiatives to enhance and improve Canada's treatment of people who live with mental illnesses. One initiative is the Opening Minds initiative, whose mandate is to change Canadians' attitudes and behaviors toward people living with mental illnesses to ensure they are treated fairly, as full citizens with equal opportunities to contribute to society (see Stuart et al. 2014a, b).

Opening Minds has taken a unique targeted approach. Building on the emerging international research at the time, we focused on programs using contact-based education as their key intervention approach. Contact-based education involves people with lived experience of a mental illness sharing their personal recovery stories. It is one of the most promising strategies in the evidence-based literature for stigma reduction (Corrigan et al. 2012), particularly when Allport's (1954) four optimal contact conditions are observed (i.e., equal status, cooperation, work toward a common goal, support from authorities) (Couture and Penn 2003; Pettigrew and Tropp 2006, 2008). Contact-based approaches are thought to lead to stigma reduction through such pathways as disconfirming stereotypes, diminished anxiety, heightened empathy, creating personal connections, and improving understanding (e.g., see Blascovich et al. 2001; Corrigan 2000; Corrigan et al. 2001; Couture and Penn 2003; Pettigrew and Tropp 2008).

Our initial target groups were youth and healthcare providers, and we reached out to organizations across the country to identify existing anti-stigma programs for these groups. We committed to evaluating programs to determine which ones were effective, with the goal of sharing new knowledge about key components and replicating successful programs as broadly as possible. A research team of academics from different universities was created, research associates were hired, and survey tools were developed to measure success related to stigma reduction for these different target groups. Subsequently, two additional targets were added: news media and the workforce. More than 100 active partners have been involved in this research to date. With much of the research now complete, particularly for youth and healthcare providers, we are able to share promising practice information and replicate successful programs. The purpose of this chapter is to provide an overview of the activities in each of the target groups, providing key examples of how teams have worked to identify best practices.

Approach to Stigma Reduction

We understand stigma as a complex social process involving labeling, stereotyping, separation, status loss, and discrimination (Link and Phelan 2001), rather than a mark of shame that an individual bears (Goffman 1963). As awareness of the effects of stigma has increased, anti-stigma work has gained momentum. Public campaigns have been used to raise awareness and spread counter-attitudinal messages to combat misconceptions about mental illnesses, and social media tools have helped to widen the reach of positive messages. However, these messages are often broad, short in duration, and restricted by context (e.g., print media) and may not have the desired impact (Sartorius 2010; Stuart et al. 2012, Stuart et al. 2014a, b, c). For example, a recent review of workplace anti-stigma programs (Szeto and Dobson 2010) suggests that knowledge and information learned from particular public anti-stigma campaigns are often tied to the context in which they were learned and that some campaigns have low public awareness (Gaebel et al. 2008). In other words, some people are not even aware that these messages exist, let alone what these messages are. Further, the individuals who attend to the campaign and learn positive and counter-stereotypic portrayals of mental illnesses may not necessarily apply these ideas to other contexts. For example, positive messages about supporting friends with mental illnesses may not be carried over to the workplace to support coworkers who may be experiencing a mental illness. To amplify the effect of anti-stigma programs, contextually specific interventions need to be implemented (Szeto and Dobson 2010).

Target Group: Youth

Youth are an important and strategic target for anti-stigma activities because of their high prevalence of mental ill health. For example, in a large 24 country study, the World Health Organization (1996) reports that Canadian youth ($n = 6758$) are among the most likely to report feeling low or depressed once a week or more. Among 11-year-olds, a quarter of boys and 27 % of girls reported depression (seventh rank among 23 countries). Among 13-year-olds, Canada ranked eighth, with 22 % among boys and 32 % among girls. Finally, among 15-year-olds, Canada ranked sixth, with 25 % among boys and 39 % among girls (World Health Organization 1996). Waddell et al. (2005) reports that epidemiologic studies conducted in countries such as Canada, the UK, and the USA have found that 14 % of children aged 4–17 have clinically important mental disorders at any given time. Moreover, when less disabling disorders are taken into account, the prevalence rises to 20 %. Over half of those children with a disorder have two or more disorders at the same time and less than 25 % receive specialized treatment services.

The high prevalence of mental health problems among youth, particularly the high prevalence of untreated disorders, means that young people may be at increased risk of experiencing mental health-related stigma. Indeed, recent research examining a national sample of Canadians ($n = 10{,}389$) has demonstrated that youth (aged 12–25) who received treatment for a mental health problem in the year prior to the survey were more likely to report being stigmatized as a result of a current or past mental or emotional problem. These results support the need for anti-stigma programs that target youth (Stuart et al. 2014c).

Toward this end, Opening Minds has partnered with more than 20 anti-stigma programs across Canada that regularly provide in-class contact-based education to youth in middle and high schools. Contact-based education in this context occurs when someone who has experienced a mental illness tells a personal story to the students and engages them in a question and answer period. In a recent meta-analysis, Corrigan and colleagues reported a statistically significant adjusted mean effect size of 0.457 (corresponding to a medium effect) for contact-based education in eight studies targeting adolescents, the highest effect size reported for any method of intervention, with little heterogeneity across studies (Corrigan et al. 2012).

Preliminary investigation showed that most programs in Canada targeting youth had not been formally evaluated so their effectiveness was unknown. Also, while staff in many of these programs regularly collected pre- and posttest data, they often did not have the expertise or resources to regularly analyze the data or ensure that findings were reported in the scientific literature where they could be used to support policy developments. To build on these grass roots initiatives and more clearly identify promising and best practices, Opening Minds funded a series of evaluation projects as the first phase of our national anti-stigma strategy (Stuart et al. 2014a).

The data collection instruments used by the various programs were unstandardized and had not been psychometrically tested. Thus, one of the first challenges was to develop and test an appropriate measure that could be used by all programs (Stuart et al. 2014b). A pool of items was generated from the existing instruments used by the programs, with additions from the literature when there were gaps related to important concepts. A draft survey was circulated to all of the programs for review and comment. A revised survey was recirculated to all programs and tested on a youth focus group. Final revisions were made; items were reworded to meet the Flesch-Kincaid reading level for sixth grade, and graphic elements were added to make the survey visually appealing.

The revised survey was field tested on approximately 600 students. Preliminary factor analysis indicated that two 11-point scales were present – one measured stereotypic content (controllability of the illness, potential for recovery, and potential for violence and unpredictability) and the other measured social acceptance (feelings of social distance and feelings of social responsibility for mental health issues). Items on the social acceptance scale are reflective of behavioral intent, which in turn is often considered to be a proxy for behavioral outcomes (albeit an imperfect one). The reliability coefficients (Cronbach's alpha) were 0.79 for the Stereotype Scale and 0.85 for the Social Acceptance Scale. Table 14.1 shows the items that were retained. A complete copy of the pre- and posttest surveys is contained in the Opening Minds Interim Report (Pietrus 2013).

Using these newly tested instruments, program partners have now collected data on approximately 10,000 school children in grades 7–12 from various parts of Canada, including one school in the far north. The schools were not purposefully selected; rather they were already receiving contact-based education and agreed to work with the research team to evaluate the results. Though data collection varied somewhat depending on the program, typically pretest data were collected approximately 2 weeks before the intervention and immediately afterward. Follow-up and comparison data were not collected as it proved to be too logistically difficult for these programs and schools.

Table 14.1 Survey items

Stereotype scale	
1	Most people with a mental illness are too disabled to work
2	People with a mental illness tend to bring it on themselves
3	People with mental illnesses often do not try hard enough to get better
4	People with a mental illness could snap out of it if they wanted to
5	People with a mental illness are often more dangerous than the average person
6	People with a mental illness often become violent if not treated
7	Most violent crimes are committed by people with a mental illness
8	You cannot rely on someone with a mental illness
9	You can never know what someone with a mental illness is going to do
10	Most people with a mental illness get what they deserve
11	People with a serious mental illness need to be locked away
Social acceptance scale	
1	I would be upset if someone with a mental illness always sat next to me in class
2	I would not be close friends with someone I knew had a mental illness
3	I would visit a classmate in hospital if they had a mental illness
4	I would try to avoid someone with a mental illness
5	I would not mind it if someone with a mental illness lived next door to me
6	If I knew someone had a mental illness I would not date them
7	I would not want to be taught by a teacher who had been treated for a mental illness
8	I would tell a teacher if a student was being bullied because of their mental illness
9	I would stick up for someone who had a mental illness if they were being teased
10	I would tutor a classmate who got behind in their studies because of their mental illness
11	I would volunteer my time to work in a program for people with a mental illness

Results were initially analyzed using the standard differences of means for matched data. However, this obscured many important item-specific differences that had relevance for program planning and delivery and left the research team with no clear threshold for judging what constituted a meaningful success. After much discussion with the Opening Minds investigators and the program partners, an a priori cutoff of 80 % correct (meaning non-stigmatizing) answers was chosen as the threshold for determining overall program success. All agreed that 80 % was a meaningful threshold for an educational intervention. The proportions of students who met or exceeded this threshold were compared before and after the contact-based education.

Figure 14.1 illustrates this analysis using results from one program. It shows the cumulative percent of the Stereotype Scale items that reflected a non-stigmatizing response. It shows observable improvements in the posttest score beginning where students got at least four items correct, and the posttest improvement increases steadily over the remaining items. In this example, 29 % of the students gave a non-stigmatizing response to 9 of the 11 stereotype items (reflecting 80 % correct) prior to the intervention. Following the intervention, this increased to 57 %, reflecting a 28 % improvement overall. When item scores were aggregated to reflect a scale value out of 55 (where a high score reflects high stigma), the average (median) difference was much less dramatic and difficult to interpret. It dropped from 24 to 21, reflecting a 5 % drop in the scale score.

Differences on the Social Acceptance Scale (not shown here) were typically smaller across most programs, indicating that it was easier to change stigmatizing attitudes than intended behaviors. In the program depicted in Fig. 14.1, for example,

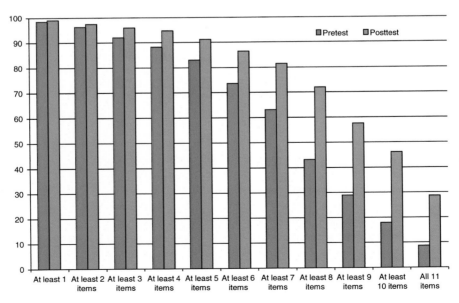

Fig. 14.1 Cumulative percent of stereotype scale items reflecting a non-stigmatizing response ($N = 376$)

47 % of students reached the 80 % threshold on the Social Acceptance Scale prior to the intervention and this increased to 57 % following the intervention, reflecting a 10 % improvement overall.

Figure 14.2 shows the proportion of students who exceeded the 80 % threshold of success across the 27 separate interventions offered by the programs with the Stereotype Scale.

The bars show the different baseline levels of stereotypic thinking (as reflected by the stereotype scale) at pretest, as well as the variability of success across interventions at posttest. The first four interventions experienced some of the largest gains, whereas interventions 23–27 were among the smallest. These results suggest that there are critical ingredients that must be implemented in order to maximize program effectiveness. They further suggest that fidelity criteria would be helpful to promote best practices in contact-based education. Mowbray and colleagues (2003) indicate that the development and use of fidelity criteria should be an expected component of quality evaluation and practice, especially in the mental health field where programs often lack model specification and rely heavily on clinical knowledge and skill.

According to Mowbray et al. (2003), the first step in creating fidelity criteria is to develop critical components of a program model, and this is often done using a process of expert consensus instead of more in-depth qualitative investigation. We conducted a qualitative study of 18 programs to produce a detailed description of the critical program elements resulting in a logic model. Representatives from each program were interviewed, including three speakers and one family member. One investigator observed several of the programs as they delivered their interventions. Detailed discussions were also held with program representatives when they reviewed their quantitative evaluation results. Based on this information, a detailed logic model was developed describing key

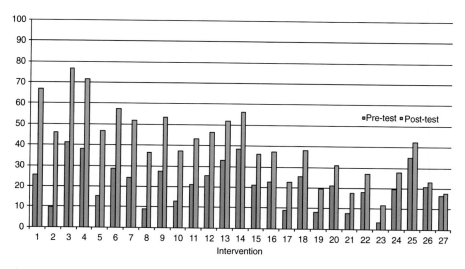

Fig. 14.2 Students meeting the 80 % threshold of success by program ($N\sim10,000$)

inputs (or program structures) that need to be in place and the key processes determining the way in which contact-based education can best be delivered (Chen et al. 2014). The resulting model was focus group tested with representatives of each program and revised accordingly. Therefore, the logic model is based on both expert opinion and qualitative research.

Regarding program inputs, the most successful programs had secure funding, had spent considerable time building their intervention team, had a strong relationship with the schools or school boards, and had actively maintained this relationship. In addition, they spent considerable time training and preparing their speakers and had worked out an efficient way of coordinating their activities.

With respect to processes, the most successful programs had engaged speakers who were living well with their illness; had good public speaking skills; were comfortable sharing their personal recovery stories in an open, confident, and genuine way; and acted as a role model for the students, thus normalizing mental illnesses. Youth engagement was also important, so the most successful programs created a safe environment for students and encouraged an open dialogue with the speakers. This typically meant having the educational sessions in small classrooms rather than larger gatherings where students were uncomfortable asking questions. In the most effective programs, teachers were also engaged and offered information and activities centered on mental health and mental illnesses in the days leading up to the contact-based education, followed by a debriefing the following day and a concerted attempt to maintain school-based mental health and awareness activities throughout the year.

The second step in developing fidelity criteria is to quantify programs' adherence to the proposed critical ingredients, usually based on ratings of experts from program documentation, observations, interviews, or survey data (Mowbray et al. 2003). Using all available qualitative and observational data, the components of the logic model were translated into a set of measurable items, and programs were systematically rated for the presence or absence of each item. Members of the evaluation team and representatives from Opening Minds who knew the programs best reviewed the ratings. All items were discussed and a consensus reached. In the next step (research underway), program ratings will be coded into the pooled quantitative data for analysis. The goal will be to empirically evaluate the importance of each item in predicting program outcomes.

One of the challenges in assessing the impact of contact-based education from existing literature has been the variability in the nature and quality of the measures used and the resulting lack of comparability across interventions (Corrigan et al. 2012; Mellor 2014). Also, there has been considerable heterogeneity in the quality and type of interventions offered. In a recent meta-analysis of the literature, Mellor (2014) concludes that there is insufficient data to determine how one might design a successful intervention. Because we are assessing the importance of different program elements across a range of programs, all of which are using the same standardized measures, there is potential to overcome this problem and contribute important best practice information to this emerging field.

Target Group: Healthcare Providers

Healthcare is one of the key environments in which people with mental illnesses experience stigma (Abbey et al. 2012; Schulze and Angermeyer 2003; Schulze 2007; Stuart et al. 2012). Research involving people with a mental illness, as well as research with healthcare providers, show stigma in healthcare settings to be a major barrier to treatment and recovery. Stigma in healthcare is associated with a greater internalization of stigmatizing beliefs and self-silence (self-stigma) among people with mental illnesses, as well as inadequate access to proper treatment, less treatment compliance, breakdown of the therapeutic relationship, and greater avoidance of healthcare services (Abbey et al. 2012; Ross and Goldner 2009; Sartorius et al. 2010; Schomerus and Angermeyer 2008; Thornicroft et al. 2007; Thornicroft 2008).

Consumers of mental health services often say they feel "patronized, punished, or humiliated" in their interactions with health professionals (Thornicroft et al. 2007, 115). Other common experiences include being excluded from decisions, receiving subtle or overt threats of coercive treatment, being subjected to excessively long waits when seeking help, being given insufficient information, being treated in a paternalistic or demeaning manner, or being told they would never get well (Corrigan 2005; Clarke et al. 2007; Schulze and Angermeyer 2003; Thornicroft et al. 2010). Negative attitudes and stereotypes, prognostic negativity (pessimism about a person's chance of recovery), diagnostic overshadowing (the tendency to misattribute unrelated symptoms and complaints to the person's mental illness), fragmentation and marginalization (not wanting to treat psychiatric symptoms in a medical setting), and insufficient skills have all been reported in empirical studies (Atzema et al. 2011; Lauber et al. 2006; Ross and Goldner 2009; Schulze 2007; Thornicroft et al. 2007).

Improving the attitudes and behaviors of healthcare providers toward people with mental illnesses is an important target for anti-stigma efforts. Our research has focused on identifying programs and program components that improve attitudes and behavioral intentions among practicing and student healthcare providers. One of the most valuable findings is the observation that key programming elements can be used effectively in different ways and with different emphases to suit the needs of different healthcare provider audiences, including the way contact-based education is used as an anti-stigma programming tool.

To date, we have identified three main programming models, each of which seems to be particularly well-suited to certain audiences, as described below.

The Intensive Social Contact or Social Contact Partnership Model: Engaging Students to See the Person Behind the Illness and Break Down the Barriers Between "Us and Them"

This first model is a particularly good fit for student healthcare providers, as program elements can be incorporated seamlessly as part of a larger course. In this type of program, student participants meet one-on-one or in small groups with a person with lived experience of a mental illness at multiple time points. In this case, the person with lived experience is often known as a "client-educator" to designate their status vis-à-vis the students as one of "teacher" or "expert" as opposed to "patient." The objective is for students to learn about the client-educator's life and experiences on a personal level, through an interactive conversational process. Typically, students are given an interview protocol to follow or are provided with directions from the instructor as to the topics that should be covered and discussed. Students are then required to complete a project that represents the client-educator's life and experiences based on what they learned from their conversations and interactions. In this program model, client-educators are involved in the project component of the program as well, either as co-constructors, presenters, and/or graders of the project itself. The involvement of client-educators in students' projects represents an incorporation of a number of Allport's (1954) ideas about optimal contact conditions for reducing discrimination, including equal status, cooperation, working toward a common goal, and the buy-in of the institutional context (see also Couture and Penn 2003; Pettigrew and Tropp 2006, 2008).

Typically, student projects are written assignments or presentations. In one program of this type (e.g., see Knaak et al. 2016), for example, students prepared a 15–20 page "recovery narrative" to describe the client-educator's life story. Client-educators reviewed and provided feedback on the content of the completed narrative. The student's grade, which was weighted at 30 % of their final course grade, was based primarily on the client-educator's evaluation and feedback. In another program of this type (e.g., see Luong et al. 2012a), students collaboratively built a presentation that shared the client-educator's story with the class. While client-educators were given a choice as to their preferred level of involvement in the presentations, most chose to attend the presentation and many actively participated in telling their stories. Presentations tended to be varied, using a wide array of media, including photography, poetry, PowerPoint slides, role-plays, fabric arts, visual arts, video, and music.

Our evaluations of programs using the partnership/intensive contact-based education model have shown them to be effective at improving attitudes and behavioral intentions toward people with a mental illness and also at sustaining those positive changes over time (Knaak et al. 2016; Luong et al. 2012a). We suspect this may be due to the personal and cooperative nature of the social contact, which according to our qualitative evaluation data, can provide a powerful and positively transformative experience for students. Specifically, our qualitative findings suggest that these programs provide a "humanizing" process whereby students come to recognize individuals experiencing severe and persistent mental illnesses just like everyone else, effectively breaking down the divide that underlies stigmatization processes (Knaak et al. 2016; Knaak and Patten 2014; Link and Phelan 2001). As one student articulated, *"it helps reduce the 'us and them' feeling that we might have … it reduces those barriers, you see them as a real person."* Another student commented on how their group chose to do their presentation sitting together on stools (along with their client-educator) as a symbol of equality and cohesion.

While this programming model also could be effective for practicing healthcare providers, we have not seen it implemented beyond student audiences and in the context of a full-term course, likely because the structure of the program (e.g., multiple meetings over time followed by a project) works particularly well in this setting. However, this programming model could be modified for inclusion in a practicum or within a modular curriculum like medicine or pharmacy, for example.

The Anti-Stigma Workshop: An Efficient and Effective Way to Combat Stigma Among Time-Strapped Healthcare Providers

The second type of program model is particularly well-suited for practicing healthcare providers working in busy hospitals or health centers, although it also can be used with student audiences. The workshop model involves participants attending a single base session or workshop on the topic of stigmatization and mental illnesses (e.g., see Kassam and Patten 2011; Knaak et al. 2013; Kopp et al. 2013; Modgill and Patten 2012). Workshops can be as short as 1 h or as long as a full day, although we have found that shorter programs (e.g., 1–2 h) seem to work best, especially for ensuring high levels of attendance. This finding comes from our qualitative research, where we learned that shorter programs tend to be more attractive and feasible for attendees given that practicing healthcare providers are often confronted with many competing demands on their time (Knaak and Patten 2014). As one interviewee commented

> You have to think about program length from a participant perspective. Obviously it has to be long enough to cover the content. But too long and it will be difficult for staff to commit … multiple shorter sessions are preferred over one long session.

The workshop model has a number of typical program elements (Kassam and Patten 2011; Kopp et al. 2013; Modgill and Patten 2012):

- An educational component focused on myth busting (i.e., correcting false beliefs about mental illness prevalence, recovery, violence, etc., typically delivered in an interactive and nonthreatening format like a multiple choice or "jeopardy"-style game).
- An educational exercise explicitly focused on mental illness stigma, which is also introduced in an interactive and nonthreatening manner (e.g., the "earache exercise," an interactive exercise that compares and contrasts the experience of having a mental illness with the experience of having a physical illness, such as an earache).
- An action-oriented component whereby participants connect what they have learned to activities and practices in their individual workplaces and declare specific commitments for behaviors they will change and/or action they plan to undertake to help reduce stigma.
- One or more contact-based education elements whereby a person with lived experience of a mental illness who is managing their illness shares their personal story. Findings from our qualitative research suggest that showing recovery in action through social contact helps to disconfirm stereotypes healthcare providers

may have about people with a mental illness – showing that they are competent, capable, and can live full and successful lives. This research also suggests that seeing someone in recovery and hearing them reflect on their experiences reminds healthcare providers that what they do does make a difference, which helps to combat feelings of helplessness, or that what they do does not matter.

While we have found that both live and video forms of social contact can be effective when assessed using quantitative metrics, our qualitative research (see Knaak and Patten 2014) suggests that having a live, personal testimony component is still preferred over video-based social contact for the following reasons:

- The personal connection is more powerful when it is live. As one interviewee commented, *"The reaction tends to be stronger when it is live. There's more of a 'wow' factor."*
- Having a live speaker allows program participants to see recovery in action. As one interviewee commented, *"Getting up there and telling your story in a positive way evokes admiration and shows competence. It allows the audience to see that recovery is real. This changes their perceptions of people with a mental illness because the stereotype is that people with a mental illness aren't supposed to be competent or capable or funny or likeable."*
- Having a person with lived experience of a mental illness in the room allows the audience to ask questions about that person's life and experiences and learn from them. As one interviewee commented, *"It has to be interactive – this is what gets people to reflect … Healthcare providers have a lot of questions about 'what can we do?' 'What is the right thing to say?' Having the speaker there to help answer these kinds of questions is really helpful for the audience."*

Our research also shows that the best performing programs tend to include multiple forms of social contact, such as a video featuring interviews or personal testimonies from people with lived experience of a mental illness, as well as a live, personal testimony (Knaak et al. 2014).

The workshop model, while shorter in total program duration and social contact exposure than the more intensive social contact model, can be equally as effective, at least for short-term stigma reduction (Pietrus 2013). An important observation we have made, however, is that this model appears to be less effective at sustaining positive attitude changes over time. As such, this model is best implemented in conjunction with a series of follow-up or booster sessions offered at various intervals after the initial workshop, whereby key learnings can be reinforced and enhanced (Knaak and Patten 2014; Pietrus 2013; Szeto and Hamer 2013).

The Skills-Based Model: Teaching Healthcare Providers "What to Say" and "What to Do" to Help

The third model for anti-stigma programming being used successfully among healthcare provider audiences is a particularly good fit for physicians, who often bypass anti-stigma workshop-style programs (Pietrus 2013). While we do not yet have a clear understanding why physicians are less inclined to attend anti-stigma workshops than healthcare provider groups (though we suspect it may be related to how they are incented and how they perceive value in educational programming), we have consistently found that programmers using the anti-stigma workshop model experience considerable difficulties recruiting physicians to attend their programs (Knaak and Patten 2014; Pietrus 2013). This has not, however, been the case for skill-based programs, where the primary objective is to teach new skills and tools for helping patients with a mental illness.

We have learned that healthcare providers often feel a sense of hopelessness and helplessness with regard to their ability to work with and treat patients with mental illnesses – they do not know what to do or what to say to help (Knaak and Patten 2014). This lack of confidence and perceived lack of competence may contribute to stigmatization creating feelings of anxiety and a desire for avoidance or social and clinical distance. To this end, the skills training programming model addresses the problem of stigmatization by focusing directly on behavior change, mainly by teaching skills that help healthcare providers know what to say and do and increase their understanding of mental illnesses as being inherently treatable and manageable.

One of the most promising programs within this model is one that teaches self-management cognitive behavioral tools (e.g., relaxation, activation, cognitions, lifestyle skills, etc.) to family physicians and other front-line healthcare providers that they can use for the care of people with mild and moderate depression and anxiety (Knaak and Patten 2013a, b; Luong et al. 2012b). The objective of the program is to improve physicians' comfort and confidence in the diagnosis and treatment of patients with mental health concerns through approaches that engage patients as partners. In addition, this approach can be used in the context of family practice appointment slots and existing payment codes (MacCarthy et al. 2013).

The program has been delivered in various formats, all of which have demonstrated positive stigma reduction outcomes in uncontrolled comparisons (Knaak and Patten 2013a, b; Luong et al. 2012b). The full program is a collection of three modules taught 6–8 weeks apart with practice-based action periods in between. Experienced physicians called peer facilitators to teach the learning modules. Training techniques include live and video demonstrations, as well as role-playing with the physician and patient working together, looking at the patient's problems with the goal of managing the problem as opposed to "fixing" the problem. Patient engagement, and patients taking part in their own solutions to their own problems, is encouraged and demonstrated throughout the training. In addition to full program delivery, the program also has been offered in condensed form as a single full day training session and in a truncated form whereby only one of the three modules (cognitive behavioral skills training) was taught.

A potentially important observation we have made with this programming model is that, similar to the intensive social contact model described above for student audiences, the skills-based model seems to work well at sustaining, and even improving, positive outcomes over time (e.g., see Knaak and Patten 2013a, b). Although more research is required, it is our hypothesis that, as healthcare providers put such skills into practice, they become more comfortable and confident in their ability to interact with and care for people with a mental illness. They may also come to have a greater belief in the likelihood of recovery. The setting in motion of such dynamics may translate over time into improved attitudes and behaviors (MacCarthy et al. 2013). However, the skills typically taught in these sessions target common mood and anxiety disorders, and the extent to which positive effects generalize to other groups, such as people with a severe and persistent mental illness, is uncertain.

Importantly, the programs we have evaluated using the skills-based model that have been shown to be effective from a stigma reduction standpoint, all emphasize an approach to care that prioritizes patient empowerment and provider/patient partnerships in the recovery process. They also teach therapeutic techniques that aim to enhance healthcare providers' abilities to communicate effectively with patients with a mental illness. This could be an important element of this type of programming model, particularly as programs within this model sometimes have limited contact-based education/personal testimony components.

Programming Models and Key Ingredients

Despite their different approaches, there are important commonalties among the three main programming models described above. Namely, they all use identified key ingredients important for maximal program effectiveness, albeit in different ways, and with different emphases. One of the most important of these key ingredients is emphasizing that recovery from a mental illness is both real and probable and showing what recovery looks like by demonstrating competence and successful living of people with lived experience of a mental illness (Knaak et al. 2014).

Other key ingredients that have been identified through our research, and which the best performing programs within each of these three programming models do, include contact-based education in the form of a personal testimony from a trained speaker who has lived experience of a mental illness; using multiple forms or points of social contact if possible (e.g., live plus video, multiple speakers with lived experience, multiple points of social contact between program participants, and people with lived experience); focusing on behavior change, often by teaching skills and providing tools that increase healthcare providers' confidence and competence in working with patients with a mental illness; engaging in myth busting (correcting false beliefs); and using an enthusiastic facilitator/instructor who models a person-centered approach (i.e., a person-first perspective as opposed to a pathology-first perspective) to set the tone and guide program messaging (Knaak et al. 2014).

Anti-stigma programming to improve the attitudes and behavioral intentions of healthcare providers toward people with a mental illness is an important tool for reducing stigmatization in healthcare contexts. The three programming models and the six key ingredients for effective anti-stigma programming have been derived from extensive evaluation research on current anti-stigma programs in Canada. The research allows organizations to capitalize on time and resources to implement effective programs across different healthcare providers and settings. While each of these models may be tailored to meet the differing needs of a variety of audiences or contexts, it would be important to keep in mind the main themes described above and, in particular, the key ingredients for maximal program success.

Target Group: The Workforce

There are several important reasons for targeting workplaces. Firstly, mental health problems and common disorders, such as anxiety and depression, are often experienced during the prime working years (Richards et al. 2003). In fact, it has been estimated that 44 % of the working population in Canada lives with or has had a mental health problem (Thorpe and Chénier 2011). Secondly, there are financial costs. Mental illnesses in the workplace can limit productivity, resulting in financial strain for companies and contributing to the overall economic burden (e.g., Langlieb and Kahn 2005; Lerner and Henke 2008). A recent study estimated the annual national economic costs of mental illnesses in Canada to be $51 billion (Lim et al. 2008), with short-term and long-term disability claims related to mental illnesses costing organizations upward of $30 billion a year (Dewa et al. 2010; Sroujian 2003).

A third reason to target the workplace is to prevent exclusion of people with mental illnesses from the workforce. As a group, people with mental illnesses experience rates of unemployment that are much higher than the general population, and stigma is considered a major contributor to this (Stuart 2006b). In addition, working is an important element of recovery, providing people with access to important social roles that can bring meaning and purpose, quality of life, social interactions, and a range of other health and well-being benefits. With the alarming financial and human costs of mental illnesses in relation to the Canadian working population, targeted workplace mental illness anti-stigma interventions make sense.

Stigma is unique in the way it presents itself in the work context. The structure of social relations within workplaces creates multiple avenues where stigma might present. For example, individuals with a mental illness may be stigmatized by coworkers, supervisors, or employees. Individuals who experience a mental illness may face stigma in the form of negative attitudes (such as feelings of distrust from others) or behavior (such as avoidance in the workplace) within these relationships (Brohan and Thornicroft 2010), which could consequently lead to termination, unemployment, underemployment, failure to advance, or alienation at work (e.g., Read and Baker 1996). Research has demonstrated that those with mental illnesses are less likely to be hired and they may have their skills devalued (e.g., Bordieri and Dremher 1986; Bricout and Bentley 2000).

As well, organizational discrimination may contribute to unequal treatment of people with mental illnesses because of workplace policies or rules. For example, absence reporting policies may prevent people with mental illnesses from taking the time away from work because the episodic nature of their illnesses is not accounted for and because there is a fear of disclosure. Many employees are reluctant to disclose a mental health problem, even if this would provide them access to their legal rights for reasonable accommodations, as they are concerned about the stigma and consequences that can result. Paradoxically, the failure to disclose can lead to delayed treatment, mounting difficulty on the job, and subsequently, more time off work, and increased disability claim costs to the employer.

This negative chain of events can happen even where the solution could be relatively simple. For example, a worker who does not disclose may not be able to access work accommodations that provide specified time off to attend health-related appointments. Consequently, this worker could experience more serious difficulties that would lead to prolonged time on leave. If interventions can help address the specific ways that stigma manifests itself in the workplace and promotes more supportive work environments among employees and employers, this could lead to environments more accepting of mental illnesses and encouraging of earlier help seeking. Such programs can be of benefit to employees, employers, and the company's overall performance.

While several workplace-based anti-stigma programs exist in Canada, few have been systematically evaluated for effectiveness (Szeto and Dobson 2010). We have partnered with organizations to evaluate different anti-stigma interventions in multiple workplace contexts across the country (private sector, public sector, telecommunications, police services, governments, etc.). Results of the evaluations will lead to recommended best practices and identify essential components of workplace-based interventions. Because of the unique ways that stigma manifests itself in the workplace, effective interventions need to be relevant to the employment context. The design or selection of workplace anti-stigma interventions needs to be guided by a good understanding of how stigma presents itself in the workplace and how stigma might also be perpetuated by the context itself (Stuart 2004). These factors also need to be considered when these interventions are evaluated and the results are interpreted.

A conceptual model of workplace stigma (Fig. 14.3), developed by Krupa and colleagues (2009), provides an understanding of how stigma presents itself in various workplace settings and how these influence the effectiveness of interventions.

The key components of the model include the consequences of stigma (which vary in range and have impact on multiple stakeholders), the assumptions that underlie the expressions of stigma (i.e., the fundamental negative beliefs and stereotypes that influence discriminatory behaviors), the salience and intensity of those assumptions, and the outside influences that perpetuate these assumptions (such as the media and organizational or government policies).

This model suggests that there are assumptions held about people with mental illnesses, specifically that they will not have the competence (related to both task and social performance) to perform the job and that these assumptions influence the disposition to act in a discriminatory manner. For example, labeling someone as "unreliable, unproductive, or untrustworthy" may lead to isolation of the labeled person or limits to recognition or promotion in the workplace. This suggests that to counteract this influence, anti-stigma interventions should identify key assumptions that exist in the workplace, identify where and how they emerge, and directly challenge them.

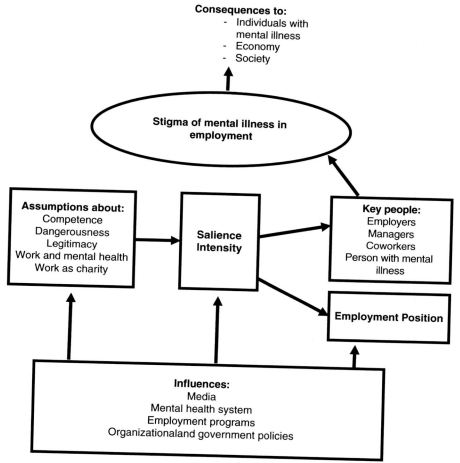

Fig. 14.3 A theoretical framework to understand stigma in employment (Reprinted from Work, 33, Krupa et al. (2009), with permission from IOS Press)

Early evaluation results support this theory. Anecdotal comments from participants who have taken training programs have suggested that when the program highlights how stigma is directly applied in the workplace, the messages have more meaning and applicability for them. Furthermore, the saliency and intensity of stigmatizing assumptions can be addressed by how relevant or customized the messages are for a particular workplace. Program feedback has suggested that the *specific* workplace (i.e., the actual organization where the intervention is taking place) is more influential than more general messages. For example, positive comments from participants have come from those attending programs that have provided the opportunity to discuss specific workplace issues, consider those issues in the light of new knowledge gained about mental illnesses, and problem solving that is respectful of both workers and workplaces.

In relation to the success of work context-specific interventions is the use of contact-based education in these initiatives. In the workplace context, contact-based education may have the ability to challenge negative assumptions and work to shift negative social dynamics. For example, in one workplace a supervisor noted that the personal narrative provided by one worker commanded the respect, attention, and commitment of other employees in a way that other educational interventions could not. This combination of counter-attitudinal messages that address assumptions specific to the workplace, customization to the context, and contact-based education is emerging as key components to successful workplace-based interventions.

Another key component of the model is that workplace stigma differentially affects the many stakeholders in a work environment. Stakeholders differ in their roles and relationships within an organization and with a worker experiencing a mental illness. Accordingly, there are different influences within the context of horizontal and vertical relationships that affect how stigma manifests itself. This premise suggests that the assumptions held about mental illnesses can vary according to the position an individual holds in a workplace. Our qualitative work has revealed some key issues that are relevant to the supervisory role. For example, one issue unique to the managerial position is providing accommodations for employees with mental illnesses while managing confidentiality within the team dynamic. This suggests that workplace interventions require targeted messages and strategies for supervisors and that these are different from those required by employees. While a deeper understanding of the distinct factors that influence stigma according to stakeholders needs further exploration, we are taking care to examine interventions targeted at supervisors versus employees to examine differences in effectiveness, to identify key issues that are likely salient for each group, and to identify program gaps.

The conceptual model described above indicates that a full understanding of the workplace environment is critical to understand the development of stigmatizing behaviors and how interventions can then effectively target these behaviors. The model also implicates overarching structural forces that are at play in the workplace and requires analysis of these factors to fully understand how a given workplace might enhance or limit emotional and mental well-being. Factors such as acceptance, promotion of diversity, and respect, particularly if they are embedded in the organizational culture and policies, reduce the likelihood of stigma (Kirsh 2000). When present, these factors also enhance the ability to successfully implement anti-stigma programs, as well as shape the uptake and overall effectiveness of these programs.

In working with dozens of workplace organizations, we have found that those with a robust and positive mental health culture have been generally more successful with implementation of initiatives. These results are particularly striking when organizational leadership demonstrates acceptance and support of initiatives (Pietrus 2013). Given these considerations, an assessment of organizational culture becomes important to understanding the work context and its relationship to stigma. While formalized culture assessment is not yet part of the systematic research we are conducting, efforts are being made to understand the broad workplace culture of each organization involved in the various evaluations to better inform the processes involved in program implementation and to interpret the results of our evaluations. To this end, a formal evaluation framework is drawn up as a first step in the evaluation process so that each step is guided by objectives and processes that are relevant and fitting to the workplace context. At a broad level, the development of the National Standard of Canada for Psychological Health and Safety in the Workplace (Mental Health Commission of Canada 2012) has contributed to the development of processes for evaluating organizational cultures and, in combination with focused anti-stigma interventions, offers a powerful approach to addressing workplace stigma.

Given the range of factors implicated in the development of stigma in the workplace, as well as in the development, design, implementation, and evaluation perspectives for anti-stigma work, there is incredible value in collaborative frameworks to combat stigma. Collaboration among program developers, workplaces, and researchers enables evaluation that is of value to all stakeholders and maximizes the potential transition between research and real life application of that research. For example, only experts within a given organization can provide researchers with background information on organizational culture, which researchers can then use to inform the level of success of a given program.

This opportunity for collaborative evaluation is providing us the opportunity to conduct meta-analyses on a range of similar organizations, such as anti-stigma programs in police services across Canada, without the assumption that organizational cultures are identical despite the similarity of the nature of the service. Conversely, while researchers can provide organizations with the results of quantitative and qualitative analyses of programs, it is individual leaders within any given organization who will ultimately determine which internal policies might be reviewed or modified, what training is provided to key staff, and ultimately how the organizational culture might evolve. The collaborative framework we are using facilitates the opportunity to make a real impact on the development of anti-stigma programs and the implementation of these programs in workplaces. The ultimate goal is to envisage and enact meaningful change in negative workplace attitudes and behaviors related to those with mental illnesses.

Target Group: The Media

A large degree of research indicates that the popular media is one of the primary sources of information about mental illnesses for the general public (Wahl 1992; Coverdale et al. 2002). This includes television, radio, newspaper, magazines, and the Internet. Studies suggest that these media combined can contribute to the construction of some of the common stereotypes and inaccuracies about people with a mental illness (Stout et al. 2004; Wahl 1995). For example, a preponderance of stories about crime and violence by people with a mental illness may lead to widespread fear of people with a mental illness among the general public (Stuart 2006a). Similarly, stories that have a tone of mockery about people with mental illness can lead to ridicule and derision. This form of stigma can be internalized by people with a mental illness. Assessing media representations of people with mental illnesses is vitally important, given that evidence suggests that the media can exert such a strong influence.

Most research on this topic has occurred in countries such as Australia, the UK, and the USA, so our team set out to systematically monitor media representations of mental illnesses. We are conducting a systematic study of news media representations of mental illnesses in Canada from 2005 to 2016 to assess patterns and trends in media coverage. The method used for this research project is described in detail elsewhere (Whitley and Berry 2013a), as are preliminary study results reporting patterns and trends from 2005 to 2010 (Whitley and Berry 2013b). Results so far indicate that 40 % of newspaper articles focus on crime, violence, or danger. Less than 20 % of newspaper articles discuss treatment for a mental illness and only 18 % have recovery and rehabilitation as themes. Less than 20 % include a direct quotation from someone with a mental illness. We did not observe any significant changes between 2005 and 2010 on any of the variables measured. These figures should be interpreted in light of evidence suggesting that recovery is a common process or outcome for people with a mental illness (Drake and Whitley 2014). Additionally, people with a mental illness have similar levels of crime and violence compared to those without a mental illness, when controlling for homelessness and substance abuse (Stuart 2003).

We also noted that stories about mental illness per se were more positive and less stigmatizing than articles about an individual with an alleged mental illness. For articles about an individual with a mental illness, stories about men were significantly more likely to have stigmatizing content and violence as themes when compared with those about women (Whitley et al. in press). Many articles about men focused on individuals who had committed a violent act. Interestingly, many of these casually linked mental illnesses to killers such as Adam Lanza or Anders Breivik. This occurred despite the fact that there was no evidence at the time of these shootings that either had a mental illness. Indeed, we analyzed the data to examine how far such incidents contributed to negative portrayals. To meet this aim, we compared data in the immediate aftermath of the actions of Lanza with baseline data.

Lanza was a 20-year-old man who murdered 20 children and six adults at Sandy Hook Elementary School on December 14, 2012. The murders received widespread media coverage in Canada and around the world. At the time of these shootings, many of the articles linked Lanza to mental illness, despite the fact that there was no

Table 14.2 Comparison of 30 days following Sandy Hook incident with 2012 baseline data

	30 days following Sandy Hook incident ($n = 247$)	Complete 12 months for 2012 ($n = 2083$)
Is the article stigmatizing?	43 % (107)	26 % (549)
Does the article negatively link mental illness to danger, crime, or violence?	76 % (188)	45 % (930)
Is recovery or rehabilitation a theme?	10 % (25)	18 % (366)

current evidence that he had a mental illness. In the 30 days following this incident, we assessed any article from a major Canadian newspaper that mentioned the terms "mental illness," "mental health," "schizophrenia," and "schizophrenic." This led to 247 articles. Of these articles, 43 % (107) were judged to be stigmatizing in tone and content by well-trained coders; 76 % (188) had danger, crime, or violence as a theme; and only 10 % (22) had recovery as a theme. For the baseline data, we examined our whole data set for the year 2012. This led to 2083 articles. Of these articles, 26 % (549) were stigmatizing in tone and content and 45 % (930) had danger, crime, or violence as a theme. Eighteen percent (366) had recovery and rehabilitation as a theme. These figures are contrasted in Table 14.2 for ease of comparison.

This analysis shows that a single well-publicized violent incident can lead to a spike in negative articles, as well as a decrease in positive articles. Our wider analysis of the data shows that these types of irregular one-off incidents lead to a massive increase in negatively oriented articles, which link, often erroneously, mental illnesses to violent events. A weakness of the study is that we did not measure audience impact; however, other research suggests that such articles may unwittingly distort the perception of the dangers posed by people with a mental illness (Stuart 2006a).

Our team is currently working with journalists and journalism students in a variety of modalities to improve coverage of mental illnesses in Canada. In this process, we are suggesting that journalists do not speculate on the mental health status of people suspected of or alleged to have committed acts of violence. We are also suggesting that they do not quote others, for example, chiefs of police or on lookers, who speculate on the mental health status of alleged perpetrators. To assist members of the news media in reporting on mental health-related items, Opening Minds has funded the creation of a media resource guide for working journalists called Mindset. It is designed to reduce stigma in new coverage (http://www.mindset-mediaguide.ca/). Such measures can lead to the reduction of articles that subtly link mental illnesses to violent crimes. While such articles may be harmless in isolation, when they are repeated and regular over a concentrated period of time, they may leave the reader with the impression that violence and criminality are the inevitable consequences of a mental illness. Reducing such potentially misleading articles must be a priority for those aiming to diminish stigmatization against people living with a mental illness. We hope further efforts will be made in other countries around the world.

Summary and Conclusion

Research teams have now spent a considerable amount of time isolating effective programs that work in local contexts and identifying their critical components. Once these active ingredients have been more rigorously validated, they can form the basis for fidelity criteria and measures that can be used to promote best practices in targeted anti-stigma programming. Supporting resources (such as guides, toolkits, and videos) can then be disseminated across Canada.

The benefits of this approach have been considerable. By working with grassroots organizations, it has been possible to identify a range of effective anti-stigma interventions, build capacity in the field to participate in evaluations and critically reflect on program activities, and engage a broad array of stakeholder groups (including policy makers, program providers, and researchers). Most importantly, we have worked to develop a scholarly evidence base that can be used to inform research and public policy in Canada and elsewhere.

Acknowledgments Opening Minds is the anti-stigma initiative of the Mental Health Commission of Canada, which is funded by Health Canada. For further information on Opening Minds, our reports and partners, go to our website: http://www.mentalhealthcommission.ca/English/initiatives-and-projects/opening-minds

References

Abbey S, Charbonneau M, Tranulis C, Moss P et al (2012) Stigma and discrimination. Can J Psychiatr 56(10):1–9

Allport G (1954) The nature of prejudice. Addison-Wesley, Reading

Atzema CL, Schull MJ, Tu JV (2011) The effects of a charted history of depression on emergency department triage and outcomes in patients with acute myocardial infarction. Can Med Assoc J 183(6):663–669

Blascovich J, Mendes WB, Hunter SB, Lickel B, Kowai-Bell N (2001) Perceiver threat in social interactions with stigmatized others. J Pers Soc Psychol 80:253–267

Bordieri JE, Drehmer DE (1986) Hiring decisions for disabled workers: looking at the cause. J Appl Soc Psychol 16(3):197–208

Bricout JC, Bentley KJ (2000) Disability status and perceptions of employability by employers. Soc Work Res 24(2):87–95

Brohan E, Thornicroft G (2010) Stigma and discrimination of mental health problems: workplace implications. Occup Med 60:414–420

Chen SP, Koller M, Krupa T, Stuart H (2014) Identifying the critical componens of youth anti-stigma education programs. Paper presented at 'sharing traditions, sharing futures,' the 16th international congress of the world federation of occupational therapists, Yokohama, Japan, 18–21 June 2014

Clark D, Dusome D, Hughes L (2007) Emergency department from the mental health client's perspective. Int J Ment Health Nurs 16:126–131

Corrigan P (2000) Mental health stigma as social attribution: implications for research methods and attitude change. Clin Psychol Sci Pract 7:48–67

Corrigan P (2005) On the stigma of mental illness. American Psychological Association, Washington, DC

Corrigan P, Backs Edwards A, Green A, Lickey Thwart S, Penn D (2001) Prejudice, social distance, and familiarity with mental illness. Schizophr Bull 27(2):219–225

Corrigan PW, Morris SB, Michaels PJ, Rafacz JD, Rüsch N (2012) Challenging the public stigma of mental illness: a meta-analysis of outcome studies. Psychiatr Serv 63:963–973

Couture S, Penn D (2003) Interpersonal contact and the stigma of mental illness: a review of the literature. J Ment Health 12:291–305

Coverdale J, Nairn R, Claasen D (2002) Depictions of mental illness in print media: a prospective national sample. Aust N Z J Psychiatry 36:697–700

Dewa CS, Chau N, Dermer S (2010) Examining the comparative incidence and cost of physical and mental health-related disabilities in an employed population. J Occup Environ Med 52:758–762

Drake RE, Whitley R (2014) Recovery and severe mental illness: description and analysis. Can J Psychiatr 59(5):236–242

Gaebel W, Zäske H, Baumann AE, Klosterkötter J, Maier W, Decker P et al (2008) Evaluation of the German WPA program against stigma and discrimination because of schizophrenia – Open the Doors: results from representative telephone surveys before and after three years of anti-stigma interventions. Schizophr Res 98:184–193

Goffman I (1963) Stigma: notes on the management of spoiled identity. Penguin, Harmondsworth

Kassam A, Patten S (2011) Quantitative analysis of the 'Mental Illness and Addictions: Understanding the Impact of Stigma' program. Mental Health Commission of Canada, Calgary, http://www.mentalhealthcommission.ca/English/node/5234. Accessed September 2014

Kirsh B (2000) Organizational culture, climate and person-environment fit: relationships with employment outcomes for mental health consumers. Work: J Prev Assess Rehabil 4:109–122

Knaak S, Patten S (2013a) BC PSP adult mental health module: key findings. Mental Health Commission of Canada, Calgary, http://www.mentalhealthcommission.ca/English/node/33741. Accessed 14 Sept 2014

Knaak S, Patten S (2013b) CBIS Program: final evaluation report. Mental Health Commission of Canada, Calgary, http://www.mentalhealthcommission.ca/English/node/22351. Accessed 15 Sept 2014

Knaak S, Patten S (2014) Building and delivering successful anti-stigma programs for healthcare providers: results of a qualitative study. Mental Health Commission of Canada, Calgary, http://www.mentalhealthcommission.ca/English/initiatives-and-projects/opening-minds) Accessed 20 Sept 2014

Knaak S, Hawke L, Patten S (2013) That's just crazy talk evaluation report. Mental Health Commission of Canada, Calgary, http://www.mentalhealthcommission.ca/English/node/19771. Accessed 12 Sept 2014

Knaak S, Karpa J, Robinson R, Bradley L (2016) They are us - we are them': Transformative learning though nursing education leadership. Healthcare Management Forum (May): forthcoming

Knaak S, Modgill G, Patten S (2014) Key ingredients of anti-stigma programs for healthcare providers: a data synthesis of evaluative studies. Can J Psychiatr 59(10 Suppl):19S–26S

Kopp B, Knaak S, Patten S (2013) Evaluation of IWK's 'Understanding the Impact of Stigma' program. Mental Health Commission of Canada, Calgary, http://www.mentalhealthcommission. ca/English/initiatives-and-projects/opening-minds. Accessed 14 Sept 2014

Krupa T, Kirsh B, Cockburn L, Gewurtz R (2009) Understanding the stigma of mental illness in employment. Work 33:413–425

Langlieb AM, Kahn JP (2005) How much does quality mental health care profit employers? J Occup Environ Med Am Coll Occup Environ Med 47(11):1099–1109

Lauber C, Nordt C, Braunschweig C, Rössler W (2006) Do mental health professionals stigmatize their patients? Acta Psychiatr Scand 113(Suppl 429):51–59

Lerner D, Henke RD (2008) What does research tell us about depression, job performance, and work productivity? J Occup Environ Med 50:401–410

Lim K-L, Jacobs P, Ohinmaa A, Schopflocher D, Dewa CS (2008) A new population-based measure of the economic burden of mental illness in Canada. Chronic Dis Can 28:92–98

Link BG, Phelan JC (2001) Conceptualizing stigma. Annu Rev Sociol 27(3):363–385

Luong D, Szeto A, Burwash S, Patten S (2012a) U of A OT client-educator program. Mental Health Commission of Canada, Calgary, http://www.mentalhealthcommission.ca/English/node/5186. Accessed 16 Sept 2014

Luong D, Szeto A, Weinerman R, Patten S (2012b) PSP adult mental health module. Mental Health Commission of Canada, Calgary, http://www.mentalhealthcommission.ca/English/node/5177. Accessed 21 Sept 2014

MacCarthy D, Weinerman R, Kallstrom L, Kadlec H, Hollander M, Patten S (2013) Mental health practice and attitudes of family physicians can be changed! Permenente J 17(3):14–17

Mellor C (2014) School-based interventions targeting stigma of mental illness: systematic review. Psychiatr Bull 38:164–171

Mental Health Commission of Canada (2012) Changing directions, changing lives: the mental health strategy for Canada. Mental Health Commission of Canada, Calgary, http://strategy.mentalhealthcommission.ca/pdf/strategy-text-en.pdf. Accessed 29 Sept 2014

Modgill G, Patten S (2012) British Columbia's Interior Health Authority's usage of the Ontario Central LHIN Anti-stigma Training Program: an independent evaluation by Opening Minds. Mental Health Commission of Canada, Calgary, http://www.mentalhealthcommission.ca/English/node/5180. Accessed 14 Sept 2014

Mowbray C, Holter M, Teague G, Bybee D (2003) Fidelity criteria: development, measurement, and validation. Am J Eval 24(3):315–340

Pettigrew T, Tropp L (2006) A meta-analytic test of intergroup contact theory. J Pers Soc Psychol 90:751–783

Pettigrew T, Tropp L (2008) How does intergroup contact reduce prejudice? Meta-analytic tests of three mediators. Eur J Soc Psychol 38:922–934

Pietrus M (2013) Opening minds interim report. Mental Health Commission of Canada, Calgary, http://www.mentalhealthcommission.ca/English/initiatives-and-projects/opening-minds/opening-minds-interim-report. Accessed 29 Sept 2014

Read J, Baker S (1996) Not just sticks & stones: a survey of the stigma, taboos and discrimination experienced by people with mental health problems. Mind Publications, London

Richards D, Bradshaw T, Mairs H (2003) Helping people with mental illness: a mental health training programme for community health workers. World Health Organization, Geneva, https://www.who.int/mental_health/policy/en/Module%20A2.pdf. Accessed 28 Oct 2014

Ross C, Goldner E (2009) Stigma, negative attitudes and discrimination towards mental illness within the nursing profession: a review of the literature. J Psychiatr Health Nurs 16:558–567

Sartorius N (2010) Short-lived campaigns are not enough. Nature 468:163–165

Sartorius N, Gaebel W, Cleveland W-H et al (2010) WPA guidance on how to combat stigmatization of psychiatry and psychiatrists. World Psychiatry 9:131–144

Schomerus G, Angermeyer MC (2008) Stigma and its impact on help-seeking for mental disorders: what do we know? Epidemiol Psychiatr Soc 17:31–37

Schulze B (2007) Stigma and mental health professionals: a review of the evidence on an intricate relationship. Int Rev Psychiatr 19(2):137–155

Schulze B, Angermeyer M (2003) Subjective experiences of stigma. A focus group study of schizophrenic patients, their relatives, and mental health professionals. Soc Sci Med 56:299–312

Sroujian C (2003) Mental health is the number one cause of disability in Canada. Insurance Journal (August):8

Stout PA, Villegas J, Jennings NA (2004) Images of mental illness in the media: identifying gaps in the research. Schizophr Bull 30:543–561

Stuart H (2003) Violence and mental illness: an overview. World Psychiatry 2:121–124

Stuart H (2004) Stigma and work. Healthc Pap 5:100–111

Stuart H (2006a) Media portrayals of mental illness and its treatments – what effect does it have on people with mental illness. CNS Drugs 20:99–106

Stuart H (2006b) Mental illness and employment discrimination. Curr Opin Psychiatr 19:522–526

Stuart H, Arboleda-Flórez J, Santorius N (2012) Paradigms lost: fighting stigma and the lessons learned. Oxford University Press, New York

Stuart H, Chen SP, Christie R, Dobson K, Kirsh B, Knaak S, Koller M, Krupa T, Lauria-Horner B, Luong D et al (2014a) Opening minds in Canada: background and rationale. Can J Psychiatr 59(10 Suppl 1):S8–S12

Stuart H, Chen SP, Christie R, Dobson K, Kirsh B, Knaak S, Koller M, Krupa T, Lauria-Horner B, Luong D et al (2014b) Opening minds in Canada: targeting change. Can J Psychiatr 59(10 Suppl 1):S13–S18

Stuart H, Patten S, Koller M, Modgill G, Liinamaa T (2014c) Stigma in Canada: results from a rapid response survey. Can J Psychiatr 59(10 Suppl 1):S27–S33

Szeto ACH, Dobson KS (2010) Reducing the stigma of mental disorders at work: a review of current workplace anti-stigma intervention programs. Appl Prev Psychol 14:41–56

Szeto ACH, Hamer A (2013) Central LHIN Phase 2 report. Mental Health Commission of Canada, Calgary, http://www.mentalhealthcommission.ca/English/document/18621/central-lhin-phase-2-report. Accessed 24 Sept 2014

Thornicroft G (2008) Stigma and discrimination limit access to mental health care. Epidemiol Psichiat Soc 17(1):14–19

Thornicroft G, Rose D, Kassam A (2007) Discrimination in health care against people with mental illness. Int Rev Psychiatr 19(2):113–122

Thornicroft G, Rose D, Mehta N (2010) Discrimination against people with mental illness: what can psychiatrists do? Adv Psychiatr Treat 16:53–59

Thorpe K, Chénier L (2011) Building mentally healthy workplaces: perspectives of Canadian workers and front-line managers. Conference Board of Canada, Ottawa, http://www.conferenceboard.ca/e-library/abstract.aspx?did=4287. Accessed 29 Oct 2014

Waddell C, McEwan K, Shepherd C, Offord D, Hua J (2005) A public health strategy to improve the mental health of Canadian children. Can J Psychiatr 50(4):226–233

Wahl OF (1992) Mass media images of mental illness: a review of the literature. J Commun Psychiatr 20:343–352

Wahl OF (1995) Media madness: public images of mental illness. Rutgers University Press, New Brunswick

Whitley R, Berry S (2013a) Analyzing media representations of mental illness: lessons learnt from a national project. J Ment Health 22(3):246–253

Whitley R, Berry S (2013b) Trends in newspaper coverage of mental illness in Canada: 2005–2010. Can J Psychiatr 58:107–112

Whitley R, Adeponle A, Miller AR (in press) Comparing gendered and generic representations of mental illness in Canadian newspapers: an exploration of the chivalry hypothesis. Soc Psychiatry Psychiatr Epidemiol

World Health Organization (1996) The health of youth: a cross-national survey. World Health Organization, Geneva

Like Minds, Like Mine: Seventeen Years of Countering Stigma and Discrimination Against People with Experience of Mental Distress in New Zealand

15

Ruth Cunningham, Debbie Peterson, and Sunny Collings

Introduction

In 1996 New Zealand was one of the first countries in the world to initiate a comprehensive national programme to combat stigma and discrimination against people with experience of mental illness. Combining national level social marketing and community-driven education and training with a range of other strategies, the programme became known as *Like Minds, Like Mine* and achieved international recognition as the 'gold standard' in stigma reduction initiatives. Serial evaluations have demonstrated success in shifting public attitudes, and there are indications that discriminatory behaviours are also reducing. A great deal has been learnt about the extent of social exclusion and discrimination experienced by New Zealanders living with mental illness and about effective strategies to change attitudes and counter discrimination. Seventeen years later the work of *Like Minds, Like Mine* to increase social inclusion and reduce discrimination continues. This chapter documents the origins, evolution and current status of the *Like Minds, Like Mine* programme (referred to as *Like Minds*).

The Like Minds, Like Mine logo and slogan (see Fig. 15.1.) were the winning entry in a consumer art competition. The slogan is a play on the phrase 'we are all of one mind'. It indicates that mental illness can happen to you, me or anyone. The Māori slogan 'Whakaitia te whakawhiu i te tangata' can be translated as 'reduce your potential to discriminate'. The mathematical symbols in the logo represent 'greater than' and 'equal to' and are used to indicate 'greater than discrimination, equal to others'.

R. Cunningham (✉)
Department of Public Health, University of Otago, Wellington, New Zealand
e-mail: ruth.cunningham@otago.ac.nz

D. Peterson
Social Psychiatry and Population Mental Health Research Group,
University of Otago, Wellington, New Zealand

S. Collings
Dean's Department, University of Otago, Wellington, New Zealand

© Springer International Publishing Switzerland 2017
W. Gaebel et al. (eds.), *The Stigma of Mental Illness - End of the Story?*,
DOI 10.1007/978-3-319-27839-1_15

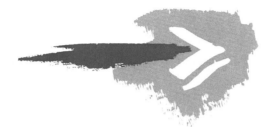

LIKE MINDS, LIKE MINE
Whakaitia te Whakawhiu i te Tangata

Fig. 15.1 *Like Minds* logo

The New Zealand Context and the Origins of *Like Minds*

In 1995 Judge Ken Mason presided over an inquiry into events occurring in New Zealand psychiatric care, and multiple submissions put the issue of discrimination squarely at the centre of problems to be addressed with urgency. The Mason Report (Mason et al. 1996) made five recommendations – one of which was the establishment of a Mental Health Commission to act as an independent monitor of changes in mental health care; another, a 'public awareness campaign' as 'a must' to support changes to mental health services themselves. The Ministry of Health subsequently allocated $12.6 million to fund a 5-year initiative – the *Project to Counter Stigma and Discrimination Associated with Mental Illness*, the project which went on to become *Like Minds, Like Mine*.

The Mason Report was also instrumental in shifting New Zealand mental health services towards a recovery approach. As in other countries, New Zealand began the process of deinstitutionalising psychiatric care in the 1970s and 1980s, but the Mason Report highlighted the under-resourcing of this transition. The Ministry of Health's *Moving Forward Mental Health Strategy* (Ministry of Health 1997) set the direction for mental health services following the Mason report and acknowledged the need for more and better mental health services. In 1998 the Mental Health Commission produced *Blueprint for Mental Health Services in New Zealand: How Things Need to Be* (Mental Health Commission 1998) which set out the Commission's view of how *Moving Forward* should be implemented and put the recovery approach at the heart of this implementation process.

The consumer movement, the social and political movement of people with experience of mental illness which has sought to change society's treatment of and approach to mental illness, has had a fluctuating voice in New Zealand for three decades. Accounts of the experience of psychiatric care such as Mary O'Hagan's *Stopovers on My Way Home from Mars* (O'Hagan 1994) were influential in bringing issues of stigma and discrimination to the attention of mental health services and the

New Zealand public in the 1980s and 1990s. The Aotearoa Network of Psychiatric Survivors (ANOPS) was set up in 1989 to foster a collective voice for people with lived experience of mental illness. However, at the time *Like Minds* began, recognition of the importance of formal consumer input into mental health policy was new. The first time that consumer input into mental health policy had actively been sought was in the National Mental Health Consortium set up in 1989 to establish national objectives and priorities, including for consumer participation. Following the Mason Inquiry, the national Mental Health Strategy (Ministry of Health 1997) included a goal to 'improve the responsiveness of mental health services to consumers'.

At the time *Like Minds* was initiated, mental illness was generally regarded as 'not my problem' by the New Zealand public. New Zealand studies of public attitudes to mental illness had revealed a lack of knowledge and uneasiness about how to relate to people with mental illness (Ng et al. 1995; Patten 1992). There was also a perception that people with mental illness were more violent, dangerous and unpredictable than others in the population (Ng et al. 1995). Research conducted in 1996 to define the baseline for public attitudes before initiating the campaign found similar results (Health Funding Authority 1999). The media were the main source of information about mental illness for the general public (Ng et al. 1995), and news media reporting in New Zealand tended to portray mental illness in a negative and stereotypical way. A 3-month review of all print media clippings on mental health in 1997/1998 found that article headlines, subject matter and treatment of the subject were all more likely to be negative than positive (Mental Health Commission 2000). There was, however, no information on the nature and extent of discrimination experienced by people with mental illness until 2004 when a survey of people with experience of mental illness was conducted (Peterson et al. 2007). This survey found that as in other countries, people with experience of mental illness in New Zealand experienced discrimination across multiple spheres of public and private life.

New Zealand is a culturally diverse country, with approximately 15 % Māori (the indigenous people of New Zealand), 7 % Pacific (the majority of whom are New Zealand born), 12 % of Asian ethnicities (principally Chinese and Indian) and 74 % identifying as New Zealand European (or 'pakeha'). The Treaty of Waitangi is the foundation document for New Zealand as a nation and sets out an agreement between the indigenous Māori people and the Crown (originally the British Monarch, now the New Zealand Government). The three articles of the Treaty guarantee Māori participation in governance at all levels, self-determination and equal rights of citizenship. A commitment to honouring the Treaty is made in all sectors of government and so Māori involvement in governance and developing appropriate approaches for Māori was a cornerstone for *Like Minds*. Moreover, approaches to increasing awareness and changing attitudes need to align with current understandings of the causes and consequences of mental illness, and so culturally appropriate approaches for different groups within New Zealand society are needed, and are often best led by people in those communities. By Māori for Māori and by Pacific for Pacific approaches have therefore been key to developing appropriate solutions.

Three key agencies were initially involved in *Like Minds*. Within government the Ministry of Health was the lead agency, responsible for national coordination and contract management. The Mental Health Commission set up in 1996 to act as an independent advisor to government had a support and monitoring role in *Like Minds*. The Mental Health Foundation, established in 1977, is the largest non-government provider funded by the *Like Minds* programme and has had a major role producing research and resources as well as currently administering national *Like Minds* communications including the website. For most of the life of *Like Minds*, these organisations have had central roles, although this is now changing, with the disestablishment of the Mental Health Commission in 2012 and coordination of *Like Minds* moving from the Ministry of Health to the Health Promotion Agency in 2013.

Overview of *Like Minds*

This section sets out the history of *Like Minds*, focusing on the key changes and the role of national plans. The key to the development of the underlying framework of *Like Minds* has always been in the process of developing the national plans. Although the plans themselves provide the map for future action, the processes of developing the plans and ensuring the commitment of stakeholders have been at the heart of ensuring success of the *Like Minds* programme. There have been five so far, each one heralding or consolidating a change in direction for the programme. All of the National Plans, along with research publications and other material, are available on the *Like Minds* website.[1]

The First National Plan (1999–2001)

The *Like Minds* programme was set up in 1996 with funding allocated for 5 years. One-third of funding sat in the Ministry of Health's public health group for a 'public education campaign', and two-thirds was allocated to the four Regional Health Authorities[2] to contract local providers for community initiatives to reduce stigma. A 'grass-roots' approach was taken, with each region developing its own approaches. Providers contracted included public health services, Māori health providers and NGOs working in mental health. Also involved from the beginning were people with experience of mental illness.

In 1998 the first National Project Manager was appointed and a series of national hui (meetings) were organised to bring together all those working on the project,

---

[1] www.likeminds.org.nz

[2] Regional Health Authorities were agencies responsible for purchasing health services, formed as part of 1993 reforms splitting purchasers and providers of health services in New Zealand. In 1997 the four RHAs were amalgamated into a single Health Funding Authority and then in 2000 into the Ministry of Health.

including specific days for people with experience of mental illness and for Māori and Pacific providers. Out of these meetings came a shared vision: 'To create a nation that values and includes people with mental illness'.

The first *Like Minds, Like Mine* National Plan was produced in 1999 (Health Funding Authority 1999), setting out this vision and the planned actions towards the vision. The two components of the first plan were:

- Project and sector development (including empowering consumers and changing attitudes in the health sector)
- Public awareness (including changing public attitudes through mass media, public relations and local mental health awareness work and changing attitudes and behaviours in those working closely with people with experience of mental illness)

The first national television advertising campaign ran in 2000–2001, focusing on raising awareness of mental illness and recovery through images of well-known people with experience of mental illness. Separate media campaigns utilising radio and print media were also instituted for Māori and Pacific audiences.

An evaluation system was also set up at this stage. A market research company was commissioned to conduct annual telephone surveys to track public attitudes and response to the television campaign and to produce qualitative and quantitative investigations of attitudes in different groups including youth, employers and health service staff. Evaluation of the early community initiatives was also undertaken, although a cohesive evaluation system for local Like Minds workshops was not set up until much later.

The Second National Plan (2001–2003)

In 2001 funding for *Like Minds* was extended and included in the Ministry of Health's public health baseline funding, giving some ongoing certainty. A second National Plan (Ministry of Health 2001) was produced, strongly aligned to the first, with the same vision, aims and principles. The plan continued the focus on building the infrastructure and networks needed for the programme, as well as the focus on health services and government agencies as priority audiences, and on changing general public attitudes through further media work. It also included for the first time an objective to develop community education to address stigma and discrimination among Māori and Pacific communities. The plan's strategic objectives were explicitly aligned with the Ottawa Charter for health promotion, providing a uniting framework for the plan's actions at different levels.

More television advertisements were produced, again focusing on awareness raising and shifting public attitudes and again using well-known faces. Local level work also continued to develop, with providers gaining knowledge and expertise. In particular, significant experience was being gained in presenting workshops designed to allow people to examine their own attitudes and behaviour towards people with experience of mental illness. Regular meetings of providers fostered sharing of this growing knowledge, and the *Like Minds* services provided in different regions continued to be very diverse. Regular newsletters also kept the providers up to date with work at national level and around the country, and in 2001 the *Like Minds* website[3] was launched, providing content for providers and the general public.

The Third National Plan (2003–2005)

In 2003 a third National Plan (Ministry of Health 2003) was launched, with a new focus directly on addressing discrimination and changing behaviour, building on the awareness raising work done in the previous phases. This plan also marked a significant shift in the philosophical foundations of the project, putting human rights and the social model of disability at its core. The objectives now included advocating for non-discriminatory policies and practices within organisations responsible for housing, education, employment and within health services. Strategies included encouraging the use of existing complaint mechanisms for addressing discrimination and providing human rights training for people with experience of mental illness.

A third series of advertisements moved away from using well-recognised people and instead told the stories of 'ordinary people', some with diagnoses such as bipolar disorder and psychosis. These advertisements also focused on the actions of others and their impacts.

Key new research was also published during this period. A major survey of extent of discrimination experienced was undertaken by the Mental Health Foundation (*Respect Costs Nothing*) (Peterson et al. 2004), to document the degree to which discrimination was occurring (in contrast to previous research which had focused on documenting public attitudes). An updated literature review on effective educational interventions to reduce discrimination (*The Power of Contact*) (Case Consulting 2005) was produced, summarising the evidence about the way in which contact with people with experience of mental illness can be used to combat discrimination, and the features of contact which are necessary for it to achieve this aim. These two reports had a major influence on the subsequent direction of *Like Minds*.

An important feature of this phase was making more formal connections between organisations involved in anti-discrimination work, both within and outside the *Like Minds* programme. Two new organisations, the Office for Disability Issues and the Human Rights Commission, were taking an increasingly prominent role in anti-stigma work. A Multi-Agency Group was formed in 2005, with a multi-agency plan (Mental Health Commission 2005) formalising the working arrangements and roles of these two organisations alongside the Ministry of Health and Mental Health Commission, to minimise duplication and increase cooperative working towards shared goals. The Mental Health Foundation and the Health and Disability Commission joined the Multi-Agency Group in 2006.

---

[3] http://www.likeminds.org.nz/

The Fourth National Plan (2007–2013)

The fourth National Plan (Ministry of Health 2007) spanned the 6 years from 2007 to 2013. The actions specified in the plan were built around the three strategies of contact, protest and education, which had been identified as the most effective in the *Power of Contact* report, and internalised stigma (or self-stigma) was for the first time made a target of the plan. The results of the *Respect Costs Nothing* survey were used to identify target groups and organisations for actions to reduce discrimination.

An outcome framework was used, mapping out the logic linking the approaches and actions of the plan to its outcomes, and performance indicators were detailed. Three outcomes were specified (in contrast to the single societal level outcome specified in the earlier plans):

- A nation that values and includes people with experience of mental illness (a societal outcome).
- All organisations have policies and practices to ensure that people with experience of mental illness are not discriminated against (an organisational outcome).
- People with experience of mental illness have the same opportunities as everyone else to participate in society and in the everyday life of their communities and whanau (extended family) (an individual level outcome).

A fourth series of advertisements continued the increasing focus on discrimination and were the first to use the word discrimination in their message: 'Discrimination is still the biggest barrier to recovery. What you do makes the difference'. A fifth series of advertisements aired in 2009 and was rerun in 2010 and 2011, focusing on practical approaches friends and extended family could take to support someone experiencing mental illness.

In 2008 the provision of workshops and other services by regional providers was reviewed, and the number of providers was cut, in an effort to increase the consistency of services provided. In 2010 the position of project manager in the Ministry of Health was disestablished, meaning that there was no longer a single person overseeing the whole programme. There was also a decrease in the funding available to the programme, as part of reductions in funding across the whole of government. However the work of *Like Minds* continued and a number of major resources were produced in the years 2007–2014, including new resources and guidelines for providers, and research work into aspects of stigma such as employment, family stigma and self-stigma (discussed in detail later in the chapter).

The Fifth National Plan 2014–2019

In 2013 and 2014 management of the *Like Minds* programme has been moved from the Ministry of Health to the newly created Health Promotion Agency. Coupled with this move is a 'refresh' of the *Like Minds* programme. The Fifth National Plan

(Ministry of Health and Health Promotion Agency 2014) covers the period 2014–2019 and again has a single (societal) outcome, which now includes social inclusion: 'A socially inclusive New Zealand that is free of stigma and discrimination towards people with mental illness'. The organisational and individual outcomes have been removed in favour of a tighter focus on specific organisations (workplaces and the media) and focus on the excluders rather than the excluded (i.e. a move away from including actions targeted at people with experience of mental illness including actions to reduce self-stigma). A part of the refresh was a move to a contestable fund for providers in 2015, which may result in significant changes in the organisations providing *Like Minds* services.

Ways of Working

There have been several key commitments which have been at the heart of *Like Minds*. These include ensuring that people with lived experience are central in the programme and a commitment to ensuring the programme is acceptable and effective for Māori and other groups.

People with Lived Experience Are Central

Since the beginnings of *Like Minds*, the involvement of people with lived experience of mental illness has been a key feature. As the programme has developed so too have the roles of those with lived experience within the programme.

Early in the project, advisory roles and groups were created for people with lived experience at national and local levels. A National Consumer Advisory Group and Māori and Pacific caucuses were convened to provide advice to the project governance group. The National Advisory Group was disestablished in 2005 and focus instead turned to ensuring that people with experience of mental illness were employed in roles reflecting their skills and expertise throughout the programme, including in leadership roles.

Contact with people with experience of mental illness was recognised as the key strategy for reducing stigma and discrimination, and so people with lived experience also had a role in sharing their personal experiences of mental illness and recovery. This was initially done at the local level through facilitating public speaking engagements as well as involving people with lived experience in 'telling their story' in education sessions. However it became apparent that support and guidance was needed to help people to tell their stories in a way that was both safe for them and also elicited reflection by their audiences on their own capacity to discriminate. For this reason training was developed to equip people to present information based on their personal experience of mental illness, stigma, discrimination and recovery, and *Speakers' Bureaux* – collectives of people with experience of mental illness trained and supported to tell their personal stories with the purpose of countering discriminatory attitudes – were established around New Zealand.

Members of the bureaux would then take part in workshops, gradually building capacity to take on more of leading role in workshop facilitation. *Speakers' Bureaux* members could also use their training to be media spokespeople for the programme and were available to journalists to provide the perspective of someone with lived experience.

Over time there was increasing recognition of centrality of people with lived experience of mental illness to the success of the project, as providers and decision makers rather than as advisors and 'storytellers'. As human rights and disability rights models became more central, the motto 'nothing about us without us' became increasingly pertinent. Moreover for those who saw eliminating stigma and discrimination as requiring a social movement similar to the civil rights movement, it was felt that the leaders and drivers of the work had to be those who had their own lived experience of mental illness.

The first National Plan identified the importance of 'well-funded strong consumer networks' both to benefit the *Like Minds* project and to improve mental health service delivery (Health Funding Authority 1999, p42). *Like Minds* went on to fund opportunities for face-to-face gatherings of people with lived experience from throughout the country, something which had not happened before, and which enabled the development of a consumer network through the shared work of the campaign. These meetings brought together an extremely diverse group with little in common but a shared experience of mental distress and service use. At times these meetings became very passionate, and they were an essential part of building a coherent consumer voice in *Like Minds* and in mental health services.

People with lived experience have had roles at all levels of the *Like Minds* programme, including many leadership positions, bringing both their own experiences and also specific skills in areas such as research, education, communications, journalism and many others. Most of the *Like Minds* training and education workshops are now provided by organisations which are either consumer led or have very strong consumer involvement.

The Programme Must Work for Māori

One of foundations of *Like Minds* has been a commitment to developing a programme that meets the needs of Māori. The approach to ensuring *Like Minds* works for Māori has included Māori involvement at all levels including in governance, providing resources for specific 'by Māori for Māori' approaches and monitoring Māori outcomes to ensure equity.

The first National Plan articulated a commitment to Māori involvement at all levels based on the Treaty relationship. At a governance level, the *Like Minds* Māori caucus (now called Te Roopu Arahi) was established in 1998 and included Māori leaders and Māori tangata whaiora (people with experience of mental illness). There has also been active encouragement of diversity on groups such as the National Advisory Group and recognition that it can be harder for the voices of Māori with experience of mental illness to be heard. The National Plans document an increasing focus on specific actions to ensure that the programme works for Māori.

There has also been a commitment to empowerment of communities to address their own needs. Māori providers have been contracted to deliver anti-stigma programmes in their local communities around the country. There has been increasing recognition of the need to support these providers with specific resources and training. Annual meetings of all Māori *Like Minds* providers were also convened from 2003, enabling providers to share their ideas, experience and growing expertise. The Māori providers have all had quite different practices, and the providers have changed over time. The use of Māori language, and tikanga (protocol), and delivering workshops in marae settings have however been important features of many providers' work. *He kakano o Rangiatea – He kete Matauranga* (Like Minds 2009), a document for Māori *Like Minds* providers intended to sit alongside the 2007 National Plan, was produced in 2009. It emphasises the importance of cultural approaches to addressing the stigma and discrimination associated with mental illness while engaging with Māori communities. This document combines a Māori model of health promotion (Te Pae Mahutonga – based on the stars of the Southern Cross constellation) with the outcomes, actions and approaches of the *Like Minds* programme.

Research has been an important mechanism by which the *Like Minds* programme has shown its commitment to Māori. Research undertaken at the outset of Like Minds explored Māori models of health and understandings of mental distress, in order to inform approaches to reducing stigma and discrimination for Māori (Cram et al. 1997). The main research streams of the programme have also endeavoured to include sufficient power (numbers) to study the results for Māori separately. For example, the tracking surveys of public attitudes which have followed the media campaigns have oversampled Māori (and Pacific) to ensure that the attitudes of Māori and Pacific communities are tracked alongside the general population which is predominantly Pakeha (European).

Appropriate Approaches for Pacific and Other New Zealanders

Like Minds also has a commitment to developing a programme that meets the needs of the other communities and cultures in New Zealand. In particular *Like Minds* has had a focus on Pacific communities, and in 2007 the Mental Health Foundation developed a specific focus on Chinese communities, recognising that the different belief systems of these groups require different approaches to stigma and discrimination.

Approaches for Pacific peoples have included both grass-roots education by Pacific providers and strategies to ensure that the mainstream parts of *Like Minds* work for Pacific, for example, with radio advertising aimed at Pacific audiences to sit alongside the television advertising, and the inclusion of Pacific people in the television advertising. Pacific communities in New Zealand are not homogenous but come from different Pacific Islands and speak different languages, and include both New Zealand born and overseas born Pacific people, and so a variety of approaches is needed. Face-to-face approaches have proven to be effective in engaging Pacific audiences, as have the use of settings such as churches which are community hubs for Pacific communities, while radio has been more effective for reaching a younger Pacific audience.

For Chinese communities, the approach taken has been principally via an online resource: the Chinese language website Kai Xin Xing Dong (KXXD).[4] The focus is on providing information and support to Chinese people with experience of mental illness and their families. The Mental Health Foundation also has Chinese speaking health promoters and works with health service providers and other professionals to help them work effectively with the Chinese community. As with other parts of *Like Minds*, KXXD utilises the power of contact, with personal stories of recovery from Chinese New Zealanders on the website. As about 80 % of the Chinese community in New Zealand are overseas born (Statistics New Zealand 2014), the work with new migrants is ongoing. The holistic Chinese view of health and the importance of tangible support for Chinese people with mental illness have been highlighted as key features.

Strategies to Combat Stigma and Discrimination

Like Minds has aligned its work to the strategies of contact, protest and education, with a strong focus on contact as the central and most effective strategy for change. These strategies have been used to work towards four key outcomes: changing public attitudes towards people with mental illness, changing the behaviour of those in most contact with people with experience of mental illness, changing policy and law to combat discrimination and empowering people with experience of mental illness to challenge discrimination and self-stigma.

Changing Public Attitudes

The Advertising Campaign

The face of the *Like Minds* programme has been a series of advertisements fronted by both well-known and previously unknown New Zealanders who have experienced mental illness. As noted earlier, the Mason report recommended a national public education campaign as 'a must' and from the outset funding was set aside for a television advertising campaign. The campaign has been built around the stories of real people with experience of mental illness, providing real stories of recovery and success. A series of five phases of advertising have run over 12 years, with the advertisements from each phase running on the major television stations for several months at a time. Some of the phases have included serial advertisements about the same person, providing opportunities for repeated contact and sense of getting to know the person. Inclusion of the stories of family and friends in the advertisements

---

[4] http://www.mentalhealth.org.nz/kaixinxingdong/page/5-Home

has also been an important mechanism for allowing people to relate to the people with lived experience featuring in the advertisements.

The advertising campaign has been backed up by a telephone help and information line which has been available whenever the advertisements have been on air. It has focused on shifting public attitudes towards mental illness, with a focus on 18–44 year olds (the rationale being that the attitudes of this group are more malleable than older adults). There has also been a careful process to ensure that the people who were so publicly telling their personal stories in the campaign were well supported. Each phase has been pretested to ensure that the messages received were as intended, and ongoing evaluation has tracked public attitudes. A mass media advisory group has also been important in ensuring that people with experience of mental illness have input into the campaign. A single advertising company has held the contract for all the advertisements produced up to 2014, and this consistency allowed the building of institutional knowledge and expertise in an area far outside the usual remit of the advertising industry.

The initial focus was on increasing awareness and putting mental health on people's personal agendas. The first and second campaigns featured well-known people and identified them as having experience of mental illness, asking the viewer 'are you prepared to judge?' and telling the viewer 'you can make the difference'. These advertisements emphasised the high prevalence of mental illness, focused on the more common mental illnesses such a depression, and aimed to increase the acceptability of mental illness disclosure. Significantly for New Zealand, a star rugby player was among the people featured in the first campaigns, as well as musicians, a fashion designer and other well-known locals.

Over time, as mental illness has become more acceptable as a topic for discussion, more challenging material has been included which shows recovery from mental illnesses generally regarded as more severe and emphasises the importance of the actions of others and the impacts of discrimination. The third campaign 'Know me before you judge me' included 'ordinary' New Zealanders, less common illnesses such as bipolar disorder and psychosis and moved the focus on to the impact of the attitudes of others towards the person experiencing mental illness ('They can live great lives. With understanding they can do even more'). The fourth campaign had the tagline 'Discrimination is still the biggest barrier to recovery for people with mental illness: What you do makes a difference', shifting the focus directly to the impact of discrimination. The advertisements focused on a single individual with experience of mental illness and his wife, friends and employer, recounting their experience of his illness and recovery and the ways in which recovery was supported. The fifth set of advertisements 'Be there, stay involved', targeted extended family and friends and aimed to equip people to stay involved as part of a support network for someone experiencing mental illness. Unlike earlier campaigns, the mental illness experienced is not named but rather the focus is on the experience and recovery and the importance of support. This phase featured the stories of Maori and Pacific New Zealanders prominently.

Alongside the advertisements running on national television, specific advertisements were made for Pacific audiences, playing on a Pacific news programme and on television in the Pacific, as well as in primary care waiting rooms and at community training events. A series of brief documentaries were also made for use in training workshops, focusing on particular issues such as employment, personal discrimination and the association between mental illness and violence. An increasing catalogue of personal recovery stories is also available. All this material can be viewed on the *Like Minds* website.[5]

Serial surveys have tracked the response to the advertising campaign. There has been generally high recall of television advertising, with over 80 % recall through phases two and three of the advertising and 65–79 % in the latter phases (Wylie and Lauder 2012). Awareness of the advertising was initially lower for Maori and Pacific people but increased to be higher than other groups in the most recent survey, perhaps reflecting the inclusion of Maori and Pacific people in the advertisements more prominently than previously. Message recall is good, with 74 % of those who had seen the advertisements recalling the main 'be more accepting/supportive/don't discriminate' messages in 2012. Of those who had seen the advertisements, over half reported discussing them at least once in 2012, with an even higher proportion having discussed them with others in earlier phases of the campaign. These surveys have also found that public attitudes to mental illness appear to be changing, and this is discussed later.

Working with Media to Change Public Attitudes

Together with the mass media campaign, multiple other strategies have been used to change the climate of public opinion. A focus has been reporting by the media, who are a major source of public information about mental illness, trying to discourage reporting which perpetuates stereotypes and encourage positive reporting about mental health issues. The strategies used for this have been a mixture of challenging and commending of reporting and education and contact initiatives for journalists.

Monitoring of media reporting and working with journalists to improve their approach has been important throughout *Like Minds*. The Mental Health Foundation currently leads this monitoring and response work, which includes working with producers and script writers and providing resources for journalists. They also run a stigma watch mailing list, which provides notifications of potentially stigmatising reporting, plus templates for letters of complaint or praise, to encourage a wider group to get involved in monitoring the media.

Growing an informed media is also important. Since 2001 awards have been available for individual journalists to do dedicated pieces of work relating to mental health issues. Initially these awards were funded by the Carter Centre in Atlanta Georgia and gave the opportunity for a New Zealand journalist to travel to their centre. After this arrangement finished in 2007, the Mental Health Foundation took over running a scheme of annual media grants for journalism and creative projects. Recent work includes an in-depth magazine feature *Speaking Out About Suicide* and a photojournalism exhibition *The Space Between Words* which chronicles the

---

[5] www.likeminds.org.nz

internal journeys of 14 individuals in the 2 years following the devastating Canterbury earthquakes (more information is available on the MHF website).[6]

Other ways to grow an informed media include working with journalism students and with local media, to raise awareness and to provide opportunities for contact with people with experience of mental illness. Some local providers have also conducted workshops with journalism students and have developed relationships with local media. *The Media Handbook*, giving advice on the use of appropriate language, the avoidance of reinforcing myths and stereotypes, as well as guidance on interviewing mental health consumers, was produced in 2001 and distributed to journalists and media outlets. More recently a video resource for media, *Working with Mental Health Stories*, has been produced by the Mental Health Foundation (Mental Health Foundation 2011).

As well as building an informed media, it is also important that the *Like Minds* workforce is able to get the attention of the media for the right reasons and encourage positive portrayals of the *Like Minds* work and of people with experience of mental illness. A series of videos entitled 'Media Savvy' were produced for *Like Minds* in 2011 to provide a resource for *Like Minds* providers on working with the media (Like Minds Like Mine 2011).

Other Work to Change Public Attitudes

There has been a variety of other work aimed at changing public attitudes run by regional providers which has occurred under the *Like Minds* banner. Some examples include arts events and community radio shows.

Community radio shows which give space for people with experience of mental illness to tell their stories of recovery have been set up in a number of centres, with eight different shows either directly or indirectly affiliated with Like Minds running in 2014 (Like Minds Like Mine 2014). These shows are for the most part hosted and produced by people with lived experience and include a variety of guests talking about mental health-related topics, with some also including a talk-back component. The shows run on community radio stations every week, including stations with mainly Māori or Pacific audiences. A number of the shows have been running for many years and are well received by their local communities. However there has been no formal evaluation of the impacts of any of the radio shows, and the limited budgets of community providers tend to preclude collecting information on the audience for such stations.

Creative arts initiatives to challenge stigma and discrimination have also been a part of the *Like Minds* work of many local providers. A recent example was the Big reTHiNK festival held in 2012, in which 12 plays from around the world were staged, interspersed with comedy acts, film, music and graphics, all dealing with topics of distress and madness. The festival was attended by around 2,000 people and was well received, and all the performances are now available on YouTube (Mind and Body 2012). Other creative initiatives have included a short film competition, art shows and theatre performances in schools. The use of the creative arts is

---

[6] http://www.mentalhealth.org.nz/page/1586-journalism-fellows

recognised as a powerful way to present recovery messages and to challenge discriminatory attitudes, and where feedback has been sought, the audience responses have been very positive. However one-off events may only reach a small audience. Social media has the potential for making such events available to a far larger audience.

Changing Behaviours

Workshops for Education and Training

Local level 'grass-roots' action for behaviour change to complement attitude change work was and is a key approach. Workshops with local organisations to provide education about mental illness and stigma and discrimination were delivered from the outset of the project and always included the voices of people with lived experience. However over time the way in which these workshops are run and the audiences they target has evolved. Initially many different kinds of workshops and education sessions were run, depending on local knowledge and expertise. There has been growing evidence about importance of behavioural orientation, not just providing information, and growing knowledge about the kinds of recovery stories and explanations which can incite reflection and behaviour change. Workshops need to be built around supporting favourable contact.

Knowledge of what works better for reducing discrimination has fed into growing guidance and consistency in training for providers, delivery of workshops and in evaluation. Best practice guidelines for delivering education and training to counter stigma and discrimination associated with mental distress have recently been produced (Jane 2012). The guidelines provide a structure for planning, designing and evaluating education and training interventions, based around the core conditions of effective contact: that it must be targeted, continuous, local and credible (see Fig. 15.2). The focus is on encouraging the active involvement of participants, providing a safe place to air concerns and ask questions.

There has also been increasing awareness of the importance of targeting workshops. Initially many workshops were delivered to community organisations and community groups who did not necessarily have a major influence on the lives of people with experience of mental illness. Workshops are now increasingly targeted at, and tailored to, specific audiences with the potential for a high impact on discrimination, for example, government agencies such as the NZ Police, Work and Income NZ (the social welfare agency responsible for benefit provision and employment assistance) and Housing NZ (New Zealand's social housing agency). Health service providers and students training for health professions are also an important target group. Research into the discrimination experienced has been very important in enabling targeting of face-to-face interventions. The current National Plan specifically targets employers.

Although evaluation was recognised as important from the outset, initially each provider was left to design and implement its own evaluation plan, which meant

WORKSHOP CRITERIA

Use the following criteria to judge whether your existing Like Minds workshops are matched to the principles of contact for countering stigma and discrimintation:

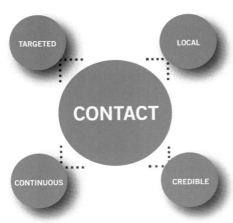

CONTACT – does your workshop include someone with personal experience of mental distress delivering the education or training?

TARGETED – is your workshop matched to one of the target groups, and relevant to specific barriers or issues for that group?

LOCAL – does your workshop meet the mutual needs of your community and the Like Minds programme?

CREDIBLE – is your 'contact' person embodying the principles of recovery at present? Are they matched to the target group, e.g. role, ethnicity, religious/spiritual belief, age, or other relevant status?

CONTINUOUS – have you planned multiple contact opportunities with your target group?

Fig. 15.2 Criteria for workshops to counter stigma and discrimination (Source: (Jane 2012). Copyright Kites Trust)

that there was little consistency and it was difficult to bring knowledge together. A consistent approach to evaluation of workshops has recently been developed by Kites Trust, and workshop evaluations now follow one of several standard templates (including options for written or facilitated verbal feedback from participants, as well as written feedback from workshop facilitators) with results collated nationally (Oakden and Jane 2013).

Changing Policy and Law

Challenging systemic discrimination, such as that existing in statute or organisational policy, has always been a part of the broad agenda of *Like Minds*. Initially emphasis was placed on developing media campaigns and the workforce at local level. By 2003, however, an explicit top level goal was created seeking 'change public and private sector policy to value and include all people with experience of mental illness' (Ministry of Health 2003). The objectives now included advocating for non-discriminatory policies and practices, both within organisations responsible for housing, education and employment and within health services.

The Government Policy Project, set up in 2000, was the first attempt to explicitly influence policymakers. However much of the work of this project ended up being research to understand the nature and extent of discrimination experienced in different aspects of life, in order to provide evidence for policymakers. Results from the *Respect Costs Nothing* survey (Peterson et al. 2004) were fed back to sectors including housing, justice and health, asking what action the agencies would take to address the issues raised.

Korowai Whaimana, a human rights training programme by and for people with experience of mental illness, was developed in conjunction with the Human Rights Commission. People with experience of mental illness were trained to run 1-day workshops on human rights and using the Human Rights Act and other legislation to challenge discrimination. The programme focused on enabling people with experience of mental illness to use the existing protest mechanisms such as the Human Rights Commission's complaints process, recognising that such mechanisms were underutilised in protesting discrimination on the basis of mental illness. An increase in complaints and enquiries to the Human Rights Commission relating to mental illness was noted after the programme was implemented in 2005 (Edwards 2007).

Local providers of workshops aimed at changing behaviour also often link in to addressing discrimination in the organisations they are working with, through developing relationships with leaders in the organisations and encouraging and aiding policy review.

Work on addressing systemic and organisational discrimination is perhaps the least developed area of *Like Minds* work but continues to be identified as a key area for making a difference.

Empowering People with Lived Experience to Challenge Stigma and Discrimination

One of the destinations in the Mental Health Commission's *Travel Guide for people on the journeys towards equality, respect and rights for people who experience mental illness* was 'A country in which people with mental illness have the personal power to gain equality, respect and rights' (MHC 1998). At a strategic level, *Like Minds* has not always included empowerment as an objective of the programme. The Fourth National Plan included an individual level objective as well as a societal one and included self-stigma as a target for *Like Minds* work. In contrast the Fifth National Plan explicitly focuses the work of *Like Minds* on the general public and those in positions of influence as those doing the excluding, rather than on those being excluded. However whether or not empowering people with lived experience is a target of *Like Minds*, it has certainly been an effect.

The *Like Minds* programme has to some extent been a vehicle for the development and growth of the mental health consumer movement in New Zealand, together with increasingly formalised roles for consumers in mental health service organisations. Involvement in *Like Minds*, and having the experience of mental illness valued, has been an important part of the recovery journey for many people with experience of mental illness and has often been a stepping stone to other careers. By funding organisations run by and focused on the well-being and rights of people with experience of mental illness, *Like Minds* has also helped to strengthen the political voice of people with experience of mental illness. However government funding also comes with restrictions, particularly on advocacy work, which can also have the effect of lessening political voice. The 'overlapping circles' of a social movement and a government funded and managed public health programme have been a source of tension throughout *Like Minds*.

Some work within the *Like Minds* programme has also focused explicitly on empowering and enabling people with lived experience, such as *Korowai Whaimana* human rights training to empower people with experience of mental illness to protest discrimination. A major piece of research on self-stigma (Peterson et al. 2008) was also completed by the Mental Health Foundation as part of the *Like Minds* programme, recognising that self-stigma must also be challenged if stigma and discrimination are to be addressed, although to date this has not been a focus of *Like Minds* work.

Where Are We Now?

Like Minds Has Been Shown to Be Effective

Throughout the life of Like Minds, public attitudes to mental illness have been assessed, with both annual telephone surveys and more in-depth research into the attitudes of particular groups including employers, mental health service providers and young people. Telephone surveys have included approximately 1,000 randomly selected respondents aged 18–44 each year from 2000 to 2012, including booster samples for Māori and Pacific, and have asked about awareness of mental health diagnoses, agreement or disagreement with positive and negative attitude statements and about willingness to accept someone with mental illness in a variety of roles, as well as awareness and perception of the advertising campaigns.

Over time there has been a general increase in positive attitudes and acceptance and a decrease in negative attitudes (Wylie and Lauder 2012). There have been some changes in perceptions about the nature of mental illness, for example, disagreement with the statement 'people with mental illness are never going to contribute much' has increased (77 % in 2000, 88 % in 2012), as has disagreement with the statement 'people with mental illness are more likely to be dangerous' (27 % in 2000, 39 % in 2012). Acceptance of people with experience of mental illness has also improved. Disagreement with the statement 'I would feel uncomfortable talking to someone with mental illness' has increased (61 % in 2000, 78 % in 2012), as has disagreement with 'If I got a mental illness I would feel ashamed' (30 % in 2000, 44 % in 2012).

There have been increases in willingness to accept a person with experience of mental illness as a workmate, as a resident of a halfway house in your street or as a babysitter (as shown in Fig. 15.3 below). Willingness to accept people with schizophrenia in these situations has also increased, albeit from a lower base. There is also some increase in awareness of what individuals can do to support someone with a mental illness, with an increase in the proportion responding that they could give support (32 % in 2008, 49 % in 2012). There has however been little change in the

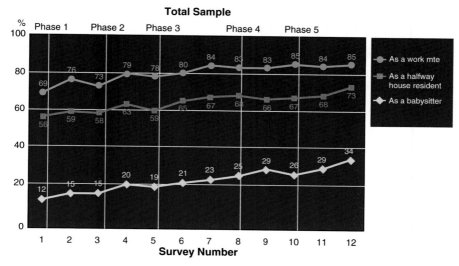

Fig. 15.3 Willingness to accept a person who has experience of mental illness (Source: Wylie and Lauder 2012)

proportion who agrees that they can see discrimination against people with experience of mental illness (74 % in 2000, 71 % in 2012).

More in-depth surveys conducted in 1997 and 2004 also showed changes in attitudes which are likely to be the result of the *Like Minds* programme (Fearn and Wylie 2005). The main changes seen in the 2004 survey were that people with mental illness were seen as more capable, there was increased social acceptance of people with experience of mental illness and increased acceptance that people with mental illness should not be denied responsibility. Those identifying as employers or managers in these surveys were also specifically examined and showed similar trends to the overall sample, showing increased agreement that a person with a mental illness is able to hold down a job and increased willingness to a employ or work with a person with specified mental illnesses, although small numbers meant that these changes were not statistically significant (Phoenix Research 2006). In-depth interviews with employers highlighted ongoing concerns about employing a person with experience of mental illness (Lennan and Wylie 2005). Research with people with experience of mental illness about employment experiences has highlighted the importance of employment and experiences of discrimination but also support and accommodation from employers (Peterson 2007).

The impact on Maori and Pacific communities has also been assessed through the serial surveys. For Maori, as with the general population, there has been an increase in positive attitudes and acceptance and decrease in negative attitudes over the 12 years of the campaign, with greater increases seen in Maori across many of the questions asked particularly in later years. For Pacific peoples there have also been improvements, particularly in acceptance of people with experience of mental illness (Wylie and Lauder 2012).

In 2010 an economic evaluation commissioned by the Ministry of Health examined the costs and benefits of the *Like Minds* programme (Vaithianathan and Pram 2010). It focused on the benefits accrued to employment rates through decreased discrimination by employers and increased use of primary care leading to better recovery outcomes and found that for the $52 million spent to that point, an economic benefit of approximately $720 million had accrued. This equates to $13.80 benefit for every dollar spent. This analysis used the results of surveys of employer attitudes in 1997 and 2004 and assumed that all change was due to *Like Minds*. However under even their most conservative assumptions of the proportion of change due to *Like Minds*, a 4:1 benefit was still accrued for every dollar spent. Benefits beyond employment are harder to put a dollar value on, but if these could be accounted for then an even greater return for investment would no doubt be seen.

There is also some evidence from people with experience of mental illness of positive changes in discriminatory behaviour. A survey of over 1,000 people with a history of mental health service use conducted in 2010 (Wylie and Brown 2011) found that 54 % reported that there had been some improvement over the last 5 years when considering all ways of being treated unfairly because of their mental illness. Conversely, there were 16 % who thought it was now worse. When considering unfair treatment by mental health staff, there were 42 % who thought it had improved over the last 5 years and 11 % who thought it was now worse.

Other Projects Have Launched from the Like Minds Platform

The *Like Minds* programme has also served as a platform for the launch of a number of other important and successful initiatives in mental health promotion and public education.

The National Depression initiative (NDI), funded by the Ministry of Health, aims to reduce the impact of depression on the lives of New Zealanders by aiding early recognition, appropriate treatment and recovery. The NDI includes a television campaign and website[7] fronted by the ex-All Black who was also involved in the *Like Minds* campaigns (a fact which means that the general public do not distinguish between *Like Minds* and NDI). It also provides health resources, online and text-based support services and research. The NDI supports primary mental health service development and the implementation of guidelines for GPs on mental health issues including depression. NDI focuses on education and encouraging help seeking and treatment (in contrast to the *Like Minds* focus on public attitudes and behaviours), but NDI nonetheless has a complementary role to *Like Minds* in changing attitudes and making mental illness more acceptable.

---

[7] www.depression.org

MH101 is mental health literacy programme, also funded by the Ministry of Health, which aims to 'give people the confidence to recognise, relate and respond to mental illness' (Blueprint for Learning 2014). MH101 is a 1-day workshop, and as with *Like Minds* MH101 utilises the power of contact, with at least one facilitator in workshops having lived experience. The workshops are tailored to front-line staff in government and social service agencies but are also provided to a wide range of other groups. The programme has been achieving good results and is highly regarded internationally.

Other mental health promotion and suicide prevention initiatives in New Zealand have also benefited from the profile and experience gained through *Like Minds* and the changes in public attitudes to mental illness which have resulted. More generally, the growth of consumer input into mental health services and the moves towards recovery orientated services have been aided by the work of *Like Minds*, particularly in growing the consumer workforce.

We Are Gaining an Increasing Understanding of Stigma, Discrimination and Social Inclusion

Research into the experience of people with mental illness has always been a key part of *Like Minds*, generating new knowledge and understanding about the issues the programme targets. Extensive research into the experience of discrimination has been conducted, as discussed earlier. The most recent project about discrimination is *Walk a Mile in Our Shoes*, which explores the experience of discrimination towards and within families of people diagnosed with mental illness (Barnett and Barnes 2010). Building on this understanding of discrimination, the recent research report *Stories of Success* (Hamer et al. 2014) also explores successful stories of social inclusion experienced by people with mental illness. Social inclusion is defined as 'the fundamental right to be recognised as equal alongside others in society', and the actions of others, alongside personal power and individual champions, are highlighted as important for social inclusion. A number of recommendations are made to enable *Like Minds* to promote social inclusion.

A new model of stigma and discrimination was developed from the *Fighting Shadows* research which investigated the experience of self-stigma among people with experience of mental illness (Peterson et al. 2008). This model describes a cycle which includes both internalised and public stigma and discrimination. Importantly, the model also identifies actions which can interrupt the cycle of stigma and discrimination and has the potential to widen the scope of anti-stigma work, showing the role of actions beyond the focus on challenging attitudes and behaviour. It emphasises the important role mental health services have in breaking the cycle of stigma through recovery-oriented practices, as well as the role of peer support and empowerment. While it may be appropriate for a programme aimed at addressing discrimination to focus on challenging behaviour and attitudes (as *Like Minds* currently does), this model serves as a reminder of all the other activities which are necessary for the cycle to be broken.

Some Reflections About What Matters

Language Matters

The language we use matters. The word discrimination has deliberately been used in *Like Minds* to keep the focus on the importance of the actions of others. The language of experience has also been a key feature. By talking about the 'experience of mental illness', mental illness does not become a permanent feature of the individual but rather something which is temporary, from which recovery is possible. Experience also implies expertise gained through that experience. The term 'lived experience' is also used to emphasise the expertise gained by living through an experience of mental illness. Moreover the term distress is often used instead of illness, in an attempt to move away from medical recognition and diagnosis as defining features. While there has been conflict about the language used, and particularly around the use of diagnostic labels, there has been general agreement on the value of talking about discrimination and experience. The language of consumers or mental health service users is also used to talk about those whose distress has brought them into contact with services, but in general *Like Minds* has focused on all those who identify as having had experience of mental illness or distress.

Consumer Leadership Matters

Like Minds has been built by consumer leaders and has built consumer leaders. It has been built around the real stories of people with experience of mental illness, stories told face-to-face and virtually, but always real stories told by real people. People with lived experience have led and innovated in all parts of *Like Minds*. This is the group for whom *Like Minds* matters the most, and continued meaningful involvement and leadership will be vital to continued success.

Do Not Be Afraid of Conflict and Passion

Finally, the lesson from *Like Minds* has been to not be afraid of conflict. *Like Minds* has been forged amidst huge amounts of passion and conflict. It has brought together a very diverse group with different world views, and different experiences, and very different ideas about how to achieve change. However, through a shared understanding of the goal of the work, it has been possible for this diverse group to work together to achieve change, bringing along the different groups they represent for the ride. It is important that the different views and voices within *Like Minds* continue to have a place, for *Like Minds* to have an innovative and successful future.

Conclusions

Like Minds, New Zealand's programme to combat stigma and discrimination, has now been in existence for 17 years. It has not been a straightforward journey but one full of twists and turns, changes in focus and direction. The underlying philosophy of the programme has drawn on health promotion and public health, on human rights and the disability movement and on the voice of lived experience. *Like Minds* has been a programme of social change, and social change evolves over time and requires commitment. Social change does not always sit easily with being a government funded programme sitting within the health sector whose core business is the provision of health services. However, *Like Minds* has been responsible for changes in the way people with experience of mental illness are viewed, and changed the New Zealand social environment for the better. The work of social change is not complete, and there remains a place for concerted and coordinated efforts focused specifically on addressing and reducing discrimination associated with mental illness.

Acknowledgements This chapter reflects the views of the authors, and does not represent the views of *Like Minds* staff or funders. The authors would like to thank the following people who have generously spoken with us about their experiences of *Like Minds, Like Mine*: Taimi Allan, Egan Bidois, Darryl Bishop, Sheldon Brown, Judi Clemments, Sonja Eriksen, Sarah Gordon, Alex Handiside, Marge Jackson, Warren Lindberg, Virginia MacEwan, Vito Malo, Dean Manley, Mary O'Hagan, Janet Peters, Fale Puka, Tane Rangihuna, Mary Strang, Gerard Vaughn, Allan Wylie, and Ivan Yeo. Thanks also to Judi Clemments, Gerard Vaughn and Janet Peters for peer review.

References

Barnett H, Barnes A (2010) Walk a mile in our shoes. He tuara, ngā tapuwae tuku iho ō ngā Mātua Tūpuna. Exploring discrimination within and towards families and Whānau of people diagnosed with 'Mental Illness'. Mental Health Foundation, Auckland

Blueprint for Learning (2014) MH101 website. From http://www.mh101.co.nz/

Mind and Body (2012) The big ReTHink. from http://www.youtube.com/playlist?list=PLJdzhW3 HIi5Z7NoSfMd0HI-igAsg5ojuT

Case Consulting (2005) The power of contact. Case Consulting Ltd. Wellington, New Zealand

Cram F, Reid P, Panapa A, Keefe V (1997) Community attitudes towards people with mental illness. Stage 1 – pre-research with Maori. Te Roopu Rangahau Hauora a Eru Pomare, Wellington School of Medicine, Wellington

Edwards G (2007) Evaluation of Korowai Whaimana: summary report. Positive Thinking Ltd, Wellington

Fearn A, Wylie A (2005) Public knowledge and attitudes to mental health and mental illness: update of 1997 benchmark survey. Phoenix Research, Auckland

Hamer H, Clarke S, Butler R, Lampshire D, Kidd J (2014) Stories of success: mental health service users' experiences of social inclusion in Aotearoa New Zealand: Na pukorero rangatira: Na tangata waiora i whaiora i enei tuahuatana. The Mental Health Foundation of New Zealand, Auckland

Health Funding Authority (1999) The project to counter stigma and discrimination associated with mental illness: national plan. Health Funding Authority, Wellington

Jane D (2012) Best practice guidelines: for delivering education and training to counter stigma and discrimination associated with mental distress. Kites Trust, Wellington

Lennan M, Wylie A (2005) Employer attitudes and behaviours relating to mental illness. Phoenix Research, Auckland

Like Minds LM (2009) He kākano ō Rangiātea, He kete Matauranga. Mental Health Foundation of New Zealand, Auckland

Like Minds Like Mine (2011) Media Savvy videos. http://www.likeminds.org.nz/resources/for-reporters/media-savvy-videos/

Like Minds Like Mine (2014) Like Minds radio shows. Retrieved 26 Sept 2014, from http://www.likeminds.org.nz/discrimination/radio-show/

Mason K, Johnston J, Crowe J (1996) Inquiry under section 47 of the Health and Disability Services Act 1993 in respect of certain mental health services. Report of the Ministerial Inquiry to the Minister of Health. Ministry of Health, Wellington

Mental Health Commission (1998) Blueprint for mental health services in New Zealand: how things need to be. Mental Health Commission, Wellington

Mental Health Commission (2000) The discrimination times: a report on an investigation into news media (re)presentation of people with mental illness. Mental Health Commission, Wellington

Mental Health Commission (2005) Reducing discrimination against people with mental illness, Te Hekenga: Whakamana i te Tangata Whaiora. Multi-agency plan 2005–2007. Mental Health Commission, Wellington

MHC (1998) Travel guide for people on the journeys towards equality, respect and rights for people who experience mental illness. Mental Health Commission, Wellington

Mental Health Foundation (2011) Working with mental health stories. http://www.likeminds.org.nz/resources/for-reporters/in-our-own-words/

Ministry of Health (1997) Moving forward: the national mental health plan for more and better services. Ministry of Health, Wellington

Ministry of Health (2001) National plan 2001–2003: project to counter stigma and discrimination associated with mental illness. Ministry of Health, Wellington

Ministry of Health (2003) Like Minds, Like Mine national plan 2003–2005. Ministry of Health, Wellington

Ministry of Health (2007) Like Minds, Like Mine national plan 2007–2013. Ministry of Health, Wellington

Ministry of Health and Health Promotion Agency (2014) Like Minds, Like Mine national plan 2014–2019: programme to increase social inclusion and reduce stigma and discrimination for people with experience of mental illness. Ministry of Health, Wellington

Ng S, Martin J, Romans S (1995) A community's attitudes towards the mentally ill. N Z Med J 108(1013):505–508

O'Hagan M (1994) Stopovers on my way home from Mars: a journey into the psychiatric survivor movement in the USA, Britain and the Netherlands. Survivors Speak Out, London

Oakden J, Jane D (2013) Evaluation manual: for the new evaluation system for Like Minds, Like Mine education and training activities. Kites Trust, Wellington

Patten D (1992) Public attitudes to mental illness. D. o. Health, Wellington

Peterson D (2007) I haven't told them, they haven't asked: the employment experiences of people with experience of mental illness. Mental Health Foundation, Wellington

Peterson D, Pere L, Sheehan N, Surgenor G (2004) Respect costs nothing: mental health discrimination in New Zealand. Mental Health Foundation, Wellington

Peterson D, Pere L, Sheehan N, Surgenor G (2007) Experiences of mental health discrimination in New Zealand. Health Soc Care Community 15(1):18–25

Peterson D, Barnes A, Duncan C (2008) Fighting shadows: self-stigma and mental illness: Whawhai Atu te Whakamā Hihira. Mental Health Foundation, Auckland

Phoenix Research (2006) Employer and manager knowledge of and attitudes towards mental illness. Phoenix Research, Auckland

Statistics New Zealand (2014) 2013 census ethnic group profiles. Retrieved 25 Sept 2014, from http://www.stats.govt.nz/Census/2013-census/profile-and-summary-reports/ethnic-profiles.aspx

Vaithianathan R, Pram K (2010) Cost benefit analysis of the New Zealand national mental health destigmatisation programme ("Like-Minds Programme"). Department of Economics, University of Auckland, Auckland

Wylie A, Brown R (2011) Discrimination reported by users of mental health services: 2010 survey. Phoenix Research, Auckland

Wylie A, Lauder J (2012) Impacts of a national media campaign to counter stigma and discrimination associated with mental illness: survey 12, response to the fifth phase of campaign. Phoenix Research, Auckland

Australian Country Perspective: The Work of *beyondblue* and SANE Australia

16

Georgie Harman and Jack Heath

Introduction

This chapter illustrates the approaches used to reduce stigma against people affected by mental illness in Australia. The work of *beyondblue, the National Depression and Anxiety Initiative*, and *SANE Australia, the National Mental Health Organisation*, will demonstrate how the voice of people with lived experience of mental illness has informed our approach. It will show how the learnings to be found in the scientific literature, the grey literature, the unpublished market research and the experiences of our international colleagues have informed our efforts. Finally, this chapter will illustrate what we know about the impact of this work, with the goal of improving the lives of people with mental illness, their families, friends and carers.

Background: The Australian Context

The Prevalence of Mental Illness in Australia

Australia is well-served by research into the prevalence and impact of mental illness. A series of major studies enable us to state with confidence that around 20 % of the adult population is affected by some form of mental health problem in a 12-month period and that the lifetime prevalence rate for all conditions is estimated at 45.5 % (Reavley and Jorm 2013).

G. Harman (✉)
beyondblue, Hawthorn, VIC, Australia
e-mail: Georgie.Harman@beyondblue.org.au

J. Heath
SANE Australia, South Melbourne, VIC, Australia
e-mail: jack@sane.org

© Springer International Publishing Switzerland 2017
W. Gaebel et al. (eds.), *The Stigma of Mental Illness - End of the Story?*,
DOI 10.1007/978-3-319-27839-1_16

Anxiety disorders and depression are the most prevalent mental health conditions in Australia. The 2007 Australian *National Survey of Mental Health and Wellbeing* (NSMHWB) estimated the 12-month prevalence rate for anxiety disorders to be 14.4 % (10.8 % in males and 17.9 % in females), affecting over two million people. The rate for affective disorders (depression, dysthymia, bipolar affective disorder) was estimated to be 6.2 % (5.3 % in males and 7.1 % in females), affecting around one million people.

Low-prevalence conditions often have the most severe and chronic impact on the lives of those affected. Twelve-month prevalence of psychotic conditions such as schizophrenia in Australia has been conservatively estimated at 0.45 % (0.54 % in males and 0.35 % in females) (Morgan et al. 2011). This estimate is restricted to clients of public mental health services aged 18–64, however, and overall prevalence may be as much as double this figure – around 1 %, affecting over 100,000 Australians.

Undiagnosed and suboptimally treated mental illness across a range of conditions is associated with higher risk of suicide. In Australia in 2011, there were 2,273 deaths from suicide (Reavley and Jorm 2013). Reducing stigma can make a significant contribution to lowering the suicide rate, through promotion of improved understanding of symptoms, awareness of risk, earlier intervention and greater willingness to seek treatment.

The Lived Experience of Stigma in Australia

Australian research confirms that most people with mental illness report experiencing stigma relating to their mental health condition. The degree, nature and experience of stigma and discrimination may be influenced by factors such as the mental health condition itself, age and gender of the person and culture (*beyondblue* Information Paper 2014). Further workplace research conducted as part of an international study found that 41 % of Australian employees would not disclose a diagnosis of depression to their employer, primarily due to the fear of putting their job at risk (SANE Australia 2014a). The impact of stigma is profound, leading to social exclusion, discrimination and reluctance to seek diagnosis and treatment, with all the negative impacts this brings, affecting family as well as the person with the illness.

The Approach of *beyondblue*, the National Depression and Anxiety Initiative

About *beyondblue*

beyondblue was established as a national initiative in October 2000, in the context of the World Health Organization's projections of an increasing global burden caused by depression. The intent was to create a community response to depression, such that it was understood, acknowledged and addressed by the community at large. By 2009, the organisation was established as a focal point for depression in Australia, with 87 % of Australians aware of *beyondblue* and its work. As it continued its work, *beyondblue* expanded its focus to include anxiety and, in 2013, suicide prevention. *beyondblue's* work is aimed at achieving an Australian community that understands depression and anxiety, empowering all Australians, at any life stage, to seek help. *beyondblue* recognises that health inequalities warrant dedicated, tailored approaches to meet the needs of groups of people at high risk. The experiences and needs of people with depression and anxiety and their families and friends underpin all *beyondblue* work.

beyondblue's key result areas have evolved as the organisation has evolved; however, common goals over its first 15 years have included:

- Increasing awareness of depression and anxiety
- Reducing stigma and discrimination
- Improving help seeking for people with depression and anxiety (and more recently, for those at risk of suicide)
- Reducing the impact and disability associated with these conditions

As such, whilst stigma reduction has consistently been identified as a key result area, it remains one of several areas for *beyondblue* to address, as opposed to being the single focus of *beyondblue*'s work.

Measuring *beyondblue's* Progress Towards Stigma Reduction

In order to assess progress towards achievement of its goals, *beyondblue* commissioned a randomly generated national telephone survey, involving 3,200 people aged 18 and older, every 2–3 years, commencing in 2004. Known as the Depression Monitor survey, this provides a snapshot of awareness, knowledge, attitudes and behaviour, relating to depression and anxiety in the Australian community.

Data collected from the Depression Monitor shows that since 2004 there has been a decline in stigmatising attitudes associated with depression and anxiety. In the most recent 2012 survey, significantly fewer participants agreed that people with severe depression were 'dangerous to others', 'have themselves to blame', 'are unpredictable', 'are unreliable', 'are weak willed' and 'should pull themselves together'. Depression Monitor data also shows that since 2004 there have been small but significant increases in the proportion of people indicating that they would be willing to make friends with someone with depression and have someone with depression marry into their family. Overall, the findings suggest the vast majority of the population is comfortable socialising and working with people with depression.

However, whilst data trends suggest that *beyondblue's* efforts to reduce stigma and discrimination associated with depression and anxiety are contributing to changes in community attitudes, there is also evidence that there is more work to be done.

In the most recent survey findings (2012), on average, one in seven people believed those with severe depression are 'weak willed', and one in four believed they should 'pull themselves together'. This suggests many people still wrongly believe overcoming depression is simply a case of 'mind over matter'. Also of concern is the finding that despite improvements from earlier surveys, one in four continued to believe that people with severe depression 'are dangerous to others'.

Further, when differences between the sexes are considered, it is evident that men are more likely than women to hold negative views towards people with depression. Compared to women, men were more likely to believe that people with severe depression 'should pull themselves together' (31 % versus 20 %) and 'have themselves to blame' (13 % versus 5 %) (*beyondblue* Depression Monitor 2014).

What Does the Published Research Say About Stigma and Depression in Australia?

Much of the published research has a focus on mental illness in its fullest definition; there has been some focus on depression and schizophrenia and very little pertaining to the effectiveness of interventions to address stigma associated with depression and anxiety. Further, there is little that is gender specific and little that is anxiety specific. *beyondblue* has prioritised the need to address these research gaps, in recognition of the evidence suggesting the lack of generalisability of research across the different mental health conditions.

Most of the improvements in stigmatising attitudes identified in the Depression Monitor are consistent with those found in research conducted by Reavley and Jorm (2012), with one notable exception. In their survey involving 6,000 Australians aged 15 years and over, Reavley and Jorm found that the belief that 'people with depression are dangerous and unpredictable' had increased since 2003. Methodological differences are noted and may account for this apparent contradiction: different questions were used to assess stigmatising attitudes, and the surveys were conducted over different time periods. *beyondblue* will continue to monitor these trends and refine the measurement tools utilised (*beyondblue* 2014a).

What People with Lived Experience Tell Us

beyondblue commissioned in-depth, targeted consultations in 2001 and again in 2010, amongst people with lived experience and carers. Although depression, anxiety and bipolar disorder were the most common mental health issues affecting the research participants in this study, a wide range of other mental health problems were also reported. The aims of these consultations were to comprehensively describe the range of needs and experiences of these people and to use this information as the basis for developing practice and policy recommendations, including how to decrease stigma and to improve treatment amongst policymakers and healthcare service providers (Sawrikar et al. 2011).

Although participants believed that awareness of mental health issues had significantly increased, stigma was not seen to have decreased to the same extent. Moreover, stigma was seen as especially prominent amongst families and, at work, amongst males and the older generation (Sawrikar et al. 2011).

Stigma was noted by the authors as 'the greatest barrier to an effective response to mental health issues, inhibiting the full potential of awareness raising campaigns, help seeking behaviour for both consumers and carers and a prioritised response to mental health issues by health care service providers and government'.

These findings are consistent with those found over time, as measured in the *beyondblue* Depression Monitor.

A Renewed Strategic Focus on Stigma Reduction

beyondblue was fast to recognise that despite that fact that stigma reduction has been a priority since its inception in 2000, its efforts had been less effective in this endeavour than was the case in raising community awareness of depression. Given the relationship between stigma and help seeking, in 2012, *beyondblue* adopted a renewed strategic focus for stigma reduction.

The elements of an effective stigma reduction approach for depression and anxiety were identified, and the implications for *beyondblue*'s work were distilled from a range of sources. These included:

- Australian market research conducted with people with an experience of depression and anxiety and their carers
- Outcomes from a national stigma summit convened by *beyondblue* in 2011
- Findings from the International Stigma Conference 2012
- A desktop review of the published literature from Australia and overseas
- Consideration of stigma reduction initiatives in areas outside mental health
- Discussion with research and programme practitioners in the UK and Canada
- Analysis of cost-effectiveness data
- International and local evaluation of interventions

These were articulated in a set of operational principles, which were adopted across the organisation.

beyondblue's renewed strategic direction supported a comprehensive, evidence informed response, utilising a combination of contact, education and protest approaches. Consistent with its public health business model, it was aimed at reaching people across the lifespan, in a range of settings and utilising a combination of approaches. The principles went beyond a focus at the individual level and acknowledged the need to address the structural inequities which serve to entrench disadvantage amongst those discriminated against, on the basis of their experience of depression and/or anxiety (*beyondblue* 2014b).

beyondblue's stigma reduction principles were based on analysis and research suggesting

- that anti stigma interventions are more likely to be successful it they focussed on individual disorders rather than on mental illness in general (Reavely and Jorm, 2011)
- the most effective stigma reduction initiatives are based on an understanding of the lived experience of people with an experience of depression and/or anxiety and their carers; that the lived experience should inform communication, goal setting and evaluation
- changes in knowledge (misinformation, ignorance) and stigmatising attitudes (stereotypes, prejudice) are a poor indicator of changes in behaviour (discrimination), and that approaches which do not address behaviours are "suboptimal" in reducing stigma in all its manifestations (Thornicroft et al, 2007)
- a characteristic of independently evaluated and effective stigma reduction initiatives is a contact-based approach, meeting the conditions outlined by Corrigan and described in the moniker "TLC3: targeted, local, credible, continuous contact" (2011)

As a result, *beyondblue*'s current suite of activities includes a greatly strengthened stigma reduction focus.

beyondblue Initiatives with a Dedicated Focus on Addressing Stigma and Discrimination

beyondblue Ambassador and Speaker Bureau

The sharing of personal stories of depression and anxiety has been a central plank in *beyondblue*'s efforts to reduce stigma over time. The lived experience, including the experience of carers, has been sensitively communicated to diverse audiences via DVD, video and face to face (one to one and one to many). Anecdotally, this perspective is often rated the most powerful aspect of our communications.

The *beyondblue* Ambassador and Speaker Bureau was formally launched in 2012, with the explicit goal of better implementing emerging evidence regarding effective contact and education approaches in stigma reduction. Members are people with a personal experience of depression and anxiety, who volunteer to assist *beyondblue* in its work by sharing their personal story. Most commonly, this takes place at a public speaking engagement, in response to a request from members of the general public or media, to address a group, be it intimate or large. Ambassadors and Speakers participate in a tailored training programme, aimed at preparing them for the experience ahead and to ensure they are equipped to deal with the range of questions they may encounter. Follow-up and support following a public speaking engagement has been welcomed by these volunteers. Care is taken in selecting a speaker who is representative of the people who make up a particular audience. *beyondblue* Ambassadors and Speakers are representative of people from all walks of life and a variety of ages and circumstance. The *beyondblue* Ambassador and Speaker Bureau also includes the contribution of people who have cared for a friend or loved one.

Audience feedback tells us that a personal story has the potential to build empathy, dispel inaccurate stereotypes about depression and anxiety and convey a sense of optimism that with the right treatment and support, recovery is possible. Key messages include the importance of disclosure and talking to friends and family, the various forms of help available and the ways to access professional help and peer support. Emphasis is also placed on approaches to staying well.

beyondblue has more than 200 Ambassadors and Speakers across Australia, 34 of whom are considered high-profile individuals (Ambassadors) and 174 are representatives of the general community (Speakers). Anecdotally, many people report that hearing the personal story of a member of the *beyondblue* Ambassador and Speaker Bureau was instrumental in their decision to let others know of their own concerns, to seek professional help or support from a family or friend. Over time, and in light of the sheer number of people reached, it has been is acknowledged that the sharing of personal stories has assisted in the normalisation of common mental illnesses in Australia.

Skills Development to 'Have the Conversation'

Overcoming the commonly cited barriers to talking about mental health is seen as an important step in facilitating increased contact between people with experience of anxiety and depression and others in their family or community. Research suggests that the Australian public's knowledge and skills in supporting individuals experiencing mental health conditions requires 'substantial improvement' (Rosetto et al. 2014). Market research commissioned by *beyondblue* has also found people with anxiety and depression commonly experience unsupportive, and emotionally invalidating, responses when talking about their anxiety or depression (Sawrikar et al. 2011).

The skills of a social network are critical, given 65 % of people turn to family and friends in the first instance when experiencing anxiety and depression (*beyondblue* Depression Monitor 2014). *beyondblue* identified a need to develop resources which promote the skills required to facilitate effective interpersonal contact and which in turn enable help seeking, social support and stigma reduction.

beyondblue's 'Have the conversation' project aims to increase people's skills and capacity to talk about anxiety and depression. It recognises that the barriers to having a conversation about a personal experience of depression and anxiety differ according to age, perspective and circumstance. In order to identify the intrapersonal and interpersonal barriers to talking about an experience of depression or anxiety, consultation was undertaken with over 200 people. The insights from this work informed 'how to' have an effective conversation, in a manner which addressed the identified barriers to doing so, from the differing perspectives of the different target groups. Participants were selected and filmed, explaining their conversation tips for what they found helps, and what doesn't, when talking about their anxiety and depression. A suite of digital resources have been produced including an app, videos, fact sheets and website content. Resources are tailored to the needs of young people (12–25), parents and guardians, older adults and people accessing health services and adapted materials for culturally and linguistically diverse communities (available at www.beyondblue.org.au/conversations).

Prior to release, the resources were tested with 230 members of the general community. Eighty-eight percent of users reported that the resources were helpful in preparing them to have a conversation about mental health. Engagement with the resources increases confidence to have conversations (up to 26 % increase) and intentions to have conversations (up to 31 % increase). Eighty-four percent of users would recommend them to someone they felt could benefit.

Online resources went live in October 2014 and were supported with a marketing campaign across social media, targeted websites and radio; printed materials were distributed in hospitals and doctors' offices. After 3 months, almost 35,000 unique visitors had accessed the 'Have the Conversation' page on the *beyondblue* website with an additional 24,645 unique visitors to the relevant area of the youth *beyondblue* website. At that time, 10,814 fact sheets had been downloaded. The project is being externally evaluated on criteria of reach, effectiveness and impact, with a focus on the extent to which the project has prompted behaviour change and facilitated emotionally supportive conversations.

The 'Have the Conversation' project is proudly funded with donations from the Movember Foundation.

Reducing Discrimination in Insurance

The Insurance Discrimination project aims to improve access to insurance products such as travel, life, income protection and total and permanent disability insurance for people who have experienced or are currently living with a mental illness.

In Australia, some people with an experience of mental illness have reported not being able to access insurance in the same way as the rest of the population. A prior history of mental illness can mean that a person is denied insurance cover, asked to pay a higher premium or has their claim rejected. Additionally, some have identified that this can act as a disincentive to discussing their mental health issues and treatment with a health professional, particularly in instances where an insurance company allows people with a mental illness to purchase cover if they have been without symptoms or have not sought treatment for a given time (Mental Health Council of Australia and *beyondblue* 2011).

The issue of unlawful discrimination in accessing insurance is a challenging one. Generally, under state and federal anti-discrimination legislation, insurance companies can legally discriminate against someone with a disability, which includes mental illness, if their actions are reasonable, having regard to actuarial data on which it is reasonable to rely. However, due to the commercial nature of actuarial judgements (decisions made by the insurance company about the risk posed by people in different categories), the data upon which these decisions are made is not accessible. Additionally, at a federal level and in some states if there is no such actuarial data, insurers can rely on other relevant factors which may be particular to the individual such as medical opinion, opinions from other professional groups, actuarial opinion and commercial judgement. Unfortunately, *beyondblue* has heard a number of stories that suggest the use of appropriate data or consideration of the full range of relevant factors may not always be occurring in practice for people accessing or claiming against insurance policies when a disclosure of mental illness has been made.

Since 2002, *beyondblue* has worked with the Mental Health Australia (formerly the Mental Health Council of Australia) to improve insurance outcomes for people who have experienced mental illness. This work initially focused on life insurance and involved mental health organisations, health professional associations and the life insurance industry signing Memoranda of Understanding (MoU) to work on the issue. *beyondblue*, as a signatory to the initial MoU in 2003 and subsequent MoUs until 2011, contributed to key outcomes including the development of the *Mental health and life insurance: what you need to know* guides which provide people with experience of mental illness and carers with information about the impact of having a mental illness on insurance applications, how risk is assessed, and rights and responsibilities when making an application and the development of industry-wide guidelines for both underwriting and claims management.

However, in 2010, a survey looking at insurance and discrimination, conducted by *beyondblue* and the Mental Health Australia (MHA), revealed people with mental health problems continued to face difficulties when applying for insurance or making claims. The survey of 424 people was the first of its kind in Australia and highlighted that over 35 % of respondents strongly agreed that it was difficult for them to obtain any type of insurance due to them having experienced mental illness. This almost doubled, increasing to 67 % for life and income protection insurance. Additionally, 45 % of people indicated their application for income protection insurance was declined due to mental illness, whilst 50 % received their insurance products with either increased premiums or exclusions specifically for mental illness (Mental Health Council of Australia and *beyondblue* 2011).

Although the insurance industry's stated intention to support change had been encouraging, the survey results indicated significant change was still needed to improve access and equity for people with a mental health condition. As a result *beyondblue* and MHA commenced alternative activities to influence change. This included developing a relationship with the Public Interest Advocacy Centre to support people with experience of mental illness, who may have been discriminated against, and to access free legal advice and, if appropriate, legal representation in relation to a complaint about their insurance policy. This was supported by a media presence calling for people with experience of mental illness who may have been potentially discriminated against to contact *beyondblue* and MHA and to share their experience and, as appropriate, supporting people to access legal advice. To build on this work and to further raise awareness of the issue, a social marketing video is being developed for release in 2015.

beyondblue awaits the outcomes of any legal precedent which may arise as a result of this process with great interest. It may be that until public scrutiny is brought to bear, progress in addressing these matters will remain slow.

Additional steps to strengthen *beyondblue*'s work regarding discrimination in insurance are currently being explored. These include how best to address the public demand for advice regarding those insurance products deemed to be 'mental health friendly'. The feasibility of producing and distributing comparative information on the mental health friendliness of a range of insurance policies and practices is under consideration.

Workplace and Workforce Stigma Reduction

People with lived experience of depression and anxiety report that the workplace is one of the most potent sources of stigma and discrimination encountered in daily life, impacting on recruitment, returning to work, promotional opportunities and acknowledging workplace-related mental health problems (Sawrikar et al. 2011). Addressing workplace stigma through a combination of educational and contact-based approaches is one of several goals in the suite of initiatives that comprise this programme.

beyondblue National Workplace Program

The *beyondblue* National Workplace Program (NWP) was developed in 2004, as an awareness, early intervention and prevention programme designed specifically for workplace settings. It is a training programme delivered face to face and online, aimed at increasing knowledge and skills of staff and managers to address mental health issues, including mental health stigma in the workplace (*beyondblue* 2014).

The NWP features tailored workshops for organisational leaders, human resources staff, managers and front-line workers. It includes the possible impacts of depression and anxiety at work, how this can be managed and accommodated, the importance of accessing professional help and how to respond to and support colleagues or subordinates. Case studies of people with lived experience of depression and/or anxiety highlight the impact of stigma on help seeking and the way stigma and discrimination can lead to discriminatory behaviours. The lived experience is incorporated in video form.

The ongoing monitoring of feedback from program participants suggests that participation results in increased awareness of the prevalence of depression in Australia, reduced stigma around depression in the workplace and increased individual confidence to assist colleagues who might be experiencing depression (*beyondblue*, 2015).

'Heads Up' Initiative

In May 2014 *beyondblue* launched the 'Heads Up' initiative (www.headsup.org.au) in partnership with the Mentally Healthy Workplace Alliance. The Alliance is a tripartite collaboration between business, government and the mental health sector, including SANE Australia. Heads Up aims to highlight the benefits of creating mentally healthy workplaces and to assist a range of individuals – from front-line employees to business owners and leaders – in managing workplace mental health issues, including their role in the creation of mentally healthy workplaces. The three key elements of the Heads Up initiative are a website (www.headsup.org.au), a communications campaign and an engagement programme.

Heads Up Website

The Heads Up website provides a central point for organisations and individuals to access an extensive range of free, practical resources developed by *beyondblue*, members of the Mentally Healthy Workplace Alliance and other organisations such as the Australian Human Rights Commission. Key features of the website include videos of business leaders and owners talking about mental health at work and the benefits of creating a mentally healthy workplace, in addition to decision-making tools to aid consideration of the issues associated with disclosing a mental health condition at work.

The website also includes a range of stand-alone online resources which incorporate educational and contact-based approaches aimed at reducing stigma:

- *beyondblue Workplace Mental Health Awareness* – explores and challenges common myths and misconceptions about depression and anxiety.
- *What it's like*: *Personal stories of depression* – features the personal stories of four men who relate their experience of getting through tough times. Representing manual and professional workers, the men also discuss the strategies they use to stay well.
- *Business in Mind* – aimed at small-to-medium business owners, to learn how to manage mental health in the workplace, and features the perspective of business owners who have a personal experience of mental illness.
- *Organisational Leadership* – built around the personal experience of an organisational leader, including how to stay well; it provides senior leaders from larger organisations with the information, tools and the necessary steps to create a mentally healthy workplace.

At December 2014, the Heads Up website had attracted over 146,000 unique visitors and 270,000 unique page views. The Heads Up online resource was awarded Best Online Learning and Education Resource at the Digital Industry Association of Australia Awards 2014.

Marketing and Engagement Activities

In May 2014, *beyondblue*, with the support of members of the Mental Healthy Workplace Alliance, commenced a national communications campaign aimed at organisational leaders. Its key focus was on the benefits of creating a mentally healthy workplace. Preliminary findings indicate that over 70 % of leaders exposed to the advertising material found it believable, an appropriate way to communicate, informative and a catalyst to them thinking about mental health in their business or organisation.

The current campaign features digital, print, TV and social media activities and will continue into 2015. The campaign will be complemented by activities which aim to establish relationships with influential businesses, industry groups and high-profile organisations who can act as exemplars and as advocates for this approach. These activities include staging, sponsoring and presenting at national events and conferences. Key messages highlight the prevalence of and normalise the range of mental health conditions.

Evaluation

An independent evaluation of the Organisational Leadership online resource found organisational leaders who completed the online resource had reduced behavioural, affective and total stigma scores, and these reductions were sustained at 6-month follow-up (Shann 2015).

An independent evaluation of the Heads Up initiative will take place in 2015. A focus of the evaluation includes the extent to which the initiatives' activities have changed attitudes and reduced stigma.

Stigma Amongst Health Professionals: *beyondblue* Doctors' Mental Health Program

People with depression and anxiety report a wide range of different experiences in their interactions with health professionals – some experiencing empathy, understanding and a sense of relief at diagnosis, whereas others reporting insensitive comments, being excluded from participation in decisions about treatment, and a lack of a sense of optimism regarding recovery, rather a focus on symptoms and medication (Mental Health Council of Australia 2011; *beyondblue* focus group research, unpublished).

Australian research on the stigma amongst different health professional groups suggests that general practitioners may be more likely to hold stigmatising attitudes relating to mental health conditions and to desire social distance, than psychologists and psychiatrists (Reavely et al. 2013). These stigmatising attitudes may also impact on the mental health and wellbeing of health professionals and their likelihood of accessing appropriate treatment for their own mental health problems (*beyondblue* 2013).

Research and media reports in Australia have highlighted the high rates of suicide, depression, anxiety, substance use and self-medication throughout the medical profession. These issues reflect the mental health of doctors and may affect their capacity to provide quality treatment and care to members of the community.

The *beyondblue* Doctor's Mental Health Program (bbDMHP) was established to address the prevalence of depression and anxiety in Australian medical students and doctors. An Advisory Committee of experts in doctors' mental health, including a doctor with a mental health condition, informs the programme's strategic directions. A number of projects have been undertaken as part of the bbDMHP including a systematic literature review examining what is known about the mental health of doctors and medical students, development of a wellbeing guide for medical students in partnership with the Australian Medical Students Association and the expansion of the Australasian Doctors' Health Network website to incorporate information for all medical practitioners.

Most significantly, in 2013, *beyondblue* launched the landmark *beyondblue* National Mental Health Survey of Doctors and Medical Students which examined the mental health of approximately 50,000 doctors and medical students. Based on the responses of 14,000 doctors and medical students (representing a 27 % response rate), key findings of the survey include:

- One in five medical students and one in ten doctors had suicidal thoughts in the past year, compared with one in 45 people in the wider community. More than four in ten students and a quarter of doctors are highly likely to have a minor psychiatric disorder, such as mild depression or mild anxiety.
- 3.4 % of doctors are experiencing very high psychological distress, a rate much greater than that found in the wider community.
- Male doctors work longer hours (46 h per week) and engage in more risky drinking, but female doctors are more psychologically distressed and think about suicide more often.
- Young doctors work longer hours (50 per week on average), are far more psychologically distressed, think about suicide more and are more burnt out than their older colleagues.
- Perceived stigma is common, with almost half of respondents thinking doctors are less likely to appoint doctors with a history of depression or anxiety.
- Four in ten doctors agreeing that doctors who have experienced depression or anxiety are perceived to be less competent by their peers.

Strikingly similar trends were found amongst medical students (*beyondblue* 2013).

Following the launch of the survey, *beyondblue* identified a number of areas for potential intervention, with the aim of improving the mental health and wellbeing of Australian doctors and medical students. *beyondblue*-led activity with a focus on stigma reduction within the medical profession since the launch of the survey includes:

- A round-table forum of senior leaders representing peak national medical bodies and training colleges convened jointly by the Australian Medical Association and *beyondblue*. The purpose of the forum was to draw on the *beyondblue* research findings and to develop an action plan for implementation by key players from within the profession itself.
- Targeted promotion of the bbDHMP and survey findings at a range of conferences (e.g. International Conference on Physician Health (2014), Health Professionals Health Conference (2013, 2011), Rural Medicine Australia (2013), Australian Medical Students' Association Conference (2013), and Royal Australian and New Zealand College of Psychiatrists Congress (2011).
- Production of video depicting the lived experience of two medical practitioners, to be accessed via the Heads Up website.

This area remains a priority for *beyondblue*; *beyondblue* will continue to work in partnership with the medical and mental health professions, in addition to monitoring the outcomes of work taking place internationally, to inform next steps.

Stigma Reduction Amongst Men

The impact of stigma in relation to Australian men's help seeking is well documented. Exacerbated by lower levels of awareness of depression and anxiety (*beyondblue* 2014), this is borne out in qualitative research commissioned by *beyondblue*, showing that whilst depression and anxiety are more openly discussed than was the case in previous generations, men are less likely (than the community as a whole) to discuss their mental health. This research identified that discussing anxiety/depression with family, partner, friends and/or workmates meant having to let go of the image men had of themselves, whether that be the 'abundant provider, the confident and supportive friend, the capable and earnest workmate, or simply the group's cheerleader' (Hall and Partners, 2012).

This same research identified that depression is perceived as a burden, and men were loath to burden themselves with that label. Despite the achievements to date in raising awareness and normalising depression and anxiety, Australian men reported that admitting to an experience of depression holds the stigma of 'not being good enough, strong enough or capable enough'. Men reported fears of perceived stigma with a key concern being what 'others' would think; frequently, 'others' referred to workmates, and notably, anticipated stigma in relation to the attitudes of health professionals was evident (Hall and Partners, 2012).

Implications for Communication

This research provided an impetus to change the way *beyondblue* communicated with men and provides a tangible example of the organisation's focus on 'stigma-mindful communications'. It identified that in order to improve help-seeking behaviours amongst men, there was a need to frame help seeking as a masculine trait: courageous, performance enhancing, a responsible course of action, self-determining and collaborative. Communications with men needed to be logical, factual and directive.

Communications were tailored to:

- Focus on tangible actionable elements.
- Point to easy-to-navigate pathways that use video, checklists and tools.
- Provide exposure to real-life examples of other men, not celebrities, who are out of reach of many men.
- Focus on naming the specific issue of depression or anxiety, not 'mental health', which does not have a clear meaning.
- Recognise the language of 'help seeking' is emasculating; 'taking action' was empowering for many men.

The full report documenting findings regarding means of help seeking can be accessed at http://www.beyondblue.org.au/docs/default-source/bw0139_mens-help-seeking-behaviour-report.

From Market Research to Practice: Man Therapy

beyondblue's response to these findings resulted in its most significant public communication initiative targeting men. Known as Man Therapy, the campaign was launched in June 2013.

Man Therapy is a multiplatform campaign (encompassing television, radio, print and online executions), aimed at raising men the understanding of anxiety and depression amongst men aged 30–54, with the campaign call to action being to visit the campaign website: mantherapy.org.au.

This campaign was based on a concept developed and successfully piloted in the USA by the Office of Suicide Prevention, Colorado, with creative agency Cactus, but with an Australianised character, Dr Brian Ironwood, developed to speak to Australian men and encouraging them to take action.

The Man Therapy website is an online resource designed to deliver three learnings:

- Know the signs of depression and anxiety
- Know the range of management options
- Know what to include in your action plan

The sharing of personal stories of people who have experienced, and effectively managed, depression and anxiety occurs via a dedicated area of the website (Tales of Triumph); this approach was further reinforced via the broadcast of a range of personal stories from the Australian Rules Football community which were broadcast during prime-time Saturday evening football games. This approach was undertaken with stigma reduction as its primary objective; a further goal was to encourage visitation to the website as a course of action.

The Man Therapy campaign was evaluated through a comprehensive evaluation framework including pre- and post-campaign surveys, conducted by Ipsos Social Research Institute (https:// www.beyondblue.org.au).

The post-campaign survey conducted in March 2014 identified that 41 % of Australian men had seen at least one Man Therapy advertisement over the 10-month period. The evaluation surveyed a sample of the 512,000 unique visitors to the website and found that 90 % had visited the website for themselves, 80 % indicated the information on the website was new to them, and there had been a direct impact on behaviour:

- Thirty-six percent had spoken to family or mates
- Twenty-nine percent had visited a general practitioner
- Twenty-one percent had looked for further information (IPSOS Social Research Institute, 2014)

Across the entire Australian man population, those who had been exposed to the Man Therapy campaign, there were a number of observed effects uniquely attributable to the campaign. Refer www.mantherapy.org.au to download full details including the most recent evaluation reports.

The STRIDE Project (Stigma Reduction Interventions: Digital Environments)

In 2012, *beyondblue* and the Movember Foundation agreed to allocate funds into research associated with the reduction of stigma associated with anxiety and/or depression amongst Australian men and for that research to focus on knowledge translation, real-world effectiveness and implementation models.

The potential effectiveness of digital technology as part of a comprehensive stigma reduction approach was identified as an area worthy of examination in a review of published and grey literature conducted for *beyondblue* by Reavely and Jorm (2013). The STRIDE project was conceived in response to this finding. STRIDE is a programme which funds action research into the use of interventions which utilise digital platforms in achieving the reduction of stigma associated with anxiety, depression or suicide amongst Australian men.

A distinguishing feature of this project is the locally identified nature of the interventions proposed.

With a project timeframe of 2 years spanning 2015–2017, phase 1 (project proposal phase) of STRIDE is now complete. Successful proposals represent a partnership between community groups and academics and comprise consortia characterised by contributions from a multidisciplinary team, ranging from evaluators to digital designers. The specific interventions are locally determined – that is, the interventions under consideration are devised at the local level, to meet local need. Each partnership demonstrates participatory design principles, with men aged 30–64 years from the target community of interest fully engaged in the proposed project. The action research findings arising are intended to demonstrate whether digital platforms realise their proposed potential in achieving stigma reduction goals and to provide insights into the most effective ways of utilising digital media/platforms in engaging men in stigma reduction interventions.

Each of the successful partnerships will, within their evaluation framework, use an appropriate stigma measure which is comparable to existing population surveys, applied to their target male population. Each successful partnership is expected to identify change in the adopted measure over time and whether there is an attribution to their specific digital intervention.

The specific questions answered through this project will depend on the nature of the work that is approved for funding, but a key question will be 'Can digital interventions, implemented at a local population level, prompt change across the knowledge, attitudinal and behavioural components of stigma experienced and/or exhibited by men aged 30–64 years?'

The synthesis of the outcomes of each partnership is intended to have practical implications for those charged with the implementation of stigma reduction strategies, will address an identified gap in the stigma reduction literature and will ultimately impact on men who are experiencing stigma associated with depression and/or anxiety.

Information on the STRIDE Project is progressively updated at http://www.beyondblue.org.au/stigma.

The STRIDE project is proudly funded with donations from the Movember Foundation.

Using Social Media to Achieve Stigma Reduction Goals

beyondblue utilises its strong social media presence to reduce the stigma of depression and anxiety. Social media is used to:

- Extend campaign reach – for example, in the 2013 *I Am Anxiety* campaign, community members used the Twitter hashtag #IamAnxiety to say they had experienced anxiety, and there was no reason to hide their experience.
- Promote stories of hope and recovery – #SmashTheStigma is used when stories of hope and recovery are posted on Twitter, particularly from high-profile individuals. Sharing and retweeting posts through Facebook and Twitter also provide a way for people to promote understanding and share experiences of depression and anxiety.
- Increase knowledge of depression and anxiety – *beyondblue's* Facebook, Twitter and Instagram communities are encouraged to share *beyondblue* image and video content which increases knowledge about depression and anxiety (e.g. infographics on the prevalence of depression and anxiety).
- Enable conversations about depression and anxiety – through *beyondblue's* online forums, Twitter and Facebook communities; there is a public place for people to share their stories of depression and anxiety and receive advice and support from others (*beyondblue* 2014).

The Work of SANE Australia

About SANE Australia

Founded in 1986, SANE Australia – http://www.sane.org – is an independent national mental health organisation. Since inception, the organisation has focused on the human impact of mental illness, extending beyond clinical symptoms to include the wider personal, social and economic effects, including the impact on family and other carers. SANE was founded on acknowledgment of the importance of this personal experience and its value in helping others. This approach continues to be integral to all of our work today, with people affected by mental illness directly involved in all of our programmes, especially members of our Speaker Bureau, the SANE Speakers.

SANE's vision is for Australia to lead the world in mental health within 10 years. Its mission is to help all Australians affected by mental illness lead a better life. It pursues this mission through three key areas of activity: support, training and education.

Support
SANE Australia supports people affected by mental illness, their family and friends with a suite of direct services providing information, support, referral and access to online peer support.

Education
SANE researches and develops resources to inform and educate the community about the impact of mental illness and to promote a fulfilling life for all those affected – guidebooks and e-books, fact sheets, podcasts, videos, guidelines for health professionals and our popular magazine, *SANE News*. All resources are available in digital and print format.

Training
SANE develops and provides innovative training programmes for the community and professionals, to promote better understanding of mental illness and services for people affected.

SANE Australia's reach has grown over the years; during 2013–2014, SANE had contact with 780,000 Australians of whom 94,000 were directly engaged with our programmes. Combating stigma has always been at the heart of SANE's work; it is integral to everything the organisation does – we believe that by changing minds, we can change lives. The organisation has deep experience and a long, proud history of fighting misunderstanding and prejudice against those affected by mental illness. It pioneered mass media work in this area in the 1980s with the 'Schizophrenia – A Treatable Illness' national advertising campaign, followed by a series of others over the past two decades, including the more recent SIGNS campaign (SANE Australia 2011b) and the 'Say no to stigma!' YouTube and social media campaign (SANE Australia 2014b). SANE launched Australia's first mental health website in 1994 and has continued this pioneering spirit most recently with the launch of online forums for people living with mental illness and for carers, using a distributed service model, making them available all around Australia via the websites of familiar local mental health organisations. Working with over 100 partner mental health organisations around the country has been essential to SANE's work – collaboration is one of the organisation's key values to ensure the maximum collective impact. It is also a member of the Global Anti-Stigma Alliance and participates actively in international gatherings on this topic.

SANE Australia's Framework: Seven Domains of Stigma

SANE Australia (2013) has identified seven domains in which stigma affects people living with mental illness, whatever their diagnosis. Each of these is therefore a target for tailored strategies to reduce stigma in that area.

General Community
Whilst there have been some improvements in the general public's knowledge about mental illness and understanding of its impact on day-to-day lives, there is still widespread misunderstanding and ignorance, particularly about some diagnoses.

Myths – such as that all people with psychotic illnesses such as schizophrenia are unpredictable and to be feared – are hurtful and harmful as well as being inaccurate (SANE Aus 2011a). Dispelling these myths is important if people with mental illness are to be fully accepted into families, workplaces and communities.

Australian and overseas surveys support the need for community education and have identified a wide range of particular misunderstandings that need to be tackled. The 2013 National Mental Health Commission report, *Can we talk … about mental health and suicide*, reinforced that we are still struggling to make sense of mental illness and suicide and that the stigma associated with accessing the mental health system is one of the biggest barriers to treatment. A Wesley Mission study (2007) found that one in three (32 %) would not feel comfortable working with a colleague who has mental illness. Two-thirds (66 %) would not be comfortable with their child sharing a unit with someone who had a mental illness, and 71 % did not believe people with mental illness could be trusted in positions of high responsibility. The Australian *National Survey of Mental Health Literacy and Stigma* found that statements with which respondents were most likely to agree included that people with mental illness were unpredictable, that those affected would not tell anyone about their diagnosis and that most other people would not employ someone with the problem (Reavley and Jorm 2011).

Information Box 16.1: SANE Australia Response

Improving community understanding of mental illness is undertaken through the SANE website and an associated and comprehensive range of information resources covering mental health issues, how they are treated and importantly what affected people can do to help themselves.

The SANE Helpline operates via three channels (1800 Freecall, Online and Chat) helping people concerned about mental illness to understand symptoms, treatments, where to go for support in their local area and self-help strategies.

In addition to rolling promotion of better understanding through social media (a dedicated position at SANE), media campaigns are also conducted, such as the 'Say no to stigma!' initiative and collaboration in wider activities such as the R U OK Day, Mental Health Week and *Mental As* week, in which national broadcaster, the ABC, dedicated a week's programming on all platforms to improving understanding of mental health issues.

Health and Other Services

When we are unwell, we have a right to be treated with understanding and respect by people working in health and community services. Unfortunately this is not always the case for people with mental illness, who frequently report that they feel stigmatised (SANE Aus 2007). A Mental Health Council of Australia study (2011) found that people with mental illness reported similar levels of stigma from health professionals as from the general community. The Australian Bureau of Statistics also reports that people who are living with a mental health problem find it harder to get and keep their own home compared to the general population (Australian Bureau of Statistics 2009). A 2008 survey of people living with mental illness found that nearly 90 % believed they had been discriminated against at some time in regard to housing, particularly private rental accommodation, forcing them to accept unsafe or substandard housing options (SANE Australia 2008). This is one of many challenges faced by older Australians with an ongoing mental illness (SANE Australia 2013).

Information Box 16.2: SANE Australia Response
Reducing stigma and discrimination, including improving understanding and attitudes amongst health and allied professionals, is the direct focus of a number of our programmes.

SANE's Suicide Prevention project aims to educate and train them in being more aware of clients' risk of suicide and to respond to any possible concerns; it also trains health and allied staff in working with those bereaved by suicide, as these are often at higher risk of taking their own lives too. SANE is a lead member of the National Coalition for Suicide Prevention.

People living with mental illness, especially those with schizophrenia, experience high levels of physical ill health and have a mortality rate up to 20 years lower than the general population. For many years there was a stigmatising attitude amongst many health professionals of ignoring this disparity. SANE's Mind + Body project works to encourage health and mental health workers to actively encourage better physical health for their clients, through improved diet, exercise, weight reduction and smoking cessation. Amongst other activities, the project is currently working with a national non-government organisation to train peer educators in this area.

Older people with mental illness are often treated as 'invisible' over the age of 65. They may be regarded as 'too old' for regular adult mental health services yet do not fit in to mainstream aged care services such as nursing homes. SANE's Aged Care project has undertaken a research study on this issue (SAE Australia 2013) and is currently preparing guidelines for health professionals in the area as well as for the person and their families.

Education

Three quarters of people who develop mental illness do so between the ages of 16 and 25 years. Reducing stigma in educational institutions is an integral part of stigma reduction work. It is also critical if we want friends, fellow students, teachers and others to provide them with understanding and support. In Australia, schools have long been a setting for attitude and behaviour change towards mental illness in students. The MindMatters programme has been in operation for over 10 years and, as part of its whole-of-school approach to mental health promotion, looks at stigma reduction in a variety of ways, including curriculum materials as well as teacher education and resources.

Information Box 16.3: SANE Australia Response
A range of resources have been developed by SANE for young people, especially focused on children and teenagers in families where a parent is affected by mental illness: *You're Not Alone* (a cartoon book for under 12s), *Joe's Diary* (for teens) and www.itsallright.org, a website for this target group. (Following a decision to focus on adult Australians, SANE transferred the website to COPMI, a federally funded initiative supporting young people in families affected by mental illness.)

Workplace

Having a job is more than a source of revenue. It helps define who you are as a person, provides friendships and gives you status in the community. Australia, along with many other countries, now has employment equity legislation in place to protect the rights of people with disabilities and to remove barriers to their economic participation. Yet despite this legislation, disabled employees in general are more likely to be paid by the hour, less likely to be a member of a union, less likely to receive benefits such as employer-provided health insurance and pension plans and less likely to be in professional, technical or managerial jobs (Schur et al. 2009). Unemployment rates remain especially high amongst people seriously affected by mental illness, with stigma a recognised factor in the reluctance of employers to appoint or retain those who are affected. Large-scale surveys have consistently estimated the unemployment rate amongst people with mental illness to be three to five times higher than the general population.

Information Box 16.4: SANE Australia Response
The national Mindful Employer programme equips managers and employees with the information and skills they need to respond to mental health issues in the workplace. The programme offers e-learning and face-to-face training to businesses of all sizes on how to manage mental health-related issues in the workplace.
   SANE Australia is also a partner in the Mentally Healthy Workplace Alliance, and drew on its experience in this area to produce a series of 12 videos for the initiative, highlighting good practice in mentally healthy workplaces across a range of industries.

Mass Media

The media is also a primary source of knowledge about mental illness. The language and images used, however, are often inaccurate, sensational, unbalanced and stereotypical (Pirkis et al 2008). These stigmatising representations have a real and profound effect on people living with a mental illness, causing great distress and distorting community attitudes. Violent or disturbed behaviours are too often linked exclusively to mental illness. A recent study found that new stories about mass shootings involving a shooter with mental illness heighten readers' negative attitudes towards persons with serious mental illness in general (McGinty et al. 2013).

In recent years there have been improvements in Australian media representation of mental illness. We still have a long way to go, however. A University of Melbourne study concluded that there is a tendency for news media to present mental illnesses in a way that promotes stigma (e.g. by conflating it with violence and crime) or perpetuates myths about mental illness (e.g. by presenting information that is inaccurate about treatment and prognosis) (Pirkis and Francis 2012). Irresponsible media reporting of suicide has been shown to trigger suicidal behaviour, but the influence of suicide reporting may not be restricted to harmful effects; coverage of positive coping in adverse circumstances, such as items about coping with suicidal ideation, may have protective effects (Niederkrotenthaler et al. 2010).

Information Box 16.5: SANE Australia Response

The SANE Media Centre promotes and supports the accurate and responsible portrayal of mental illness and suicide in the Australian media. The Centre provides a 'one-stop' service of information, expert comment, advice and referral for journalists reporting on mental illness and suicide. It also provides advice and support to organisations in the mental health sector on how to deal with the media.

Incorporated in the Centre is the StigmaWatch programme, which voices community concern about representations in the media that stigmatise mental illness or inadvertently promote self-harm and suicide. Established over 15 years ago, this award-winning programme is now part of the Mindframe initiative to improve media reporting of mental illness and suicide, supported by the Australian government. It relies on hundreds of StigmaWatchers throughout Australia – people with a mental illness, family, friends and others – who care about how mental illness and suicide are represented in the Australian media and forward their reports to StigmaWatch. When a report is received, the submission is researched and analysed using the Mindframe guidelines and media industry codes of conduct. If a report is inappropriate, StigmaWatch informs the media or business of the reason for complaint and encourages the amendment or removal of the item. Positive, accurate stories are also highlighted and commended to encourage the media to act responsibly.

Incorporated in the Centre is the StigmaWatch programme, which voices community concern about representations in the media that stigmatise mental illness or inadvertently promote self-harm and suicide.

Governments and Other Decision-Makers

Governments in Australia have been supportive of improved mental health services in recent years. At a national level, the Better Access and Personal Helpers and Mentors programmes, headspace and early intervention centres are all welcome initiatives. However, much of the planning and spending allocation seems ad hoc, and the 2012 *Report Card* from the National Mental Health Commission concluded there is little or no accountability for the $6.3 billion Australia spends on health annually (National Mental Health Commission 2012). Whilst mental health spending increased by 4.5 % per annum between 2005–2006 and 2009–2010, overall health expenditure increased by around 8.5 % per annum over the same period, meaning that mental health's share of the health budget is shrinking not growing (Rosenberg 2012).

Information Box 16.6: SANE Australia Response

As well as making individual representation and regular submissions to enquiries and draft documents, SANE works in partnership with other leading mental health organisations to advocate for improved mental health services and support, presenting a consistent and evidence-based case to government. Recent examples include the federal government's review of mental health services undertaken by the National Mental Health Commission and how the National Disability Insurance Scheme (NDIS) will operate for people affected by mental illness.

Research to improve understanding of the best treatments and support for mental illness is also regularly supported by SANE. Examples include partnerships with Griffith University and with Mental Illness Fellowship Australia regarding suicide prevention and with the Study of High Impact Psychosis (SHIP) consortium regarding optimisation of treatment modes and improvement of physical health.

Self-Stigma

Just because someone has a mental illness doesn't mean they don't share common community attitudes to mental illness. When someone self-stigmatises, they take on negative and inaccurate stereotypes and accept that 'people with mental illness are of less value to society or to themselves'. The fear of being rejected can then stop someone from going out, socialising, looking for a job or taking part in their local community.

Self-stigma is common. It also causes harm. Studies have shown that people with mental illness who self-stigmatise are more isolated, alienated and socially withdrawn than those who are not self-stigmatising. Social isolation often involves withdrawal from, and problems with, friends and family. It also includes avoiding employment seeking for fear of rejection and 'failure'. Having fewer social support networks then means that people who self-stigmatise are less likely than others to receive support just when they need it. Another consequence for people with mental illness and self-stigma is that they are less likely to seek treatment for symptoms than are people without self-stigma, less likely to cooperate with treatment and are more likely to experience worsening of symptoms and problems with recovery (Peterson et al. 2008).

> **Information Box 16.7: SANE Australia Response**
>
> SANE Speakers are a team of people affected by mental illness who talk candidly in public about their personal experience – providing unique, authentic input to our campaigning and other work. Trained and supported by SANE, Speakers talk to the media and employers and contribute to advocacy, research and new information resources to help break down the barriers of misunderstanding.
>
> Positive role models for people living with mental illness are also provided through the snapshots area of sane.org, where interviews and photographs provide vivid, authentic evidence that those affected can live 'a life worth living' and inspire others.
>
> The SANE Forums initiative – delivered in partnership with mental health organisations around Australia – provides a safe, anonymous online space for people living with mental illness and for carers to exchange experiences, tell stories and provide support and information to each other.

SANE Australia: What Works Best

SANE's 2013 report, *A life without stigma*, identifies the following ten principles for best practice in stigma reduction, drawing on the research, international anti-stigma programmes, advice from research and programme experts and a valuable literature review by the Queensland Alliance (2009).

1. *Direct personal contact with people who experience mental illness is the best approach.*
   Direct contact is the best approach to changing attitudes and behaviours, particularly when there is a relationship of equal status, a context of cooperation, an opportunity for discussion and credible presenters who disabuse myths of dangerousness, incompetence and incapacity.
2. *Information alone does not change attitudes.*
   The goals of education are to increase understanding of the challenges real people face (including discrimination), how difficulties are overcome, what helps and how others can be supportive and to include messages of equality, hope and recovery. Use of creative arts and multimedia increases impact.
3. *Mental health problems are best framed as part of our shared humanity.*
   Mental health problems are an understandable response to a unique set of circumstances and not purely as biomedical, genetically based illnesses or a diseased state of the brain.
4. *Create a simple and enduring national vision.*
   A vision that promotes human rights, social inclusion, full citizenship and a shared responsibility for change will be most effective, using multimedia and social marketing tools to create clear programme outcomes and benchmarks.

5. *Support grass roots, local programming.*

A national campaign that increases contact and education and builds consumer leadership from the grass roots up is essential. Change happens at the local level. Encourage bold, creative programming and evaluate carefully.

6. *Plan strategically at the national level.*

Develop a national strategic plan that works in partnership with government and stakeholders to develop and deliver a multilevel plan targeting transformative systemic change at a service system, legislative, policy and practice level. Ensure that funding is multi-year and with specific targets in reducing levels of stigma and discrimination over a 10-year period.

7. *Support people living with mental health issues in active leadership.*

Consumer leadership should be encouraged to define issues, design programmes, undertake research and evaluate programme success. Protest, disclosure and group identification are cornerstones of empowerment. Support consumer leadership and empowerment through the national programme.

8. *Target programmes at influential groups.*

Influential groups could include emergency response, policing and corrections, social service providers, employers, educators, friends, family and religious leaders.

9. *Assist media to play a significant role.*

Require media to have a special focus on increasing depictions of people as competent, capable and productive citizens and utilise 'first-person' narratives. Challenge inaccurate or discriminatory portrayals of people with mental health issues.

10. *Utilise evidence.*

Programmes must use evidence-informed approaches. Informed programming should also be evaluated to allow for course correction. Build knowledge through research and findings shared through programme networks.

An Ongoing Priority for *beyondblue* and SANE Australia

Reducing stigma and discrimination is a key goal in Australian mental health policy. The work of *beyondblue* and SANE Australia illustrates the translation of research and tailoring of international best practice to the Australian context. A willingness to adapt this practice to accommodate emerging technologies and the preferences of young people, coupled with a focus on ensuring that the published evidence translates to effectiveness in the 'real world', is posed as critical to any future successes. Yet despite the current investment of effort and resources, much work remains to be done, particularly in the coordination of effort to facilitate sustainable population level change.

Both *beyondblue* and SANE Australia will continue to participate in international forums and to monitor improvements in practice, with the ultimate goal of reducing experiences of discrimination amongst those with mental illness as our most effective gauge of progress.

Acknowledgments *beyondblue* and SANE Australia would like to acknowledge the work of Judy Finn and Paul Morgan in the preparation of this chapter.

References

Australian Bureau of Statistics (2009) National Health Survey 2007–2008. Australian Bureau of Statistics

beyondblue (2014) *beyondblue* depression monitor: independent findings from 2004 to 2012. Melbourne

beyondblue (2014) http://www.beyondblue.org.au. Accessed 9 Dec 2014

beyondblue Information Paper (2014) Stigma and discrimination associated with depression and anxiety. Melbourne

beyondblue (2015) Mental Health in the Workplace: beyondblue National Workplace Program. Accessed online 2016, https://www.headsup.org.au

Corrigan P (2011) Strategic Stigma Change (SSC): five principles for social marketing campaigns to reduce stigma. Psychiatr Res 62(8):824–826

Hall & Partners Open Mind, Men's Help-Seeking Behaviour Report of Research Findings, September 2012

Ipsos Social Research Institute, Beyond Barriers Evaluation, Benchmark Survey, May 2013

McGinty E et al (2013) Effects of news media messages about mass shootings on attitudes toward persons with serious mental illness and public support for gun control policies. Am J Psychiatry 170(5):494–501, 1

Mental Health Council of Australia (2011) Consumer and carer experiences of stigma from mental health and other health professionals. Mental Health Council of Australia

Mental Health Council of Australia and beyondblue (2011) Mental health discrimination and insurance: a survey of consumer experiences 2011. Canberra

Morgan V et al (2011) People living with psychotic illness 2010: report on the second Australian national survey. Commonwealth of Australia

National Mental Health Commission (2012) A contributing life: the 2012 national report card on mental health and suicide prevention. National Mental Health Commission, Sydney

National Mental Health Commission (2013) Can we talk … about mental health and suicide. National Mental Health Commission, Sydney

Niederkrotenthaler T et al (2010) Role of media reports in completed and prevented suicide: Werther v. Papageno effects. Br J Psychiatry 197:234–243

Peterson D, Barnes A, Duncan C. (2008) Fighting Shadows: Self-stigma and Mental Illness: Whawhai Atu te Whakama Hihira. Auckland: Mental Health Foundation of New Zealand

Pirkis J et al (2008) The Media Monitoring Project: changes in media reporting of suicide and mental health and illness in Australia: 2006–07. Commonwealth of Australia

Pirkis J, Francis C (2012) Mental illness in the news and information media: A critical review. Canberra, ACT: Commonwealth Department of Health and Aged Care - See more at: http://www.mindframe-media.info/for-media/reporting-mental-illness/evidence-and-research/evidence-about-mental-illness-in-the-media#sthash.KGNAIE46.dpuf

Queensland Alliance for Mental Health (2009) From Discrimination to Social Inclusion A review of the literature on anti stigma initiatives in mental health, http://qldalliance.org.au/resources/discrimination-social-inclusion/ Accessed at 2 Feb 2016

Reavely N, Jorm A (2011) Stigmatising attitudes towards people with mental disorders: findings from an Australian National Survey on Mental Health Literacy and Stigma. Aust N Z J Psychiatry 45:1086–1093

Reavley N, Jorm A (2012) Stigmatising attitudes towards people with mental disorders: changes in Australia over 8 years. Psychiatry Res 197(3):302–306

Reavely N, Jorm A (2013) Community and population-based interventions to reduce stigma associated with depression, anxiety and suicide: a rapid review. Accessed online 9 Dec 2014:

https://www.saxinstitute.org.au/publications/interventions-to-reduce-stigma-associated-with-depression-anxiety-and-suicide/

Reavley N, Mackinnon AJ, Morgan AJ. & Jorm AF (2013) Stigmatising attitudes towards people with mental disorders: a comparison of Australian health professionals with the general community. Australian and New Zealand Journal of Psychiatry, 48(5):433–441

Rosenberg S (2012) What's missing from the first national mental health report card <blogs.crikey.com.au/croakey/2012/11/27/whats-missing-from-the-first-national-mental-health-report-card>. Accessed 20 Feb 2015

Rossetto A, Jorm A, Reavley NJ (2014) Quality of helping behaviours of members of the public towards a person with mental illness: a descriptive analysis of data from an Australian national survey. Ann Gen Psychiatry 13:2

SANE Australia (2007) Research bulletin 4: stigma and mental illness. SANE Australia

SANE Australia (2008) Research bulletin 7: housing and mental illness. SANE Australia

SANE Australia (2011a) People living with psychotic illness: a SANE response. SANE Australia

SANE Australia (2011b) http://www.sane.org/projects/signs. Accessed 20 Feb 2015

SANE Australia (2013) Growing older, staying well. SANE Australia

SANE Australia (2014a) Research bulletin 14: working life and mental illness. SANE Australia

SANE Australia (2014b) http://www.sane.org/projects/say-no-to-stigma. Accessed 20 Feb 2015

Sawrikar P, Muir K, Craig L (2011) Focus group research for beyondblue with consumers and carers: final report. Social Policy Research Centre University of NSW, Sydney

Schur L et al (2009) Is disability disabling in all workplaces? Workplace disparities and corporate culture. Ind Relat 48(3):381–410

Shann C. (2015). Workplace Mental Health and the Role of Organisational Leaders: A training needs analysis and evaluation of an online program to reduce depression-related stigma (Doctoral Dissertation, University of Tasmania)

Thornicoft G, Rose D, Kassam A, Sartorious N (2007) Stigma: ignorance, prejudice or discrimination? British Journal of Psychiatry 190:192–193

Wesley Mission (2007) Living with mental illness; attitudes, experiences and challenges. Wesley Mission, Sydney

17

Johanne Bratbo and Anja Kare Vedelsby

Why an Anti-Stigma Campaign in Denmark?

Denmark is known to be among the most egalitarian countries in the world with a well-organised welfare state providing social security, free access to health and social services and a policy of education for all. Still, the stigma of mental illness remains a challenge to us as a society, as it is in countries we usually compare ourselves to.

Mental illness is a public health challenge with a remarkable increase in the number of people suffering from stress and nonpsychotic disorders such as anxiety, depression, borderline and ADHD. Of a population of 5.6 million people, at least 500,000 people are estimated to have a mental illness – equalling approx. 9 % of the population including young people – of which several have more than one diagnosis.[1] The employment rate for people with a handicap or prolonged health problems is significantly lower than the general population. Like everywhere else, mental illness is the most frequent cause of exclusion from the labour market. Danish labour market statistics underline the call for action (see Table 17.1).[2]

Research estimates the societal expenses connected to mental illness to amount to about 7.26 million euro annually of which currently only 10 % constitutes treatment expenses. The remaining 90 % is spent on sickness, unemployment, incapacity benefits, loss of earnings, etc.[3] Part of the explanation is stigma, taboo

---

[1] The Danish Mental Health Fund and The Department of Clinical Epidemiology
[2] OECD: Sick on the Job? Myths and Realities about mental Health and Work, 2012
[3] The National Research Centre for Working Environment, 2010

J. Bratbo (✉) • A.K. Vedelsby
The National Campaign for Anti-stigma in Denmark,
Danish Committee for Health Education,
Carl Nielsens Allé 9D, Underetagen, Copenhagen DK-2100, Denmark
e-mail: jb@en-af-os.dk; akv@en-af-os.dk

© Springer International Publishing Switzerland 2017
W. Gaebel et al. (eds.), *The Stigma of Mental Illness - End of the Story?*,
DOI 10.1007/978-3-319-27839-1_17

Table 17.1 Employment rate

General population	People w/ mobility impairment	People w/ mental illness
77.5 %	43.9 %	24.2 %

and a lack of knowledge about mental illness – with major implications on everyday life for individuals affected by this.

The number of people excluded from the labour market who receive incapacity benefits due to mental illness has increased to 50 % over the last 10 years, and among young people aged 19–39, the number adds up to an alarming 80 %.[4]

Within the past few years, the government therefore has passed reforms on the educational system, incapacity benefits, social welfare, sick leave and subsidised employment schemes all with the common goal to increase the education and employment rate for vulnerable groups, including people with mental illness. The underlying principle is to prevent exclusion, maintain employment and increase acceptance of inclusion on the labour market as well as increase focus on the psychological work environment.

The Setup of a Danish Anti-Stigma Campaign

In 2007 a major structural public sector reform was implemented changing the division of responsibilities, financing and services between national, regional and local authorities. This led to several initiatives in 2009 from the main actors in the field of health, psychiatry and psychosocial rehabilitation, e.g., the umbrella organisation for the five Danish regions, presenting eight fundamental visions for a future psychiatry, emphasising the ambition to cure more patients and reduce stigma. The Danish Health and Medicines Authority followed with an action plan emphasising rehabilitation and recovery. The service users and relatives' organisations formed a network – The Psychiatry Network – and developed a policy also emphasising the reduction of stigma. Add to this an increasing interest on international developments in the field of anti-stigma initiatives, especially Time to Change, launched in England that same year.

One of the positive outcomes of these initiatives was the formation of a large and strong partnership consisting of the Danish Health and Medicines Authority; the philanthropic foundation TrygFonden; the umbrella organisation of Danish Regions including the five regions; the Psychiatry Network; the Danish Ministry of Children, Gender Equality, Integration and Social Affairs; Local Government Denmark and The Danish Mental Health Fund. To create a baseline and a framework for the funding of an anti-stigma campaign, the partnership launched a public survey of the state of stigma of mental illness in Denmark. On the positive side, essential findings of the study were

---

[4] Annual statistic from the Danish Ankestyrelsen (National Social Appeals Board) 2012 on incapacity benefits

- A relatively high level of knowledge among the population. Many are acquainted with a person with a mental illness within their personal network, neighbourhood or workplace.
- Readiness to contact. About nine in ten are willing to associate with a person with a mental illness within their personal network, workplace or neighbourhood.

On the negative side, the findings calling for anti-stigma efforts were

- Significant hierarchy of diagnoses: Schizophrenia is the most stigmatised illness.
- Lack of specific knowledge. One in ten is not able to mention just one mental illness and only four in ten can mention three or more.
- Stigma is expressed through silence, avoidance, rejection and anger.
- Fear of stigma restricts openness. Four in ten prefer to hide their mental illness and one in five will avoid disclosure even in relation to a partner, close friends and family.

On the basis of the baseline survey and the awareness of the increasing exclusion of people with mental illness, the partnership decided to establish a Danish anti-stigma campaign over a 5-year period from 2011 to 2015[5] based on funding from the Danish Health and Medicines Authority, Danish Regions, the philanthropic foundation TrygFonden and a financial framework of 4.32 million euro was granted. In 2013 the budget was increased to a total of 5.92 million euro for the project period. In addition to the financial funding, the Psychiatry Network added 1.98 million euro worth of volunteer work. At regional level, funding was allocated for a part-time regional coordinator located in each of the five regional psychiatric information units amounting to 0.99 million euro over the 5-year period.

Five target areas were set out (see section "The five target areas of ONE OF US and their main activities" with description of the target areas and essential activities):

1. The public and the media
2. Service users and relatives
3. Staff in health and social sectors
4. Labour market
5. Young people

Key objectives, messages and target groups have been identified along with a number of main activities for each target area. The overall strategy is to start with the primary target groups and working our way out, e.g., starting with psychiatric staff and then move on to staff in psychosocial rehabilitation, etc. In section

---

[5] 2011–2015 made up the first phase of ONE OF US. At the end of 2015, the campaign received funding for a second phase 2016–2020

"The five target areas of ONE OF US and their main activities" you will find a description of selected activities and results from each of the target areas.

On World Mental Health Day October 10th 2011 ONE OF US[6] – the national campaign for anti-stigma in Denmark – was launched officially with name, logo and graphical identity with national and regional outdoor events. The payoff reading 'No more silence, doubt and taboo'.

Main Objectives

The objectives across the five target areas can be summarised in four main points:

- Increased recognition and involvement of service users' and relatives' knowledge and competencies
- Increased knowledge of recovery – and a call to seek timely help
- Increased reflection on culture and language
- Combating self-stigma, guilt and shame

The Mandate of ONE OF US

An action plan defines objectives and key messages within each of the target areas outlining the scope of the campaign. It is not within this scope to engage in structural issues of treatment capacity for mental illness or other political perspectives concerning this, including forced treatment, funding and organisation. The joint focus is on stigma in everyday life caused by lack of knowledge, prejudice and discriminatory behaviour.

The ONE OF US Organisation

The overall vision for the Danish anti-stigma campaign was formulated in spring 2011 and is originally inspired by the vision for Time to Change in England: 'To create a better life for all by promoting inclusion and combating discrimination related to mental illness', combined with the wording from the overall mission:

- Enhancing the knowledge about mental illness among the Danish population.
- Reducing social isolation and exclusion that leads to stigmatisation, prejudice and social exclusion.
- Creating a better understanding of mental illness in schools, workplaces and in everyday life situations.

---

[6] In Danish: EN AF OS. Væk med tavshed, tvivl og tabu om psykisk sygdom.

Furthermore, the set-up of the project model for the Danish anti-stigma campaign is basically inspired by the Time to Change model from England operating with three interacting levels (national, regional and local) which define the main tasks and focal points for each of the levels (see Fig. 17.1).

The organisational model reflects the three levels and allows all partners to be represented on both a national, regional and local level in a complex working organisation (see Fig. 17.2).

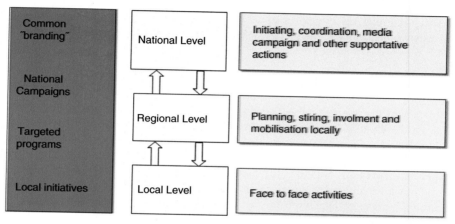

Fig. 17.1 Organisational levels

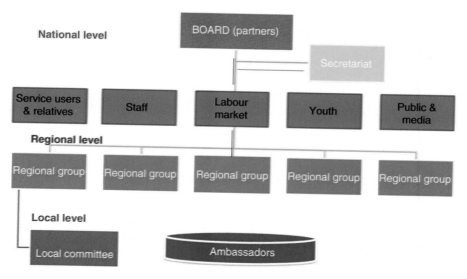

Fig. 17.2 Organisational model

National Level

On the Board, all partners are represented by people in leading positions in their system, fund or network. The national secretariat consists of four full-time employees and a part-time student-employee and, until the end of 2014, an external part time communications consultant. Resource groups were established in August 2012 and replaced a broad subcommittee representing all target areas and partners at a professional or practical level. The aim of this change was to work more focused with representatives interested in a specific target area and to include more service users and relatives as well as to ease networking with relevant partners. A recent evaluation carried out end of 2014[7] shows that this goal has been fulfilled.

Regional and Local Level

In each of the five regions in Denmark, a regional group is established and located at the Psychiatric Information centres, and management resources allocated for at least a part-time coordinator (funded and managed by the regions).The five coordinators cooperate both with the national secretariat on the implementation of programmes and tools targeting different groups within the five target areas and act on their own when it comes to prioritising and developing local activities. The regional groups have representation from psychiatry, some municipalities and user- and relatives' organisations and meetings are held to inspire and stimulate plans and activities at regional and local level.

Furthermore, people with or without lived experiences are encouraged to join the campaign as volunteers through the website. By December 2014, 966 people have registered so far. From this group approximately 90 adults and 30 young people – called Ambassadors – have received special training in oral performance to improve their communication skills when speaking publicly about their personal experiences so they are better equipped to participate in social contact activities.

Means and Strategies

What Works and What Does Not in an Anti-Stigma Effort?

The approach of ONE OF US is based on means and strategies which have been developed and tested by national anti-stigma campaigns in other countries; the effect of which has been documented scientifically.[8]

ONE OF US activities are based on two main strategies: (1) Like other anti-stigma campaigns, ONE OF US organises activities at a national, regional and local level – all having anti-stigma as their starting point – matching messages and target groups to

---

[7] Berger et al.: Status på afstigmatiseringskampagnen EN AF OS 2014 KORA (Danish Institute for Local and Regional Government Research)

[8] E.g. Henderson and Thornicroft 2013; Thornicroft 2006; Stuart et al. 2012.

those of the campaign. (2) The campaign latches on to other relevant stakeholders' activities (ambushing). The latter brings the campaign into contact with people that would not otherwise seek information on mental illness and thus spend fewer resources trying to reach these target groups and increase the possibility of implementation.

The campaign gives priority to both strategies because combined they allow the campaign to follow the focused action plans at the same time as maintaining a flexibility to 'seize the moment' when opportunity arrives.

Another important aspect is evidence of the methods which work and the ones that do not in regard to reducing stigma. Traditional communication about mental illness and its symptoms cannot stand alone as this can lead to overstating the diagnosis rather than seeing the individual expression or the person with the mental illness. Similarly, comparing mental illness to a broken leg or diabetes does not take into account the psychological aspect that the individuals' perception of him- or herself and of others and the relation between them is significantly affected during periods of mental illness and the fact that this is where silence, doubt and taboo stem from.

On the other hand, effective anti-stigma methods should contain the following:

- Facilitation of identification and empathy through, e.g.,
  - Using social contact where people with lived experience of mental illness engage in dialogue with people without prior knowledge or who hold prejudices (see section "Ambassadors – a key instrument to ONE OF US" about ambassadors).
  - Videos, images, TV, radio, plays, etc. portraying people with personal experience of mental illness in a respectful manner.
  - Dialogue on social media.
- Challenging myths with facts
- Intruding without being intrusive and never moralising

Ideas, materials and designs are tested in focus groups with the target audience and carried out both by external consultants and internally to make sure that ONE OF US remains respectful and relevant.

The list of outgoing activities is diverse but can be categorised as follows:

- Presentations, information and training
- Festivals, happenings, creative and cultural events
- Workshops and conferences
- Systematic use of toolkits and materials

Ambassadors: A Key Instrument to ONE OF US

There are two types of ambassadors:

- The primary ambassadors in ONE OF US are people with personal experience of mental illness.
- The secondary ambassadors are celebrities who support the campaign – some of them by sharing their personal story with mental illness.

The celebrities attract attention to the cause and legitimise the social importance of fighting stigma and discrimination. They mainly appear at larger public events or in PR activities and are valued in the campaign. However, the ambassadors who most effectively change attitudes are the people with lived experience of mental illness, and we refer to them in the following:

The ONE OF US ambassadors – people with lived experience – are recruited among people who volunteer for ONE OF US through the website, the national secretariat or the regional coordinators. Being an ambassador requires an ability to put one's personal experiences into perspective. It is therefore vital that the ambassadors are well on the way in their recovery process or in a good place in their lives.

ONE OF US ambassadors receive a three-day oral presentation course developed and carried out by external communications consultants with expertise both in rhetoric and journalism as well as disability and psychosocial rehabilitation. During the training programme, the ambassadors learn to structure their personal stories and to adapt it to different target audiences. They also receive training in dealing with the media and an introduction to ONE OF US. Part of the training also deals with protecting personal boundaries and maintaining one's integrity when disclosing. By the end of 2014, ONE OF US has trained about 120 ambassadors, including 30 young people (18–25 years). Currently about 70 of these are active in the campaign and more people are joining.

The ambassadors are organised at the regional level and attached to the coordinator in the region they live in. It is the responsibility of the regional coordinator to maintain and develop the corps of ambassadors. This is carried out differently in the five regions. Also the regional coordinator prepares ambassadors for activities and debriefs them afterwards. Exceptions to this rule are when ambassadors participate in national level activities organised by the national secretariat which then is responsible for the preparation and debriefing.

A part of the ONE OF US evaluation carried out in November 2014 by an independent agency investigated the ambassadors' outcome of their volunteer work in the campaign by (1) a quantitative electronic survey to all current and previous ambassadors and (2) focus groups among a selection of ambassadors. The response rate was 68 % and the results very positive. When asked to point out the most important factors for upholding their commitment to the campaign, the highest-rated answers were as follows:

1. To be involved in the campaign (84 % replied 'very important' or 'important')
2. Getting the experience that their contribution makes a real difference to others (83 % replied 'very important' or 'important')
3. Being appreciated (90 % replied 'very important' or 'important')

As in evaluations by the Swedish campaign (H)järnkoll from 2014[9] and the English Time to Change from 2013[10], the Danish evaluation also clearly documents

---

[9] Hjärnkoll – psykiska olikheter lika rättigheter, Myndigheten för delaktighet 2014
[10] Time to Change: Phase 1. Sharing the learning from England's biggest mental health anti-stigma and discrimination programme, 2007–2011

that being an ambassador has a strong empowering impact on the ambassadors' personal life. The main and important findings are

1. Disclosure has been of great significance to me (94 % replied 'very important' or 'important').
2. Being an ambassador has improved my self-esteem (71 % replied 'very important' or 'important').
3. Being an ambassador has given me greater hope for the future (70 % replied 'very important' or 'important').
4. I have improved my capacity to deal with prejudices from others (70 % replied 'very important' or 'important').
5. Being an ambassador has made me more confident deciding when to disclose and when not to (67 % replied 'very important' or 'important').

Another item in the questionnaire concerned how much having a mental illness dominated the person's self-perception **before** attending the role of ambassador and **currently**. The significance of this item is documented in the ONE OF US discrimination survey which pointed out that the more the illness dominates a person's self-perception, the bigger the risk of self-stigma and discrimination (see section "The public and the media" about service users and relatives) (Table 17.2).

The results clearly state a reduction in how much having a mental illness dominates the ambassadors' self-perception after attending the role of ambassador from 82 % to 61 % stating 'to a high degree' and 'to some degree' thereby indicating a reduced risk of self-stigma.

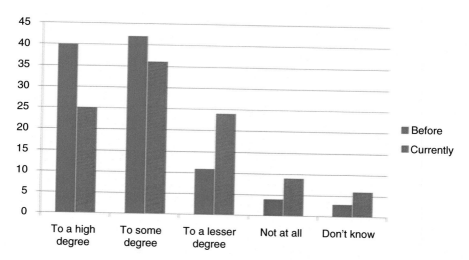

Table 17.2 How much does having a mental illness dominate your self-perception <u>before</u> attending the role of ambassador and <u>currently</u>?

PR Agency

ONE OF US closely cooperates with the PR agency PrimeTime Kommunikation in relation to strategies for press releases, social media and campaigning for different target areas as well as graphic design, key messages and campaign material. See also section "The public and the media".

The ONE OF US Panel

In the spring of 2012, the ONE OF US panel was established as an electronic survey panel and counts by the end of 2014 more than 2,000 people with lived experience of mental illness. One can join the panel through the ONE OF US website or surveys posted on ONE OF US' Facebook. Every two months the panel participants fill out an electronic questionnaire from ONE OF US about different themes related to stigma of mental illness. The survey data are mainly used in press stories consistent with the campaign focus at the time. The panel is also asked to test new material and evaluate specific activities. The press has shown quite a remarkable interest in these surveys which are not representative of the general public but give a fair indication of important aspects of life with mental illness.

Press stories are shared on Facebook along with posts thanking the survey participants for their contribution thereby maintaining commitment. Furthermore, the panel is an opportunity for people with lived experience of mental illness to contribute in a meaningful way even if they are not able to physically engage in activities or disclose publicly.

Social Media

ONE OF US is present on several social media platforms: Website, Facebook, Twitter, YouTube, Instagram and Spotify. Facebook is the primary platform for the campaign because

- Facebook is the preferred social media of the Danish population (68 % have a profile).
- Posts can be segmented to target specific groups.
- It entails a golden opportunity to engage in dialogue with the users.

This corresponds well with the campaign values and intentions of openness and communication. Facebook represents a community for likers of ONE OF US and is used to recruit for the ONE OF US panel, new likers and for advertising creating traffic for the website. The Facebook profile has developed into a dynamic and caring community with high activity and engagement from the likers. The campaign has managed to create an environment where the nonprofessional

Table 17.3 Main statistics from the ONE OF US media monitoring

Year	Number of mentions	Readers/unique users	Estimated ad value
2013	331	30,980,921	735,429 euro
2014	344	37,197,754	891,429 euro

Facebook-user plays an important part in ensuring an including atmosphere that reduces the need for the campaign staff to actively moderate negative comments and debates. The number of likers is steadily increasing and by the end of December 2014 passed 29.000.

The ONE OF US secretariat and the PR agency continuously monitor and evaluate social media activities for ongoing development, refinement and adjustment of the social media strategy.

Media Monitoring and Analysis

The campaign cooperates with Infomedia – a provider of media intelligence, i.e. media search, media monitoring and media analysis covering a wide range of Danish print media, broadcast media and online media. This helps the campaign follow developments and activities in the field of mental illness and especially follow mentions of ONE OF US in the media. Semi-annually the campaign receives data on the coverage of ONE OF US both nationally, regionally and locally distributed over time, geographical area and subjects enabling the secretariat to identify fluctuations and the estimated ad value (Table 17.3).

This data forms the basis of a yearly analysis of the media coverage of mental illness covering the entire campaign period. In the spring of 2011, before ONE OF US was officially launched, four topics dominated the data: psychiatric services, mental illness, policy and crime. The latter subject taking up one-sixth of unique stories but cited so frequently that it dominated more than one-third of the overall coverage. Consequently, maintaining the prejudice of connecting mental illness to danger and crime. The analysis of October 2013 documents a positive development regarding this with a much wider variety of subjects covered including taboo, personal stories and the labour market.

The Five Target Areas of ONE OF US and Their Main Activities

The Public and the Media

Internationally, the media is notorious for stigmatising presentations of mental illness emphasising violence and crime and thus maintaining a perception of danger. There is a pressing need to challenge the myths and spread the message of recovery. In few words, the campaign name – ONE OF US – signals the objective of the campaign namely that mental illness is everybody's business, and everybody should be included and feel part of the community.

Working with the press is therefore a core activity within this target area, and the focus is on telling personal stories of hope and recovery to inspire and to show the wide variety of people and lives with a mental illness.

In 2014 at the annual four-day democracy festival in Denmark with 80,000 participants including politicians, decision-makers, PR and communication agents, a wide variety of organisations as well the general public, ONE OF US had a panel debate with representatives from the Danish Union of Journalists, editor-in-chief for one of the largest tabloid newspapers, the national Danish broadcasting network, the political level and the service user movement. Data from the media analysis (see section "Media monitoring and analysis") formed the base for the debate focusing on ethical principles[11] and language and depictions of mental illness. An indication of the outcome is found in the final statement made by the editor-in-chief: 'Today I'm taking something with me; no one is only their diagnosis!' Subsequently the vice president of the Danish Union of Journalists remarked in an article that he had participated in the event, and that the media should pay attention to language and ethics when dealing with mental illness.

Early 2011 ONE OF US was fortunate to establish a collaboration with DR – Danish Broadcasting Corporation, the national public service network resulting in an adapted Danish version of the British BBC show 'How Mad are You?' aired in May 2012 with financial contribution from ONE OF US. Out of a population of 5.6 million people, 700,000 people watched the show with overwhelmingly positive response.

This created an increased awareness of the importance of an anti-stigma effort within the broadcasting network and consequently created the onset of a much more comprehensive strategy titled 'Invisibly Ill' consisting of several TV series, radio programmes, online news stories and several features in news and entertainment shows.

The objectives of the TV network were

- To combat prejudice related to mental illness.
- To humanise people who have personal experience with mental illness.
- To investigate society's treatment of people with mental illness.
- To make clear that a psychiatric diagnosis is not necessarily for life and that a mental illness is only part of someone's personality. You are not your diagnosis.

'Invisibly Ill' was first aired on March 31 2014 and continued throughout most of April with great success. 2.8 million people – that is half of the Danish population – watched at least one of the programmes. The response was extremely positive and supportive, and all the aired programmes were rated between 4.1 and 4.5 on a scale from 1 to 5 in a survey conducted by the broadcasting network. This is an exceptionally high ranking. Moreover, the ONE OF US campaign received a great

---

[11] Referring to the material from Canadian Journalism Forum 'Mindset. Reporting on Mental Health' from 2014.

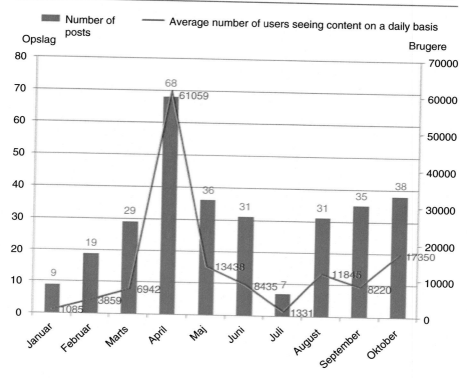

Table 17.4 Posts and exposure on ONE OF US' Facebook site 2014

deal of attention as a result. The ONE OF US Facebook got 10,000 new likers in April alone (Table 17.4).

In a ONE OF US panel survey with 1,235 respondents with lived experience of mental illness, 93 % stated that their general impression of 'Invisibly Ill' was 'very positive' or 'positive'. When asked to describe it using words from a list, the majority ticked off 'informative', 'interesting' and 'thought-provoking'. 88 % of the respondents thought that the TV shows gave good insight into living with mental illness, and 62 % stated that the programmes had made them want to be more open about their own mental illness.

In 2011, 2012 and 2014, ONE OF US carried out representative population surveys on different topics relating to mental illness, and the most recent from June 2014 also contained questions about 'Invisibly Ill'. Interestingly, the respondents ticked off the same words from the list describing their personal rating as the ONE OF US panel respondents. This strongly indicates that it is possible to depict mental illness and the people affected by this in a way which is perceived as respectful and relevant to both people with lived experience of mental illness and people without.

In the population survey from 2012, 26 % indicated to 'have seen or heard information' about the campaign which in 2014 (3 years into the campaign) had risen to 37 %. This is very satisfactory – also compared to similar campaigns.

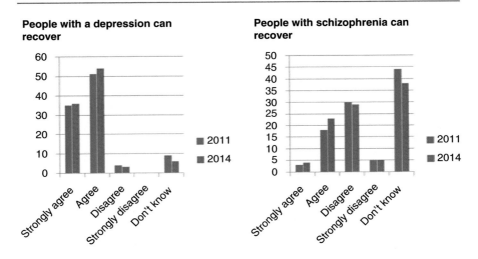

Table 17.5 Population survey 2011 and 2014

The baseline survey from 2010 pointed out that in Denmark, as in other countries we compare ourselves to, schizophrenia is the most stigmatised illness. Consequently this has been a focal point in the campaign, e.g., with a targeted use of ambassadors with the illness in different stages of recovery and willing to disclose publicly – also on TV. This has also been a topic in the population surveys. Table 17.5 illustrates a positive change regarding this and also demonstrates the contrast regarding knowledge about recovery from depression and schizophrenia, respectively (21 % strongly agree/agree in 2011 and 27 % in 2014).

On the World Mental Health Day in 2014, ONE OF US sent out a press release based on the results of the work on renaming schizophrenia in Japan.[12] The story was picked up by the Danish Radio Broadcasting Corporation and resulted in representatives from the campaign being interviewed about the issue.

Service Users and Relatives

It is well known that service users experience stigma connected to mental illness resulting in exclusion from the labour market, education and social life. Being a relative of a person living with mental illness can be associated with shame because of the perception that the parents are the cause of mental illness. This can lead to self-stigma which adds to the mental illness.

One of the main activities of this focus area is therefore a major discrimination survey among people with lived experience of mental illness first carried out in 2013 and to be repeated in 2015. The survey method is the internationally recognised scale DISC-12 translated and validated into Danish and carried out as an

---

[12] Sartorius et al. (2014)

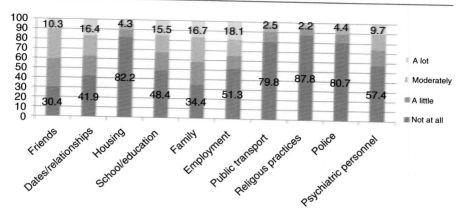

Table 17.6 Experienced unfair treatment (selected results): Have you been unfairly treated due to mental illness within the past year?

electronic or postal self-completed questionnaire with 1,561 respondents instead of a phone interview as originally prescribed in the manual. About 300 of the respondents lived in social service housing facilities.

The questionnaire was separately supplied with questions concerning background variables and a very important question concerning how much having a mental illness dominates the person's self-perception at the time of the survey.

The results indicate that the level of stigma is in line with parallel international surveys based on DISC-12 (e.g. England, Sweden, New Zealand). It is worth noticing that as regards the target area staff in the social and health sectors, about 30 % have experienced unfair treatment 'a lot' or 'moderately' by psychiatric staff (Table 17.6).

The data also documents that self-stigma is a major problem and that experienced unfair treatment increases the risk of self-stigma in line with parallel international surveys based on DISC-12 (e.g. England, Sweden, New Zealand) which can be interpreted as an indication that we are dealing with a 'universal problem'. Furthermore the data clearly indicate that the more the illness dominates a person's self-perception, the bigger the risk of self-stigma and discrimination. This emphasises that everybody can make a positive difference to a person's experience of stigma by 'seeing the person behind the diagnoses' which has become a fundamental statement in the ONE OF US dialogue material targeted psychiatric staff (see section "Staff in health and social sectors").

The survey was supplemented by three focus groups: one with women, one with men and one with both men and women. Table 17.7 illustrates an example of a person counteracting stigma.

Staff in Health and Social Sectors

Research documents that health sector staff, including psychiatric staff, does not differ from the general population when it comes to stigmatising attitudes towards

Table 17.7 Quote from focus group

Woman, 36 years, counteracting stigma

But when I got this diagnosis [schizophrenia] and we left the psychiatrist (…), she [my contact person] looks at me and says: 'So listen, you have schizophrenia. You'll need medication for the rest of your life, you won't be able to work, you'll have to apply for early retirement, you won't have children and you won't get married.' You might say that was a death sentence – but actually, for me it wasn't – because I remember looking at her thinking: 'You know what, you stupid cow. That's not up to you to decide (…).' [Later on, my husband is given the same contact person]. So I take my kid in the pram, go to the hospital and stand right in front of her and say: 'Hi there (…) Yeah, what do you know, this is my son. I also work a little and just got my HF-degree [Higher Preparatory Examination]. Now we have a boy and you know what? I'm not on medication anymore. And I'm married and we have our own house.'

people with mental illness and their relatives. Through their close contact with patients, the staff holds a position of power and can affect the patients' self-perception and thereby play a major role in adding to or reducing self-stigma. This also applies to the social and employment sector, including rehabilitation and employment services.

In the autumn of 2011, an attitudes survey based in MICA-2 and MICA-4 was carried out at two psychiatric units in Copenhagen. 61 psychiatrists and 487 mixed staff (166 nurses, 52 physical and occupational therapists, 112 nurse assistants, 28 psychologists, 65 administrative staff, 30 social counsellors, 15 from other groups/+ 19 not registered) filled in the questionnaire anonymously. The scale was translated, validated into Danish and adjusted so the focus was on 'schizophrenia' instead of 'mental illness' as recommended by Kassam et al.[13] Separately, four questions were added, one of them being 'The tone at the work place and the way we speak about patients affect our perception of their possibility of recovery'. Table 17.8 clearly shows that the majority of the staff strongly agrees or agrees with this statement thus indicating the relevance of the objective to increase reflection on culture and language – also at psychiatric units (Table 17.8).

A key initiative within this target area is the 'Dialogue Kickstarter' toolkit aimed at psychiatric staff with the objective to increase reflections on culture and language in everyday practice. The objectives of the toolkit are

- To create awareness of communication.
- To motivate staff to enter into a dialogue based on respectful language and acknowledging culture and social conventions.
- To inspire staff to work in a more goal-oriented manner to promote anti-stigma.

The Dialogue Kickstarter manual is structured and designed to be accessible and easy to use even when time is limited. The manual comprises

---

[13] Kassam et al. (2010)

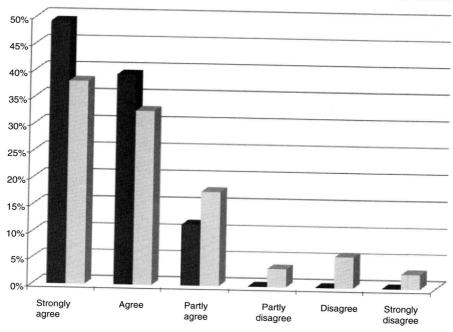

Table 17.8 The tone at the work place and the way we speak about patients affect our perception of their possibility of recovery (The dark columns are psychiatrists and the light columns are mixed staff.)

- Videos 'Maybe I'm just a unique human being' with ambassadors sharing their experience of both stigma and empowerment in psychiatric treatment, including questions for debate.
- Case vignettes based on real-life examples, including questions for debate.
- Videos 'Plain talk' humorously illustrating common situations of miscommunication in the health system, including questions for debate.
- An appeal to invite an ambassador in to share his or her personal story.
- Memo to be filled in to maintain focus on anti-stigma.
- Exercise: 'Have you encountered these attitudes?'
- Electronic evaluation questionnaire.

Additional material (poster, information card and stickers) has been produced to create attention among staff, patients and relatives in psychiatric units working with the toolkit.
Statements on this material are

- See the person behind the diagnosis
- No one is just a diagnosis
- Hope is always part of recovery
- Have you asked your patient for his/her experiences of prejudice?
- Have you asked your patient for his/her opinion?

The management level of all five regions in Denmark have committed to action plans implementing the Dialogue Kickstarter adapted to their strategy of competence development and organisation. An evaluation carried out in November 2014 document that 75 % of the staff working with the toolkit responded that they 'strongly agree' or 'agree' that the toolkit increases their knowledge on the importance of prejudices in their daily work as well as their attention to the importance of communication and use of language.[14]

Similar toolkits targeted the psychosocial rehabilitation services and employment services are currently being developed.

The Labour Market

In Denmark mental illness is a common cause for people to leave or never to gain foothold in the labour market. A better understanding of mental illness would contribute to greater inclusion and job retention, and in this respect both employers and colleagues have the potential to play a pivotal part. This could reduce sick leave due to mental illness and create better conditions for making the adjustments necessary for the inclusion of people with mental health problems in the labour market.

ONE OF US-tools like short humorous videos illustrating men's behavioural patterns when it comes to mental illness, flyers and leaflets on inclusion of employees with mental health problems in the work place along with specially trained ambassadors with lived experience are key to starting the dialogue with employers and colleagues.

Within this target area, ONE OF US has been particularly successful using the ambush strategy, e.g., setting up stalls manned by ambassadors and campaign staff at conferences on HR, work environment and employment as well as trade unions' meetings and other conferences, etc.

Young People

Adolescence and early adulthood are a vulnerable period to many. It is also the period where mental illness often begins. In the prevalence of mental illness among young people between the age of 15 and 25 is 8 %. Stigma of mental illness is of significant importance during this period of time. It may have the effect that young people abstain from seeking help and thus delay treatment. As a consequence they risk exacerbating their mental health problems and adding to self-stigma which may have life-long effects.

Schools and festivals are some of the venues ONE OF US seek out to meet young people and start talking with our youth ambassadors and handing out material. For this group, the social media is an important platform to distribute short videos along with a wide range of other material.

---

[14] Berger et al. (2014)

In the spring of 2013, ONE OF US carried out a coordinated national and regional initiative highlighting the target area of young people focusing on four topics, each promoted over the course of a month:

- Help from the educational system (March)
- Help from family (April)
- Help from friends (May)
- Help from mental health professionals (June)

Each topic was supported by ONE OF US panel surveys among young people under the age of 25 (250–500 respondents). The surveys gave important information, e.g., 72.2 % of the respondents pointed out that teachers should be more aware of students with mental health problems and support them in getting help, 47.1 % wanted young people with lived experience of mental illness to visit their school which supports the idea of ambassadors, 43 % replied they did not know where to go for help when needed and 70 % reported their health care professional/therapist had not discussed prejudice towards mental illness with them.

The findings created the basis for an intensive media effort supported by personal stories from ambassadors related to each subject. The topics received national coverage by national radio stations, TV networks and national papers. A series of short videos were produced with actors and ambassadors and distributed strategically on the social media and the campaign website. The videos were viewed up to 180,000 times and had 450,000 viewers when they aired as public service announcements on national TV.

In the spring of 2015, ONE OF US will carry out a new campaign initiative focusing on young men in vocational colleges based on the experiences from the spring 2013 campaign and activities targeting the labour market aimed at male dominated workplaces.

Lessons Learned: So Far

Realistic Preparation Time Important

The Danish anti-stigma campaign was initiated early autumn 2010 and the Board was established. The campaign opted for a framework similar to the English campaign Time to Change which operates on a national, regional and local level, however, not fully adapted to a Danish context. From January to April 2011, staff for the national secretariat was recruited and established comprising three employees. From the very start, the secretariat was expected to

- Handle the challenge of setting up a complex organisation.
- Initiate and facilitate cooperation between all partners involved.
- Meet expectations from the Board to be visible and carry out activities.
- Develop the overall vision.

- Develop an overall action plan in setting out objectives, target groups and basic activities for the five target areas.
- Prepare a call for tenders together with the Danish Health and Medicines Authority in order to find PR agency in charge of creating a campaign identity, website, graphic design in respect to materials, merchandise, etc.
- Prepare public launching of the campaign in September-October 2011.

The many parallel processes and expectations created an extreme work load on the national secretariat of three people. On this basis, a recommendation would be to plan for a realistic preparation time.

Interaction Between National, Regional and Local Levels

Planning and time schedules for activities are crucial to secure a red thread and joint actions for all parties involved and, on the other hand, leave room for a high degree of flexibility, motivation and capability to 'seize the moment' if opportunities arise and new contacts show interest and capacity to offer an 'open door'. The culture of operation at regional levels embedded in the psychiatric services has been challenged by expectations to show more flexibility over time as part of a campaign culture.

The processes and time needed to facilitate joint ownership of the campaign by service users' and relatives' organisations should not be underestimated. The organisations have different member groups, organisational culture, political agendas and practises regarding activities and acceptance of evidence-based methods for anti-stigma interventions and activities.

Complex Financial Conditions

ONE OF US is based on a complex budget as explained in section "The set-up of a Danish anti-stigma campaign" consisting of a mixture of real money, indirect manpower and user organisations' voluntary manpower resulting in an uneven balance of power, joint ownership and decision-making power. In the event of a possible new campaign phase, it would be desirable to have funds allocated for activities carried out by the service users' and relatives' organisations to support their voluntary involvement and joint ownership.

Criterion for Success

In many anti-stigma campaigns, criterions for success are based on mainly quantitative measures using validated scales measuring changes in attitudes. However, to measure actual and sustainable behaviour changes remains a common challenge.

The original baseline of ONE OF US indicated a high level of politically correct responses from the Danish population. Due to this finding, we choose not to use a percentage improvement criteria as opposed to Time to Change and the Swedish campaign (H)järnkoll. Instead, the priority has been to document improvements of more specific issues related directly to each target area and target groups as described in the above sections.

Ambassadors Are Vital

Like other anti-stigma campaigns, ONE OF US has had great success using ambassadors with lived experience of mental illness in social contact activities creating identification and empathy to facilitate dialogue and break down barriers of prejudice. In this respect, systematic training of the ambassadors' communication skills as well as preparation and debriefing related to activities are very important.

Most of the ambassadors and other volunteers are not active members of any of the service users' and relatives' organisations but have chosen to join ONE OF US because of the campaigns overall vision and goals.

Indications exist to the fact that extended use of ambassadors at all levels of the campaign in itself contributes to the desired development in psychiatric services to include people with lived experience as well as relatives in treatment and in employment of staff.

Synergy Between Different Professional Competences

To a national campaign, a PR agency can play a vital and facilitating role and help develop a detailed communication strategy which optimises synergy. However, it should also be taken into consideration that it may take time for an external agency to grasp the soul of an anti-stigma programme as well as the complexity of the field of mental illness. It requires very clear communication from campaign agents as regards professional knowledge and the tone desired. The same challenges apply to external evaluation institutes.

Future Perspectives for ONE OF US

The first phase of ONE OF US was funded till the end of 2015. The evaluation report released in January 2015 documents both a high level of activity at national, regional and local level, effective campaign strategies, a growing network nationally and internationally, a growing awareness of the campaign in the public and increasing readiness to 'open up doors' and invite people in for a talk about mental illness. In October 2015 ONE OF US received state and regional funding once more for a second phase 2016–2020.

Further support of the need to continue the campaign is the government's release of a new national action plan for the development and quality of psychiatric treatment in spring 2014. The national action plan contains objectives of more systematic involvement of patients/service users and relatives as well as increased knowledge about recovery among health professionals and the public. ONE OF US is explicitly mentioned in the plan as one of the ongoing initiatives which supports openness and anti-stigma.

References

Berger N et al. (2014) Status på afstigmatiseringskampagnen EN AF OS 2014 KORA (Danish Institute for Local and Regional Government Research)

Borg W (2010) White paper Hvidbog om mentalt helbred og sygefravær, The National Research Centre for Working Environment

Bracken R (2014) Hjärnkoll – psykiska olikheter lika rättigheter, Myndigheten för delaktighet. Can J Forum Mindset. Reporting on Mental Health

Henderson C, Thornicroft G (April 2013) Reducing stigma and discrimination: evaluation of England's time to change programme. Br J Psychiatr 202(Suppl 5)

Kassam A et al (2010) Development and responsiveness of a scale to measure clinicians' attitudes to people with mental illness. Acta Psychiatr Scand 122:153–161

OECD report Sick on the Job? Myths and Realities about mental Health and Work, 2012

Sartorius N et al (2014) Name change for schizophrenia. Schizophr Bull 40(2):255–258

Stuart H, Arboleda-Flórez J, Sartorius N (2012) Paradigms lost. Fighting stigma and the lessons learned. Oxford University Press, New York

Time to Change (2013) Time to Change: Phase 1 Sharing the learning from England's biggest mental health anti-stigma and discrimination programme, 2007–2011

Thornicroft G (2006) Shunned. Oxford University Press

www.ast.dk Annual statistics on incapacity benefits, Ankestyrelsen, 2012

The Time to Change Programme to Reduce Stigma and Discrimination in England and Its Wider Context

Claire Henderson, Sara Evans Lacko, and Graham Thornicroft

Introduction

Stigma and discrimination against people with mental illness have substantial public health impact in England as demonstrated by a range of health, social, and economic indicators: poor access to mental and physical health care (Mai et al. 2011), reduced life expectancy (Laursen et al. 2007; Gissler et al. 2013), exclusion from higher education (Suhrcke and de Paz Nieves 2011; Lee et al. 2009) and employment (Social Exclusion U 2004), increased risk of contact with criminal justice systems, victimisation (Clement et al. 2011a), poverty, and homelessness. Goffman's seminal definition of stigma written in the 1960s as 'an attribute that is deeply discrediting and that reduces the bearer from a whole and usual person to a tainted, discounted one' is still relevant (Goffman 1968). More recent conceptualisations include labelling, stereotyping, separation, status loss, and discrimination (Link et al. 1989) and incorporate experiences of discrimination; traditionally work on stigma has tended to focus on public attitudes and knowledge about mental illnesses.

C. Henderson (✉) • S.E. Lacko • G. Thornicroft
Institute of Psychiatry, Psychology and Neuroscience, King's College London,
Box P029, De Crespigny Park, London SE5 8AF, UK
e-mail: claire.1.henderson@kcl.ac.uk; Sara.Evans-Lacko@kcl.ac.uk;
graham.thornicroft@kcl.ac.uk

© Springer International Publishing Switzerland 2017
W. Gaebel et al. (eds.), *The Stigma of Mental Illness - End of the Story?*,
DOI 10.1007/978-3-319-27839-1_18

Internationally, public attitude data suggest that there has been little spontaneous improvement over time (Schomerus et al. 2012); however there is growing evidence for the effectiveness in high-income countries of anti-stigma interventions, both national programmes and those targeted to specific groups (Stuart et al. 2014). As a result, more countries are investing in national anti-stigma programmes targeted at both the general public and specific target groups (Borschmann RG et al. 2014; https://www.time-to-change.org.uk/news/global-meeting-anti-stigma-programme--london 2013). The National Institute for Health and Clinical Excellence emphasises the inclusion of knowledge, attitude, and behavioural components when developing and evaluating behaviour change interventions (National Institute for H & Clinical E. Behaviour Change. NICE 2007). Applying this to anti-stigma interventions requires the evaluation of lack of knowledge and misinformation such as stereotypes, prejudicial attitudes and emotional reactions such as fear and anger, and discriminatory behaviour, as evidenced by the indicators listed above and by the experiences of people with mental illness (Thornicroft 2006; Thornicroft et al. 2007).

Key Current Issues

Surveys of mental health service users show that experiences of discrimination pervade many areas of life (Corker et al. 2013; Lasalvia et al. 2012; Thornicroft et al. 2009) and that anticipation of discrimination is even more frequent, leading people to avoid possible opportunities for employment and relationships (Ucok et al. 2012). In this chapter we focus on three areas of life in which the impact of discrimination has a significant public health impact: health care, employment, and citizenship.

Evidence from the first year of the Time to Change anti-stigma programme in England (Henderson et al. 2012a) showed significant improvements in life areas in which relationships are informal, i.e. family, friends, and social life. In some areas where discrimination may occur at a structural level, there were no improvements, including mental and physical health care and welfare benefits; in others including those in seeking and gaining employment, early improvements have since plateaued or been lost (Corker et al. 2013). This chapter therefore takes account of discrimination at both the structural (Schomerus et al. 1464, 2006) and the interpersonal level.

Population Level Interventions

A review from the National Institute of Mental Health England (Gale et al. 2004) identified six principles of an effective anti-stigma campaign:

1. Service users and carers should be involved throughout the design, delivery monitoring, and evaluation of the campaign.
2. Campaigns should be monitored and evaluated.
3. National campaigns should be supported by local grass-roots initiatives.
4. Campaigns should address behaviour change.
5. Clear specific messages should be delivered in targeted ways to identifiable audiences.

6. Long-term planning and funding should be in place to ensure campaign sustainability.

In a more recent consensus development study on effective types of messages to use in population-level campaigns, experts recommended messages which were recovery oriented and those which sought to remove the distance between 'us' and 'them' (Clement et al. 2010). Other research has demonstrated that enhancing public understanding of the biological correlates of mental illness is not accompanied by reduced levels of stigma (Schomerus et al. 2012; Mehta et al. 2015; Thornicroft et al. 2015; Semrau et al. 2015).

Several population-level programmes have shown evidence of effectiveness. Evaluation of the Nuremberg Alliance Against Depression (Hegerl et al. 2003, 2006; Dietrich et al. 2010) found a significant reduction in the number of suicidal acts over each of the 2 years of the campaign when compared to a control-comparison region. In Australia, survey respondents in states and territories which funded the beyondblue programme (Jorm n.d.) showed greater recognition of depression and more frequent recognition of depression in people they knew; this may be due to both greater awareness and greater openness on the part of those affected. In Scotland, the 'See Me' campaign was launched in 2002 (Mehta et al. 2009; Dunion et al. 2005). Since then, there has been a significant reduction (30 % vs. 19 %) in the proportion of survey respondents who agreed that people with mental illness are often dangerous and a significant increase in willingness to interact with someone who had a mental illness (Henderson et al. 2013). The proportion of people with a mental illness who reported experiencing discrimination also dropped significantly between 2002 and 2008 (Davidson. S et al. 2009). Survey data from 1993 to 2003 suggest that public attitudes in England worsened between 2000 and 2003, but changed less in Scotland (Laursen et al. 2007). In England, Time to Change (http://www.time-to-change.org.uk/), run by Mind and Rethink Mental Illness, is the largest ever programme to reduce stigma and discrimination against people with mental health problems; details are provided as a case study.

Interventions to Specific Target Groups

The three strategies most commonly used to address the stigma and discrimination related to mental illness at the individual level are (1) education (to replace preconceived myths and stereotypes with facts), (2) contact (direct interactions with persons who have mental illness), and (3) protest (to change behaviour and challenge attitudes) (Corrigan et al. 2001). A meta-analysis of studies in 2012 revealed that, while contact was more effective than education at reducing stigma in adults, the opposite was true for adolescents (Corrigan et al. 2012), while evidence for protest is weak and less well studied.

Health Care

While anti-stigma interventions with health-care students may have a positive short-term impact (Clement et al. 2011b), there is no evidence for longer-term behavioural change, either from targeted interventions for medical students

(Friedrich et al. 2013) or from the overall evaluation of Time to Change (Corker et al. 2013). This has shown no significant reduction in reported discrimination by mental health service users from either health professionals (30 % in 2008 and 29 % in 2011) or mental health professionals (34 % in 2008 and 30 % in 2011). The TTC social marketing campaign may be ineffective among health professionals, for example, because they do not recognise their role as stigmatisers (Schulze 2007) or because the 'clinical fallacy' means their attitudes and behaviour are resistant to change, as they most often see cases with the worst course and outcome. Medical students exposed to this bias during training may not benefit from anti-stigma training. Thus, initial treatment seeking for mental health problems may increase if public attitudes and behaviours improve, but negative experiences with health professionals may deter people from seeking further help.

Employment

A significant improvement in employment-related attitudes (a significant reduction in the proportion of employers who endorsed the view that people with mental health problems are less reliable than other employees and that employees with mental health problems are unlikely to ever fully recover) was observed between 2006 and 2010 (Henderson et al. 2012b). Employers also report the use of workplace accommodations for people with mental health problems with increasing frequency, and this can be important for facilitating openness and disclosure by employees (Evans-Lacko et al. n.d.). There was an initial improvement after the start of Time to Change in terms of frequency at which mental health service users reported unfair treatment in both finding and keeping work (Henderson et al. 2012c), but the magnitude of this change was no longer significant by 2011 (Corker et al. 2013). This may be due to economic problems; European data (Evans-Lacko et al. 2013a) suggest that the gap in unemployment rates between individuals with and without mental health problems significantly widened during the recent economic recession and that the disadvantage facing people with mental health problems was greater in countries with higher levels of stigmatising attitudes.

Citizenship

The 2013 Mental Health (Discrimination) Act removed sections from several pieces of legislation and abolished any common law rule which had disqualified people on the grounds of mental health from a number of offices and roles: member of parliament and membership of devolved bodies, jurors, and company directors. Exclusion from jury service is now based on being currently detained under the Mental Health Act or residing in hospital. This legislation sends an important message, that no one should be automatically excluded from playing their part as a UK citizen due to having, or having had, a mental illness. However, in terms of the experiences of mental health service users' daily lives, there is no evidence that the ability to take part in any area of life besides contact with friends, family, and neighbours (Corker et al. 2013) has got any easier. Besides employment and health care, examples where no reduction in unfair treatment has been observed include welfare benefits, personal safety, and parenting. 'Unfair treatment' covers a range of experiences in these different life areas (Hamilton et al. 2014).

In the area of welfare benefits, this can include the behaviour of job centre staff and problems getting entitlements. Discriminatory experiences in terms of personal safety encompass disability hate crime and victimisation more broadly. A review (Choe et al. 2008) found 2–13 % of outpatient attenders with mental health problems had perpetrated acts of violence in the previous 6 months to 3 years, compared with 20–34 % who had been the victims of violence. The authors conclude that victimisation is a greater public health problem than perpetration, and focusing on perpetration may contribute to negative stereotypes. In the area of parenting, the problems most commonly reported are being assumed to be an unfit parent and a lack of understanding of how the mental illness could affect the parenting role (Jeffery et al. 2013).

The Time to Change Programme in England: Policy Framework

Reducing mental health-related stigma and discrimination is one of the six objectives of the government's mental health strategy, No Health Without Mental Health (https://www.gov.uk/government/publications/the-mental-health-strategy-for-england). This was launched in 2011, the same year as the UK Department of Health became the largest funder of the second phase of Time to Change (TTC) in England (2011–2015). The Department of Health requested that TTC include campaigns targeted at children and young people, so that the programme covers all ages. The outcomes dashboard for monitoring progress on No Health Without Mental Health (https://www.gov.uk/government/uploads/system/uploads/attachment_data/file/265388/Mental_Health_Dashboard.pdf) uses the surveys undertaken to evaluate TTC (Corker et al. 2013) to track progress towards its objective to reduce stigma and discrimination. The importance of reducing discrimination is reiterated in 'Closing the Gap: Priorities for Essential Change in Mental Health' (Department of Health 2014). Anti-stigma programmes are also ongoing in Wales (Time to Change Wales/Cymru) and Scotland (See Me), but not in Northern Ireland.

Experiences of Discrimination Among Mental Health Service Users in England

Figure 18.1 presents findings from a national sample of service users on their reported experiences of discrimination across the areas of employment, health, and citizenship during 2012.

Trends in Public Stigma in England

Public Stigma in Relation to Employment

The majority of the public agrees that most people with mental health problems want to work and that they have equal rights to employment, and this trend seems to be improving slightly in recent years; however, more than 30 % of the population appear to question these statements (Fig. 18.2).

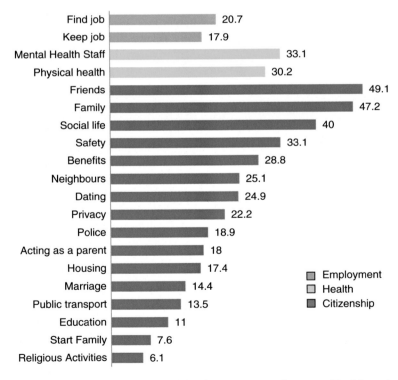

Fig. 18.1 Prevalence of experienced discrimination among secondary mental health service users across life domains of employment, health, and citizenship in England (2012) (Source: Henderson et al. 2014)

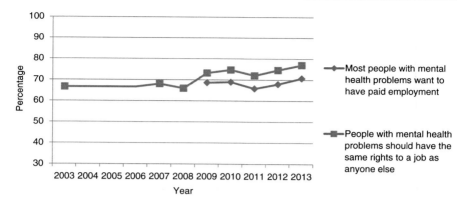

Fig. 18.2 Trends in public stigma in relation to employment (Source: Department of Health Attitudes to Mental Illness Survey. No data were collected from 2004 to 2006)

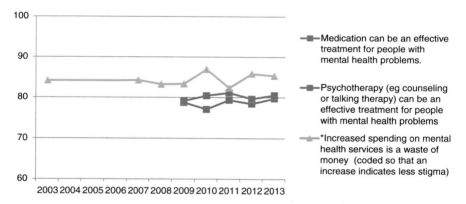

Fig. 18.3 Trends in public stigma in relation to mental health (Note: all items are coded so that trends going up indicate a favourable direction and less stigma) (Source: Department of Health Attitudes to Mental Illness Survey. No data were collected from 2004 to 2006. *Item was reverse coded so that all results could be calculated in a way where going up is the favourable direction)

Public Stigma in Relation to Mental Health

Figure 18.3 suggests that there is a high level of agreement that medication and psychotherapy are effective treatments for mental health problems and that spending on mental health services is not a waste of money; however, there was not much change in public views in relation to these statements. While agreement with these statements may be associated with increased likelihood of help-seeking for mental health problems and confidence in services, they may not directly

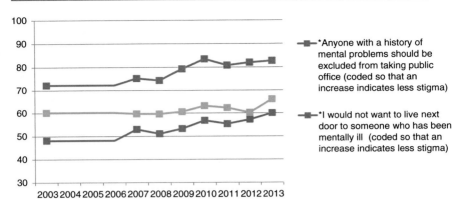

Fig. 18.4 Trends in public stigma in relation to citizenship (Note: all items are coded so that trends going up indicate a favourable direction and decreasing stigma) (Source: Department of Health Attitudes to Mental Illness Survey. No data were collected from 2004 to 2006. *Item was reverse coded so that all results could be calculated in a way where going up is the favourable direction)

translate to greater inclusion of people with mental health problems in other contexts (i.e. employment and citizenship) (Gissler et al. 2013; Suhrcke and de Paz Nieves 2011).

Public Stigma in Relation to Citizenship

The trends presented in Fig. 18.4 regarding public views of people with mental illness in relation to citizenship also seem to be improving in recent years. Although a clear majority responded positively about living next door to someone who has been mentally ill, indicators were less positive in relation to marriage and holding public office. In 2013, only one half to two thirds of respondents gave a positive (non-stigmatising) response to including people with mental illness in public office or when considering marriage.

Time to Change (TTC): Summary of Intervention and Evaluation

Question	Answer
What problem does TTC address?	Mental health-related stigma and discrimination in England; its impact on people with mental health problems and their supporters

Question	Answer
What is the intervention?	Phase 1 of TTC (2007–2011) consisted of several interventions, including a social marketing campaign, programmes for specific target groups including medical students and trainee teachers and head teachers and employers, local anti-discrimination initiatives, exercise programmes for people with mental health problems to promote social contact, social contact events organised by a range of stakeholders, and the use of social media such as Twitter and Facebook. Phase 2 (2011–2015) has built on the experience and evidence from phase 1 to deliver an even more evidence-based programme. Findings from phase 1 showed that, across England, there were significant improvements in intended behaviour and a positive (but nonsignificant) trend in attitudes towards mental illness (Evans-Lacko et al. 2013b); cumulative data including the first survey from phase 2 show further improvements such that the changes in both attitudes and intended behaviour are significant (Department of Health HMG 2013). There was a significant (3 %) increase in the proportion of service users who reported having experienced no discrimination during the previous year and a reduction in the median number of life areas in which discrimination was reported, from five to four (Corker et al. 2013). An improvement in employment-related attitudes (indicated by a significant reduction in the proportion of employers endorsing the view that people with mental health problems are less reliable than other employees and that employees with mental health problems are unlikely to ever fully recover) was observed among senior employers between 2006 and 2010 (Henderson et al. 2012b). Analysis of a sample of newspaper coverage showed 10 % proportional increases in articles coded as anti-stigmatising and in the use of people with experience of mental health problems as sources and a significant increase in the use of mental health charities as sources (Thornicroft et al. 2013). The TTC programme is innovative in terms of its long-term approach, use of evidence-based methods and significant investment in rigorous evaluation, use of social media both to amplify its message and empower people to tackle stigma, and involvement of people with lived experience at every level of both programme delivery and evaluation. The projected long-term benefits are improved quality of life for people with mental health problems and increased social capital as a result of better access to employment and services such as health care
How is TTC evaluated?	The evaluation comprises the following:
	Annual surveys of the general public, to assess mental health-related knowledge, attitudes, and intended behaviour; mental health service users, to assess experienced discrimination; responses to anticipated discrimination; perceived stigma; stigma coping responses; and social capital
	Content analysis of newspaper reporting on mental illness
	Awareness of each burst of the social marketing campaign; associations between campaign awareness and mental health-related knowledge, attitudes, and intended behaviour; and pre-post burst changes in these outcomes in the target population (aged 25–45 in middle income groups)
	Economic evaluation: costs of discrimination; costs of the campaign per point change in mental health-related knowledge, attitudes, and intended behaviour; return on investment

International Comparisons

In addition to higher rates of poverty and lower incomes, people with mental illness face a considerable employment disadvantage (Quinn et al. 2013). We know that the majority of people with mental illness want to work and that it is important for recovery; however, Fig. 18.5 demonstrates the significant disparity in employment rates between individuals with and without mental health problems. In the UK, although overall employment rates are relatively low, those with both moderate and severe disorders appear to have substantially lower rates of employment.

As employment rates are influenced by level of education, it is also important to investigate involvement among individuals in higher education. Figure 18.6 demonstrates that individuals with moderate and severe disorders tend to have much higher rates of stopping full-time education before age 15. Importantly, in the UK, overall rates seem to be higher, and the disparity between those with no mental disorder compared to those with severe mental disorder is greater than in any of the other high-income countries.

Economic Modelling

Epidemiological data demonstrates the adverse consequences for individuals with mental illness in terms of education and employment; however, there are limited data available on the economic costs of stigma (Evans-Lacko et al. 2014). The

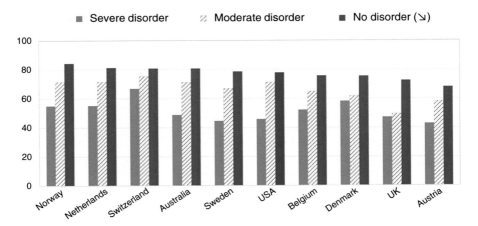

Fig. 18.5 Employment rates by mental health status across ten high-income countries. OECD (2012)

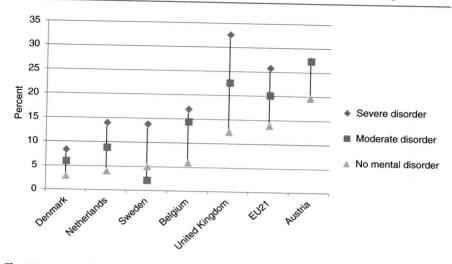

Fig. 18.6 Proportion of individuals who stopped full-time education before age 15 by mental health status across six high-income countries. Note: EU21 refers to all EU countries prior to the accession of the ten candidate countries on 1 May 2004, plus the four Eastern European member countries of the OECD, namely, Czech Republic, Hungary, Poland, and Slovak Republic (Source: OECD (2012)

economic evaluation of Time to Change builds on an evaluation of the See Me campaign examining the cost of the campaign in relation to the estimated number of people in the population with improved stigma outcomes (McCrone et al. 2010). Figures 18.7, 18.8, and 18.9 show that based on average social marketing campaign costs associated with Time to Change, and assuming that the campaign was only responsible for 50 % of the difference in responses to those who were aware vs. not aware of the Time to Change campaign, the cost for change in *knowledge* would be between £2.95 and £8.56. The cost for a change in *attitudes* would range from £2.50 to £10.96, and the cost for a change in *intended behaviour* would range from £2.24 to £3.86. Moreover, return on investment analysis suggested that the economic benefits of the campaign outweighed the costs even if the campaign resulted in only 1 % more people with depression accessing services and gaining employment if they experienced a health improvement (Evans-Lacko et al. 2013c).

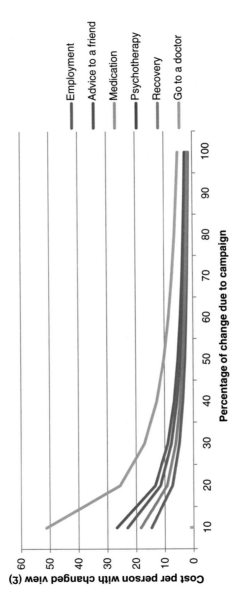

Fig. 18.7 Cost per person with changed knowledge associated with the Time to Change anti-stigma campaign. © [2013] The Royal College of Psychiatrists. Reference: (Evans-Lacko et al. 2013c) http://bjp.rcpsych.org/content/202/s55/s95.full

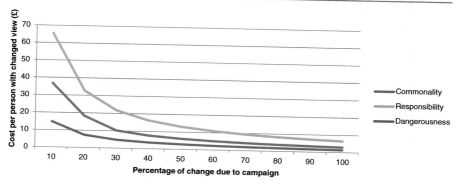

Fig. 18.8 Cost per person with changed attitudes associated with the Time to Change anti-stigma campaign. © [2013] The Royal College of Psychiatrists. Reference: (Evans-Lacko et al. 2013c) http://bjp.rcpsych.org/content/202/s55/s95.full

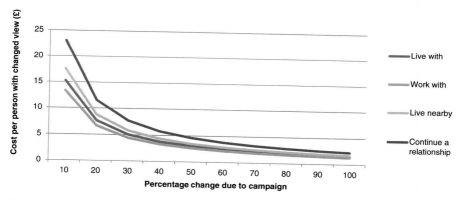

Fig. 18.9 Cost per person with changed intended behaviour associated with the Time to Change anti-stigma campaign. © [2013] The Royal College of Psychiatrists. Reference: (Evans-Lacko et al. 2013c) http://bjp.rcpsych.org/content/202/s55/s95.full

Conclusion

The following points are clear from this summary of the relevant evidence. Stigma and discrimination are major barriers to full citizenship in England. They reduce the opportunities for people with mental illness to gain employment, to receive the quantity and quality of mental and physical health care needed, and to form important social relationships. We therefore recommend the operationalisation of the Equality Act 2010 with respect to mental illness with respect to all areas of life, including the workplace, health and social care, education, the justice system, sports and leisure, and political participation. Significant, but modest, gains have been made in the reduction of stigma and discrimination during the period of the Time to Change programme, but most people with mental illness still experience these toxic reactions, and many then internalise these forms of rejection in ways that diminish their life opportunities. Hence another key recommendation is to support and evaluate projects aiming to empower mental health service users to respond to stigma and discrimination. The evidence increasingly clearly shows that carefully delivered interventions, both local and national, do reduce stigma and discrimination, if sustained over a sufficiently long term; hence our third key recommendation is to develop evidence-based social contact programmes to reduce stigma and discrimination among target groups prioritised by mental health service users. It is clear that the progress made in stigma reduction in England, in which in many ways we now lead the world, needs to redoubled to ensure further progress to eradicate what some have called 'the last taboo'.

Summary

This chapter presents information to (i) define stigma and discrimination; (ii) present evidence on their severity and toxic impact on the lives of people with mental illness; (iii) describe population-level and target-group level interventions and their effects; (iv) examine the particular detrimental effects of stigma and discrimination on health care, employment, and citizenship; (v) compare progress in England with other similar countries; (iv) examine the relevant health economic evidence; and (vi) make recommendations for further stigma reduction in England in the future. Our key recommendations are to (1) operationalise the concept of reasonable adjustments as per the Equality Act 2010 with respect to mental illness with respect to all areas of life, including the workplace, health and social care, education, the justice system, sports and leisure, and political participation; (2) support and evaluate projects aiming to empower mental health service users to respond to stigma and discrimination, e.g. through addressing self-stigma, training in self-advocacy, and peer support; and

Key Points
1. In a survey of mental health service users across England in 2011, 87 % reported experiencing discrimination in at least one aspect of life in the preceding 12 months (Corker et al. 2013).
2. Three studies have found that about 70 % of mental health service users feel the need to conceal their illness (Corker et al. 2013; Lasalvia et al. 2012; Thornicroft et al. 2009).
3. An annual survey of mental health service users in England held 2008–2011 (Corker et al. 2013) found that while there was a significant fall in those reporting being shunned by others, this was still common, at 50 % in 2011 (down from 58 % in 2008).

4. Articles that contribute to stigma are the commonest type of newspaper article on mental illness, accounting for nearly half of all coverage (Thornicroft et al. 2013).
5. A review (Choe et al. 2008) found 2–13 % of outpatient attenders with mental health problems had perpetrated acts of violence in the previous 6 months to 3 years, compared with 20–34 % who had been the victims of violence.
6. National Labour Force Survey figures reveal that in 2003, employment in the whole adult population was about 75 %, for people with physical health problems about 65 %, while for people with long-term mental health problems, it was 24 % (Social Exclusion U 2004).
7. A survey of mental health service users in 2011 (Corker et al. 2013) found that 19 % reported experiencing discrimination in seeking work; 17 % had experienced discrimination while in employment; and 46 % reported not looking for work due to the anticipation of discrimination.
8. Legal analysis of cases brought to employment tribunals under the Equality Act 2010 shows failure to make reasonable adjustment is the commonest type of mental health discrimination claim (Lockwood and Thornicroft in press); this type of claim also has the highest win rate, at 72 %.
9. Legal analysis of cases brought to Employment Appeal Tribunals on the basis of mental health discrimination shows that 58 % were based on an error in the application of the law/procedure; such appeals also have the highest win rate at 60 % (Lockwood and Thornicroft in press). This reflects insufficient detail and quality of employment tribunal judgements.
10. An annual service user survey held 2008–2011 (Corker et al. 2013) showed no significant reduction in reported discrimination from either health professionals (30 % in 2008 and 29 % in 2011) or mental health professionals (34 % in 2008 and 30 % in 2011).

(3) develop evidence-based social contact programmes to reduce stigma and discrimination among target groups prioritised by mental health service users in surveys such as Viewpoint (Corker et al. 2013) and Stigma Shout (Change 2008) and summarise the evidence for the effectiveness of England's most recent anti-stigma programme, Time to Change.

Acknowledgements This research was supported by the National Institute for Health Research (NIHR) Collaboration for Leadership in Applied Health Research and Care South London at King's College London Foundation Trust. The views expressed are those of the author(s) and not necessarily those of *the NHS, the NIHR, or the Department of Health. GT is supported by the*

European Union Seventh Framework Programme (FP7/2007–2013) Emerald project. The authors acknowledge financial support from the Department of Health via the National Institute for Health Research (NIHR) Biomedical Research Centre and Dementia Unit awarded to South London and Maudsley NHS Foundation Trust in partnership with King's College London and King's College Hospital NHS Foundation Trust. This chapter draws upon material in Thornicroft G., Evans-Lacko S., & Henderson C. (2014) Stigma & Discrimination. In Davies, S., Mehta, N., Murphy O, ed. Annual Report of the Chief Medical Officer 2013. Public Mental Health Priorities: Investing in the Evidence. Department of Health, London.

References

Borschmann R, Greenberg N, Jones N, Henderson RC (2014) Campaigns to reduce mental illness stigma in Europe: a scoping review

Change Tt. Stigma Shout (2008). Time to Change. Stigma Shout. Mind and Rethink, 2008

Choe JY, Teplin LA, Abram KM (2008) Perpetration of violence, violent victimization, and severe mental illness: balancing public health concerns. Psychiatr Serv 59(2):153–164

Clement S, Jarrett M, Henderson C, Thornicroft G (2010) Messages to use in population-level campaigns to reduce mental health-related stigma: consensus development study. Epidemiol Psichiatr Soc 19(1):72–79

Clement S, Brohan E, Sayce L, Pool J, Thornicroft G (2011a) Disability hate crime and targeted violence and hostility: a mental health and discrimination perspective. J Ment Health 20(3):219–225

Clement S, van Nieuwenhuizen A, Kassam A, Flach C, Lazarus A, de Castro M et al (2011b) Filmed v. live social contact interventions to reduce stigma: randomised controlled trial. Br J Psychiatry 201:57–64

Corker E, Hamilton S, Henderson C, Weeks C, Pinfold V, Rose D et al (2013) Experiences of discrimination among people using mental health service users in England 2008–11. Br J Psychiatry 202:s58–s63

Corrigan PW, River LP, Lundin RK, Penn DL, Uphoff-Wasowski K, Campion J et al (2001) Three strategies for changing attributions about severe mental illness. Schizophr Bull 27(2):187

Corrigan PW, Morris SB, Michaels PJ, Rafacz JD, Rüsch N (2012) Challenging the public stigma of mental illness: a meta-analysis of outcome studies. Psychiatr Serv 63(10):963–973

Davidson. S, Sewel K, Tse D, Ipsos M, O'Connor R (2009) Well? What do you think? (2008). The fourth National Scottish survey of public attitudes to mental wellbeing and mental health problems. Scottish Government Social Research

Department of Health HMG (2014) No health without mental health: mental health dashboard. Department of Health, London gov.uk/dh. https://www.gov.uk/government/uploads/system/uploads/attachment_data/file/281250/Closing_the_gap_V2_-_17_Feb_2014.pdf

Dietrich S, Mergl R, Freudenberg P, Althaus D, Hegerl U (2010) Impact of a campaign on the public's attitudes towards depression. Health Educ Res 25(1):135–150

Dunion L, Gordon L (2005) Tackling the attitude problem. The achievements to date of Scotland's 'see me' anti-stigma campaign. Mental health today (Brighton, England) 22

Evans-Lacko S, Knapp M (in press) Importance of social and cultural factors for attitudes, disclosure and time off work for depression: findings from a seven country European study on depression in the workplace. PLoS ONE

Evans-Lacko S, Knapp M, McCrone P, Thornicroft G, Mojtabai R (2013a) The mental health consequences of the recession: economic hardship and employment of people with mental health problems in 27 European countries. PLoSONE 8(7):e69792

Evans-Lacko S, Henderson C, Thornicroft G (2013b) Public knowledge, attitudes and behaviour regarding people with mental illness in England 2009–2012. Br J Psychiatry 202(s55):s51–s57

Evans-Lacko S, Henderson C, Thornicroft G, McCrone P (2013c) Economic evaluation of the anti-stigma social marketing campaign in England 2009–2011. Br J Psychiatry Suppl 55:s95–s101

Evans-Lacko S, Clement S, Corker E, Brohan E, Dockery L, Farrelly S et al (2015) How much does mental health discrimination cost: valuing experienced discrimination in relation to healthcare care costs and community participation. Epidemiol Psychiatr Sci. 2015;24(5)423–34

Friedrich B, Evans-Lacko S, London J, Rhydderch D, Henderson C, Thornicroft G (2013) Anti-stigma training for medical students – the Education Not Discrimination project. Br J Psychiatry 202;S55:s89–94

Gale E, Seymour L, Crepaz-Keay D, Gibbons M, Farmer P, Pinfold V (2004) Scoping review on mental health anti-stigma and discrimination: current activities and what works. National Institute of Mental Health England. NIMHE, Leeds

Gissler M, Laursen TM, Ösby U, Nordentoft M, Wahlbeck K (2013) Patterns in mortality among people with severe mental disorders across birth cohorts: a register-based study of Denmark and Finland in 1982–2006. BMC Public Health 13:834

Goffman E (1968) Stigma: notes on the management of spoiled identity. Penguin, Harmondsworth

Hamilton S, Lewis-Holmes E, Pinfold V, Henderson C, Rose D, Thornicroft G (2014) Discrimination against people with a mental health diagnosis: qualitative analysis of reported experiences. J Ment Health 23(2):88–93, 2014

Hegerl U, Althaus D, Stefanek J (2003) Public attitudes towards treatment of depression: effects of an information campaign. Pharmacopsychiatry 36(06):288–291

Hegerl U, Althaus D, Schmidtke A, Niklewski G (2006) The alliance against depression: 2-year evaluation of a community-based intervention to reduce suicidality. Psychol Med 36(9):1225–1234

Henderson C, Williams P, Little K, Thornicroft G (2012) The time to change programme against stigma and discrimination. Mental health problems in the workplace: changes in employers' knowledge, attitudes and practices in England 2006–2010. Br J Psychiatry 202(suppl 55): s70–s76

Henderson C, Corker E, Lewis-Holmes E, Hamilton S, Flach C, Rose D (2012b) Reducing mental health related stigma and discrimination in England: one year outcomes of the Time to Change Programme for service user-rated experiences of discrimination. Psychiatr Serv 63(5):451–457

Henderson C, Corker E, Lewis-Holmes E, Hamilton S, Flach C, Rose D et al (2012c) England's time to change antistigma campaign: one-year outcomes of service user-rated experiences of discrimination. Psychiatr Serv 63(5):451–457

Henderson RC, Evans-Lacko S, Thornicroft G (2013) Evidence for reducing discrimination in mental health: results of public awareness campaigns undertaken in the U.K. Seishin-Igaku. Clin Psychiatry (in press)

Henderson RC, Corker E, Hamilton S, Williams P, Pinfold V, Rose D et al (2014) Viewpoint survey of mental health service users' experiences of discrimination in England 2008–2012. Soc Psychiatry Psychiatric Epidemiol 49(10):1599–1608. https://www.time-to-change.org.uk/news/global-meeting-anti-stigma-programme-london 2013. Global Alliance Against Stigma

Jeffery D, Clement S, Corker E, Howard LM, Murray J, Thornicroft G (2013) Discrimination in relation to parenthood reported by community psychiatric service users in the UK: a frame-work analysis. BMC Psychiatry 20;13:120

Jorm AF, Christensen H Fau – Griffiths KM, Griffiths KM. Changes in depression awareness and attitudes in Australia: the impact of beyondblue: the national depression initiative. (0004-8674 (Print))

Lasalvia A, Zoppei S, Van BT, Bonetto C, Cristofalo D, Wahlbeck K et al (2012) Global pattern of experienced and anticipated discrimination reported by people with major depressive disorder: a cross-sectional survey. Lancet 381:55–62

Laursen TM, Munk-Olsen T, Nordentoft M, Mortensen PB (2007) Increased mortality among patients admitted with major psychiatric disorders: a register-based study comparing mortality in unipolar depressive disorder, bipolar affective disorder, schizoaffective disorder, and schizophrenia. J Clin Psychiatry 68(6):899–907

Lee S, Tsang A, Breslau J, Aguilar-Gaxiola S, Angermeyer M, Borges G et al (2009) Mental disorders and termination of education in high-income and low- to middle-income countries: epidemiological study. Br J Psychiatry 194:411–417

Link BG, Cullen FT, Struening E, Shrout PE, Dohrenwend BP (1989) A modified labeling theory approach to mental disorders: an empirical assessment. Am Sociol Rev 54(3):400–423

Lockwood GH, C, Thornicroft G (in press) Challenging mental health discrimination in employment: comparison of claimant win percentage. J Work Rights

Mai Q, D'Arcy C, Holman J, Sanfilippo FM, Emery JD, Preen DB (2011) Mental illness related disparities in diabetes prevalence, quality of care and outcomes: a population-based longitudinal study. BMC Med 1;9:118

McCrone P, Knapp M, Henri M, McDaid D (2010) The economic impact of initiatives to reduce stigma: demonstration of a modelling approach. Epidemiol Psichiatr Soc 19(2):131–139

Mehta N, Kassam A, Leese M, Butler G, Thornicroft G (2009) Public attitudes towards people with mental illness in England and Scotland, 1994–2003. Br J Psychiatry 194(3):278–284

Mehta N, Clement S, Marcus E, Stona A-C, Bezborodovs N, Evans-Lacko S et al (2015) Systematic review of evidence for effective interventions to reduce mental health related stigma and discrimination: medium and long-term effectiveness and interventions in low- and middle-income countries. Br J Psychiatry; In press

National Institute for H, Clinical E. Behaviour Change. NICE (2007)

OECD (2012) Sick on the Job?: Myths and realities about mental health and work, mental health and work, OECD Publishing, Paris

Quinn N, Knifton L, Goldie I, Van Bortel T, Dowds J, Lasalvia A et al (2013) Nature and impact of European anti-stigma depression programmes. Health Promot Int 29(3):403–413

Schomerus G, Lucht M, Holzinger A, Matschinger H, Carta MG, Angermeyer MC. The stigma of alcohol dependence compared with other mental disorders: a review of population studies. (1464–3502 (Electronic))

Schomerus G, Matschinger H, Angermeyer MC (2006) Preferences of the public regarding cutbacks in expenditure for patient care: are there indications of discrimination against those with mental disorders? Soc Psychiatry Psychiatr Epidemiol 41(5):369–377

Schomerus G, Schwahn C, Holzinger A, Corrigan PW, Grabe HJ, Carta MG et al (2012) Evolution of public attitudes about mental illness: a systematic review and meta-analysis. Acta Psychiatr Scand 125(6):440–452

Schulze B (2007) Stigma and mental health professionals: a review of the evidence on an intricate relationship. Int Rev Psychiatr 19(2):137–155

Semrau S, Evans-Lacko S, Koschorke M, Ashenafi L, Thornicroft G (2015) Mental health stigma and discrimination in low and middle income countries. Epidemiol Psychiatr Sci 24(5):382-94

Social Exclusion U (2004) Mental health and social exclusion. London Office of the Deputy Prime Minister, London

Stuart H, Chen SP, Christie R, Dobson K, Kirsh B, Knaak S et al (2014) Opening minds in Canada: background and rationale. Can J Psychiatry 59(10 Suppl 1):S8–S12

Suhrcke M, de Paz Nieves C (2011) The impact of health and health behaviours on educational outcomes in high-income countries: a review of the evidence. WHO Regional Office for Europe, Copenhagen

Thornicroft G (2006) Shunned: discrimination against people with mental illness. Oxford University Press, Oxford

Thornicroft G, Rose D, Kassam A, Sartorius N (2007) Stigma: ignorance, prejudice or discrimination? Br J Psychiatr 190:192–193

Thornicroft G, Brohan E, Rose D, Sartorius N, Leese M (2009) Global pattern of experienced and anticipated discrimination against people with schizophrenia: a cross-sectional survey. Lancet 373:408–415

Thornicroft A, Goulden R, Shefer G, Rhydderch D, Rose D, Williams P et al (2013) Newspaper coverage of mental illness in England 2008–2011. Br J Psychiatr 202(suppl 55): s-64–s69

Thornicroft G, Mehta N, Clement S, Evans-Lacko S, Doherty M, Rose D et al (2015) Evidence for effective interventions to reduce mental health related stigma and discrimination: narrative review. Lancet; In press

Ucok A, Brohan E, Rose D, Sartorius N, Leese M, Yoon CK et al (2012) Anticipated discrimination among people with schizophrenia. Acta Psychiatr Scand 125:77–83

See Change: The National Mental Health Stigma Reduction Partnership in Ireland

Kahlil Coyle, Sorcha Lowry, and John Saunders

See Change is Ireland's national programme working to positively change social attitudes and behaviour so that there is a reduction of stigma and discrimination associated with mental health problems, ensuring that everyone in Ireland enjoys the same rights on an equal basis. See Change works within a number of interrelated settings: finding the conversation, joining in and working with people and communities on the ground. This is Ireland's first ever national stigma reduction partnership and exists to inspire a disruptive social movement in Ireland to reduce the stigma and discrimination of mental health problems so that mental health problems are viewed as part and parcel of being human – in the workplace, at home, out and about, in the media and everywhere else.

The See Change vision is that every person in Ireland can be open and positive about their own and others' mental health.

See Change aims to:

- Create an environment where people are more open and positive in their attitudes and behaviour towards mental health
- Promote greater understanding and acceptance of people with mental health problems

K. Coyle (✉) • S. Lowry • J. Saunders
See Change and Shine – Supporting People Affected by Mental Ill Health,
38 Blessington Street, Dublin, Ireland
e-mail: kthompson@shineonline.ie, kthompson@seechange.ie; sorcha@seechange.ie; jsaunders@shineonline.ie

© Springer International Publishing Switzerland 2017
W. Gaebel et al. (eds.), *The Stigma of Mental Illness - End of the Story?*,
DOI 10.1007/978-3-319-27839-1_19

- Create greater understanding and knowledge of mental health problems and of health services that provide support for mental health problems
- Reduce the stigma associated with mental health problems and challenge discrimination

See Change values are:

Inclusion: Mental health experts, through lived life experience, are at the heart of the development and implementation of all elements of the See Change programme at national and local levels.

Collaboration: To work closely with like-minded groups from every sector of society in order to seed change across the broadest audience in Ireland.

Community: To be committed to delivering our message and initiatives at a grassroots level to empower local communities to be the change.

Invention: To look for ways to break new ground and work together to maximise the impact of our combined resources. To evaluate our impact and to learn by experience, drawing on international best practice.

At the cornerstone of the See Change approach is social contact theory, which has been shown to be successful in reducing the social distance between stigmatised groups and the rest of society. See Change passionately believes that the stories of those who have experienced mental health problems and the associated stigma have the power to help change peoples' attitudes and positively influence behaviour change.

The target audience for the campaign includes:

- Young males 18–24
- People in the workplace
- Farmers and people living in rural communities
- People who have been negatively impacted by the economic recession in Ireland

The Stigma Picture in Ireland

People with mental health problems and their relatives in Ireland, like in many countries, consistently identify stigma and discrimination as major barriers to health, welfare and quality of life. In fact, the 2012 See Change study into mental health attitudes in Ireland found that while 94 % of people in Ireland feel that mental health problems can affect anyone, one in two people would not want anyone to know if they had a mental health problem. This sentiment was particularly strong among young males, farmers and people in the workplace, identifying three key target audiences for the campaign (See Change 2012).

How Did It All Start?

The See Change campaign started to take shape in February 2010. Within the Irish mental health voluntary sector, there had been a long-standing desire to have a national stigma reduction campaign. See Change was initiated by the mental health

NGO, Shine – Supporting People Affected by Mental Ill Health, as well as from other NGOs from the mental health voluntary sector, the Department of Health and Children and the then Minister for Equality, Disability and Mental Health, John Moloney.

After the department hosted a series of round table meetings on how best to approach the issue, a formal proposal was put forward by Shine, outlining the possible steps to take. Through the National Lottery Fund, the Department of Health and Children allocated core funding for See Change over an initial 2-year pilot period (March 2010–March 2012), and Shine was given the responsibility of being the coordinating organisation for See Change, including leveraging further funding for campaign activities.

The National Context

By 2010, Ireland had witnessed recent developments that influenced the direction of the Irish mental health sector that had favourably set the scene for the commencement of a national stigma reduction campaign (Stigma background mapping work of Ireland and Internationally 2010). These included, inter alia:

- The publishing of the national mental health policy, *A Vision for Change*, which was formulated by the Mental Health Expert Group and launched in 2006, replacing the country's 1984 policy. The expert group included, for the first time, representatives from not only within the statutory services or government but also from the NGO sector.
- NGOs working closely together for the first time in a cohesive and organised manner (the Irish Mental Health Coalition, Action on Suicide Alliance and Amnesty's mental health campaign).
- Ireland's National Disability Authority launching of a nationwide campaign to challenge public attitudes to disabilities, including mental health in 2007.
- Creation of Ireland's National Service User Executive.
- The National Office for Suicide Prevention, part of Ireland's Health Service Executive, had invited representation from the NGO sector to contribute to their positive mental health campaign.
- Ireland's Mental Health Act 2001 becoming legislation.
- The establishment of Ireland's Mental Health Commission in 2002.
- Research being conducted on attitudes in Ireland by St Patrick's Hospital and the College of Psychiatry of Ireland.
- Establishment of organisations that complimented a stigma reduction programme, for example, Headline which is Ireland's national media monitoring programme for mental health and suicide.

Therefore, by 2009 when the discussions were kicked off by the minister to scope out the feasibility of initiating an Irish stigma reduction campaign, there were significant drivers already in existence to encourage organisations to work closely together to tackle stigma.

The timing was also considered to be right, given the NGO work in the area and the significant statutory investment in the National Office for Suicide Prevention's positive mental health awareness campaign, *Your Mental Health*, which focused on disseminating a positive mental health message through a mainstream social-marketing campaign.

Against this background, the Irish mental health sector was also positively encouraged to pursue a national stigma reduction campaign by watching and learning from the well-received international stigma reduction programmes within the English-speaking world. In particular, and not surprisingly, Ireland was greatly influenced by the Scottish *See Me* campaign as well as the English *Time to Change* campaign.

The First Steps

The first step towards initiating See Change was the drafting of a programme plan setting out the stigma case, programme description, operations, communications strategy, research and evaluation strategy and funding requirements.

This was a crucial first step as it helped to facilitate discussions with the Department of Health and to secure the initial funding for the pilot phase of the campaign. Additionally, it was this document that was used to help inform potential partner organisations. From the outset, the vision was to ensure that the stigma reduction efforts in Ireland would harness existing and potential new resources to bring about stigma reduction, and it was viewed that pursuing a partnership model was the only way to move forward.

An initial meeting of interested partner organisations, now referred to as the founding partners, was held in early February 2010 to float the idea of a national mental health stigma reduction programme built on a foundation of partnership and collaboration. The response was favourable by those present, the name of the programme 'See Change' was decided, and initial steps in deciding on a logo was taken. There was keen interest to have a logo that acted as a kind of 'stamp' on literature, websites, etc.

Next, a meeting was organised and held in the Department of Health, bringing together all of the partners who had already commenced signing up and some partners who were interested yet wanted to learn more about the process. A 1 day programme was established whereby discussions on establishing the agreed vision, aims and values were discussed along with research and evaluation and next steps. Crucially, the day was facilitated by the former and founding director of the Scottish campaign, *See Me*, which also offered a 'master class' element to the day where we could explore the lessons learned from the Scottish experience.

Subsequent to this meeting the See Change coordinating organisation went about drafting the *See Change Partner Manifesto* and coordinated the suggested changes and final agreement with the founding partners.

Once the initial procedures were in order, the then minister with responsibility for mental health took the unprecedented step of commencing a nationwide town hall meeting tour to highlight the start of the See Change programme and partnership. The meetings were also intended to promote greater awareness of mental health problems, stigma and discrimination, to provide information on local and national supports to people, to encourage organisations to become part of the partnership and to invite people to contribute to the campaign, either through sharing their stories or by becoming involved with the various advisory panels. Overall the feedback from the town hall meetings was positive with 84 % of attendees indicating that they had a greater awareness of mental health problems and 73 % of attendees indicating that they had a greater awareness of the stigma and discrimination people with self-experience of mental health problems face.

The Partnership Approach

The work of See Change is underpinned and driven by a partnership model. See Change recognises that the job of challenging stigma and changing attitudes and behaviours needs concerted effort and collaboration with groups from every sector of society. Therefore, from the outset, See Change went about building a coalition of organisations (currently over 90 organisations) to work together in a united approach in order to end mental health discrimination. For See Change, the task is focused on helping them to spark a social movement for change. See Change partners include a broad range of organisations who have signed up to at least one major action to support the movement.

However, the idea of partnership is also rooted in practical feasibility. To commence a major national stigma reduction programme as the country fell into a severe economic recession was both daunting and challenging – particularly due to the obvious budget constraints that the campaign faced from the very outset. Despite having government and statutory buy in to the See Change concept, financial resources were going to be a major issue from day 1. The financial backdrop, therefore, further necessitated the need to take a partnership approach – which ultimately has proven to be a tremendous strength of the campaign.

By each partner organisation committing to undertake actions under the See Change banner, this empowers the organisation to take ownership of the campaign, which has ultimately strengthened the approach and facilitated the work at the grass-roots level, especially with key stakeholders whose constituents are the campaign's target groups.

It goes without saying that when people choose to belong to an organisation in society, whether it be a sporting group, a local club, a professional body, etc., the powerful part is that they choose to become a part of that group. When those groups or organisations help to carry the See Change message, the experience of the campaign is that the messaging takes on a different dimension because the person is coming into contact with the campaign through an organisation or group that they **choose** to belong to, rather than consuming the messaging through the usual media advertising channels.

The partner organisations, truly the backbone of the programme, represent every sector of society, from the mental health sector, education, arts, general health, business, public affairs, sports, government and representative organisations of people with self-experience of mental health problems.

The Partnership Framework

The *See Change Partner Manifesto* was devised in consultation with the See Change partner organisations and steering committee and is regularly updated – by agreement – to reflect current practice and procedure. Specifically, it provides information about See Change, the partnership framework, the role of the coordinating organisation (secretariat), responsibilities of the coordinating organisation, the role of partner organisations, responsibilities of partner organisations, role of the steering committee, role of advisory panels; role of stakeholder forum, guiding principles for stigma reduction and key messages for stigma-reduction activity (Figs. 19.1 and 19.2).

What Now? When a New Government Takes Power

One major concern for the campaign was that See Change was closely linked with John Moloney TD, the government minister responsible for mental health in the Irish government from 2008 to 2011. Minister Moloney had been a forthright advocate for See Change and publicly highlighted his own personal experience of having a mental health problem.

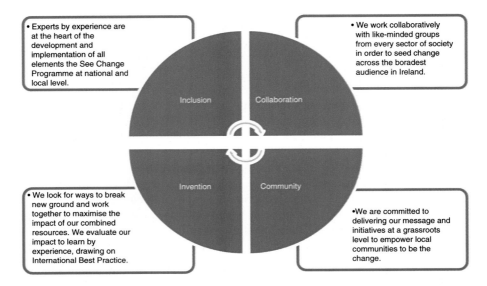

Fig. 19.1 Partnership values

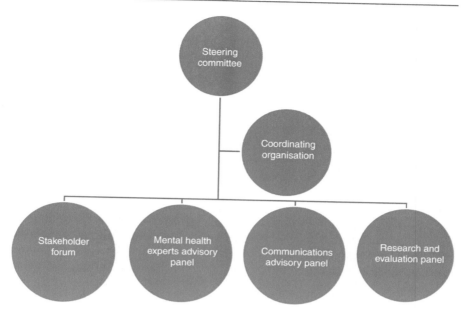

Fig. 19.2 Partnership framework

The subsequent minister responsible for mental health, Kathleen Lynch TD, who was from a different political party, warmly welcomed the See Change partnership and continues to be a strong advocate for the campaign. This kind of crosspolitical party support has been invaluable to the See Change partnership.

Current Practice: Where Have Efforts Been Focusing On?

Where We Work (Table 19.1)

Workplace

While awareness of the scale and impact of mental health problems at work is increasing in Ireland, the timing for See Change to work with partners focused on the workplace has proven to be very positive. See Change has identified the workplace as a key setting for stigma-reduction activity, working with partners to create honest discussion and understanding of mental health problems in the workplace and collaborating with various groups to find ways to support employers and employees in launching this all-important conversation.

The 2012 See Change survey into Irish attitudes towards mental health found that 57 % believe that being open about a mental health problem at work would have a negative impact on job and career prospects, up from 48 % in 2010. Forty-seven per cent believe that being open about a mental health problem at work would have a negative effect on a person's relationship with colleagues, up from 36 % in 2010 (See Change 2012).

Table 19.1 Where we work

Key channels	Partnership Grass roots Arts and entertainment Media and online	Targeted initiatives	Young men Farmers People in the workplace
		Flagship public engagement campaign	Green Ribbon month (every May)

The workplace has been one of the areas where See Change has, to date, made a significant impact with partner organisations. By forging an early alliance with organisations such as the Irish Business and Employers Confederation (IBEC), which represents its 7,500 member companies, the Equality Authority, the Irish Congress of Trade Unions (ICTU), Business in the Community Ireland and various other organisations and companies, the See Change partnership has been received positively. Against this background, See Change has developed, in consultation and at the request of a multinational company with an office in Ireland, a six-step 'See Change in your workplace' programme, guiding employers and employees towards creating open workplace cultures, supporting each other and working to their full potential.

See Change in Your Workplace Workshop

As part of the workplace programme, See Change has, again collaboratively, developed a half-day 'See Change in your workplace' workshop, providing information on mental health and mental health problems for employers, managers and employees as well as offering best practise advice on creating workplaces that are free of stigma and discrimination and equipped to support the mental health needs of the organisation. The workshops are delivered in collaboration with some of the See Change partner organisations, bringing a tremendous richness to the discussions. The workshops are funded by the Irish Health Service Executive's National Office for Suicide Prevention and have proven popular with companies. The workshop came about after a major multinational tech company with offices in Ireland asked See Change to develop such a training workshop for line managers in their company. The company agreed to do a pilot and helped See Change to fine-tune the training and operationalise it within their Irish office.

This workshop provides a practical approach to mental health, highlighting the workplace as a key setting in addressing stigma. Attendees hear personal stories and learn about mental health, mental health problems and wellness tools. This workshop is valuable for employers, staff and in professional services working with clients. Attendees come away with useful tools and information.

Overview of the workshop:

1. The session begins with an introduction to mental health, mental health problems and how they relate to the workplace context followed by an opportunity to discuss the myths that surround mental health problems, prevailing Irish attitudes to mental health and strategies to reduce stigma.

2. A See Change ambassador with a professional background shares their personal experience of a mental health problem, including strategies to support positive mental health.
3. Topics covered include how best to support an employee, colleague or client who is experiencing a difficulty with their mental health, through information on relevant equality legislation, examples of reasonable accommodation in practise, recommendations on responding to a crisis, how to broach the subject and deciding whether or not to disclose.
4. The session concludes with a discussion on practical resources, wellness tools and how people can proactively look after their own mental health.

A Q&A session and opportunity to speak personally with the speakers closes the workshop. The 3 hour workshop is designed to be participative and interactive in nature.

The feedback from companies who have brought the workshop into their workplace indicate that:

- 98 % said that they would feel more comfortable addressing a colleague's mental health disclosure.
- 87 % would feel more comfortable raising mental health as a workplace issue.
- 78 % said that it would change the way they behave.

Other Areas of Work in the Workplace

Other key aspects of work in this area have included teaming up with Business in the Community Ireland to cohost a national conference. Over 300 employers, managers, HR specialists and community leaders attended this conference aimed at sparking a national discussion on how each of us as individuals can play a role in creating an open culture towards mental health in Irish workplaces and communities.

Each year in Ireland, there is a National Employment Week, and See Change has worked with partners to ensure that mental health and stigma reduction have become part of the week's annual programme. The Mental Health and Employment Day as part of National Employment Week offers a breakfast briefing aimed at providing employers with the practical tools to support employees who may be experiencing difficulties and to promote a culture of openness towards mental health in Irish workplaces.

Another significant step for the workplace strand of work was when IBEC, the group that represents Irish business, launched *Mental health and wellbeing: A line manager's guide*, a resource for employers to promote mental wellbeing in the workplace (IBEC 2012). Produced in collaboration with See Change, the guide is directed at line managers who are key to promoting a culture that is positive towards mental health and supporting individuals with mental health problems in the workplace.

The guide has a range of information and practical advice on recruitment, wellbeing, disclosure as well as a large reference section directing employers to where there is expertise from a range of specialist organisations and online resources that can offer further assistance. The guide can help managers facilitate conversations about mental health problems, understand what issues may arise and put in place support so employees can stay well and in work – meaning they perform at their best and the employer retains talent and expertise.

Equality Authority Guides

In 2011, the Irish Equality Authority and See Change published two guides including *Equality and mental health: What the law means for your workplace* (Equality Authority 2011), which provides information for employers on their responsibilities towards employees and potential employees with experience of mental health issues. The guide explains the legal requirement for employers to provide reasonable accommodation for employees and potential employees with experience of mental health difficulties. The companion guide, *Equality and mental health: How the law can help you* (Equality and Mental Health: What the law means for your workplace n.d.) provides practical information for people with experience of mental health difficulties on their equality rights in employment and access to services.

In 2014, See Change received Equality Authority/EU funding which led to the publishing of a 'Case Law Review on Mental Health in the Workplace' and a 'Mental Health in the Workplace Policy Document' to provide information and guidance on how to develop and implement a comprehensive workplace mental health policy. The project proposal originated from the need to equip managers and employers with legal and policy guidance to support people with personal experiences of mental health problems in the workplace. An invaluable consultation with partners and HR managers from various companies was held to discuss concerns, blockages, legal issues and human resource implications when it comes to mental health in the workplace. See Change also benefitted from the advice of a number of key partner organisations on the project. These included the Equality Authority, Irish Business and Employers' Confederation (IBEC), Business in the Community Ireland (BITCI), the Irish Congress of Trade Unions (ICTU), Suicide or Survive (SOS), Sigmar, St John of God Hospital and Employment Health Advisors (EHA). The project's funding was provided by the Equality Mainstreaming Unit in the Equality Authority.

Young People

See Change has collaborated with various partner organisations to engage with the young male target group on reducing the stigma of mental health problems and promoting open discussion. College campuses and student groups have proved very effective channels to reach the young male target group while also providing invaluable testing grounds for pilot projects and initiatives that can be used among other groups and settings. Beyond on-campus activity, the potential of embedding our message within sporting organisations to reach those outside of third level education is a focus that is currently being developed by the campaign.

See Change research has shown that 72 % would not want others to know if they had a mental health problem, 56 % would hide a diagnosis of a mental health problem from friends (increased from 39 % in 2010) and 35 % would delay seeking help for fear of someone knowing about it (See Change 2012).

College Roadshows

In the initial phases of the campaign, See Change and partners embarked on a social contact-based tour of college campus to screen a documentary entitled 'I See A Darkness' in partnership with two suicide prevention organisations (Suicide or Survive and Save Our Sons and Daughters) and host a postshow discussion with the documentary's participants who have personal experience of suicide and suicide bereavement.

See Change and partners staged a successful Guinness World Record Challenge for 'most people to write a story' on the campus of Trinity College, Dublin. More than 800 students were actively engaged in the initiative but it also led to national acclaim for the partnership and the message.

Chats for Change Initiative

Since 2013, the annual Chats for Change initiative has seen thousands of 'tea and chats' packs being distributed by students' unions across campuses nationwide. The pack contents provide a clear behaviour change call to action: two tea bags, tips on taking the fear out of talking about mental health and useful support service contacts. It aims to encourage students to make time and space to chat about their mental health over tea – a veritable communal ritual in an Irish context. Chats for Change has also been successfully transferred to the workplace setting.

Youth Advisory Panel

In addition to the campaign advisory panels on research, communications, etc., See Change established a Youth Advisory panel to provide feedback and guidance on all youth-related engagement. The Youth Advisory Panel also serves as an extension of the volunteer and ambassador programmes where appropriate.

Suite of Stigma Reduction Activities

See Change has developed a suite of activities that organisations and individuals can run as stigma-reduction initiatives, including a mental health themed magic show, table quiz, comedy set and various promotional materials. In collaboration with our partners, ambassadors and volunteers, this range of engaging and thought-provoking stigma-challenging activities were devised to help spark discussion of mental health. These specially commissioned activities were piloted in collaboration with Union of Students in Ireland as part of on-campus mental health weeks and transferred successfully to other key settings such as workplaces and community groups.

Third Level Stigma Reduction Programme

In collaboration with the staff and students of Dublin Business School, See Change developed a Third Level Stigma Reduction programme in 2013. With workshops, training and initiatives involving staff, students and the wider community, this integrated approach is aimed at creating an openness around mental health on college campuses and empowering the entire college community to play a direct role in challenging stigma. The programme was also expanded to UCD College of Agriculture, Food Science & Veterinary Medicine.

Farming Community

Since our baseline study identified Irish farmers as a key target group for stigma reduction, See Change has continued to collaborate with our partners who have a presence on the ground in rural communities to explore ways in which farmers can be supported and stigma can be addressed.

Our research showed that 72 % of Irish farmers would not want others to know if they had a mental health problem, 39 % of farmers would hide a diagnosis of a mental health problem from friends and 33 % would delay seeking help for fear of someone knowing about it (See Change 2010).

Speaking Tour of Regional Members Meetings

A crucial first step in establishing the partnership among our farming partnership and embedding the message at grass-roots level was a speaking tour of many of the regional members meetings of our farming partners.

Annual Presence at National Ploughing Championship

See Change and partners have developed free wallet-sized 'Talking Cards' to distribute the 279,500 National Ploughing Championships attendees that feature straight-talking advice aimed at taking the fear out of talking about mental health and encouraging open discussion.

Farming Partner Organisations' Activity

See Change established a working group of all partner organisations working in the agricultural or rural setting to share learnings, research and to find ways to collaborate on stigma-reduction activity across the agricultural sector. This includes representatives from the Irish Farmers Association, Macra na Feirme, the Irish Cattle and Sheep Farmers Association, the Irish Creamery Milk Suppliers Association, the Irish Countrywomens' Association and Teagasc. It should be noted that this is the first time all of the farming and rural sector organisations have joined together to discuss and prioritise the issue of mental health for their members. The addition of the Department of Agriculture to the partnership is considered as invaluable in terms of legitimacy and reach.

Grass roots

The partnership model best befits the grass-roots approach, allowing us to reach our target audiences in the communities, groups and clubs with which they identify. Outside of the partnership structure, See Change's approach has been to 'find the conversation and join in', taking our message to the major events on the Irish corporate, social and agricultural calendars such as the Electric Picnic Festival and Volvo Ocean Race Festival. In terms of maximising our impact and capacity however, our role as the spark that supports and empowers others to carry the message to the grass-roots level is our strongest methodology.

Volunteer Strategy

See Change developed a volunteer programme to recruit and train volunteers to help roll-out See Change's stigma-challenging campaigns on the ground and create that ripple effect in their own families, circle of friends, towns, communities, workplaces or colleges. Volunteers are also supported in hosting their own initiatives to start a conversation about mental health or support the campaign's activity at a community level.

Pop-Up Café Programme

See Change successfully piloted a weeklong grass-roots engagement of a rural community with the road-testing of the Time to Talk pop-up series in Clonmel, County Tipperary. The joint objectives of the project were firstly to encourage increased conversation and engagement on mental health among the local population and secondly to embed stigma-reduction activity within the local community.

The 4 day programme took place in a disused commercial premises on a pedestrianised street. The location befitted our target audiences (those with a rural base and those who have been negatively affected by the financial recession).

From conception to roll-out, we employed the catalyst approach, seeing the campaign team's role as to empower and support the local community to devise and deliver the programme content. We teamed up with a variety of local organisations, volunteers and community groups to host various events throughout the week including health and wellbeing workshops and talks, story-sharing and stigma-reduction focussed entertainment and arts exhibitions. The café was run by local volunteers who were on hand to meet and greet members of the public. The people of Clonmel were openly invited to come in and explore and enjoy the space and make the time and space for conversation about mental health.

Over the course of the 4 days, 950 conversations about mental health were recorded in the pop-up cafe. The local group of volunteers and organisations have since completed a second event together for World Mental Health Day and are already planning a second weeklong festival under the stigma-reduction banner.

Arts and Entertainment

From thought-provoking cinema, disarming comedy to initiate theatre pieces the arts have been an invaluable channel to encourage discussion about mental health problems and provide a platform for social contact.

First Fortnight Arts and Mental Health Festival

Since 2012, See Change has been a presenting partner of the First Fortnight Festival. Taking place in the first 2 weeks of every new year, the festival continues to offer ground-breaking programme of mental health-themed arts events, acclaimed theatre pieces, music, cinema, visual art and spoken word nights to get Dublin audiences talking about mental health.

Mad*Craic* Comedy Show

See Change commissioned Irish comedians John Moynes and Carol Tobin to bring new comedy set 'Mad*Craic*' to the stage to get people talking about mental health. Informed by the comedians' own experiences, Mad*Craic* takes an irreverent look at stigma and how it impacted on their own journeys through college and life thereafter. A Q&A with the performers takes place after the show. Mad*Craic* was successfully piloted at Trinity College Dublin Mental Health Week, toured college campuses in 2013 and subsequently workplaces, community groups and colleges.

Demystify This: The World's First Mental Health Magic Show

Acclaimed conceptual magician Shane Quilty created a new show that was specially commissioned by See Change to help change attitudes to mental health. Audiences can expect mind-bending illusions and thought-provoking stunts where the take-home message is that far from the realms of mysticism, experiencing a mental health problem is in fact quite an ordinary experience of everyday life while the lengths that we go to hide it are actually quite the magic trick.

Box of Frogs National Theatre Tour

Box of Frogs is a highly successful theatre piece commissioned by See Change and based on the authentic content of three people's real-life experiences to spark open conversation about mental health problems and challenge stigma in Ireland. Actress Mary McEvoy, comedian John Moynes and broadcaster Dil Wickremasinghe have teamed up to share their stories of personal experience with a mental health problem in a mixture of stories, comedy sketches and songs to demystify, debunk and ultimately have a laugh with what really goes on inside our heads.

On evaluation, 91 % of people who attended the play said that they would change their behaviour towards their own mental health and openness to others.

Media and Online

Media and the online space are a crucial setting for creating discussion of mental health problems. See Change sees its role here is to empower others and support media professionals to share the stories of real people's experiences of mental health problems.

Ambassador's Programme

See Change has established a vibrant and fully supported ambassador's programme of people with personal experience of mental health problems who are willing to share their experiences at events, media interviews and blogs and add their voice to conversations in social media and in their own spheres of influence. Ambassadors receive comprehensive briefings and training on how to share their story in a way that is most beneficial to them and their audience and receive full support throughout the year.

By giving the issue a voice and a human face, See Change ambassadors can be the catalyst to real and lasting attitude and behaviour change in how Irish people view their own and others' mental health. Our aim is that audiences will be not only be touched but inspired to take a personal role in challenging stigma, making ripples from one individual to the next until a large community of people are engaged on the issue.

Make a Ripple Online Portal

In May 2010, See Change launched 'Make a Ripple', an online story-sharing portal as an innovative way of using social contact theory through social media and starting a conversation about mental health with the online community. Here people can post messages of support for the campaign, speak out against stigma or share their personal stories of experience with a mental health problem in the hope of creating a shared understanding of the mental health problems that touch all of us. People can engage with this online campaign in a number of ways, by posting directly on the portal, through Twitter or Facebook using the hashtag #makearipple or displaying a Twibbon – all in the hope of creating online momentum around the campaign's key messages of openness and understanding.

My Ripple Radio Awareness Campaign

The 'My Ripple' radio awareness campaign involved a series of audio advertisements aired on local and regional radio. This series of 60 s audio pieces featured the personal stories of 22 people's real-life experiences with mental health problems, recovery, stigma, seeking help and becoming open about their personal experience in their own voice. Each advertisement in the series was bookended with a voice-over containing the See Change message and call-to-action by the recognisable voice of RTE broadcaster and See Change ambassador Eileen Dunne; 'Break the silence of stigma; see change'.

Supporting Irish Media

- *Awards*: See Change partners with Headline, the national media monitoring programme for mental health and suicide to run an annual Voice Media Award to recognise those media outlets who use social contact theory in their coverage and give voice to mental health problems.
- *Empowerment*: In 2013, See Change began sponsoring the only dedicated mental health slot on Irish radio; The Feel Good slot on Newstalk FM'S Global Village.
- *Training*: See Change and partners have devised a series of training sessions for media professionals combining content aimed at media professionals on responsible coverage and content that focussed on their roles as employers, managers and employees in creating workplaces that have an open culture towards mental health.

Flagship Campaign: Green Ribbon

Changing minds about mental health, one conversation at a time

Although it had been long established as a symbol for mental health in North America, the Green Ribbon first came to our attention from our partners at HSE West Mental Health Services when we were looking for an effective engagement tool to reach out to the potential audience of 800,000 at our collaborative pop-up at the Galway Volvo Ocean Race Festival in 2012. The symbol was very successfully piloted in Galway so we set out to create a flagship mass engagement campaign to make the month of May every year synonymous with challenging the stigma of mental health problems to lay groundwork for real and lasting change in Irish attitudes and behaviours to mental health.

Thousands of ribbons are distributed nationwide, free of charge and in conjunction with various partner and community events with the aim of sparking a national conversation about mental health in Ireland's boardrooms, break-rooms, chatrooms, clubhouses, arts venues, college campuses and around kitchen tables.

The second Green Ribbon in 2014 saw 300,000 ribbons distributed (double the amount from year 1) and 500 events and initiatives took place in communities and workplaces across the country in collaboration with our partner organisations, volunteers and ambassadors to achieve 1.6 million conversations about mental health.

Information Box 19.1: 2014 Green Ribbon Campaign Overview

Here's how one simple ribbon achieved 1.6 million conversations about mental health:

1,201,783 was the potential reach of national media pieces alone (of a total of 149 media pieces including 75 ambassador stories).

116,484 conversations started by volunteers and supporters (who organised 282 community events and initiatives).

112,951 Green Ribbon promo materials distributed nationwide.

103, 484 conversations started by See Change partner organisations (who organised 116 Green Ribbon events and initiatives).

58,083 online conversations.

31,380 conversations started in workplaces (where 107 Green Ribbon events and initiatives took place).

984 gifted outdoor advertising spots by our distribution partners Irish Rail, Citizens Information as well as Dublin Bus and Frangos Dundrum.

505 Green Ribbon events and initiatives in May 2014.

How did we measure this? *One interaction, attendee or green ribbon = 1 conversation.*

According to research conducted by Millward Brown Landsdowne on the 2014 campaign, a growing number of Irish adults have been hearing conversations about mental health among family, friends and at work since the Green Ribbon campaign:

- Seven in ten say they now feel more comfortable in having a conversation about mental health.
- 66 % say the Green Ribbon campaign has encouraged them to start conversations about mental health.

Table 19.2 Green Ribbon 2014 campaign overview

Campaign aim	To encourage open conversation of mental health problems in Ireland
Target groups	General population and also encompassing See Change target groups of young males, farmers and people in the workplace
Campaign duration	May 2014
Principle activity	Distribution of 300,000 green ribbons free of charge
Key messaging	It's time to talk about mental health
	You don't have to be an expert to start talking about mental health problems or have all of the answers
	Sometimes the most simple thing you can do is let someone know you are there for them and simply listen
Campaign partners	See Change in collaboration with 90 partner organisations
Distribution partners	Irish Rail and Citizens Information Centres nationwide
Media partner	Newstalk FM
Grassroots activity	505 community events organised nationwide by 90 See Change partner organisations, workplaces and growing network of hundreds of volunteers and over 50 ambassadors
Conversations	1,656,654 conversations started on mental health during Green Ribbon 2014
Online elements	Greenribbon, i.e. social media platforms and engagement tools totalling 58,083 online conversations
Media and advertising:	984 advertising spots outdoor and on partners' public-facing property and 149 media pieces

- 62 % have been hearing conversations about mental health among family and friends since the campaign (up from 52 % in 2013).
- 53 % have been hearing mental health conversations in their workplaces since the campaign (up from 44 % in 2013) (Table 19.2).

The Development of the See Change Programme (Table 19.3)

The campaign's structure as a partnership lends itself naturally to the catalyst model, creating the spark that empowers others to embed change within their organisations. To bolster the effectiveness of this approach, phase 2 made considerable progress in developing the ambassadors and volunteers strand and creating an active social movement. To further progress this approach, phase 3 has focused on developing training packages and campaign suites that can be adopted internally and embedded at grass-roots level.

See Change has developed its messaging strategy alongside developments in international research about what is most effective. In phase 2, behaviour change rather than attitude change became a key priority in any external communications.

In terms of targeting, the introduction of the Green Ribbon campaign in phase 2 allowed for a whole population approach solely for the month of May. This approach is instrumental in establishing awareness on a national level and most

Table 19.3 Green Ribbon 2014 campaign overview

Phase 1	2010–2012	*Key messaging*: Raising awareness of stigma, mental health problems *Developments*: Developing the partnership, establishing the brand and replicable programmes among key targets (young men, farmers, workplace)
Phase 2	2012–2014	*Key messaging*: Behaviour change and the catalyst model – how to have the conversation *Developments*: Green Ribbon mass engagement campaign and engagement resources, toolkits. Development into a social movement with recruitment of ambassadors and volunteers
Phase 3	2014–2016	*Key messaging*: Refine behaviour change message around specific blockages and the catalyst model *Developments*: Focus on sources of discrimination; embed grass-roots programmes

importantly, allows the message to gain traction beyond the key target groups that are the focus of activity throughout the year: young men, farmers and people in the workplace.

In phase 3, in-line with best practise, messaging and campaigns should also focus on the sources of stigma, prejudice and discrimination as well as addressing the high levels of fear and misconception that surround certain mental illnesses. With the recently published national suicide prevention strategy for Ireland, connecting for life See Change welcomes the inclusion of stigma reduction as a key objective.

Current Knowledge: The Important Lessons Learned

Partnership

A partnership approach has been at the heart of the See Change programme and has enabled it to reach far more people than the budget would have dictated. See Change has a democratic approach, but, this has not always been easy and there has not always been agreement, a case in point is in terms of what wording to use in terms of mental health (e.g. mental illness, mental health problems, mental health difficulties, etc.). However, with strong and committed leadership with a clear vision, it is possible to bring like-minded organisations together to work together in different ways, yet with the same goal of ending mental health discrimination. Having an open door policy has also been key to the campaign.

Social Contact Theory

Mental health experts, through lived life experience, are at the heart of the development and implementation of all elements of the See Change programme at national and local levels.

Volunteers

Volunteers have brought a tremendous enthusiasm to See Change, as well as many helpful contacts and links.

Ambassadors

Ambassadors have given voice to ending mental health discrimination, sharing stories that resonate and inspire. Ambassadors that also work within the media have been a very positive experience for the campaign.

Community Activation

Pulling any national campaign through to the local level is paramount. See Change is committed to delivering our message and initiatives at a grass-roots level to empower local communities to be the change.

Strategic Planning

The strategic planning stage was so important, and thankfully the campaign invested wisely in getting the right kind of expertise to assist in mapping out the initial start of the campaign. Though we have had many limitations and challenges along the way, the strategic planning phase has helped to keep us firmly on the right path.

Learning from other campaigns internationally was and continues to be vital – what works and what does not and the sharing of information and materials.

Targeted Approach

Focusing our efforts on the campaign's target groups has also enabled us to stay focused and clear on the campaign's priorities.

Political Support

Getting political buy in has also been key, including at the government level, cross party and with Ireland's Health Service Executive.

Framing the Discussion

See Change takes great care in conveying the notion that while one in four of us will experience a mental health problem at some point in our life, four out of four of us will experience mental health dips, the day to day struggles that are an ordinary part of life. By framing the discussion in this way and using the concept of the *mental health continuum model*, it seems to be more accessible that this is all of us, not just the one in four of us – which in some ways may reinforce the notion of stigma.

Moving Forward

Since its inception in 2010, the See Change campaign has grown beyond the confines of a traditional public health campaign into a partnership of over 90 partner organisations, 200 volunteers and 50 campaign ambassadors. Four years on, the founding approaches of Ireland's stigma reduction campaign remain strongly backed by the evidence base; the campaign is structured around the partnership model, takes a targeted approach and social contact theory is the cornerstone of campaign activity. The campaign has also benefitted from the insight and experience of our international counterparts; the adoption of behaviour change messaging is a strong example of this.

In 2012, Stuart et al. called for a paradigm shift in stigma-reduction programming and research requiring an inversion of the most widely used social change model of the knowledge to behaviour continuum (*increased knowledge leads to attitude change which leads to behaviour change*) to a focus on behaviour change first. Basing their theory on the evidenced impact of stigma reduction programmes internationally, Stuart et al. suggest that 'attitude change is not a good predictor of behavioural change... and a focus on attitudes will not yield meaningful improvements in social inclusion and equity' for people with personal experience of a mental health problem.

As detailed by Stuart et al., the ultimate goal of stigma-reduction programmes and the focus of related research 'should not be knowledge or attitude change but improved quality of life for people with personal experience of a mental health problem'. The most apt measure here is to seek changes in discriminatory behaviours and structural inequities.

The limitations of focussing on attitude change alone were clear from See Change's evaluation results of phase 1 of the campaign, whereby awareness, attitudes, knowledge of mental health problems and even willingness to seeking professional help increased dramatically in the first 2 years of the campaign, but there was sustained reluctance to actively disclose a mental health problem to a friend, family member or colleague (See Change 2012).

It is on this basis that See Change would like to bring into future focus discrimination and prejudice as direct consequences of stigma as stigma itself is a rather theoretical concept to engage audiences on. There are opportunities for the partnership to address structural and institutional arrangements that propagate stigma such as insurance, contract law, government policy and also social norms.

See Change recognises that real change happens at local and community level. With this in mind, we will continue to work closely with grass-roots networks to embed our message and programmes among local communities, campus communities, membership organisations and representative bodies.

Rooted in the behaviour change message, the Green Ribbon campaign has proven to be See Change's flagship campaign. One month in the Irish calendar is now earmarked for helping to the end the stigma of mental health problems with more than 90 partner organisations helping to spread the messaging and taking ownership of the campaign.

The concept of going back to basics, back into communities with a simple and effective approach of the Green Ribbon has proven very popular with the Irish public and organisations. This is something that See Change will be working hard on building on taking the Green Ribbon campaign from strength to strength, ensuring that everyone has heard about the importance of ending mental health discrimination.

References

(2010) Stigma background mapping work – of Ireland and internationally. Amnesty International – Ireland, Ireland

Equality Authority (2011) Equality and mental health: how the law can help you. Equality Authority, 2011. http://www.equality.ie/Files/Equality%20and%20Mental%20Health%20-%20How%20the%20law%20can%20help%20you.pdf

Equality and mental health: what the law means for your workplace. http://www.equality.ie/Files/Equality%20and%20Mental%20Health%20-%20What%20the%20law%20means%20for%20your%20workplace.pdf

IBEC (2012) Mental health and wellbeing: a line manager's guide. http://www.ibec.ie/IBEC/DFB.nsf/vPages/Social_affairs~Resources~mental-health-and-wellbeing-a-line-manager's-guide-04-10-2012/$file/Mental%20health%20and%20wellbeing%20-guide.pdf

See Change (2010) Irish attitudes to mental health problems; a population survey

See Change (2012) Irish attitudes to mental health problems; a population survey

See Me: Scotland Case Study

20

Judith Robertson

Background

Scotland's mental health anti-stigma campaign was launched in 2002. One of the first of its kind around the world, the campaign focused on using social marketing techniques to shift negative public attitudes to mental health problems. The approach taken by See Me included national publicity campaigns including paid for advertising and general media work aimed at the whole population, targeted publicity campaigns aimed at groups such as children and young people or workplaces, specific focus on the media and journalists to change the way metal health issues were covered and increase awareness of the effects of stigma and discrimination and support for local awareness-raising activity through the provision of materials and small grants to fund local action.

The campaign was fully funded by the Scottish Government (Scottish Executive at that time) and was led and managed within the voluntary sector. Five Scottish organisations made up the management group of the campaign with a small staff team delivering the bulk of the work.

The Strategic Review of Anti-stigma Approach in Scotland of the programme undertaken at the end of the first 10 years found near unanimity in those surveyed that See Me had 'succeeded in raising awareness of mental health stigma and had developed a fund of goodwill. The majority of interviewees saw See Me as an original international trendsetter that had established a model for others to follow' (Pilgrim and Corry 2013).

The Strategic Review through its literature review found that:

- The campaign's advertising 'bursts' achieved their aim of putting the issue of mental health stigma on the public's agenda. Awareness was raised.

J. Robertson
"See Me", Scottish Association for Mental Health, 51 Wilson Street, Glasgow, Scotland
e-mail: info@seemescotland.org

© Springer International Publishing Switzerland 2017
W. Gaebel et al. (eds.), *The Stigma of Mental Illness - End of the Story?*,
DOI 10.1007/978-3-319-27839-1_20

379

- The campaign acted as a catalyst for existing stigma reduction efforts to adopt a more strategic approach which helped to co-ordinate activities as well as reach new areas, such as football clubs.
- Existing groups and activists were encouraged and new activists were recruited to the cause.
- Sustained exposure to campaign advertising and broader anti-stigma activity at local and national levels could be linked to improved public attitudes across a range of measures, but not all.
- It is also possible that improved public attitudes may merely reflect learnt responses and are therefore weakly correlated with behavioural change.
- There is little or no evidence, in part because none has been sought, that the campaign has led to sustainable behavioural change.
- The campaign does not seem to have had a major impact on some groups, for instance, people diagnosed with schizophrenia.
- The campaign found it difficult to engage with some target audiences, for instance, health service professionals.

The Review devised an aspirational template that a refounded programme in Scotland could work to. Presented as a '21st-century ideal', the template includes such components as:

- A vision that expresses the ending of discrimination through the perspective of a civil or human rights movement
- Aims that set out to mobilise the people directly affected as leaders of the movement to target the behaviours and organisations that most stigmatise and discriminate
- Delivered by nongovernmental organisations through a model of bursts of strategic national umbrella activities such as advertising to create the space and confidence for aligned local activities that facilitate social contact with people with and without the lived experience of mental health stigma and discrimination
- Underpinned by policy commitments, legal rights enforcement and sustained, multisource funding (Pilgrim and Corry 2013)

This analysis of the campaign led to a refocusing of the work in 2013. The Scottish Government, now in partnership with the UK-funding body, Comic Relief, renewed its commitment to the mental health anti-stigma work and committed a further 3 years of funding to a newly refounded programme. The Scottish Government's Mental Health Strategy 2012–2015 had already committed to support the ending of stigma and discrimination in Scotland and had also charged the Scottish Human Rights Commission and the Mental Welfare Commission to 'develop and increase the focus on rights as a key component of mental health care in Scotland' (Scottish Government 2012).

In this context the Scottish Government sought partnership bids to run the programme from the voluntary sector in Scotland, and the joint programme plan created by a partnership between the Scottish Association for Mental Health (SAMH) and the Mental Health Foundation (MHF) became the refounded programme, launching in November 2013.

The refounded programme contained many of the elements of the '21st-century ideal' recommended in the Strategic Review.

The programme focus on behaviour change and the commitment to building a knowledge base of what works in ending stigma and discrimination are key elements of the refounded programme as is an underpinning equality- and human rights-based approach that brings the lived experience of people with mental health problems to the front and centre of the development and delivery of the refounded programme. The concluding recommendations of the European anti-stigma network's research on stigma and depression, known as ASPEN, were a key building block of the refounded programme:

- Planning, development, execution and evaluation of activities to reduce stigma must involve people with mental illness and carers at every stage.
- The primary target of anti-stigma work is not a change of attitudes but a change of behaviour. This is a major shift in emphasis.
- The reduction of discrimination is more important than the elimination of stigma that produced it. It is important also that it can be measured in meaningful terms and achieved faster.
- Short-lasting campaigns against stigma are not particularly useful; long-term programmes incorporated into other efforts are needed to make a difference.
- Making society tolerant to people with mental illness is an obsolete goal which should be replaced by their inclusion in society despite the fact that they might be different.
- Fighting stigma and discrimination with success is possible regardless of the size of the national income or of the coexistent problems in that nation.
- Programmes against stigma should adopt general principles, but their activities should be tailored to fit local circumstances.

(*53EU Conference on Stigma and Discrimination, Lisbon 2010*)

Programme Approach and Strategy

The 2013–2016 Programme Strategy is described as a theory of change. (See Table 20.1 for full model). The overall programme aim is that *people who experience mental health problems will lead more fulfilled lives.*

To achieve that aim, the programme works to three strategic goals and seven programme outcomes.

Table 20.1 Programme goals, outcomes and related activities

Strategic goal and related outcomes	Related work programme
Strategic goal 1: Self-stigma amongst people with mental health problems will be reduced *Outcome 1* People with lived experience increasingly imagine a life without stigma and discrimination and demand their rights *Outcome 2* Concerns about stigma and discrimination become less of a barrier to talking about mental health problems	See Me Now – conference Outreach programme Community champions Media volunteers Engagement of people with lived experience in decision-making Local grants Scottish mental health arts and film festival
Strategic goal 2: Stigma and discrimination is reduced within communities and organisations to have a positive impact on the lives of people with mental health problems *Outcome 3* The rights of people with lived experience are increasingly met *Outcome 4* Diverse leaders and organisations champion elimination of stigma and discrimination *Outcome 5* Negative stereotyping is reduced in targeted settings and communities	Community innovation fund Change networks Partnership development National campaign Speakers bureau Workplace strategy Children and young people's strategy Health and social care strategy Ongoing communications and media work
Strategic goal 3 Recovery from mental health problems will be more widely understood and more people believe that recovery is possible *Outcome 6* National and local policies increasingly and explicitly address stigma and discrimination *Outcome 7* Increased understanding of nature, source and effects of stigma and discrimination and what works in tackling it	Policy work SNAP Evaluation Plans going forward

The activities of the programme reflect a shift of emphasis from changing attitudes and improving knowledge at society level to changing behaviour across all levels particularly within targeted communities.

Equalities and Human Rights Framework

Fundamental to the See Me programme approach is a focus on equalities and human rights. The rights of people experiencing mental health problems come under the protected characteristics of equalities and human rights legislation including the UN Convention on the Right of Persons with Disabilities, the UN Convention on the Rights of the Child and the Universal Declaration of Human Rights, all of which the UK has signed up to and the Scottish Parliament is committed to endorsing.

See Me has taken as its approach the application of PANEL principles in line with recommendations from Scottish Human Rights Commission (SHRC, www.scottishhumanrights.com).

*P*articipation – Everyone has the right to participate in decisions which affect their human rights. Participation must be active, free, meaningful and give attention to issues of accessibility, including access to information in a form and a language which can be understood.

*A*ccountability – Accountability requires effective monitoring of human rights standards as well as effective remedies for human rights breaches. For accountability to be effective, there must be appropriate laws, policies, institutions, administrative procedures and mechanisms of redress in order to secure human rights.

*N*on-discriminatory – A HRBA means that all forms of discrimination (such as age, gender, sexual orientation or ethnicity) in the realisation of rights must be prohibited, prevented and eliminated. It also requires the prioritisation of those in the most marginalised or vulnerable situations who face the biggest barriers to realising their rights.

*E*mpowerment – Individuals and communities should understand their rights and be fully supported to participate in the development of policy and practices which affect their lives. Individuals and communities should be able to claim their rights where necessary.

*L*egality of rights – A HRBA requires the recognition of rights as legally enforceable entitlements and is linked in to national and international human rights law.

See Me Equalities and Human Rights Framework

This framework will define how these PANEL principles apply to the See Me programme, what steps we will take to improve our practice in relation to the principles and how we will go about monitoring our progress in relation to that work.

Participation People with lived experience of mental health problems will be involved in all key See Me decisions that determine what the programme does and how it does it. Key means of achieving this are through our partnership working with VOX, Scotland's national service user organisation, through effective engagement of people with lived experience in the Programme Advisory Group, through ongoing engagement of people with lived experience in programme planning, design and delivery and through the implementation of key programme processes: grants programme, change networks, innovation labs, workplace pledge, training and national campaign work. All of these will incorporate their own equality- and human rights-based approach and will ensure that we implement any required reasonable adjustments to involve and engage people from a wide range of equalities groups.

Accountability See Me itself has structures in place to support the programme accountability to people with lived experience; the Programme Advisory Group meets quarterly and reviews plans and progress and sits on the biannual monitoring meeting with our funders. But See Me also has a role to play in ensuring that people with lived experience have access to a wide range of rights and if their rights are undermined, then there will be recourse to justice. At the moment in Scotland effective, accessible means of gaining justice are only available in limited ways, and we will be working across the mental health sector to improve results for people in this area.

Non-discrimination See Me is committed to ensuring we have in place suitable and accessible programme processes and activities that include people from across society; that we understand the different ways different groups are affected by inequality in relation to mental health stigma and discrimination and work to ensure the programme is giving appropriate emphasis to them. We will also focus resources on promoting the interests of the most marginalised people in Scottish society and advocating through our policy agenda for a similar response from public sector bodies.

Empowerment See Me's goal is to empower people with lived experience of mental health problems to achieve their rights. We will work with groups across Scotland to increase understanding of rights and how different groups and organisations can gain access to them in fairer, more empowering ways. The programme recognises that we all have rights and that a rights-based approach brings all views, opinions and needs to the table to address them fairly and in balance, where possible.

Legality See Me will seek to increase understanding and awareness of the legal frameworks that support the rights of people with lived experience of mental health problems and put a spotlight on where those rights are being eroded or where the impacts of aspects of legislation and policy are undermining peoples' rights. We will promote good practice case studies to give evidence of the effectiveness of a different, fairer and more empowering approach.

The programme is also in the early stages of scoping out the potential for a Scottish Mental Health Charter of Rights developed by people with lived experience of mental health problems and potentially designed to be a tool of empowerment and enablement.

Evaluation Framework
Introduction (Excerpt from See Me Programme Evaluation Framework 2013)
Prior to the refounding of See Me, comprehensive evaluation was not integral to the programme structure and there are considerable gaps in knowledge and learning from programme work. Going forward it is clear that current measurement models and scales will need to be supplemented by testing different means of drawing learning from the evidence base.

The evaluation team has generated a series of reviews of the literature to inform the programme, a social movement survey has been developed, our monitoring systems are in place and significant work has been done to support the Community Innovation Fund award organisations to develop their own evaluations of the See Me-funded work and to support the evaluation of the Community Champions Programme. This activity is intended to support a culture of learning in relation to this work and will create new knowledge about what works in tackling stigma and discrimination in Scotland and will make an important contribution to international debates.

This evaluation framework outlines the aims and guiding principles of the evaluation for the See Me programme along with suggested methodology.

Evaluation Aims
The evaluation will:

- Assess progress towards achieving the national outcomes for the See Me programme.
- Guide strategic developments for the See Me programme in the longer term.
- Produce valid evidence of change by capturing data that will demonstrate intended and unintended impacts (the what) of the See Me programme.
- Increase depth of understanding (the where, how and why) of the effectiveness and value of vehicles for change used in the See Me programme by exploring the process and contextual factors that contribute to their success.
- Contribute to the evidence base of what works.
- Guide anti-stigma practice development within the See Me programme in the short and medium term.
- Support funder accountability requirements.

Underpinning Principles of the Evaluation
- The evaluation will adopt a theory-driven approach which is appropriate to the challenges of evaluating complex interventions for social and behaviour change that target significant social problems. The theory-driven approach will not seek to judge the See Me programme in its entirety; rather it will determine whether the programme has been delivered as intended and what aspects of the programme work, for whom and in what circumstances.
- The evaluation will have transparency of the rationale behind approach and method. This will involve fully engaging with existing knowledge and research evidence and stakeholders on the evaluation approach and methods. The evaluation should operate as a critical 'friend', taking a formative rather than summative approach to work collaboratively and developmentally with all stakeholders throughout the delivery of the See Me programme.

- The evaluation will be embedded in the See Me programme. The evaluation team will be considered part of the programme team, and the work will be overseen by the See Me Director. The evaluation report to the See Me management team in the first instance with findings being shared with the advisory group and wider stakeholders on a regular basis.
- The evaluation team will have the freedom to report all findings (positive and negative) constructively by seeking and representing the range of differing interpretations of evaluation findings and implications for policy and practice. This relationship will require specific written agreement from the two lead agencies (SAMH and MHF) at outset.
- All findings should be viewed as learning opportunities for the See Me programme (and wider anti-stigma movement) with an ethos of innovation and 'constructive failure' permeated throughout. This means embracing all findings from the evaluation including where initiatives show to be successful with significant impact or where they show to be underperforming with no significant impact and supporting continual improvement. Any reporting of evaluation findings will be sensitive and respectful to the stakeholders involved.
- The evaluation methodologies will be robust and seek to produce valid evidence of impact and change, as well as an audit trail of activity, outputs and value for money. The balance will sway towards impact over penetration data. Most of which can be collected by the See Me team and grant funded projects as output monitoring information using a framework developed by the evaluation team.
- The evaluation will be guided by the principles underpinning the entire See Me programme.

Conceptual Framework
The evaluation will be informed by the application of a theory of change (TOC) methodology to the See Me programme. In essence TOC is a way of planning a process for change through the articulating of causal linkages between actions and desired outcomes. The TOC should work backwards from long-term goals demonstrating how a pathway of short-, intermediate- and longer-term outcomes will lead to the achievement of the long-term goals. The desired outcomes should, as far as possible, be based on a set of assumptions that have an evidence base (drawn from research and experience) and explain the connections between the programme activities and the short-, intermediated- and longer-term outcomes.

The success of a TOC can be demonstrated by evidencing progress on the achievement of outcomes through the measurement of outcome indicators that support the measurement of change. Indicators can be seen as items of information that allow you to know that you've reached or made progress towards reaching an outcome. Each outcome developed for the See Me programme should have at least one indicator. A key role of the evaluation is to gather data that will enable those involved in See Me understand why activities have worked and might work in different situations and/or how they need to be adjusted to gain better results. Key to this is understanding how context influences the delivery and outcomes of an activity.

The evaluation will focus on answering an agreed set of research questions which will be based on propositions/hypotheses developed from the literature and the See Me programme TOC and the attached indicators. The research questions will be submitted to the management team and the advisory group for discussion and sign off.

The evaluation will focus on the measurement of three core areas:

Outputs With support from the evaluation team, the See Me staff team and those who receive grants will be expected to systematically and routinely collate monitoring data to gather descriptive information about the activities' reach and penetration of the programme. This will involve gathering quantitative data of factors including, for example, numbers and demographics of participants, audience, community volunteers, media volunteers, pledge+ signers, the numbers of schools using the curriculum pack, numbers of training programmes delivered and delegate numbers, etc. We will also identify where there are links between societal and community-based approaches (as is the intention of the new programme) and consider this in the evaluation design.

Outcomes Outcome measurement will occur at three levels: individual (empowerment, knowledge, behaviour), community (empowerment, knowledge, behaviour) and societal (knowledge, attitudes, behavioural intent and behaviour, national and local policy and practice change). The evaluation team will facilitate the development of short-, medium- and long-term outcomes for the See Me programme as a whole (and potentially for each distinct aspect) by the See Me team, partners and other stakeholders. As part of this process, clear outcome indicators will be also developed that will relate to each level and type of vehicle of change. The evaluation will also measure the impact of the See Me programme on individuals within delivery teams who have lived experience (LEPN members, etc.) as well as partners and recipients of the programme.

Process We will fully describe the partnerships, vehicles for change and mechanisms used to develop and implement programmes of work, involve communities and those with lived experience and the contexts within which they occur. This data will be used in conjunction with output and outcome data to attribute outcomes to specific vehicles for change and their alignment with See Me values and underlying principles will be assessed.

Programme Activities to Date

The programme is organised into two teams – the *communities team* which primarily focuses on engaging people with and without lived experience of mental health problems in community-based behaviour change activities and in building the social movement and the *national team* which primarily focuses on reaching the target audiences of the programme: the wider public, workplaces, children and young people and health and social care settings and in developing the programme communications work including social marketing.

Communities Team

See Me Now

In April 2014 the programme brought people together from all over Scotland to a large-scale agenda-setting event to generate participation, ownership and engagement in the refounded programme. The rationale was to engage with a wide range of sector stakeholder to ensure that the refounded See Me programme had all of See Me stakeholders, but most especially people with lived experience, at the heart of planning and delivery of programme objectives.

The event had a number of objectives:

- To provide a visible demonstration of the refounded See Me that establishes new ways of working and new programme direction
- To develop clarity about the key themes that See Me will work to over the 3-year period of the programme
- To provide an opportunity to engage stakeholders in a co-production process on a range of issues: key themes, the development of the refreshed See Me brand, the development of the social movement and change networks
- To enable a wide range of stakeholders to think, talk, network and plan for change in relation to the rights of people with mental health problems

A steering group of the key programme delivery partners was established to develop and organise the event.

Three hundred people applied to attend from all over Scotland, 250 people were offered places and 195 people attended the event. Of those we invited, 70 % self-nominated as having lived experience of mental health problems. On the day, 45 % of the audience chose to describe themselves as attending the event in the capacity of having lived experience.

Outreach Programme

Following See Me Now, the communities team embarked on a series of local meetings and roadshows around Scotland to further engage people in a discussion about building the social movement and what kind of activity people would like to be involved in. Often in partnership with other organisations, the programme consulted people about the social movement and how people thought they might become involved in it. Again in this process, the programme highlighted the focus on equalities and human rights and has made several local grants which target equality groups in their work.

This outreach work has now been developed into an outreach strategy which includes work with volunteers, community champions, regional staff networks and potentially regional action plans.

Over a series of 38 different events around Scotland, the programme has engaged around 2,000 people, gathering their views on how stigma and discrimination affects them and how they can contribute to tackling it.

Community Champions

Most recently the Community Champions programme was launched, focusing the first phase on South West Scotland. The programme was developed with a small team of contributors including people with lived experience, See Me staff, partner staff and a consultant who is supporting the community champions programme. Community Champions are volunteers with lived experience who take part in a 4–6 month training process around local leadership and building the social movement to take action to bring about behaviour change. The interactive training programme will build skills and capacities for people to engage other people and organisations locally. Eleven people were recruited through an open process from across four health board areas in Scotland and will complete their training early in 2015.

The next phases of the Community Champions programme will be focused on South East Scotland and the Highlands and will run during year 2 of the programme.

Grants Programme

The programme grant fund was allocated in two ways: local grants and the Community Innovation Fund (CIF).

The local grants were maintained this year to generate easier-access activity to the new focus of the programme. Key programme priorities were emphasised in the criteria, leadership of people with lived experience, focus on stigma and discrimination and supporting one of more of the programme themes: workplace, health and social care and children and young people.

The programme made 18 local grants totalling £63,000 to organisations from all over Scotland.

Community Innovation Fund/Change Networks

Partly to stimulate activity and partly to ensure change network development was progressed in year 1, the programme decided to integrate the planning and development of the Grants Programme and the change networks.

A three stage process for the Community Innovation Fund was developed which incorporated the development of change networks, the integration of an equality- and human rights-based approach and the full engagement of people with lived experience in change network development.

The decision-making group remained relatively constant throughout made up of people with lived experience, staff from See Me, staff from the managing partner organisations SAMH and MHF and staff from one of the programme delivery part- ners, the Scottish Mental Health Co-operative.

CIF grant criteria were strong, ensuring that people's work would be led by peo- ple with lived experience and would focus on mental health stigma and discrimina- tion behaviour change within specific settings: workplace, health and social care, children and young people with an emphasis on equalities groups, rights and those whom services do not reach.

The grant awards have stimulated six change networks; two focused on the crim- inal justice system, one on students in further and higher education, one on increas- ing access to mental health services in the Polish Community in Scotland, one on informal workplace conversation with people with lived experience and one social contact site-specific art project. The change network participants recently attended a workshop held by MHF on evaluating their projects and building that into their work so that the programme can establish what works. The programme made six grants totalling £120,000.

Two potential thematic change networks have been identified; criminal justice and further and higher education where the programme believes the potential impact of the funded projects could be made greater by bringing together a strategic net- work to learn from and compliment the work on the ground.

National Programme

Brand Development

The brand development process has been a major piece of work which contributes to all our strategic goals. The programme commissioned independent quantitative and qualitative research which generated considerable new knowledge and insight into current perceptions of See Me and the extent to which these align with the pro- posed new vision, mission and values.

Main Findings (Porter 2014)

Original Brand

The original brand had strong support from those who knew the brand well, but for those who were not aware of the brand, it had little meaning or salience. For those who knew the brand, they recognised it as being about raising awareness in relation to men- tal health stigma and discrimination and as being dependable and trustworthy in its work, but for those more critical supporters, that sense of credibility was diminishing.

See Me Looking Forward

Overall, the general public, active-engaged and professional audiences seek a more dynamic and determined positioning for the brand compared to that perceived to be communicated by the draft vision, mission and values. Potential beneficiaries and service users tended to be more cautious in how they wished to see the brand, looking for a positioning which feels more reserved and less exposing for themselves as individuals.

Next Steps

This research went on to inform the brief for brand agencies of See Me's brand identity and whether a new name should be chosen. As the result of an intensive research process, the programme decided to maintain the name, strengthen the strapline and use our campaign messages to strengthen the impact of our communications. The new brand identity was launched on 28th October as part of our new campaign launch. Following the feedback on the draft version of the vision, mission and values, this new statement below was crafted to better reflect the expectations of our varied audiences.

New Programme Vision, Mission and Values

Vision

To end mental health stigma and discrimination, enabling people who experience mental health problems to live fulfilled lives.

Mission

- We will mobilise people to work together and lead a movement to end mental health stigma and discrimination.
- We will work with people to change negative behaviour towards those with mental health problems.
- We will ensure that the human rights of people with mental health problems are respected and upheld.

Values

- We are *determined* to stop mental health discrimination at the source and will do everything in our power to *challenge* and prevent it.
- Our position is based on using the best evidence available. We are *informed* by and are *inclusive* of the voices of people with lived experience. We act inclusively to enable everyone to *participate* at the level they feel comfortable with.

- We talk *confidently*, *passionately* and in an appropriate manner.
- We understand the challenges that those with mental health problems face and we're *sensitive* to their situation.

See Me launched the new brand and campaign 'People like YOU will end mental health stigma and discrimination' at a high profile event attended by over 100 people in October 2014. The campaign advertised on radio, online, outdoor digital sites, trains, the Glasgow Underground and in shopping centres for 5 weeks. The campaign aimed to raise awareness and encourage people from all over the country to take action to end mental health stigma and discrimination. Through the campaign the programme encouraged people to visit the new website and join the movement. The campaign will be evaluated by the end 2014 but early signs of impact are encouraging.

Media and Social Media

Programme media and social media work has taken on a new scale and is much more targeted in its reach and delivering on a wide range of messages. Bringing the media capacity in-house has ensured the programme has much more control over activity and impact with the output. Success has been identified in getting not only increased numbers of followers and supporters but also increased engagement of the people who are following the programme through social media.

Media Volunteers

The strategy of working with people with lived experience and supporting them to tell their stories in the media has gone from strength to strength. The programme has become much more focused on what we are able to offer media volunteers, supporting them to be very clear in the messages they are generating and tailoring their input to the outlet they are talking to. The programme has also been clear in setting out the expectations of the role of being a media volunteer and has refreshed how people have been trained. Fifteen people this year have been trained by a media professional, 16 volunteers have told their story and contributed to media articles and 42 articles have been generated from this work.

The programme will be evaluating the impact of this work with the volunteers who take part and monitor the impact through social marketing processes.

Scottish Mental Health Arts and Film Festival (SMHAFF)

See Me has supported the Scottish Mental Health Arts and Film Festival for many years, seeing that the role that the arts played in breaking down stigma and increasing social contact was a significant one. The refounded programme increased the investment in the SMHAFF and committed to generating consistent and rigorous evaluation of its impact.

The 2014 festival saw over 320 events throughout October 2014 with attendances totalling over 20,000, compared to attendances for 2013 of over 17,000. The final figure does not include many of the exhibitions where it was not possible to accurately record attendances.

See me supported the recruitment of a regional SMHAFF development worker to promote the festival in local communities, build the capacity of local organisations to fund their work and ensure that stigma and discrimination in relation to mental health features prominently in that work. The partnership will also ensure a year-round component to the festival and that SMHAFF events are integrated into other festival schedules.

Workstreams

In keeping with the programme model, the programme is designed to reach both the general population through media activity and social contact development and targeted populations. The three principle target audiences are that of employers and workplaces, children and young people and health and social care settings. The objectives of working on each of these target audiences vary, but all are underpinned by the equality- and human rights-based approach and by seeking to build effective behaviour change in relation to mental health stigma and discrimination.

Workplace Workstream

Background
The overall aim of the workplace workstream is to bring about meaningful changes in behaviour in and around workplaces, as well as in attitude and awareness and to evidence this through the generation of a rigorous evidence base.

To date See Me has engaged over 500 companies who have pledged to work with the programme to eliminate the stigma and discrimination of mental ill-health. The pledge has been a public commitment (seen by employees, customers, wider public, etc.) that the pledging organisation will tackle the stigma experienced by people with mental health problems. However, there has been a lack of clarity on what action/standards accompanies the pledge in terms of the expectations and requirements this commitment places on the organisation, and little documentation exploring how signing the pledge has made any impact on staff or working practices.

Stakeholder Engagement

In addition to working in partnership, and importantly communicating, with the employers who have already showed their support to 'See Me', via the pledge, the programme is expanding their partnerships to include those who have not previously worked with 'See Me'. This includes:

- Employers (particularly SMEs and those employers not engaged with health at work and similar programmes)
- Business forums and support organisations
- National training and CPD organisations
- Colleges and universities (vocational courses)
- Employee rights organisations, e.g. unions

The Approach

The programme is now reviewing the pledge to make it more meaningful in its aspirations and focus and ensure it incorporates the rights-based approach and can support effective evaluation. A short review was conducted which highlighted that the pledge was mainly being used to raise awareness of stigma in workplaces and there was appetite to see a stronger process which helped hold people account for effective behaviour change.

The programme has developed a workplace programme theory of change which will be put to the advisory group for comment and has brought together a short-life pledge review group to devise the new pledge.

Workplace discrimination was highlighted as part of the media coverage of first campaign which highlighted the difficulty of effective recourse for employees when their rights are undermined but also the demand amongst employers for improving their practice.

Workplace activity was also highlighted within the local grants and the Community Innovation Fund grant guidelines as priority areas of focus. We funded one workplace CIF change network based on lived experience engagement in workplace settings using social contact theory to build relationships and empathy. A further two local grants focused on changing behaviour in the workplace – one with bus drivers in a Scottish town and the other in a power station.

The national work place workstream will be supported by a 'national campaign' and will link to local level activity implemented by the workplace change network.

The integration of people with lived experience is crucial to the success of this aspect of the programme – the experiences of workplace stigma and discrimination have often cost people their jobs and undermined their recovery so the programme is committed to ensuring that those with direct experience will be the key advisers in developing programme strategy and supporting delivery. This approach is informed by the emerging evidence base that highlights that 'contact' is particularly effective when the individual with lived experience has common traits and backgrounds to the target audience, e.g. experience or working in the same industry, industry leader, etc.

Children and Young People's Workstream

Background

Involving and targeting young people has been a key factor in the development of anti-stigma campaigns across the world. Addressing attitudes and behaviours at an early age has been associated with reducing the damaging effects of self-stigma and exclusion of young people experiencing mental ill health, helping to shape citizenship that includes understanding and awareness of mental health and discrimination and creating a ripple effect to influence adults and other people in young people's lives.

'See Me' prioritised stigma and discrimination in young people from the early days of the campaign, working with young people and a range of professionals to develop the cartoon based 'Cloud Boy/Cloud Girl' campaign which launched in 2006. Alongside this, 'See Me' supported the development of local initiatives, including the Positive Mental Attitudes Curriculum Pack developed by the Glasgow Anti-Stigma Partnership.

With the proliferation of social media and the rapid pace of change in young people's lives, the campaign started to consider a new approach to young people in 2009. Extensive research, codesign and testing was conducted with teenagers aged 13–15, in school and informal learning environments, yielding a range of useful data and suggested routes forward. 'See Me' developed the 'What's on Your Mind' campaign which was launched in February 2012, including an interactive DVD and printed activities pack and a web presence.

Stakeholder Consultation

The programme is currently consulting with wide range of stakeholders including children and young people over the priorities for this area of work. Given that young people's interests in mental health go beyond stigma and discrimination, the programme is looking to build links with other allies who can support the wider agenda in relation to mental health awareness and understanding how to get help.

The 'What's On Your Mind' teachers' resource pack remains the principle engagement vehicle for our work with children and young people. It is heavily used by teachers and youth workers and in consultation with Education Scotland, and the pack is currently being updated ready for relaunch in the next teaching year. Over 125 schools have actively engaged with the pack and it is well used by youth groups.

As part of the children and young people's workstream, there is also scope for exploring the potential for digital mainstreaming of its activities in its digital strategy and for young people with lived experience to assist with addressing access and self-stigma concerns in relation to technology which prevent other people with mental health problems from enjoying these benefits.

Again our grants programme also stimulated activity in this area – the programme funded one children and young people-oriented Community Innovation Fund project with the NUS to establish student-led anti-stigma and discrimination campaigns in three universities and colleges in Scotland, and five of our local grants were focused on working with young people on issues such as body image, young people's engagement and empowerment, mental health awareness and stigma reduction.

Policy Work

Our policy work has been focused on increasing awareness of the refounded See Me programme, engaging in UK level and international conferences and other programmes and some focused political engagement around rights.

The programme worked with the Scottish Government over the publication of the Social Attitudes Survey Mental Health Module. A successful See Me parliamentary reception was held in January 2014 with excellent engagement from members of the Scottish Parliament and people with lived experience, the Minister for Public Health spoke to 200 delegates on mental health stigma and discrimination at See Me Now Conference, the programme director shared a platform with the new Minister for Sport, Health Improvement and Mental Health at the recent Scottish National Action Plan Health and Social Care Action Group parliamentary launch and participated in the Mental Welfare Commission's strategy development day on the development of Commitment 5.

The programme is in the process of recruiting a person with lived experience to take part in the Global Alliance/WPA conference in San Francisco in February next year and has successfully submitted workshop proposals for the World Association of Psychiatry anti-stigma symposium to take place in San Francisco early next year.

Scottish National Action Plan for Human Rights (SNAP)

See Me is involved in two of the implementation groups for SNAP, Health and Social Care and Establishing a Human Rights Culture, and the Programme Director is a member of the SNAP leadership panel. This work runs alongside the programme's own human rights-based approach which is informed by engagement with SNAP and contributes to it.

Evaluation to Date

The evaluation covers all aspects of the programme and takes a theory-driven approach which ultimately focusses on gathering impact data that can be strongly attributed to the activities of the See Me delivery team. So the key role of the evaluation is to gather data that will enable those involved in See Me understand why activities have worked and might work in different situations and/or how they need to be adjusted to gain better results.

The first year of the evaluation has involved a wide range of activities to set in place the foundations required to respond to measuring change as the various elements of the See Me programme have begun to take shape. The evaluation team has worked alongside the delivery team to understand and support their planning and delivery process. This work, alongside substantial literature review, has been necessary to develop the See Me theory of change both for the overall See Me programme and the specific work themes within it. The first year of the evaluation has been very much focussed on establishing what should be evaluated and how and setting up a range of baseline data collection processes.

Progress (Excerpts from See Me Evaluation Report 2014)

The evaluation is designed to use specific measures to capture the relevance and impact of the See Me programme on those known to be most likely to experience stigma and discrimination (e.g. those with diagnosed mental health problems, their families, etc.) as well those who are not using mental health services but living with mental health problems (who are currently underrepresented in anti-stigma research and evaluation). It will be important to capture both the day-to-day community-based experiences of these two groups as well as the norm of collecting data from mental health service users related to their care and treatment.

People's Panel

This involves working closely with the programme and wider networks to develop innovative approaches such as a virtual 'people's panel' used by One of Us in Denmark which consists of people with lived experience recruited anonymously. The See Me peoples' panel will be accessed to produce evaluation data as well as primary research to inform the practice and campaigns of the See Me team and other stakeholders. The panel can also be used to evaluate social media campaigns in part.

It is anticipated that we would run up to two topic specific surveys of the panel yearly (i.e. six surveys) with the response rate increasing as recruitment builds up (approx. 1,000 responses).

Recruitment for the people's panel has been ongoing. The people's panel was invited to participate in the social movement survey (see below). Further involvement of the people's panel is planned for year 2. It is also intended to conduct survey work with the people's panel in the new year to support the development of See Me workstreams.

See Me Social Movement Survey

A survey of those on the contacts databases of See Me and each of the partner organisations was undertaken in October 2015. The survey intended to gather data on who is involved in tackling stigma and discrimination, what they are doing, what motivates them and how connected they feel to the See Me social movement and how effective they feel it is. Seven hundred forty-eight responses were received. The first descriptive report of the findings is due in February 2015 and substantive in-depth statistical analysis will be undertaken by August 2015. A factor analysis will be run with the intention of developing a social movement scale. The survey will repeat in October 2015 and October 2016.

See Me Events

The evaluation team are ensuring that all See Me events are evaluated. Evaluation forms are tailored to each events aims and objectives to ensure that relevant and attributable impact data is collected. This is intended to maximise the value of the findings for the See Me team in terms of reviewing their effectiveness. The See Me team are using this data to build on the approaches that are effective in realising the impacts they want to achieve and to address any less helpful outcomes directly with delegates or in future planning of events. Findings from events in year 1 are summarised below.

See Me Now

Event delegates were supplied with an evaluation form on the morning of day one and invited to set three personal goals for the event. At the end of day two, delegates were invited to rate their own goals as well as answering questions about their experiences and the See Me team's event objectives. Over half of the respondents completed the evaluation forms (54 %, $n = 106$) and submitted their evaluation forms: 81 delegates set and rated 3 goals, 14 set and rated 2 goals and 2 set and rated 1 goal.

Taking a combined rating of 4 and 5 as achieved (with 5 as fully achieved and 1 as not achieved), 74 % of respondents had achieved their first goal, 70 % had achieved their second goal and 67 % had achieved their third goal. Only two goals were rated as not achieved at all. These personal goals were coded into 12 categories. The most common goal category was 'to learn about how delegates could contribute to the See Me programme'. However, this was the third lowest rated goal with an average rating of 3.5. This perhaps reflects that the focus of the conference design was around engaging, learning and prioritising. The fact that the conference did not focus on more tangible action planning was a frustration for some delegates.

The highest rated personal goal categories were 'to learn from other people's experiences and knowledge', 'to contribute meaningfully, to have a voice and influence' and 'to be motivated and inspired'. This probably echoes the focus of the conference design. Delegates articulated that achieving these goals involved increasing their confidence and self-esteem as well as developing and maintaining a positive self-perception of their own value. One delegate set a goal to have their own attitudes challenged and rated this as achieved indicating that not all delegates came to the event as one of the 'converted' but were positively influenced by the experience.

> .. finally freeing myself of self-stigma and openly saying – 'I'm a professional and have had difficulties with mental ill health'. Thanks! (event evaluation respondent).

The highest rated See Me team objective for the event was that people were able to think, talk, network and plan for change (81 % felt this was achieved). The second most highly rated was that participants engaged in a shared planning process (77 % achieved) followed by developing clarity over the key themes for the new See Me programme and providing a visible demonstration of new ways of working and programme direction (both 62 %). Taking a combined rating of 1 and 2 (with 5 as fully achieved and 1 as not achieved) an average of 17 % of respondents rated the above goals as not being achieved.

Finally 97 % of delegates felt that they had the opportunity to participate (82 % fully felt this), 96 % able to contribute (75 % felt fully able), 93 % felt listened to (67 % felt fully listened to) and 76 % felt that Ketso was helpful (48 % felt it was fully helpful). The final comments reflected that delegates felt safe and respected in contrast to other mental health events they had attended. Staff and delegates worked hard at the event, and some difficult issues such as challenging personal testimonies and the timing and content of the theatre piece arose; however, the vast majority of criticism was constructive and welcomed by the See Me team throughout the event:

> Long, tiring but inspiring (event evaluation respondent).

Roadshows

A total of 93 people attended the roadshows in Glasgow, Inverness, Stirling and the Borders. The participants at the roadshows were asked to complete evaluation forms at the end of their sessions to feedback on the aims of the roadshows. Fifty-three people completed them. The questions asked whether they felt:

- Listened to
- Included in the group
- Able to participate
- Valued for their contribution
- Respected
- Part of a movement for change
- Inspired to challenge stigma and discrimination
- That they got what they were hoping to achieve from the group

The majority of the participants answered fully or mostly to all of the above. Those who did not answer this way usually selected 'don't know'. One participant answered 'partially' or 'not at all' to most of the questions. These results overall demonstrate that the workshops included people who generally feel part of a movement for change against mental health stigma and discrimination. The workshops seem to have been effective at involving people and inspiring them to challenge stigma and discrimination.

Innovation Lab

Twenty one of those attending the Innovation Lab completed the evaluation (53 %). The feedback on the whole was very positive, but with constructive criticism.

The majority of evaluation respondents strongly agreed or agreed that participating in the Innovation Lab had the following impacts:

- I felt empowered to share my ideas (100 %).
- I feel more confident that I can contribute to reducing mental health stigma and discrimination (91 %).
- The Innovation Lab has stimulated new ideas for me in reducing stigma and discrimination (86 %).
- I feel more confident about producing a project that will have a significant impact in reducing stigma and discriminatory behaviour (81 %).
- I feel more confident that I can apply the best available evidence about what works to effectively reduce stigma and discrimination in the development of my project (81 %).

The concept development sessions were reported to be the most helpful aspect of the Innovation Lab for the majority of evaluation respondents. The marketplace and networking with others were also mentioned as helpful by some. Speed dating was the least helpful aspect of the Innovation Lab. A few people also mentioned the intro session, acoustics and human rights-based approach as less helpful.

Some examples of the constructive criticism offered by participants are given below:

I think more info and chance to engage with human rights approach would be helpful – stand alone sessions? its a new approach and we need to find a collective way of moving it forwards. (Innovation Lab delegate)

More led by people with experience e.g. groups. (Innovation Lab delegate)

The Innovation Labs has been a good way of networking and learning. The speed dating was maybe least useful but OK. (Innovation Lab delegate)

Great to have this level of interest and support from a funding body. Thank you. (Innovation Lab delegate)

Champions Evaluation

Phase 1 evaluation plan developed and implementation has begun. Baseline data has been collected from the Champions to assess where they were on the eight champions programme outcomes. Repeat data on the outcomes will be collected at the end of the training programme in March 2015 and then in November 2015 following the field work experience. Qualitative interviews will be conducted with the Champions facilitators (Rebekah and Sarah) in February 2015 and each champion will also be interviewed in March 2014 prior to their field work. Staff and the champions will all be interviewed once again in November 2015.

In addition to the above, Champions will all be invited to share their personal journey of working with See Me with the evaluation. This will explore in depth the personal impact the experience has had on them. This may be written, acoustic, filmed, photographed or any other means by which the Champions wish to convey their story.

The evaluation process above will repeat for all future Champions recruited to the programme.

Change Networks and Grants Programme Evaluation

A CIF Grant Holders Evaluation workshop was held in November 2014. At the workshop, each project created their own theory of change and generated research questions for their evaluations. The evaluation team are working with the CIF project leads to develop and implement their evaluation plans in December, January and February.

One evaluation has already begun. This is for Bun and a Blether, a workplace project. A full evaluation questionnaire has been piloted at their first workplace workshop in November. Questions were drawn from various sources but adapted to be specifically tailored to this project.

A series of peer support and evaluation skills development sessions will be held between the CIF grant holders and the evaluation team throughout 2015.

SMHAFF Evaluation

There have been various studies over the years of SMHAFF. These have usually focussed on the impact on audiences. There are three key gaps that the See Me evaluation can address:

1. Understanding the longer-term process of impact, particularly behavioural change amongst audiences
2. The extent, quality, reach and impact of media coverage of the festival
3. The impact in of participating in the festival process on artists, activists, delivery partners and people with mental health problems, particularly from an empowerment perspective

It is proposed to tackle all three of these gaps between 2014 and 2016. In 2014 (year 1), it is proposed to focus on the third gap, not least because the theme for the festival this year is power.

Immediate plan is to conduct a small piece of scoping research to explore who is involved with the festival and the impact that is has on them, which could then inform a larger piece of work.

Development of Monitoring and Mapping Systems

Within the context of the See Me programme, monitoring serves a number of functions:

- To provide evidence of the amount and type of See Me activity (outputs)
- To gauge the reach of See Me activity and change in this over time, including partners, geographies, settings and themes
- To influence decision making and future programme activity
- To contribute evidence to the wider See Me evaluation
- To support financial and resource management
- To provide feedback to funders.

The See Me evaluation team have developed a monitoring framework and associated tools to help the See Me team address these functions in a clear and consistent way, supporting them to systematically record, retain and report the most relevant data available.

Activity Mapping

The See Me team was tasked with mapping current anti-mental health stigma activity in Scotland using a set of fields developed by the evaluation team. Retrospective data was collected from the following sources:

- Previous See Me evaluation and monitoring reports
- Current See Me funded project monitoring data held by See Me
- Internet searches
- A call for evidence of projects that fit criteria to See Me contacts and other key stakeholders

The evaluation team is now working alongside the See Me team to progress this work to the point where a comprehensive data set has been collated which can be used as a baseline from which changes and developments in activity type can be tracked. The data will also be used to produce an analysis of the spheres of influence of See Me on anti-stigma and discrimination activity in Scotland.

An analysis of the extent to which current activity matches with the aims and outcomes of the new See Me programme will be undertaken for April 2015 with specific emphasis on promising activities and gaps.

Change Network Systems Mapping

A map of the mental health stigma and discrimination network in Lanarkshire, one area of Scotland has been produced. The map explores:

- How the system works (what's going on and where are the connections).
- What has really made a difference (for whom, in what circumstances and why).
- Barriers.
- Challenges.
- Facilitators.
- How See Me fits in/adds value.
- Where See Me could add value in the future.
- What is transferrable to other change networks/localities.
- The key factors that contribute to success.

The map is currently available for Lanarkshire and the See Me community team and will be used as a prototype to explore and evaluate change networks as the programme moves on to create them. In Lanarkshire, real leadership by people's lived experience has been a key strength and the See Me pledge has been the main link in to See Me.

References

McLean J (2013) See Me programme evaluation framework. Available from See Me – internal document

McLean J (2014) See Me year one evaluation report. Available from See Me – internal document

Pilgrim D, Corry P (2013) Strategic review of anti-stigma approach in Scotland, University of Liverpool

Porter S (2014) Review of branding, phase 1 report

Samh and Mhf (2013) Partnership documents for re-founded See Me Programme. Available from See Me – internal documents

Scottish Human Rights Commission. http://www.scottishhumanrights.com/humanrights/human rightsbasedapproach

The Scottish Government (2012) Mental health strategy for Scotland 2012–2015. The Scottish Government, Edinburgh

The German Mental Health Alliance

Astrid Ramge and Heike Becker

Introduction

The German Mental Health Alliance is currently the only cross-diagnosis, Germany-wide network in the field of mental health that unites a large proportion of the national nongovernmental and public stakeholders in this field. Both the Declaration of Helsinki from the European ministers of health and the so-called Green Paper from the EU Commission demand a sustainable improvement in the status of information and knowledge about mental health and the promotion of social integration of mentally ill people. The German Mental Health Alliance takes this as the starting point for its work and makes active contributions with concrete projects to implement the Green Book process in Germany.

The origins of the Alliance go back to the global program "Open The Doors," which was launched by the World Psychiatric Association (WPA) in 1996 to work against the stigmatization and discrimination of people with schizophrenia (Sartorius and Schulze 2005). The objectives of this program were to involve different stakeholders in society, affected people, and family members in long-term activities to destigmatize people with schizophrenia. In Germany, the program was coordinated by the eponymous association "Open The Doors e. V." (Baumann and Gaebel 2005). In the period that followed, the discussion among professionals in Europe broadened from the stigma of schizophrenia to the stigma of mental illnesses in general. The diagnosis-specific orientation of "Open The Doors e. V.," however, limited the further development of the content

A. Ramge (✉)
German Mental Health Alliance, Reinhardtstrasse 27B, 10117 Berlin, Germany
e-mail: Ramge@seelischegesundheit.net

H. Becker
Department of Psychiatry and Psychotherapy, Medical Faculty, Heinrich-Heine-University, LVR-Klinikum Düsseldorf, Bergische Landstrasse 2, 40629 Düsseldorf, Germany
e-mail: Heike.Becker@lvr.de

© Springer International Publishing Switzerland 2017
W. Gaebel et al. (eds.), *The Stigma of Mental Illness - End of the Story?*,
DOI 10.1007/978-3-319-27839-1_21

of anti-stigma activities and the involvement of self-support and professional organizations related to other disorders. To allow itself to open up to additional diagnoses and to facilitate the involvement of self-support and professional organizations, in 2004 "Open The Doors e. V." and the German Association for Psychiatry, Psychotherapy and Psychosomatics (DGPPN) initiated the German Mental Health Alliance (Gaebel et al. 2004). The Alliance was presented to the public for the first time in 2006. Meanwhile, it has about 80 members, including self-support groups and initiatives for those affected and relatives of people with mental illnesses as well as scientific organizations, professional associations, and charitable organizations.

Objectives

The objectives of the German Mental Health Alliance are to promote mental health in our society, prevent mental illnesses, and reduce anxiety about and prejudices towards people with mental illness. To this end, the German Mental Health Alliance wants to create links between relevant stakeholders in politics and society in order to influence the public and political dialogue through joint positions. This cause is being implemented primarily through joint informational and anti-stigma projects of the Alliance members. These projects focus on providing information for the public and on organizing events and meetings for important disseminators such as media professionals, employers, and occupational groups that deal with mentally ill people through their work.

Structure

The Alliance has adopted the following structures:

The *Steering Group* of the German Mental Health Alliance (chair Prof. W. Gaebel, German Association for Psychiatry, Psychotherapy and Psychosomatics (DGPPN); joint vice-chairs Gudrun Schliebener, Federal Association of Relatives of Mentally Ill People ("Bundesverband der Angehörigen psychisch erkrankter Menschen," BApk), and Ruth Fricke, Federal Association of People with Experience of Mental Illness ("Bundesverband Psychiatrie-Erfahrener," BPE); and 10 alliance members) are responsible for the ongoing coordination of the activities of the Alliance.

The annual *General Assembly* is attended by representatives of the individual member organizations; at this meeting, topics are presented and jointly discussed and fundamental issues are voted upon.

The work on content and concepts is performed in *Working Groups*, which are responsible for implementing the projects defined in the Steering Group and General Assembly.

The *Administrative Office* supports the Steering Group and is responsible for project management, financial management, and public relations.

The Alliance is in trusteeship of the DGPPN (German Association for Psychiatry, Psychotherapy and Psychosomatics), which is the legal representative of the Alliance.

Projects and Other Activities

Concept and Implementation of Interventions to Destigmatize Mental Illness: Results of Research and Practice

For many years, several organizations and institutions had implemented anti-stigma interventions in Germany. These interventions usually focused on only a few target groups, were mostly not implemented nationwide, and often were not evaluated (Gaebel et al. 2010). The anti-stigma project of the German Mental Health Alliance described by Gaebel et al. (2010) aimed to counteract these deficits: The aims of this project were to serve as a framework for conceptualizing and implementing interventions on the basis of scientific facts, to address a broader range of relevant target groups, and to include an evaluation of sustainable effects in reducing stigma and discrimination because of mental illness. As a first step, an international literature review was conducted and a national survey performed to assess current anti-stigma activities in Germany. Besides service users, also family members were surveyed for their needs.

Box 21.1: Interventions to Reduce Mental Illness Stigma: Results of a National Survey 2010 in Germany (Gaebel et al. 2010)
One hundred eighty-one projects were identified. Most interventions addressed the public, pupils and teachers, health professionals, or people with mental illness and their families. Many interventions focused on several of the mentioned target groups. However, often neither the target groups nor the interventions' objectives were well-defined, and there were no quantitative, measurable aims.

More than one-third of all projects were performed by psychiatric and psychotherapeutic institutions.

Box 21.2: Demands Regarding Content and Target Groups for Anti-stigma Interventions: Results from Interviews with Members of Self-Help Organizations and People with Mental Illness (Gaebel et al. 2010)
Stigma experiences because of mental illness were mostly related to the workplace, families, and friendships. Psychiatric care and government agencies were considered as other important areas of stigmatization. As a consequence, health professionals and staff of both health insurances and government agencies were identified as important target groups and disseminators.

Participants saw the necessity to advance psychiatric care structures through anti-stigma activities that should be designed in cooperation with the respective professional associations.

According to Gaebel et al. (2010), these investigations yielded the following recommendations for anti-stigma interventions:

- Interventions to destigmatize mental illness should work on different levels at the same time.
- Interventions should combine different methods (education, personal contact).
- To achieve sustainability, both education strategies and structural changes are required.
- Different areas of life are associated with different target groups and different forms of stigmatization. Consequently, different interventions are required for specific target groups, and these interventions should be interlinked.
- Interventions should be evaluated to control for sustainable effects.

Furthermore, the investigations yielded three specific areas perceived as particularly relevant for anti-stigma activities: public/media, workplace, and psychiatric care. This led to the media and workplace subprojects described in the following paragraphs, along with additional activities pursued by the German Mental Health Alliance.

Information About Mental Illnesses Provided in the Media

The presentation of mental illnesses in the media is an important factor in the perpetuation of the stigma of people with mental illnesses (Corrigan et al. 2013), whereby in particular the high proportion of negative representations is criticized (Whitley and Berry 2013). This situation has manifold negative consequences for those affected and their relatives: The stigmatization of mentally ill people reduces their participation in society (Stuart 2006; Corrigan et al. 2009) and their chances for treatment and recovery (Henderson et al. 2013). Therefore, a fundamental concern of the German Mental Health Alliance is to work towards a more balanced representation of mentally ill people in the media.

Educational Activities and Press Service

Since 2012, the German Mental Health Alliance has been implementing a comprehensive media concept as part of a 3-year media project funded by the Federal Ministry of Health (Bundesministerium für Gesundheit, BMG) in collaboration with the BApK and BPE (Fig. 21.1).

The content of the media concept covers three core messages that the Alliance wants to spread: (1) "Information" includes factual information about individual disorders, for example prevalences, symptoms, and illness courses, as well as possibilities for prevention, diagnostics, and treatability; (2) "Self-perception" refers to positive and person-related representations of people with mental illness and their

Content : 3 core messages :	Information		
	Self-perception		
	Positioning in society		
Procedures : 3 fields of work :	Press service	Training for media professionals	Training for people working in self-support

Fig. 21.1 Components of the media concept

relatives; (3) "Positioning in society" includes political demands for better care and inclusion of people with mental illness.

The concept is based on educating media representatives and people who are active in self-support. In addition to educational measures, a press service provides media professionals with background information on a monthly basis.

The trainings for media representatives are composed of the following elements:

- Experience reports from co-moderators (affected people and relatives)
- Information on the symptoms of and treatment possibilities for various illnesses
- Information on the consequences, for affected people and relatives, of the current media reporting
- Discussions of example media reports
- Practical advice for working together with affected people

The trainings for screenwriters included additional modules on typical treatment procedures, because films are particularly well suited to clearly presenting disease courses and recovery processes. For this reason, the target group was particularly interested in relevant information.

The content of the trainings for media representatives was conveyed in the form of short presentations, film contributions, and panel discussions.

The trainings for people working in self-support groups consisted of the following modules:

- General framework of media law
- How editors and journalists work
- Technical knowledge about creating and publishing contributions for different media (newspapers, newsletters, web pages, social media, and self-produced radio broadcasts)

In addition to short presentations, mainly practical exercises were used.

Box 21.3: Results of the Press Service (Becker 2015a)

The press service proved to be a suitable instrument for spreading factual information to the press and thus for promoting the information about mental illnesses among the public, but not for conveying the self-perception of affected people and their relatives.

In the period 2013 until the end of the 1st quarter 2015, 153 reports were identified that traced back to the activities of the press service and that reached over 18,075,000 people. Most of the reports fell into the following thematic categories: 68 % "Causes of illness/prevention/recognition" and 10 % "Stereotypes & inclusion." Eighty-one percent of the articles were neutral in their statements about people with mental illness, and only 3 % were positive. Over 99 % of the articles dealt with factual information and not the representation of people.

Box 21.4: Results of the Workshop for Journalists and Screenwriters (Becker 2015a)

Two 1-day trainings were conducted for journalists and two for screenwriters. The main outcome was increased awareness of opportunities to avoid stigmatizing representations in their work. The evaluation was performed with a pre/post design and self-evaluation questionnaires. In one journalist training and one screenwriter training, the participants in each training perceived significantly more possibilities to avoid stigmatizing representations in their work; in the other two trainings, the response rates were so low that possible effects could not be proven.

Screenwriters in particular have a considerable interest in realistic details and can be persuaded to give a realistic representation of people with mental illness; this was proven by qualitative responses from participants about the use of the workshop content 6 months after the workshop.

Box 21.5: Results of the Trainings for Affected People and Relatives to be Interview Partners (Becker 2015b)

The Federal Association of People with Experience of Mental Illness ("Bund der Psychiatrie-Erfahrenen," BPE) offered four 1-day trainings on interviews with journalists. They recorded the perceived self-competence as an interview partner, the self-care in dealing with media inquiries, the willingness to have contact with the media, and the knowledge about preparing for an interview. The analysis was conceived as a pre/post comparison and based on self-evaluation questionnaires.

Perceived self-competence and self-care when dealing with media contacts increased significantly immediately after the training, and a significant improvement in perceived self-competence was still present 3 months after the training. No changes were found in the willingness to have contact with the media or in knowledge about how to prepare for an interview.

In order to ensure continuity of the media project and to support the journalists in their daily work beyond the duration of the project, recommendations for journalists were developed on the basis of the workshop outcomes and published in brochures and a web portal. Here, in addition to background information, media professionals can find recommendations on correct expressions, balanced imagery, and tips for conversations with affected people and their relatives. Subject dossiers, experts, and contact addresses complete the offerings. The use of this information source is continuously promoted among media representatives through the communication campaign "Fair media – for the people, against exclusion." In this way, a joint instrument was created for the Alliance to point out the dangers of stigmatization in the media.

The Open Face Peer Interview Project

Although a large number of media reports on mental illnesses are published, only a few media reports portray the perspective of those affected and their relatives (Whitley and Berry 2013; Nairn and Coverdale 2005). This situation is only partially the fault of the actions of media representatives, because often when there are inquiries from the media no affected people or relatives can be found who are willing to present themselves to the public. Therefore, the Open Face Project, which was conducted in cooperation with the BApK, was conducted in order to find a group of affected people and relatives as contacts for the media. Additionally, the project intended to collect and publish first-hand accounts to present differentiated and person-centered portrayals as well as portrayals that previously had been under-represented in the media.

To this end, the Open Face Project followed a peer interview approach: Affected people and relatives were jointly trained as interviewers so that subsequently they could find and interview other affected people and their relatives in their circle of acquaintances. Three objectives should be achieved with this approach:

- Affected people and relatives who would like to be contacts for the media and previously had not had the opportunity to do so would have the chance to describe their experiences and, if desired, also to publish them.

- Relatives and affected people who could imagine being a contact for the media would be given the opportunity to practice an interview situation without any obligation.
- The experiences of relatives and affected people would be collected and serve as suggestions for self-support groups and their members.

The interviewers were recruited among the members of the BapK and other self-support organizations with the help of flyers and internet announcements and received a 1-day schooling from the BApK that introduced them to the use of the interview guide. The guide contained predefined thematic blocks. For each thematic block, suggestions for questions were provided that served as ideas and did not have to be adhered to.

The thematic blocks dealt with contacts with self-support and the care system, the perception of the media representation of people with mental illness, and any involvement in public relations as an affected person or relative. As part of the evaluation, the following questions were considered: What motivates relatives and affected people to become publicly involved, how do they react to media reports that they find particularly positive or negative, and who supports them in case of public protest?

Meanwhile, the interview phase has been completed, and the interviews have been subjected to a qualitative analysis of their content; the results are presented in Box 21.6.

Box 21.6: Results of the Open Face Peer Interview Project (Becker 2015b)

The Federal Association of Relatives of Mentally Ill People ("Bundesverband der Angehörigen psychisch erkrankter Menschen," BApk) collected a total of 62 interviews. The current media representation of mentally ill people often is rated negatively in the interviews, whereby negative representations repeatedly provoke anger or indignation. The most common reaction involving others is to seek a conversation in the self-help group or with other contacts.

Important reasons for refusing to have contact with the media are consideration of the family and the emotional effort and pain that can be associated with a media appearance. One interview partner expressed also the concern about being put at a disadvantage in future dealings with medical providers after publicly criticizing treatments.

The motivation to have contact with the media originates from the desire for clarification in the sense of a correct representation of mental illnesses, the desire to help other people, and also the gratefulness for the own recovery and the need to be able to pass on these positive experiences to other people.

Mental Health at the Workplace

Mental health problems have become one of the leading causes of sick leave from work and early retirement all over Europe (Järvisalo et al. 2005; Office for National Statistics 2014). Therefore, maintaining good mental health is crucial for individuals, employers, and society as a whole.

The German Mental Health Alliance pursues this objective mainly by offering training for relevant target groups and promoting both the professional dialogue and the formulation of political demands through conferences and meetings.

Joint Conference on Mental Health and Well-Being at the Workplace in Close Cooperation with the WHO and European Commission

In 2009, the World Health Organization (WHO) Regional Office and the German Mental Health Alliance held a joint conference on "Mental health and well-being at the workplace – Protection and inclusion in challenging times" in Berlin. The conference was organized in cooperation with the European Commission and DG Health and Consumers and supported by the German Federal Ministry of Health. The scope and purpose of the conference was to discuss the challenges of mental health and well-being at the workplace in the face of difficult economic times, thereby focusing on the social integration and empowerment of vulnerable people. The aims were to identify best practices and to make policy recommendations for employers and the political institutions concerned.

Management Trainings

The thoughtfully selected target groups were managers and human resources staff. These groups were chosen because they make employment decisions, shape working conditions, and usually are the direct contact for employees in a company. However, many managers are not sufficiently prepared for dealing with employees who encounter mental strain or illness. In a survey among managers in Germany, 85 % of the participating managers stated that they inadequately recognize mental stresses among employees; 87 % felt unsure about suitable behavior when dealing with people with mental problems (DGFP 2011).

Therefore, the German Mental Health Alliance conceived a target group-specific intervention to destigmatize mental illnesses. The intervention consisted of training for managers and accompanying information on the topic "mental health at the workplace." The project was implemented in collaboration with the BApK and the German Depression League and comprised the following topics:

- Explanations about selected mental illnesses and their causes
- Information on the needs of mentally ill employees
- Suitable behavior during personal contact with affected employees

Additional areas were reintegration into the workplace and the prevention of mental illness as part of the company's health management. A core component of the seminar was the inclusion of a speaker with a mental illness, who spoke about lived experiences.

To enable early help, in all parts of the training, great importance was placed on overcoming inhibitions about addressing affected employees personally. The content was illustrated through talks, group exercises, and a specially developed educational film that depicted discussions with employees and the reintegration process through personal examples.

For the model project, trainings were performed in public administrations and in a large German steel company. As a result of the model project, the German Mental Health Alliance meanwhile has developed a generally accessible training option for companies. The 1-day seminars are held regularly at interested companies and supplemented with additional offerings in the form of action guidelines, information brochures, and evaluation discussions with a view to preventative health management.

> **Box 21.7: Findings from an Anti-stigma Intervention with Managers**
> One-day trainings for managers were held at three companies, and the managers were surveyed. The evaluation was a simple control-group comparison with two conditions: the intervention group received the trainings whereas the control group did not participate in any such measures.
>
> In the intervention group, the social distance was decreased, and in comparison with the control group this decrease was still present after 3 months. With respect to the treatment methods, after the intervention the role of both medications and psychiatric care was viewed more optimistically.

Mental Health Awareness Weeks

On the occasion of the World Mental Health Day on October 10th, initiated by the World Federation for Mental Health (WFMH) and the WHO, awareness weeks or days take place in all major cities across Germany. One of the largest events is the Berlin Week of Mental Health, which is organized by the German Mental Health Alliance with the support of the Berlin Senate. More than 200 events take place, at which laypeople and professionals obtain information on new developments in mental health, gain insight into the comprehensive help system, and learn about treatment options for people with mental health problems. Since 2006, the German Mental Health Alliance has set the main topic, coordinated the individual events, and taken care of the main advertising and communication activities.

Anti-stigma Award

Once a year since 2003, the German Mental Health Alliance together with the DGPPN (German Association for Psychiatry, Psychotherapy and Psychosomatics) has awarded the DGPPN Anti-stigma Award, endowed with € 10,000. The award acknowledges initiatives that advocate in an exemplary manner the destigmatization and inclusion of people with mental illness and whose commitment exceeds the scope and content of the societal or professional mission of the applicant organizations. For years, the jury has recorded an increasing number of applications from self-support initiatives, psychosocial facilities, and care and research institutions and also from private companies, so that the award has become an instrument for identifying and promoting new and exceptional approaches to anti-stigma work in Germany.

Conclusions and Perspectives

Networks of different civic and public players can make manifold contributions to the destigmatization of people with mental illness, particularly in countries with no national campaigns and predominantly local anti-stigma work.

The large base of heterogeneous organizations allows the Alliance to handle a wide range of activities and inquiries from third parties. Smaller member organizations leverage from the Alliance's central press work resources and thereby promote nationwide efforts on a local level.

Future anti-stigma efforts will have to further differentiate the different target groups and address them with more custom-tailored offerings. Particularly in the field of the media, this implies a distinction between journalists who report about current events and those who provide their audience with background information. Furthermore, anti-stigma efforts directed at the media will have to consider major changes happening in the media industry: (1) a growing proportion of freelance part-time journalists, (2) the financial pressure on editorial offices, and (3) the growing importance of social media also in the field of classical journalism. Altogether, these trends call for significantly shorter interventions, including virtual and video formats that could reach larger numbers of individual journalists and whole editorial teams. Also, social media interventions will require more interactive and collaborative strategies to target journalists and the general public.

Anti-stigma efforts regarding the workplace should continue to promote changes in management and employee behavior. However, they also should include more and more networking between employers, job centers, authorities, and care facilities. Apart from these demands, suitable interventions are needed for small and medium-sized businesses, which then have to be disseminated, particularly within this specific business segment.

In general, future projects should create more structures within the participating organizations, allowing for a routine continuation of completed projects. The individual partners of the German Mental Health Alliance can contribute in manifold ways to solving these persisting and new challenges.

References

Baumann A, Gaebel W (2005) "Open The Doors" in Deutschland ["Open The Doors" in Germany]. In: Gaebel W, Möller H-J, Rössler W (eds) Stigma – Diskriminierung – Bewältigung. Der Umgang mit sozialer Ausgrenzung psychisch Kranker. Kohlhammer, Stuttgart, pp 249–260

Becker H (2015a) Medienprojekt – Evaluation der ABSG-Workshops und des Pressedienstes [The Media Project – an evaluation of the ABSG workshops and news services]. Unpublished report, Dusseldorf

Becker H (2015b) Stärkung der Medienkompetenz der Selbsthilfe - Evaluation der Partner-Teilprojekte 2013/2014 [Strengthening the medias competence for self-help organizations – an evaluation of the partner projects 2013/2014]. Unpublished report, Dusseldorf

Corrigan PW, Larson JE, Rüsch N (2009) Self-stigma and the "why try" effect: impact on life goals and evidence-based practices. World Psychiatry 8(2):75–81

Corrigan PW, Powell KJ, Michaels PJ (2013) The effects of news stories on the stigma of mental illness. J Nerv Ment Dis 201:179–182

DGFP (2011) DGFP Studie: Psychische Beanspruchung von Mitarbeitern und Führungskräften. Praxispapier 2-2011 [DGFP Study: Psychological strain in employees and supervisors. Paper 2-2011]. Retrieved from: http://www.dgfp.de/wissen/praxispapiere

Gaebel W, Zäske H, Baumann A (2004) Stigma erschwert Behandlung und Integration [Stigma complicates treatment and integration]. Deutsches Ärzteblatt 48:A3253–A3255

Gaebel W, Ahrens W, Schlamann P (2010) Konzeption und Umsetzung von Interventionen zur Entstigmatisierung seelischer Erkrankungen: Empfehlungen und Ergebnisse aus Forschung und Praxis [Conception and implementation of interventions to destigmatize mental illness: recommendations and results of research and praxis]. Aktionsbündnis Seelische Gesundheit, Berlin

Henderson C, Evans-Lacko S, Thornicroft G (2013) Mental illness stigma, help seeking, and public health programs. Am J Pub Health 103(5):777–780

Järvisalo J, Andersson B, Boedeker W, Houtman I (eds) (2005) Mental disorders as a major challenge in prevention of work disability: experiences in Finland, Germany, the Netherlands and Sweden, Social security and health reports 66. KELA, Helsinki

Nairn RG, Coverdale JH (2005) People never see us living well. Aust N Z J Psychiatry 39:281–287

Office for National Statistics (2014) Sickness absence in the labour market, February 2014. Retrieved from http://data.gov.uk/dataset/sickness_absence_in_the_labour_market

Sartorius N, Schulze H (2005) Reducing the stigma of mental illness. A report from a global programme of the Word Psychiatric Association. Cambridge University Press, New York

Stuart H (2006) Mental illness and employment discrimination. Curr Opin Psychiatry 19(5):522–526

Whitley R, Berry S (2013) Trends in newspaper coverage of mental illness in Canada: 2005–2010. Can J Psychiatry 58(2):107–112

Stigma in Midsize European Countries

22

Alina Beldie, Cecilia Brain, Maria Luisa Figueira,
Igor Filipcic, Miro Jakovljevic, Marek Jarema,
Oguz Karamustafalioglu, Daniel König,
Blanka Kores Plesničar, Josef Marksteiner, Filipa Palha,
Jan Pecenák, Dan Prelipceanu, Petter Andreas Ringen,
Magdalena Tyszkowska, and Johannes Wancata

A. Beldie
Department of Psychiatry Middelfart, Region of Southern Denmark, Middelfart, Denmark

C. Brain
Institute of Neuroscience and Physiology, Department of Psychiatry and Neurochemistry,
Sahlgrenska Academy, University of Gothenburg, Gothenburg, Sweden

M.L. Figueira
Department of Psychiatry, University of Lisbon, Lisbon, Portugal

I. Filipcic • M. Jakovljevic
Department of Psychiatry, University Hospital Center Zagreb, Zagreb, Croatia

M. Jarema • M. Tyszkowska
3rd Department of Psychiatry, Institute of Psychiatry and Neurology, Warsaw, Poland

O. Karamustafalioglu
Psychiatry Department, Sisli Etfal Teaching and Research Hospital, Istanbul, Turkey

D. König
Clinical Division of Social Psychiatry, Department of Psychiatry and Psychotherapy, Medical
University of Vienna, Vienna, Austria

B.K. Plesničar
University Psychiatric Hospital Ljubljana, 1260 Ljubljana-Polje, Slovenia

J. Marksteiner
Department of Psychiatry and Psychotherapy A, LKH Hall, Hall in Tirol, Austria

F. Palha
Association Encontrar+se (Association to Support Persons with Severe Mental Disorders),
Faculty of Education and Psychology, Portuguese Catholic University, Lisbon, Portugal

J. Pecenák
Clinic of Psychiatry, Faculty of Medicine, University Hospital, Bratislava, Slovakia

D. Prelipceanu
Department of Psychiatry, Carol Davila Medicine and Pharmacy University,
Bucharest, Romania

© Springer International Publishing Switzerland 2017
W. Gaebel et al. (eds.), *The Stigma of Mental Illness - End of the Story?*,
DOI 10.1007/978-3-319-27839-1_22

417

P.A. Ringen
Specialized Inpatient Department, Gaustad, Division for Mental Health and Addiction, Oslo
University Hospital, Oslo, Norway

J. Wancata (⊠)
Clinical Division of Social Psychiatry, Department of Psychiatry and Psychotherapy, Medical
University of Vienna, Währinger Gürtel 18-20, Vienna 1090, Austria
e-mail: johannes.wancata@meduniwien.ac.at

Introduction

Since many decades it is known that persons suffering from mental disorders are stigmatised. Several authors consider stigma as one of the most important obstacles to the provision of mental health care, and to the development of mental health programmes, it has been increasing in parallel with the improvement in treatment of mental disorders (Fabrega 1990; Schulze and Angermeyer 2002; Schöny 1998).

Numerous authors suggested that changes in mental health care and new treatment options for mental disorders would automatically reduce stigma. Since the old and large mental hospitals segregated mentally ill persons from the community, some authors had the idea that the closure of these hospitals and development of community psychiatric services would decrease stigma automatically. The development of community psychiatric services resulted in numerous advantages for persons with severe mental illness. Similarly, the development of psychiatric inpatient departments in general hospitals has a lot of advantages for their patients. Some authors had the idea that the introduction of effective medications with less observable side effects (e.g. extrapyramidal symptoms of antipsychotics) would reduce the false idea that mental disorders are incurable.

Unfortunately, stigma is present until now, and we do not know if and how much these developments in the health-care system and treatments influenced the amount of stigma and discrimination. We had to learn that stigma is a relevant problem until now. This led mental health workers as well as policymakers to undertake a variety of activities, hoping that these would reduce the stigma of mental illness (Paykel et al. 1998; Meise et al. 2000).

The present paper attempts to briefly report the situation and activities in some selected midsize European countries. From each of these countries, authors selected some aspects which they consider to be important in this context.

Austria

In Austria, the past decades have seen a continuing effort to reduce the stigmatisation of mentally ill patients in the society. Besides aiming to reduce the burden placed upon patients in general, these campaigns often especially focus on stigma reduction regarding patients suffering of schizophrenia. Austria was one of the countries joining the global programme of the World Psychiatric Association (WPA)

"Open the Doors" against the stigmatisation and discrimination due to schizophrenia from the very beginning (Schöny 1998).

Several organisations conducted programmes either in a regional effort, within a federal district or nationwide. These activities aimed either at the general population, on pupils and teachers, on health-care professionals or on mentally ill persons and their families. The organisations included the Austrian Association of Psychiatry and Psychotherapy, the Austrian Schizophrenia Association, the Austrian Association of Family Caregivers (HPE) and *pro mente Austria* (umbrella organisation of numerous community service providers).

The relevance of the aforementioned focus on the anti-stigma campaigns on persons suffering from schizophrenia is shown by a study conducted 5 years after completion of the World Psychiatric Association (WPA) "Open the Doors" programme. The authors demonstrated that nearly a quarter (22.3 %) of the study, population did not know the meaning of "schizophrenia", 81.3 % did not want to receive information about this illness and 64.1 % agreed with a statement that patients with schizophrenia are dangerous. This indicates the importance of activities against stigma, but shows that the effect of past programmes was rather limited (Grausgruber et al. 2009).

Educational methods specifically addressing children and adolescents have been shown to have the potential to reduce stigmatisation. This study was part of the WPA programme. Two educational units in a secondary school were successful in reducing stigmatisation towards patients with affective disorder as well as patients with schizophrenia. It has been shown that especially the personal contact with mentally ill patients was effective in reducing stigma (Kohlbauer et al. 2010).

Since 2009 several large health-care providers initiated a regular information day about mental illness in the capital city of Austria, Vienna. The enterprise including most of the hospitals in Vienna (Wiener Krankenanstaltenverbund), the largest provider of community psychiatric services in Vienna (Psychosozialer Dienst Wien) and the municipal coordination for services treating addiction (Sucht- und Drogenkoordination Wien) are organising this information day ("Tag der seelischen Gesundheit"). The fact that it is located in the city hall of Vienna shows the relevance of this activity.

During this event the general public is being informed about mental illness in the form of lectures, personal talks with experts, panel discussions and advisory groups. In the last 5 years, themes included prevention and treatment of mental illness such as depression, eating disorders, schizophrenia, substance abuse and addiction. In addition, short courses on relaxation techniques and becoming more active were offered. Furthermore, numerous psychiatric health-care providers, specialised clinics, treatment programmes and self-help groups offered more than 50 information desks. The purpose of these information desks was to provide informal and personal contact in order to encourage help seeking. Each year, thousands of citizens are attending this information day.

In 2011, well-known journalists, politicians, actors, artists and health professionals initiated a platform to initiate discussion and information in the general populations about mental health. The name of this platform "ganznormal.at" means "completely normal" and should be a hint that mental illness is very common and everybody can develop a mental disorder at some time in his or her life. The goal is to raise the level of acceptance for persons suffering from mental illness and thus reduce stigma. Further, the members of this platform try to inform the public that mentally ill should not be treated different from physically ill persons.

Finally, for two decades the "World Mental Health Day" is being used to inform mass media and the population about mental illness in order to reduce its stigma. In the year 2014, its theme was "Living with Schizophrenia in Austria".

Croatia

Stigmatisation against those suffering from mental illnesses is still a large problem in Croatian society. This finding is independent of age or gender as reported from a study in the year 2003. A lower level of education was a predictor of stigmatisation (Filipcić 2003).

The Croatian Society for Clinical Psychiatry as well as the Section for Psychotherapy and Psychosocial Treatment of Psychoses (ISPS Croatia) of the "Croatian Medical Association" initiated one of the country's first programmes against stigmatisation, the "Patient Empowerment Programme". Since 1998 the goal of the programme has been to help patients suffering from mental illnesses to develop coping skills for overcoming negative consequences of stigma, especially self-stigmatisation. Stigmatisation and self-stigmatisation of the participants of a group were evaluated before and after intervention, showing a significant decrease (Ivezic et al. 2009).

In 2002, "the programme to reduce stigma and discrimination of mental patients" was started by the "Ministry of Science, Education and Sports" of Croatia. Developed according to the guidelines of the WPA "Open the Doors" programme, it was led by the "Department of Psychiatry of the University Hospital in Zagreb" in collaboration with the "School of Medicine of The University of Zagreb" and the "Croatian Psychiatric Association".

This programme, lasting for 6 years, was targeted at the general population, as well as specific groups such as patients with schizophrenia and their families, medical professionals, medical students and secondary school students. In the first 3-year period, the programme focused on stigma related to schizophrenia and psychotic disorders, while in the next 3 year the focus widened, also including affective disorders.

As part of the nationwide campaign, the general public was informed with educational lectures, workshops and seminars. Newspapers and radio and television stations participated in these activities.

One of the results was to revise the undergraduate and postgraduate curricula at the School of Medicine, which now include lectures on the stigmatisation of people suffering from mental disorders.

Norway

The Norwegian society has some strength such as open-mindedness, informality and equality, possibly making stigmatisation of mentally ill patients a smaller problem than in other societies. This assumption seems to be supported by the fact that the prime minister announced that due to a depressive episode, he intends to take a 2-week sick leave and the public reaction were mostly not negative, but rather positive. Yet the rise in high-profile members of society publicly speaking about their mental illnesses as well as substance abuse has put the need for a better treatment of mentally ill on the public agenda as well as gathered media attention.

After the rise of the institutionalisation of mentally ill in the mid of the nineteenth century in Norway, society grew ever less accustomed to interact with people suffering from mental disorders. Starting in the 1960s of the twentieth century, the Norwegian society became more and more concerned about aspects of inhumanity in the mental health-care system. Inspired by the changes in other countries at the same time, the public opinion changed. As a result multidisciplinary community treatment was developed in Norway instead of the traditional mental hospitals. Even for people with severe mental disorders living within a normal housing situation was established.

This paradigm shift was however accompanied by a paradox in media coverage: On the one hand, psychiatric services were being criticised for setting possibly dangerous people loose and, on the other hand, for not reducing compulsory treatment and use of force fast enough.

The man who performed the terror attacks in the Oslo area on July 22, 2011, drew massive public attention to the suspected dangerousness of persons with mental illness. The terrorist was deemed psychotic in the first forensic psychiatric evaluation, but the verdict, after the second psychiatric evaluation, found him not to be so at the time of the killings and thus responsible for his actions. This case has spurred several new laws with the intention to improve control of severely mentally ill who might have the potential for violent acts.

A study intended to survey the attitudes as well as the beliefs in the population demonstrated that Norwegians commonly believe psychiatric patients to be dangerous and in need of hospitalisation. These beliefs were especially prevalent amongst the younger age groups (Hamre et al. 1994). In line with this study are findings of a qualitative study surveying psychiatric patients living in rural communities, showing that they suffer from isolation and loneliness, low self-esteem, no paid work, lack of money, discrimination and harassment (Thesen 2001).

In 2007, the Norwegian Directorate for Public Health launched the anti-stigma campaign "Et åpent sinn" ("An Open Mind") targeting first the younger age groups as a continuation of a previously launched school-based mental health information campaign ("Mental Health in Schools" [2004–2008]) and the general adult population later. Students were educated about possibilities to provide support for each other, where to seek help and about ways to safeguard their own mental health. Participants included the Norwegian Directorate for Health and Social Affairs, the Directorate for Education and Training, the Mental Health Organization, the

Norwegian Council for Mental Health, the Psychiatric Educational Foundation and the Adults for Children Organization. The effort included advertisements in magazines, cinemas and the Internet highlighting the fact that "everyone may get mental health problems". Due to the higher threshold for communication and help-seeking behaviours, men were targeted in particular in the "Adults and Men" part of the campaign.

To further reduce discrimination against members of society, the Equality and Anti-Discrimination Ombudsman was established as an independent contact in case of discrimination. Administratively, this position is within the Ministry of Children and Equality. For the supervision of public administration agencies, the Parliamentary Ombudsman is responsible.

Poland

In Poland, the prevalence of the serious mental disorders is similar to that in other countries. Hence, about 1.2–1.5 million people are affected by depression and 400,000 people suffer from schizophrenia. On the other hand, approximately 50–60 % of individuals with mental health problems who should seek help in psychiatric services do not do it for various reasons.

The public knowledge of mental health problems is definitely unsatisfied in Poland. It is changing very slowly. In the last years, since 2000, few surveys on public opinion about mental health and mentally ill persons in society were conducted by CBOS, the independent public opinion research agency. The results found amongst a representative group of Polish adults confirmed a low awareness of mental health disorders. At the same time, 61 % of the respondents observe in the close community swearwords and negative stereotypes in description of mentally ill persons, while only 25 % witness positive attitudes. In Poland, a mental illness is often perceived as a reason for shame for the persons who suffer as well as for their families. Therefore, the fact that somebody suffers from mental health problems is often kept as a secret from others. The distance or ignorance towards people suffering from mental disorders reaches also employment and law issues.

Unquestionable, breakthrough in anti-stigma activities in Poland started with "Schizophrenia: Open the Doors" programme launched in the year 2000. That particular anti-stigma campaign has raised the awareness of the problems mentally ill patients encounter in their life. The Board of Polish Psychiatric Association and Institute of Psychiatry and Neurology in Warsaw have patronised the campaign. "Schizophrenia: Open the Doors" has permanently grown into Polish public reality. Nevertheless, it was transformed from national range campaign about schizophrenia to general anti-stigma campaign, locally specific projects of people with mental health problems and disabilities. At present, the size and range of the programme depend on the source of local funding, as well as local needs. There is no formal data on the results of this anti-stigma campaign and others performed locally. Without strong local initiative how to find the financial resources and without general governmental involvement in mental health problems, we should not expect bigger progress in the nearer future.

Portugal

Amongst other reasons, lack of investment and the resulting absence of specialised services were cited in the report of the Mental Health Plan 2007–2016 as reasons why only a small percentage of the people experiencing mental health problems have access to mental health services, concluding that "mental health services have severe deficits in terms of accessibility, equity, and quality of care" (Ministério da Saúde 2007). The consequences of this situation have been reported year after year, and in the 2014 report, it was once more highlighted the great burden resulting from mental illnesses (assessed in terms of YLD and DALY) when compared to other health problems (Saúde 2014). Stigma has been identified as one of the reasons for the mental health situation in Portugal (Foreword of the Secretary of State Assistant to the Minister of Health in ENCONTRAR+SE's latest edition, by Rosalynn Carter (Carter 2014)).

Until 2007 no national anti-stigma campaign had been implemented in Portugal. It was then that ENCONTRAR+SE (ENCONTRAR+SE – Associação para a Promoção da saúde Mental, Association for the Promotion of Mental Health) started its first national anti-stigma campaign, which gave birth to a movement to combat stigma and discrimination of mental illnesses: "Movimento UPA – Unidos para Ajudar. Levanta-te contra o stigma e a discriminação das doenças mentais" (United to Help Movement. Stand up against stigma and discrimination towards mental disorders). In a positive and constructive way, UPA aims to help people move one step forward in the acceptance and understanding of mental disorders. It is addressed both for those who do not accept having a problem, who delay help seeking, and who suffer because of a mental disorder and for everyone who deals badly with this reality. UPA aims to bring hope and promote change.

The first project, "UPA08 – a song for mental health", brought together 20 bands, 10 songs, 10 film directors and 10 illustrators. For 10 months, on the tenth of each month, a song, a film and a poster were available for download in the ENCONTRAR+SE website. These musicians have translated the causes we defend into poetic lyrics and sounds. Each song represents a thematic polarity that alerts to the impact of stigma and what needs to be changed. In partnership with radio stations and other media, the UPA movement was disseminated and commented on TV, newspapers and blogs, around the country. The CD was released exclusively at FNAC stores and sold out in a few weeks. Hundreds of people worked on this project. Thousands joined in, and about 3,000,000 were exposed to the campaign (Beldie et al. 2012).

In 2009, the UPA movement started "UPA Makes a Difference", a school-based initiative to improve mental health literacy amongst young people. Twelve schools and more than 1,000 students participated. A website was also created where students could find information regarding mental health and could exhibit the interventions they did in the context of the project. In only 1 month, the website registered 17,000 visits (http://upafazadiferenca.encontrarse.pt). It was followed by "UPA Teachers Make a Difference", targeting school teachers (Campos et al. 2012). ENCONTRAR+SE is also a partner in the "Finding Space to Mental Health – Promoting mental health in adolescents (12–14 year-olds): Development and evaluation of an intervention" project, developed by the Faculty of Education and Psychology, Catholic University of Portugal, and funded by Science and Technology Foundation (Campos et al. 2014).

In 2010, an informative website providing quality contents and the possibility to clarify doubts by a health-care professional was launched (UPA INFORMS). Since then, more than 24,000 people have visited it. In 2011, we launched the "UPA Office", a community-based facility that provided clinical and social support to 75 individuals. In 2011, UPA Movement promoted the "UPA Walk" against stigma in which more than 700 people participated. In 2014, the UPA Movement started the "UPA Recognition Award" to honour national and international personalities with active voice in the fight against stigma and discrimination of the mental illnesses and to pay tribute to all that joined us.

Romania

Negative stereotypes about persons with mental illness, such as patients who are dangerous, need seclusion from society and are incurably sick, are still prevalent in the Romanian society. Media still routinely use stigmatising terms such as "mad people" or "madness". Similar to other countries, this stigma is mostly associated with schizophrenia and less with other mental illnesses such as depression or addiction.

This stigmatisation by society might result in delayed help seeking and trying to hide they have ever been ill or have been admitted to a psychiatric hospital. Even more crucial is the fact that nonpsychiatric medical doctors frequently neglect their duties and avoid contact with patients suffering from mental illness and refuse advice for or treatment of their physical illness. These prejudices against members of society suffering from mental illnesses also lead to a reluctance of family members of patients meeting in associations, leading to such groups becoming inactive and sometimes ceasing to exist.

After Romania joined the European Union (EU), a number of anti-stigma campaigns were cooperatively initiated. But when national mental health activities ended, so did the joint programmes.

The Ministry of Health, through the National Mental Health Programme, initiated a programme in four high schools in Bucharest in the first quarter of 2008 entitled "Schizophrenia Should Not Be a Reason for Discrimination". Students were directly involved in the organisation and implementation of the programme and campaign directed at increasing their knowledge of mental health and illness and the discrimination and stigmatisation associated with it.

"Trust My Mind! STOP the Prejudices Against Mental Illness" was a campaign in Targu Mures between November of 2007 and January of 2008 to increase the general population's tolerance towards patients suffering from mental illness. It focused on the qualities of people with mental illnesses and their right to work, stressing the idea of social inclusion and thus showing the benefits of interaction instead of asking for pity.

In 2007, the EU-funded programme "Confide in Their Mind" took place in six cities (Iaşi, Cluj, Timişoara, Craiova, Constanţa and Targu Mures) focusing on the evaluation of discriminatory attitudes and on the need to form a correct image about people with mental health problems.

Slovakia

Stigmatisation of members of society with mental illnesses is very common in Slovakia, as is stigmatisation of mental health disciplines. Although research into this subject is proposed in Slovakia's National Programme of Mental Health, data is still sparse.

In a study analysing 150 reports within three weekly magazines in two separate 20-month periods, the most frequent association made with mental disorders was "criminal activities" (André and Čaplová 2000).

After the publication of the first epidemiological study on depression within the Slovakian adult population, the associated Internet discussion on the article was analysed. The generally negative and dismissive consensus was that "Depression is a myth", "a weak construct", "something everybody can pretend to have" and "a diagnosis developed by pharmaceutical companies" (Heretik and Mullerovzá 2005). Amongst medical student who had previously undergone the training in psychiatry, the most frequent attributions to characterise patients with schizophrenia were "unstable", "uncritical" and "unpredictable" (Čaplová et al. 1997).

From 2001 onwards nice campaigns focusing on the de-stigmatisation of psychiatric illness have been started. They include interviews on radio and television, posters in public places, commercials, concerts and other activities.

Annually on the World Mental health Day, a large fundraising event organised by non-governmental organisation League for Mental Health (www.dusevnezdravie. sk) is taking place, called the "Day of Forget-Me-Nots" with people displaying forget-me-not flowers on their lapels and young people collecting money on the street which will then be divided amongst organisations committed to helping the members of society suffering from mental illnesses.

Slovenia

We have come a long way, yet, despite our wishes, stigma and discrimination unfortunately still exist in Slovenia. Like in many other countries, Slovenian psychiatric patients are underprivileged when it comes to schooling, employment, inclusion in social networks and nonpsychiatric health care. However, true, this strong statement is unfortunately scientifically and statistically unsupported due to the lack of properly conducted studies.

In the article published by the Economist Intelligence Unit in 2014, the EUI's Mental Health Integration Index measures the degree of governmental support regarding the integration of people with mental illnesses into society in 30 European countries (Unit T.E.I. 2014). Overall, Slovenia reached a reputable ninth place. Regarding the *access to health services* index, Slovenia ranked second, while the assessments of *providing stable home and family*, *improving work and education opportunities* and *reducing stigma and increasing awareness* put our country in the middle of the scale. These data should serve as the basis for improving critical and/or thus far neglected areas, including fighting against stigma and anti-stigma programmes.

The most common mental disorders in primary care settings in Slovenia are a cluster of anxiety, acute stress and adjustment disorders and depression (Unit T.E.I. 2014). Slovenia has one of the highest suicide rates in the world (21.2 per 100.000 in the year 2011) and is currently ranking third amongst 17 EU countries (Trdič et al. 2012). Every third person that committed suicide in 2011 was over 65 years.

The most frequent reasons for hospitalisation in a psychiatric facility are alcohol addiction and related problems and schizophrenia (21.8 % and 12.7 % of all psychiatric hospitalisations, respectively). Alcohol and drug addictions represent a serious public health problem (Trdič et al. 2012). Psychiatric disorders account for more than a quarter of all disability retirements (Trdič et al. 2012).

These are good reasons why Slovenia actively participates in various European projects. The ACTION-FOR-HEALTH project includes ten European countries. Its aim is to improve health and quality of life of the population and to reduce health inequality. Slovenia is an important partner in the EMCDDA (European Monitoring Centre for Drugs and Drug Addiction) project, which monitors the incidence of both known and new psychoactive substances in the EU. In the RARHA (Joint Action on Reducing Alcohol Related Harm) project, Slovenia and Germany jointly lead the part of the programme concerned with the tasks of recognising the examples of good practice in reducing alcohol-induced damage and identifying the criteria for the assessment of approaches regarding their efficacy, comparability and applicability (Trdič et al. 2012). Due to the aforementioned high suicide rates, Slovenia is very active also in the EUREGENAS (European Regions Enhancing Action Against Suicide) project. We marked the World Suicide Prevention Day with the "Let's cycle the world" initiative and outdoor concerts for raising awareness about this problem and reducing stigma.

The topics of stigma and de-stigmatisation are not left out completely; occasionally, opinions of leading Slovenian psychiatrists are published, usually as interviews in local newspapers and magazines. However, up to date only one research on the significance of stigma in the mental health area has been published. It compared the attitudes of psychiatric patients and students towards stigma of mental illness (Strbad et al. 2008). The outcome of the study surprised the researchers, as the results showed that the attitude of psychiatric patients suffering from severe mental illnesses towards their own group was much more negative compared to the students' views. The former were also prone to self-stigmatisation (Strbad et al. 2008). This finding was the exact opposite of the expected outcome – one would think that the patients would be more understanding of their peers since they share the knowledge and the common experience of the illness. It turned out that these patients were already suffering enough from their illness and stigmatisation; therefore they were not keen on reinforcing it by socialising with others like themselves.

In 2015, Slovenia will host the 25th Alzheimer Europe Conference. Hosting the anniversary conference is an affirmation of numerous anti-stigma activities of the Slovenian Dementia Association Spominčica. One of the most important goals of the association is raising public awareness about dementia and dementia-related problems by counselling phone lines and Alzheimer Cafés where at designated times professionals provide free advice and help.

One of the cornerstones of de-stigmatisation in Slovenia should have been the new Mental Health Act, adopted by the Slovenian parliament in 2009 (Slovenia 2009). However, to active partners in the treatment of mental disorders, the act has been a disappointment and is now awaiting amendments.

Resolution on the National Mental Health Programme 2014–2018, the first national strategic document pertaining to mental health, is being debated at national level (Slovenia 2014). Its mission is to maintain and improve the mental health of the entire population by offering support to vulnerable groups. Its final goal is to increase the quality of life of all Slovenian residents – from the public health point of view, maintaining and improving mental health are of key importance for the entire population and not only for individuals with mental health problems. The resolution is based on the principles of interdisciplinary and intersectoral cooperation at the political and legislative level. It incorporates protection of human rights; the rule of law; the welfare state; promotion and protection of mental health; positive discrimination of vulnerable population groups; de-stigmatisation; inclusion of persons with mental problems; decentralisation and accessibility of mental health services; community care and rehabilitation of persons with mental disorders; safety, quality, professionalism, efficacy, accessibility and continuity of treatment that meets users' expectations and abides by professionally approved methods and internationally confirmed standards; continuous education and training of professionals; updating methods of mental health promotion, protection and prevention; adjustment to users' actual needs; the use of the least restrictive treatment methods; coordination of needs and resources; cost efficacy; and evidence-based activities.

Hopefully, the adoption of the resolution and the financing of the abovementioned activities will gradually start to change the face of mental health in Slovenia. The National Mental Health Programme offers the possibilities of the implementation of de-stigmatisation measures that should be applied promptly, but also wisely. Despite new legislation and the active involvement of individual experts, the battle against the stigma of mental illness in Slovenia is only just beginning since good anti-stigma programmes still need to be developed. Sadly, verbalised wishes often cannot materialise on their own.

Sweden

Stigma of and suffering from mental illness have been on the agenda of the Swedish government during the last years. The public awareness of stigma has increased but there are still quite a few remaining obstacles (Beldie et al. 2012). To date there has been little research done about stigma in Sweden, and only a few studies explore the actual experiences of people with mental illness. A recent study showed that almost two-thirds of the included persons with schizophrenia ($n=111$) had experienced stigma and discrimination in social relationships in making/keeping friends and in the neighbourhood (Brain et al. 2014). About half of the participants reported discrimination by their families, in intimate relationships, concerning employment and by mental health staff. Most patients (88 %) felt a need to conceal their mental illness and avoided close personal relationships due to anticipated stigma and discrimination.

Prior to a large mental health-care reform in Sweden in 1995, an investigation concluded that individuals with mental illnesses had less social interaction compared to patients with other disorders. Therefore an important goal for the health-care reform was the integration of patients with mental illness into society. The practice of providing individual housing solutions for patients was later strongly criticised for contributing to increased social isolation and exclusion. Placing mentally ill members of society in apartments without sufficient social and occupational support may also have contributed to increased stigma and discrimination.

The Swedish Schizophrenia Fellowship initiated the first national anti-stigma campaign in 1997. The aims were to inform the general public about schizophrenia and to reduce stigma and prejudices regarding such afflictions. Family members of mentally ill persons were also acknowledged as in need of help and places to meet. All together the campaign led to more phone calls at the Schizophrenia Fellowship as well as roughly 1,000 additional memberships. Other than that, no measurable effects were reported, and no scientific studies investigated the results of the campaign.

The second campaign, "Psykekampanjen" (1999), lasted for a year and was conducted by the Equality Ombudsman, DO (a government agency that works against discrimination and for equal rights and opportunities for everyone), the user organisation "The National Association of Social and Mental Health" (RSMH) and the Schizophrenia Fellowship. By improving the attitudes towards mental illness in general, the aim was to improve the possibilities of employment as well as social inclusion. Opinions of patients themselves were considered more genuine than the opinions of health-care professionals only. Emphasis was put on involving patients in the society by enhancing interaction amongst health-care providers, social service providers and others. Much effort was put into media contacts, art exhibitions and performances aimed at changing the attitudes towards mental illness. The final evaluation of the project showed contradictory results. Supporters of the campaign claimed that it was highly credible due to the involvement of user organisations as well as artists. Others claimed that is was doubtful whether the message actually reached persons other than those already involved in anti-stigma activities and convinced of its importance. The final conclusion was that the main goal to reach the general public was not met.

The third national campaign, "Hjärnkoll" (2010–2014), was carried out by the Swedish Agency for Disability Policy Coordination (Handisam) and the network of user organisations (NSPH) (Hansson 2009). The aim was to work for developing a society in which everyone can participate on equal terms, regardless of functional capacity. The aim of "Hjärnkoll" was to increase knowledge and change attitudes about mental illness and mental disability in the general public by using national and regional public discussion forums. People with personal experience of mental illness ("attitude ambassadors") were trained to inform the public about mental illness. Additionally, a special focus was put on working with journalists, health-care professionals and social workers (i.e. "focus groups").

CEPIs (Centre for Evidence-Based Psychosocial Interventions for people with severe mental illnesses) conducted a study (Hansson 2009) before the start of "Hjärnkoll". Overall, 2,053 participants were surveyed about their attitudes towards people with mental illness. More than 25 % had a negative or partially negative attitude towards patients with mental illness or disability because of mental impairment. Most often this involved an aversion to close contact with somebody who is mentally ill. Of the participants 32 % did not think that a psychiatric illness is comparable to any other illness, and 61 % thought that persons who had been treated in a psychiatric hospital were unfit to be trusted as babysitters.

Yearly follow-ups (Myndigheten för delaktighet 2014) were performed (2009–2013) and showed a significant positive shift in attitudes towards persons with mental illness in the campaign counties. Approximately one-third to one-fifth of the general public who had a negative attitude towards mentally ill in 2009 did not report negative attitudes in 2013. The positive changes concerned decreased social distance; increased tolerance; an altered view of the expected risk of violence and in general a more positive view of the need for social integration of persons with mental illness. The attitudes towards having a person with a mental illness as a neighbour, colleague or friend also improved (relative changes 18–25 %). Still, the knowledge about people with mental illnesses only changed marginally.

The latest anti-stigma campaign ("Hjärnkoll") in Sweden was followed-up and evaluated, contrary to the previous campaigns. Other ongoing efforts such as through the Swedish Psychiatry Fund (www.psykiatrifonden.se), the Swedish Psychiatric Association (www.slf.se) and anti-stigma seminars about the perception of psychiatry, "Jonsered seminars" (www.gupea.ub.gu.se), attempt to raise awareness about mental illness. Finally, continuous efforts and further studies are needed as stigma and discrimination change not only in the course of the mental disorder (Corker et al. 2015) but might also vary in different cultures and socio-demographic settings.

Turkey

Efforts to reduce stigmatisation of mentally ill patients in the Turkish society are in their infancy. Until the end of the twentieth century, mental health-care problems were all but ignored even though the "Green Crescent" as an organisation to protect society and its young members in particular against tobacco, alcohol, drugs, gambling and technology addictions without discrimination through rehabilitative and preventive public health work had been established at the beginning of the said century (Crescent; Alliance).

Alcohol dependence is common in the Western part of Turkey and in those regions is not considered a mental illness. Abuse of other substances in contrast may be stigmatised, as is seeing a psychiatrist. Reported suicide rates, being a behaviour, which is condoned by religion, are very low in Turkey.

Newspapers still tend to report on events involving patients suffering from mental illnesses in a dramatic manner further fostering the public opinion that all psychiatric patients are very dangerous. Nevertheless, in the last 3 years, the number of community mental health centres increased rapidly. People hope that this will decrease the prejudice about mental illness.

Anti-stigma programmes mainly rely on WPA initiatives and efforts by local schizophrenia associations. One of such examples is the "Association of Friends for Schizophrenia" with family groups having had the leading role in its formation. In the last decades, local associations were founded in Turkey's main cities. Local programmes organised usually last several days and include appearances on radio, television and newspapers. The activities often take place in the second week of October as part of the Mental Health Week. However, the general public's participation as well as interest is limited.

Discussion

These reports from midsize European show that stigma is continuing to be a major problem in all of these countries. Experiences between countries differ markedly. While in some countries media frequently used stigmatising terms such as "mad people", in other countries well-known politicians reported about suffering from depressive illness. These descriptions are examples of what have been experienced, giving insight into everyday life of countries. Nevertheless, in larger countries there might be relevant differences between regions and subgroups of the population.

In all these countries, various activities have been performed in order to fight against stigma. Some countries had national campaigns supported by national governments, while others had more local activities. Some provided information about mental illness and its treatment, while others focussed on stigma and its negative consequences. Some initiatives organised fundraising events and collected money. Further, activities differed by the size and duration of campaigns. Target groups were heterogeneous. For example, school children or university students were frequently included. The topics ranged from all mental illness to single disorders like schizophrenia, depression, eating disorders or substance abuse. In some countries, potential consequences of mental disorders such as suicide were on the agenda additionally. Considering the fact that stigma is an enormous major problem until now, we must question about the effects and effectiveness of these various activities.

Recently, it was mentioned that it is sometimes difficult to define what should be counted as an anti-stigma programme (Beldie et al. 2012). Changes in legislation, national campaigns, collecting money, providing information leaflets and various other activities might influence public opinion about mentally ill. We must not exclude the possibility that the organisation of mental health care (e.g. large state mental hospitals versus small psychiatric units in general community hospitals, focus on outpatients mental health care versus inpatient care) influences peoples' views (Ghodse 2011; Rittmannsberger et al. 2004; Meise et al. 2006).

Since in some countries such as Norway, school programmes focussed on providing information to pupils, it is surprising that in Norway especially younger people believe that mentally ill are dangerous. Evaluations of ant-stigma activities were rather rare. In Austria, activities addressing children and adolescents have been shown to have the potential to reduce stigmatisation (Kohlbauer et al. 2010), while the effects of the population campaign were rather limited (Grausgruber et al. 2009). A study in Croatia showed that a programme helping patients with mental illnesses to develop coping skills resulted in a significant decrease of self-stigmatisation. In Sweden, the final evaluation of the campaign showed contradictory results. Some claimed that it was highly credible due to the involvement of user organisations; others claimed that is was doubtful whether the message really reached others than those already involved. The final conclusion was that the main goal to reach the general public was not met.

Overall, our knowledge about what is working against stigma is very limited. Further, we do not know if the effects of interventions vary in different cultures and socio-demographic settings. Thus, it is not surprising that mental health stigma is a continuing problem. Change of information like provided in this chapter might help to learn from each other. Nevertheless, sophisticated research on anti-stigma interventions seems to be essential to understand what might help to reduce stigma and discrimination.

References

Alliance EAP (2014). Available from: http://www.eurocare.org/about_us/membership/turkish_green_crescent_society_tuerkiye_yesilay_cemiyeti

André I, Čaplová T (2000) Obraz psychicky chorého v masmédiách [The image of people with mental illnesses in mass media]. Psychiatra 7(Suppl 1):94–95

Beldie A et al (2012) Fighting stigma of mental illness in midsize European countries. Soc Psychiatry Psychiatr Epidemiol 47(Suppl 1):1–38

Brain C et al (2014) Stigma, discrimination and medication adherence in schizophrenia: results from the Swedish COAST study. Psychiatry Res 220(3):811–817

Campos L et al (2012) Mental health awareness intervention in schools. J Hum Growth Dev 22(2):259–266

Campos L, Dias P, Palha F (2014) Finding space to mental health – promoting mental health in adolescents: pilot study. Educ Health 32(1):23–29

Čaplová T et al (1997) Názroy poslucháčov niektorých vysokých škôl na chorých s diagnózou schizofrénie [Opinions of university students from selected schools on patients with the diagnosis of schizophrenia]. Psychiatra 4(1–4):110–113

Carter R (2014) Ao nosso alcance. Acabar com a crise na saúde mental. ENCONTRAR+SE

Corker EA et al (2015) Experience of stigma and discrimination reported by people experiencing the first episode of schizophrenia and those with a first episode of depression: the FEDORA project. Int J Soc Psychiatry 61:438–445

Crescent TG (2014). Available from: http://www.yesilay.org.tr/en/

Ministério da Saúde, L (2007) Coordenação Nacional Paraa Reestruturaçãodos Serviços de Saúde mental, in Relatório. Proposta de Plano de Acção para a Reestruturação e Desenvolvimento dos Serviços de Saúde Mental em Portugal 2007–2016. Ministério da Saúde, Lisboa

Myndigheten för delaktighet (2014). Available from: http://www.mfd.se/

Fabrega H Jr (1990) Psychiatric stigma in the classical and medieval period: a review of the literature. Compr Psychiatry 31(4):289–306

Filipcić I (2003) Testing attitudes of the Croatian population towards schizophrenic patients using an anti-stigma questionnaire. Socijalna Psihijatrija 31(1):3–9

Ghodse H (2011) International perspectives on mental health. The Royal College of Psychiatrists Publications, London

Grausgruber A et al (2009) "Schizophrenia has many faces" – evaluation of the Austrian Anti-Stigma-Campaign 2000–2002. Psychiatr Prax 36(7):327–333

Hamre P, Dahl AA, Malt UF (1994) Public attitudes to the quality of psychiatric treatment, psychiatric patients, and prevalence of mental disorders. Nord J Psychiatry 48(4):275–281

Hansson L (2009) Psykiskohälsa – attityder, kunskap, beteende. En befolkningsundersökning [Mental illness – attitudes, knowledge, behaviour. A public opinion survey]

Heretik A, Mullerovzá Z (2005) Depresio ocami obcanov Slovenskej republiky. Sociálne reprezentácie pojmu depresia u prispievatelov v on-line diskusii v clánku o výsledkoch EPID štúdie v denníku SME [Depression among citizens of the Slovak Republic. Social representation of depression among contributors of an on line discussion on an article about the results of the EPID study in the daily SME]. Psychiatra 12(1):15–27

Ivezic S, Mužinić L, PA (2009) Evaluacija antistigma programa dnevne bolnice. In: 2. kongres socijalne psihijatrije. Split

Kohlbauer D et al (2010) Does education focusing on depression change the attitudes towards schizophrenia? A target-group oriented anti-stigma-intervention. Neuropsychiatr 24(2): 132–140

Meise U et al (2000) "…not dangerous, but nevertheless frightening". A program against stigmatization of schizophrenia in schools. Psychiatr Prax 27(7):340–346

Meise U et al (2006) Psychische Gesundheitsversorgung in Österreich. Neuropsychiatr 20:137–139

Paykel ES, Hart D, Priest RG (1998) Changes in public attitudes to depression during the Defeat Depression Campaign. Br J Psychiatry 173:519–522

Rittmannsberger H et al (2004) Changing aspects of psychiatric inpatient treatment. Eur Psychiatry 19(8):483–488

Saúde D.-Gd (2014) Saúde mental em números – 2014. 14.12.2014. Available from: http://upafazadiferenca.encontrarse.pt

Schöny W (1998) Schizophrenia – an illness and its treatment reflected in public attitude. Wien Med Wochenschr 148(11–12):284–288

Schulze B, Angermeyer MC (2002) Perspektivenwechsel: Stigma aus der Sicht schizophren Erkrankter, ihrer Angehörigen und von Mitarbeitern in der psychiatrischen Versorgung. Neuropsychiatr 16:78–86

Slovenia PO (2009) The Mental Health Act. 27.12.2014. Available from: http://fra.europa.eu/sites/default/files/fra_uploads/2162-mental-health-study-2009-SI.pdf

Slovenia GO (2014) Resolucija o nacionalnem programu duševnega zdravja 2014–2018 (Resolution on the National Mental Health Programme 2014–2018). 08.02.2015. Available from: http://www.sent.si/fck_files/file/NOVICE/NPDZ_3_J.pdf

Strbad M et al (2008) Stigma of mental illness: comparison of patients' and students' attitudes in Slovenia (Stigma Duševne Bolezni: Primerjava Stališč Bolnikov in Studentov V Sloveniji). Zdrav Vestn 77:481–485

Thesen J (2001) Being a psychiatric patient in the community – reclassified as the stigmatized "other". Scand J Public Health 29(4):248–255

Trdič J, Pribakovič Brinovec R (2012) Zdravstveni statistični letopis (Health Statistic Yearbook). Nacionalni inštitut za varovanje zdravja Republike Slovenije (National Institute of Public Health of the Republic of Slovenia), Ljubljana

Unit, T.E.I (2014) Mental health and integration. Provision for supporting people with mental illness: a comparison of 30 European countries. 08.02.2015. Available from: http://mentalhealth-integration.com/media/whitepaper/EIU-Janssen_Mental_Health.pdf

Part III

"Fighting" Stigma and Discrimination: Strategic Considerations

Fields of Intervention

23

Richard Warner[†]

Introduction

Efforts have been made since the 1950s to reduce the prejudice toward people with mental illness (Cumming and Cumming 1957; Nunally 1961). Despite these attempts, stigma (Hall et al. 1993; Brockington et al. 1993), prejudice (Sayce 1998; Thornicroft 2006), and misconceptions about mental illness (Corrigan et al. 2002; Thompson et al. 2002; Corrigan et al. 2004) continue to be pervasive. Surveys reveal that people with schizophrenia around the world experience high rates of discrimination (Thornicroft et al. 2009), and public attitudes toward the mentally ill in the developed world may be worsening rather than improving (Mehta et al. 2009). Citizen-driven not-in-my-backyard campaigns obstruct the placement of residential facilities (Boydall et al. 1989; Repper et al. 1997). The perception of stigma by people with psychosis is associated with enduring negative effects on their self-esteem, well-being, mental status, work status, and income (Link et al. 1997; Leff and Warner 2006). Public and professional opinions about mental illness adversely affect its detection and outcome (Link et al. 1999; Jorm 2000; Stuart and Arboleda-Florez 2001; Magliano et al. 2004). Both the U.S. Surgeon General's Report (NIMH 2000) and the WHO World Health Report (WHO 2001) cite stigma as one of the greatest obstacles to the treatment of mental illness.

In recent decades, we have witnessed an increase in the will to combat stigma. We have also seen the application of a well-developed tool, social marketing, to this task. This chapter describes how two sites of the World Psychiatric Association (WPA) Programme to Reduce Stigma and Discrimination Because of Schizophrenia—Calgary, Alberta, and Boulder, Colorado—harnessed this tool to combat stigma.

[†]Deceased on August 27th, 2015

R. Warner
Mental Health Center of Boulder County, Colorado Recovery,
2818 13th Street, Boulder, CO 80304, USA

© Springer International Publishing Switzerland 2017
W. Gaebel et al. (eds.), *The Stigma of Mental Illness - End of the Story?*,
DOI 10.1007/978-3-319-27839-1_23

Social Marketing

Social marketing campaigns have been used successfully around the world in AIDS prevention, smoking cessation, and in many other causes. Effectiveness is increased by audience segmentation—that is, partitioning a mass audience into sub-audiences that are relatively homogeneous and devising appropriately targeted promotional strategies and messages. For example, if one were launching an AIDS prevention campaign in San Francisco, a target group such as Asian sex workers would require a very different set of media and messages than those directed at gay, white males. In developing such campaigns, it is useful to conduct a needs assessment that gathers information about the groups' cultural beliefs and the media through which they could best learn about the topic. The needs assessment may incorporate focus groups, telephone surveys, or information from opinion leaders. Specific objectives, audiences, messages, and media are selected, and an action plan is drawn up. The messages and materials are pretested with audiences and revised. The plan is implemented and, with continuous monitoring of impact, constantly refined (Rogers 2003).

> **Box 23.1**
> Social marketing campaigns have been used successfully around the world in AIDS prevention, smoking cessation, and in many other causes. Effectiveness is increased by audience segmentation—that is, partitioning a mass audience into sub-audiences that are relatively homogeneous and devising appropriately targeted promotional strategies and messages.

Implementing a Local Antistigma Program

The WPA global antistigma program, launched in 1996 (Sartorius and Schulze 2005), established projects to fight the stigma of schizophrenia in 20 countries having created a process for setting up antistigma projects in local communities that follow these steps: establish a local action committee, conduct a survey of sources of stigma, select target groups, choose messages and media, and evaluate the impact of interventions while continuously refining them.

> **Box 23.2**
> The WPA global antistigma program created a process for setting up antistigma projects in local communities that follow these steps: establish a local action committee, conduct a survey of sources of stigma, select target groups, choose messages and media, and evaluate the impact of interventions while continuously refining them.

Establishing a Local Action Committee

The composition of the action committee is critical in establishing a local project. Committee members should include representatives of groups that the campaign is considering targeting; however, these groups will not be known when the action committee is formed. Therefore, the initial planning group should select committee members from walks of life that are likely to become target groups, such as the police, employers, or clergy, and add members later as needed. Some of the most valuable members of the action committee will be mental health service users and family members who have a firsthand understanding of discrimination.

Members of the action committee must be willing to devote substantial time to the project, as most of the work will be accomplished by their volunteer effort. It is valuable to include prominent citizens, such as legislators, on the committee. When requesting a meeting with the editorial board of the local newspaper, for example, the inclusion of someone with name recognition increases the impact of the request. Prominent individuals may have less time to commit and can be given affiliate status.

An action committee should comprise 10–20 members—neither so small as to burden members with too much work nor so big as to be unwieldy. A large group can split into task forces to refine action plans for different target groups. Action committees commonly meet monthly, distributing minutes and an agenda at each meeting.

Selecting Target Groups

It is helpful to conduct a survey of local consumers, family members, and others to determine where stigma is seen to be prevalent—for example, in hospital emergency departments or among employers. The action committee can use this information to select a manageable number of target groups, preferably no more than three. It is inadvisable to target the general population. To do so is expensive and unlikely to have a measurable impact. In the Calgary project, random pre-post telephone surveys revealed that a radio campaign targeted at the general public produced no change in attitudes toward people with mental illness or knowledge of mental illness (Stuart 2002). Target groups should be homogeneous and accessible. Landlords, for example, are not an accessible group because they do not meet as a group or use a common media outlet. Employers are more accessible because the project can identify the largest local employers and target their human resource departments. The police are also an accessible group, because they receive regular in-service training.

> **Box 23.3**
> It is helpful to conduct a survey of local consumers, family members, and others to determine where stigma is seen to be prevalent. The action committee can use this information to select a manageable number of target groups, preferably no more than three. It is inadvisable to target the general population. To do so is expensive and unlikely to have a measurable impact.

Action Plans

The action committee develops an action plan that includes specific goals and objectives for each target group. The goals might include, in increasing order of difficulty, developing awareness, increasing knowledge, changing attitudes, and changing behavior—for example, reducing discrimination in housing. For a target group such as high school students, the goals might be to increase awareness of stigma, increase knowledge about schizophrenia, and reduce stigmatizing attitudes. To meet these goals, measurable objectives might include giving a presentation about stigma and mental illness to 50% of the students in the district, achieving 25% improvement in the average scores on mental illness knowledge and a 10% reduction in the average scores on social distance among participating students. (Social distance refers to the respondents' expressed preference regarding their association with people with mental illness.)

Objectives should be realistic so that project members are not disappointed by small gains. On the basis of the project's goals and objectives, the action committee can select key messages and determine the media that will be used to distribute the messages. The action plan should specify who will accomplish each step and by what date.

Working with Schools

Secondary-school students were a popular target group in the WPA global anti-stigma program; this group was selected by at least a dozen projects, from Calgary to Ismailia, Egypt. The popularity of the target group has less to do with the likelihood that students will stigmatize people with mental illness and more to do with their ready accessibility and the opportunity to influence the attitudes of a coming generation. When meeting with school principals, project members can frame the effort to reduce stigma as an important component in diversity training and point out that mental illness is often neglected in health education.

Box 23.4
Secondary-school students were a popular target group in the WPA global antistigma program; this group was selected by at least a dozen projects, from Calgary to Ismailia, Egypt. The popularity of the target group has less to do with the likelihood that students will stigmatize people with mental illness and more to do with their ready accessibility and the opportunity to influence the attitudes of a coming generation.

Examples of messages that were used in the secondary-school antistigma programs in Calgary and Boulder include "No one is to blame for schizophrenia,"

"People with schizophrenia are people with schizophrenia," and "Watch your language"—that is, don't use derogatory terms to refer to people with mental illness.

Media that were used included speakers with mental illness, the Web page of the WPA program (www.openthedoors.com), a teaching guide on schizophrenia, and an art competition for students to produce antistigma materials. In Calgary, students were often invited to participate in simulation of the effect of auditory hallucinations: two students spoke into the ears of a seated pupil who was asked to focus on what an interviewer in front of him was saying. The approach, which has been used in several school antistigma projects, is designed to increase empathy, but some researchers have questioned whether the discomfort that the approach creates may have unintended negative consequences (Ando et al. 2011).

To mount the art competition in Boulder, organizers obtained the support of the school principals and art teachers. A consumer speakers' bureau and a project coordinator with a background in visual arts made presentations in art classes. The presenters announced a juried competition, with money prizes, for students to produce artwork dealing with stigma and mental illness. A public art show with an awards ceremony was mounted after each annual competition, and an exhibit of all the entries was displayed in participating high schools.

The impact of a social marketing campaign is increased if the target group receives the same message from different sources (the media multiplier effect) (Clow and Baack 2005). In Boulder, interior bus advertisements reach a predominantly younger audience and are free for public service announcements. The WPA project in Boulder installed several bus advertisements with antistigma messages, including one that used student art with the statement, "Sometimes those that are different are the most amazing." Cinema patrons are also predominantly younger people. The Boulder project ran slides with three different antistigma messages among the advertisements that preceded the main feature on 16 local cinema screens. One message read, "Don't believe everything you see at the movies: mental illness does not equal violence." Exit surveys revealed that 18% of cinema patrons recalled the content of at least one of the three messages displayed. Thus, during 3 months of displaying the slides, more than 10,000 people would have been able to recall one message 2 h after seeing it. The total cost was 36 cents for each person who recalled seeing a message, which compares very favorably with usual commercial media costs (Farris et al. 2010).

Outcomes from secondary-school interventions have been positive throughout the WPA project. In Calgary, more than 3,000 students participated in the intervention. Post-testing was conducted at different times, from minutes to weeks after the intervention, depending on the classroom. The proportion of students who answered all the questions about mental illness correctly increased from 12 to 28 % on pre-post testing, and the proportion who expressed no social distance between themselves and someone with schizophrenia increased from 16 to 30 % (24). An example of a social distance question is "Would you be upset to be in the same class with someone with schizophrenia?". In Vienna, positive changes in attitudes were evident 3 months after the intervention (Ladinser 2001). At three sites in Egypt, students were tested about their knowledge about schizophrenia and its treatment before and after the intervention. The students' scores doubled after the intervention, and the proportion of students who believed that someone with schizophrenia would be likely to commit a crime decreased from 56 to 29 % (El-Defrawi et al. 2001). In Leipzig, Germany, students were tested about their attitudes toward a person with schizophrenia; scores improved substantially during a 3-month follow-up in the group of 90 students that received the intervention but not in the control group of 60 students (Schulze et al. 2001). Large educational workshops for secondary-school children in Britain were shown to be effective in improving positive attitudes toward people with mental illness—benefits that were sustained over a 6-month period (Pinfold et al. 2003a).

An interesting antistigma intervention in Staffordshire, England, did not use a classroom approach but relied instead on work experience. Secondary-school students were placed in mental health treatment facilities to gain experience of the work of those programs. One of the goals of the placement effort was to assess the effect of the work experience on adolescents' attitudes toward mental illness. The experience was shown to reduce the student's categorical thinking and perceptions that people with mental illness are likely to be violent or out of control (Kennedy et al. 2014).

Published reviews of the broader field of research on school-based antistigma interventions have rendered various opinions. A 2008 review of 40 such studies concluded that the quality of the research was inadequate to draw firm conclusions (Schachter et al. 2008). A subsequent review of 12 studies reported that the results indicated a positive impact on attitudes toward mental illness and improvements in knowledge among secondary-school children (Sakellari et al. 2011). A 2014 systematic review of 17 classroom-based interventions published between 1998 and 2011 found that only a minority of the studies demonstrated a positive effect on stigma or knowledge at follow-up and again highlighted the methodological shortcomings of the published studies (Mellor 2014). The most comprehensive review of antistigma interventions, conducted by Corrigan and colleagues (2012), applied a meta-analysis to the data from 79 studies conducted in 14 countries in four continents: the studies used a variety of approaches from social activism to education to personal contact with people with mental illness. A quarter of the studies dealt with interventions with secondary-school children. Corrigan's team concluded that education and contact with people with mental illness had positive effects in reducing stigma among both adolescents and adults. Adolescents responded most strongly to education: personal contact with someone with mental illness produced more positive change in attitudes than video testimonials.

Box 23.5
Corrigan's team concluded that education and contact with people with mental illness had positive effects in reducing stigma among both adolescents and adults.

Working with the Criminal Justice System

Criminal justice personnel are under-recognized partners in the management of mental illness. The police bring people who are acutely disturbed into care or protective settings. Jail officers struggle to manage people with acute psychosis in environments that are totally unsuited to the task. Judges wrestle with the disposition of mentally ill offenders. Probation officers supervise people with mental illness, even though the officers do not have access to a consultation about the person's capacity to respond to directives. Yet, there are few programs that attempt to provide criminal justice personnel with the education necessary to perform these essential parts of their jobs. For this reason, the Boulder antistigma project, and other WPA program sites, selected criminal justice personnel as a target.

Police Training

Mental health professionals, consumers, and police officers collaborated in developing a 1-day, 8-h pilot training course, which was pilot tested with seasoned officers and rookies in the county's largest city (population 100,000). Applying lessons learned from pre-post testing in the pilot program, the project undertook the training of the entire police department in the county's second largest city (population 70,000). To minimize the disruption of police services to the community, the training was delivered six times to a portion of the department's officers each time at change of shift in the afternoon or evening before the officers went on duty.

The training, an abbreviated form of the pilot course, comprised two 2-h sessions on adult and child disorders and was presented by psychiatrists, consumers, and their family members. The content included the features, course, treatment, and outcome of psychotic disorders, the diagnosis of childhood disorders, myths about schizophrenia, the diverse characteristics of people who attempt suicide, and a discussion of why people with psychosis should not be kept in jail. The classes discussed why people with borderline personality disorder are often not admitted to a hospital. This topic is important if the training is to be successful, because police officers everywhere are likely to complain about bringing someone in for evaluation after a suicide attempt, only to learn later, as commonly phrased, "She got home before I did!"

Pre-post testing of the officers conducted immediately before and after the training revealed no improvement in attitudes toward people with psychosis, but it revealed a 48% improvement in scores of knowledge about adult and child mental disorders. The proportion of officers who held inaccurate beliefs about the causes of schizophrenia fell from 24% to 3%, but another misconception scarcely changed. The proportion who held a mistaken belief about the usual behavior of people with schizophrenia fell only from 82% to 71%. After training, 71% of the officers still believed one or more of the following statements: people with schizophrenia are (a) always irrational, (b) much more likely to be violent than the average person, or (c) usually unable to make life decisions. Officers retained these beliefs, even though they heard a presentation by a quietly eloquent, middle-aged woman with schizophrenia who was working full-time as a university library supervisor.

Continued police training in Boulder County ranged from 4 to 7 h a session, achieved modest improvements in attitudes and substantial gains in knowledge of mental illness, and reached all the county's officers by the end of 2005. A police training program in the WPA antistigma project in Kent, England, achieved the same results—minimal improvements in attitude, more extensive knowledge gains, but no change in the perceived link between mental illness and violent behavior (Pinfold et al. 2003b). On reflection, it becomes apparent that police encounters with people with psychosis nearly always occur when the person is acutely disturbed, and that officers have little opportunity to meet people with schizophrenia who are working, in stable relationships, or rarely hospitalized. The Boulder research team concluded that police training should intensively expose officers to people who have recovered from psychosis if it is to effect attitudinal change.

> **Box 23.6**
> After training, 71% of the officers still believed one or more of the following statements: people with schizophrenia are (a) always irrational, (b) much more likely to be violent than the average person, or (c) usually unable to make life decisions.... On reflection, it becomes apparent that police encounters with people with psychosis nearly always occur when the person is acutely disturbed, and that officers have little opportunity to meet people with schizophrenia who are working, in stable relationships, or rarely hospitalized.

A more extensive police training program in the United States—the Crisis Intervention Team (CIT) training—has shown greater gains. In this model, which is available in many communities across the country, self-selected police officers participate in 40 h of training provided by local mental health professionals, family advocates, and psychiatric service users. Upon completion of the training, officers are certified as first-line responders for calls involving people in crisis. The program supports relationships between hospital emergency departments and the police, increasing the likelihood that people with psychiatric difficulties will be taken to a hospital rather than jail. The CIT program has been shown to reduce unnecessary arrests and the use of force, while increasing rates of referral to emergency care and reducing incarceration (Compton et al. 2006). These are the kinds of outcomes antistigma workers and researchers rarely achieve—improvements in knowledge, attitudes, and, most difficult of all, behavior. They point the way toward a general conclusion: intensive efforts to provide education about mental illness to those who are closely involved in serving this population but have not been adequately informed about the effects of and the treatment of these conditions could bear the greatest rewards in terms of changes in behavior and outcomes. This would include other criminal justice personnel such as judges, attorneys and probation officers, and emergency room staff and physicians. The Calgary antistigma project successfully took on the task of developing criteria for the management of people with mental illness in emergency rooms. The criteria were eventually adopted across Canada (Thompson and Bland 2001). In Boulder, an education plan was developed for other criminal justice personnel in addition to the police.

> **Box 23.7**
> The CIT program has been shown to reduce unnecessary arrests and the use of force while increasing rates of referral to emergency care and reducing incarceration. These are the kinds of outcomes antistigma workers and researchers rarely achieve—improvements in knowledge, attitudes, and, most difficult of all, behavior.

Judges, Attorneys, and Probation Officers

Psychiatrists, people with mental illness, and family members provided a series of three training sessions on adult disorders and one training session on child disorders to judges, attorneys, and probation officers (approximately 12 in each category). Nearly all the county court judges attended. A pre-post test conducted directly before and after the training revealed that the judges' accuracy of knowledge about schizophrenia improved from 47% to 74%, and some judges reported immediate changes in sentencing practice. After the training sessions were completed, the judges requested two more training sessions on juvenile disorders.

The passage of time has taken the training of judges dealing with people with psychiatric disorders to a new level. The development of a system of Integrated Treatment courts across the United States has brought about a dramatic change in the management of offenders with substance abuse problems. The first Integrated Treatment Court began in 1989, when Miami courts decided to try a different approach to managing drug-abusing offenders in Florida. According to the National Drug Court Institute (http://www.ndci.org/), there are now 3,000 active drug/treatment courts in the United States. These courts have now been adapted to deal with a broader range of behavior problems including coexisting mental illness and juvenile behavior disorders.

Prior to each day of hearings of the Integrated Treatment Court, multiple treatment providers, criminal justice personnel, and attorneys gather for a meeting with the judge and present information about how well the offender has met goals since the last appearance in court, often just a week or two prior. The judge determines whether the offender should receive an award (such as free groceries or cinema tickets) or a sanction (such as days in jail) as a result of his or her performance. In Boulder and elsewhere, the judges working in the Integrated Treatment Courts attend motivational interviewing courses and use that technique in their court work. Using these time-tested, evidence-based, collaborative approaches, the treatment courts in Boulder are achieving better outcomes for adolescents and adults with coexisting mental illness and substance use disorders in terms of long-term sobriety and reduction of recidivism. The judges' regular exposure to the details of treatment information about people with mental illness and substance abuse disorders increases their understanding of the psychosocial stresses that affect the progress of the disorders and provides ongoing education about how to respond to these offenders when they appear in court. There are clear benefits in terms of knowledge, attitudes, and behavior.

Setting Up a Service-User Speakers' Bureau

A speakers' bureau is valuable for addressing students, police, and other groups. It often comprises people who have experienced mental illness, family members, and a mental health professional whose function is to answer factual questions—for example, what causes schizophrenia? People with mental illness can react to the stress of public speaking by experiencing an increase in symptoms shortly after the event. To minimize this possibility, service users with good tolerance of stress should be selected. They should be gradually be introduced to speaking in front of audiences by first observing and then speaking briefly until they can participate fully without experiencing stress. Speakers should be debriefed after each presentation to learn what they found stressful. Several speakers should be trained so that the demand on any one person is not too great.

> **Box 23.8**
> People with mental illness can react to the stress of public speaking by experiencing an increase in symptoms shortly after the event. To minimize this possibility, service users with good tolerance of stress should be selected. They should be gradually introduced to speaking in front of audiences by first observing and then speaking briefly until they can participate fully without experiencing stress.

Speakers who are service users demonstrate the reality of recovery, generating optimism and compassion. A study conducted in Innsbruck, Austria, revealed that high school students addressed by a psychiatrist and a consumer reported significant changes in social distance attitudes, whereas those who were addressed by a psychiatrist and a social worker did not (Meise et al. 2001). Other research has indicated that previous contact with someone with mental illness decreases stigma and fear of dangerousness (Link and Cullen 1986; Penn et al. 1994). Service users can talk about discrimination in employment, housing, and law enforcement, but they should try to avoid generating defensiveness in the audience.

The coordinator of the speakers' bureau can be a consumer, family member, or enthusiastic citizen. The coordinator should maintain a diary of engagements, select speakers for each event, debrief them afterwards, and ask the host to provide an assessment. The speakers and the coordinator commonly receive remuneration. A successful speakers' bureau—such as the Partnership Program operated by the Calgary branch of the Schizophrenia Society—will develop a strong sense of a shared mission, which is nurtured through regular meetings.

Setting Up a Media-Watch Group

Local and national advocacy groups can lobby news and entertainment media to exclude negative portrayals of people with psychosis. Such groups are known as "stigma busters" or "media-watch" groups. A local antistigma project can establish the media-watch function in several ways. Members can inform national media-watch organizations about negative portrayals that are distributed nationally, respond to calls to action from national advocacy groups, and contact local media outlets about stigmatizing messages.

> **Box 23.9**
> Local and national advocacy groups can lobby news and entertainment media to exclude negative portrayals of people with psychosis. Such groups are known as "stigma busters" or "media-watch" groups.

National media-watch bodies in the United States have become quite effective. The National Stigma Clearinghouse, which began in 1990 by the New York State chapter of the National Alliance for the Mentally Ill (NAMI), collects examples of negative portrayals of people with mental illness from a variety of US media. The staff writes or calls the journalists, editors, or others responsible for the negative portrayal, explaining why the material is offensive and providing accurate information about the mental illness. In one instance, the Clearinghouse was successful in getting DC Comics to change the story line that dealt with Superman's death, so that his killer was no longer "an escapee from an interplanetary insane asylum." The group distributes a monthly newsletter that summarizes recent actions and educates local advocates about the kinds of negative media portrayals to look for and how to correct them (Wahl 1995). NAMI has also used its national membership effectively to combat stigma. In 1999, in response to the airing of the TV series Wonderland in which mentally ill people were seen committing numerous violent acts, NAMI coordinated a mailing to ABC and the show's commercial sponsors. The program was pulled from the air after two episodes, even though 13 had been filmed.

Local action can also be effective. In Boulder County, a local newspaper carried an advertisement for an apartment rental that depicted a man in a straitjacket with bulging eyes and distorted features; the advertisement included the text, "Driven crazy by cramped housing?" A polite letter to the advertiser, along with a copy to the newspaper editor, led to the immediate withdrawal of the advertisement and a letter of apology.

Local media-watch groups do not need to be large or complex. One or two coordinators can establish links to a broader group of members who report stigmatizing items. The coordinators forward items of national scope to a national media-watch group or respond directly to a local newspaper or business about local items. A gradual escalation approach is generally effective. Begin with a polite request, perhaps suggesting that the stigmatizing reference was inadvertent. A positive response should be rewarded with a letter of thanks. Often those guilty of the offense are appropriately concerned and may later become supporters of the media-watch group. If the offender is unresponsive, increasing pressure can be applied, such as writing a letter for publication in the local newspaper (Wahl 1995).

Funding and Sustainability

Attempts to influence the general public through mass advertising are expensive and unlikely to prove effective, but targeted interventions, such as police training and classroom presentations, can be conducted and assessed with modest expense. Total expenditures during the first 3 years of the Boulder project were <US$10,000.

A local campaign cannot run forever (3 years is a reasonable length of time), but permanent structures and partnerships can be developed. On the basis of experiences in Boulder, Calgary, and elsewhere, these might include changing the secondary-school health curriculum to include mental illness, adapting school diversity programs to include education about mental illness, forming a service-user speakers' bureau, creating a media-watch group, and changing institutional policy, such as emergency department procedures for dealing with people with mental illness (Thompson and Bland 2001).

> **Box 23.10**
> A local campaign cannot run forever, but permanent structures and partnerships can be developed. These might include changing the secondary-school health curriculum to include mental illness, adapting school diversity programs to include education about mental illness, forming a service-user speakers' bureau, creating a media-watch group, and changing emergency department procedures for dealing with people with mental illness.

The project director should evaluate which components of the campaign will require ongoing funding and find support for these elements. Local advocacy groups or agencies may be willing to assume responsibility for some components.

Conclusions

Local antistigma projects should involve a broad array of community representatives in the planning and action committee. They should focus on a few specific target groups in which a change in knowledge, attitudes, or behavior would be likely to reduce discrimination and improve the quality of life of people with mental illness. The project should aim to establish some permanent changes that will allow sources of stigma to be monitored and modified on an ongoing basis. Attempts to target the general public are likely to be expensive and ineffective and are not encouraged.

References

Ando S, Clement S, Barley EA, Thornicroft G (2011) The simulation of hallucinations to reduce the stigma of schizophrenia: a systematic review. Schizophr Res 133:8–16

Boydall KM, Trainor JM, Pierri AM (1989) The effect of group homes for the mentally ill on residential property values. Hosp Community Psychiatry 40:957–958

Brockington IF, Hall P, Levings J et al (1993) The community's tolerance of the mentally ill. Br J Psychiatry 162:93–99

Clow KE, Baack D (2005) Concise encyclopedia of advertising. Routledge, New York

Compton MT, Esterberg ML, McGee R et al (2006) Crisis intervention team training: changes in knowledge, attitudes and stigma related to schizophrenia. Psychiatr Serv 57:1199–1202

Corrigan PW, Rowan D, Green A et al (2002) Challenging two mental illnesses stigmas: personal responsibility and dangerousness. Schizophr Bull 28:293–309

Corrigan PW, Watson AC, Warpinski AC et al (2004) Implications of educating the public on mental illness, violence, and stigma. Psychiatr Serv 55:577–580

Corrigan PW, Morris SB, Michaels PJ et al (2012) Challenging the public stigma of mental illness: a meta-analysis of outcome studies. Psychiatr Serv 63:1176

Cumming E, Cumming J (1957) Closed ranks: an experiment in mental health education. Harvard University Press, Cambridge

El-Defrawi MH, El-Serafi A, Ellaban M (2001) Medical students' involvement in health education about schizophrenia: a campaign in secondary schools in Ismailia, Egypt. Presented at Together Against Stigma conference, Leipzig, 2–5 Sept

Farris PW, Bendle NT, Pfeifer PE, Reibstein DJ (2010) Marketing metrics: the definitive guide to measuring marketing performance. Pearson Education, Upper Saddle River

Hall P, Brockington IF, Levings J et al (1993) A comparison of responses to the mentally ill in two communities. Br J Psychiatry 162:99–108

Jorm AF (2000) Mental health literacy: public knowledge and beliefs about mental disorders. Br J Psychiatry 177:396–401

Kennedy V, Belgamwar RB (2014) Impact of work experience placements on school students' attitude towards mental illness. Psychiatric Bulletin, 38(4):159–163

Ladinser E (2001) Students and community psychiatry: changes in attitudes towards people with mental illness and community psychiatry resulting from an anti-stigma programme in schools. Presented at Together Against Stigma conference, Leipzig, 2–5 Sept

Leff J, Warner R (2006) Social inclusion of people with mental illness. Cambridge University Press, Cambridge

Link BG, Cullen FT (1986) Contact with the mentally ill and perceptions of how dangerous they are. J Health Soc Behav 27:289–303

Link BG, Struening E, Rahav M et al (1997) On stigma and its consequences: evidence from a longitudinal study of dual diagnoses of mental illness and substance abuse. J Health Soc Behav 38:177–190

Link BG, Phelan JC, Bresnahan M et al (1999) Public conceptions of mental illness: labels, causes, dangerousness, and social distance. Am J Public Health 89:1328–1323

Magliano L, Fiorillo A, De Rosa C et al (2004) Beliefs about schizophrenia in Italy: a comparative nationwide survey of the general public, mental health professionals, and patients' relatives. Can J Psychiatr 49:171–179

Mehta N, Kassam A, Leese M (2009) Public attitudes towards people with mental illness in England and Scotland, 1994–2003. Br J Psychiatry 194:278–284

Meise U, Sulzenbacher H, Kemmler G, et al (2001) A school programme against stigmatization of schizophrenia in Austria. Presented at Together Against Stigma conference, Leipzig, 2–5 Sept

Mellor C (2014) School-based interventions targeting stigma of mental illness: systematic review. Psychiatr Bull 38:164–171

NIMH (2000) Mental health: a report of the surgeon general. Center for Mental Health Services, National Institute of Mental Health, Rockville

Nunally JC (1961) Popular conceptions of mental health: their development and change. Holt, Rinehart, and Winston, New York

Penn DL, Guynan K, Daily T (1994) Dispelling the stigma of schizophrenia: what sort of information is best? Schizophr Bull 20:567–575

Pinfold V, Toulmin H, Thornicroft G, Huxley P (2003a) Reducing psychiatric stigma and discrimination: evaluation of educational interventions in UK secondary schools. Br J Psychiatry 182:342–346

Pinfold V, Huxley P, Thornicroft G et al (2003b) Reducing psychiatric stigma and discrimination – evaluating an educational intervention with the police force in England. Soc Psychiatry Psychiatr Epidemiol 38:337–344

Repper J, Sayce L, Strong S et al (1997) Tall stories from the backyard: a survey of "Nimby" opposition to mental health facilities experienced by key service providers in England and Wales. Mind, London

Rogers EM (2003) Diffusion of innovations, 5th edn. Free Press, New York

Sakellari E, Leino-Kilpi H, Kalokerinou-Anagostopolou A (2011) Educational interventions in secondary education aiming to affect pupils' attitudes towards mental illness: a review of the literature. J Psychiatr Ment Health Nurs 18:166–176

Sartorius N, Schulze H (2005) Reducing the stigma of mental illness: a report from a global programme of the world psychiatric association. Cambridge University Press, Cambridge

Sayce L (1998) Stigma, discrimination, and social exclusion: what's in a word? J Ment Health 7:331–343

Schachter HM, Giradrdi A, Ly M et al (2008) Effects of school-based interventions on mental health stigmatization: a systematic review. Child Adolesc Psychiatry Mental Health 2:18

Schulze B, Richter-Werling M, Matschinger H, et al (2001) Crazy? So what! Effects of a school project on students' attitudes towards people with schizophrenia. Presented at Together Against Stigma conference, Leipzig, 2–5 Sept

Stuart H (2002) Stigmatisation: Leçons tirées des programmes de réduction. Santé Mentale Québec 28:37–53

Stuart H, Arboleda-Florez J (2001) Community attitudes towards people with schizophrenia. Can J Psychiatr 46:245–251

Thompson AH, Bland RC (2001) Canadian national standards for emergency rooms changed following WPA anti-stigma survey. Presented at Together Against Stigma conference, Leipzig, 2–5 Sept

Thompson AH, Stuart H, Bland RC et al (2002) Attitudes about schizophrenia from the pilot project of the WPA worldwide campaign against the stigma of schizophrenia. Soc Psychiatry Psychiatr Epidemiol 37:475–482

Thornicroft G (2006) Shunned: Discrimination against People with Mental Illness. Oxford University Press, Oxford

Thornicroft G, Brohan E, Rose D et al (2009) Global pattern of experienced and anticipated discrimination against people with schizophrenia: a cross-sectional survey. Lancet 373:408–415

Wahl OF (1995) Media madness: public images of mental illness. Rutgers University Press, New Brunswick

WHO (2001) Mental health 2001—mental health: new understanding, new hope. World Health Organization, Geneva

Strategies to Reduce Mental Illness Stigma

24

Nicolas Rüsch and Ziyan Xu

Introduction

As outlined in other chapters of this book, the stigma and discrimination associated with mental illness remain a major burden on people with mental illness, their families, and society. Reducing the stigma and increasing the empowerment and well-being of people with mental illness should therefore be a priority for health services and society in general. In order to achieve these goals, effective anti-stigma strategies and interventions are needed. In this chapter, we will discuss strategies to tackle three types of stigma: public stigma, self-stigma, and structural discrimination. Briefly, public stigma refers to members of the general public endorsing negative stereotypes and discriminating against people with mental illness (Corrigan 2005; Rüsch et al. 2005; Thornicroft 2006); self-stigma occurs if people with mental illness internalize negative stereotypes, leading to diminished self-esteem, self-efficacy, and demoralization (Corrigan et al. 2009); and structural discrimination implies rules and regulations in society that intentionally or unintentionally disadvantage stigmatized individuals (Hatzenbuehler and Link 2014); see Chap. 3 for further details. This chapter is based on recent original articles, systematic reviews cited in the relevant sections, as well as previous narrative reviews (Rüsch et al. 2011; Rüsch and Corrigan 2012; Thornicroft et al. 2016).

N. Rüsch (✉)
Clinic for Psychiatry II, Section Public Mental Health,
University of Ulm, Parkstraße 11, 89073 Ulm, Germany
e-mail: nicolas.ruesch@uni-ulm.de

Z. Xu
Department of Psychiatry II, University of Ulm,
Parkstraße 11, 89073 Ulm, Germany
e-mail: ziyan.xu@uniklinik-ulm.de

Interventions to Reduce Public Stigma

Strategies

Three strategies can be used to reduce public stigma: protest, education, and contact (Corrigan and Penn 1999) (Table 24.1). Protest, by stigmatized individuals or members of the general public who support them, is often applied against stigmatizing public statements, such as media reports or advertisements. Anecdotally, protest interventions, for example, against stigmatizing advertisements or television series, have successfully suppressed negative public statements, and therefore this strategy may be useful for this purpose (Wahl 1995). However, protest is unlikely to improve attitudes toward people with mental illness (Corrigan and Penn 1999).

Education interventions aim to diminish stigma by replacing myths and negative stereotypes with facts and have reduced stigmatizing attitudes among members of the public. Research on education interventions suggests that behavior changes are often not evaluated, and the degree of change achieved may be small and relatively brief (Corrigan 2005). There are, however, more comprehensive approaches to improve the knowledge about mental health – also called mental health literacy (Jorm 2012) – in certain target groups as well as the general population. One such approach is "Mental Health First Aid," a program developed by Betty Kitchener and Tony Jorm in Australia and implemented widely there and increasingly in other parts of the world (Jorm et al. 2010; Kitchener and Jorm 2006; Kitchener et al. 2010). Research shows that this program does not only improve knowledge on how to respond to people with mental health problems but also decreases some aspects of stigma (Hadlaczky et al. 2014; Jorm et al. 2010).

The third strategy is personal contact with persons with mental illness which is based on intergroup contact theory and has shown to be an effective way to reduce prejudice against various minorities (Pettigrew and Tropp 2006). In a number of interventions in secondary schools, education and personal contact have been combined (Pinfold et al. 2003). Contact appears to be the more efficacious part of the intervention. Factors that create an advantageous environment for interpersonal contact and stigma reduction include equal status among participants, cooperative interactions, and institutional support for the contact initiative (Pettigrew and Tropp 2006). Contact is also more likely than education to improve implicit attitudes, because pleasant and constructive contact, unlike abstract information, can strengthen automatic associations between members of the stigmatized group and positive characteristics (Rudman et al. 2001).

For both education and contact, the content of anti-stigma programs matters. Biogenetic models of mental illness are often highlighted because viewing mental illness as a biological, mainly inherited problem, was thought to reduce the associated shame and blame. Evidence supports this optimistic expectation in terms of reduced blame. However, focusing on biogenetic factors may strengthen the perception that people with mental illness are fundamentally different, increasing

Table 24.1 Strategies for challenging public stigma

Strategy	Method and efficacy
Protest	Organizations or individuals protest against stigmatizing public statements, for example, in TV or commercials
	Anecdotal evidence that after protest such statements are withdrawn (e.g., a TV series stopped), but no evidence for improvement of attitudes
Education	To correct erroneous and stigmatizing assumptions/stereotypes, replace myths with facts about mental illness
	Evidence from RCTs that education improves knowledge and attitudes and reduces discriminating behavior
Contact	Cooperative, small-group contact between people with mental illness in recovery and target group members (e.g., local employers); can be combined with education (e.g., a person with mental illness providing information)
	Evidence from RCTs that contact improves attitudes and reduces discriminating behavior

social distance, perceptions of mental illness as persistent, serious and dangerous, and pessimistic views about treatment outcomes (Phelan et al. 2006). Genetic models also seem to have negative consequences for people with mental illness themselves, increasing fear of other individuals with mental illness and leading to implicit self-blame (Rüsch et al. 2010a). Therefore, a message of mental illness as being "genetic" or "neurological" may be overly simplistic and unhelpful for reducing stigma (Angermeyer et al. 2011; Schnittker 2008; Schomerus et al. 2014).

Examples

Anti-stigma initiatives can take place nationally as well as locally. National campaigns often adopt a social marketing approach, whereas local initiatives usually focus on target groups. An example of a large multifaceted national campaign is *Time to Change* in England (Henderson and Thornicroft 2009). It combines mass media advertising and local initiatives. The latter try to facilitate social contact between members of the general public and mental health service users as well as target specific groups such as medical students and teachers. A series of evaluations of the program's first years provides evidence for positive effects, although some of them do not seem to be stable over time, suggesting the need for continuous initiatives (Henderson and Thornicroft 2013; Evans-Lacko et al. 2013a, b, c; Friedrich et al. 2013). Similar initiatives in other countries, for example, *See Me* in Scotland (Dunion and Gordon 2005), *Like Minds, Like Mine* in New Zealand (Vaughan and Hansen 2004), *beyondblue* in Australia focusing on depression and anxiety (Jorm et al. 2006; Sawyer et al. 2010; McCabe et al. 2013), or the international World Psychiatric Association anti-stigma initiative (Sartorius and Schulze 2005), have also reported positive outcomes.

Efficacy and Implementation

A recent meta-analysis looked at the efficacy of contact and education to reduce public stigma while there were not enough data to examine the effects of protest (Corrigan et al. 2012). Both education and contact appear to be effective to improve attitudes. For adults, contact had stronger effects than education. Interestingly, for adolescents, a reverse pattern emerged, education having stronger effects than contact. Regarding the method of delivery, face-to-face contact was more effective than virtual contact, for example by video. This has important implications for implementation: There may be a trade-off, since virtual contact can be delivered more easily and cost-effectively to large audiences, for example online, but with reduced efficacy. It should be noted, though, that another systematic review could not replicate the superiority of live as compared to virtual contact (Griffiths et al. 2014).

Another meta-analysis specifically examined the efficacy of mass media interventions (Clement et al. 2013) that are delivered by regular or electronic mail, by audio or video recordings, or via the internet. The authors found positive effects on prejudice, but no effects on discrimination. Finally, a meta-analysis focused on the medium- and long-term effects of interventions to reduce public stigma and on data from low- and middle-income countries (Mehta et al. 2015). For both questions, very few data are available, limiting the conclusions that can be drawn. However, in the latter analysis, contact was not superior to education and there was virtually no information available from low-income countries (Mehta et al. 2015).

Researchers have tried to collect systematic evidence regarding interventions to reduce stigma either in specific settings or with respect to certain disorders. Many interventions have been applied to improve attitudes among adolescents and college students in schools, colleges, and universities. Systematic reviews conclude that these programs have positive effects; however, there is insufficient information on the stability of these effects over time and of effects on behavior (rather than just on attitudes) (Mellor 2014; Yamaguchi et al. 2013). Substance use disorders are among the most stigmatized health conditions and effective interventions in this domain are therefore particularly important. Fortunately, there is initial evidence that interventions can improve attitudes of members of the general public as well as of health professionals toward individuals with these disorders (Livingston et al. 2012).

Future Directions

On average, interventions to reduce public stigma had only small to moderate effect sizes, underlining the need to develop more effective interventions in this domain. The findings of different meta-analyses highlight the need for thorough research and high-quality trials, especially those that measure effects on behavior/discrimination rather than self-reported attitudes as well as interventions that have stable medium- and long-term effects. An important outcome should be discrimination as experienced by people with mental illness. Since implicit, automatically activated reactions are relevant especially for more subtle, spontaneous, and nonverbal stigmatizing behaviors (Greenwald et al. 2009), the role of implicit mental illness stigma (Rüsch et al. 2010a, b) and the efficacy of interventions to change it (Gawronski and Bodenhausen 2006) should be investigated. Finally, the cost-effectiveness of anti-stigma campaigns is relevant to justify the resources spent (McCrone et al. 2010).

Interventions to Reduce Self-Stigma

Self-stigma occurs when people with mental illness are not only aware of public negative stereotypes about themselves and their group, but agree with them ("Yes, people with mental illness are stupid") and apply them to themselves ("Yes, that's right, I have a mental illness and therefore I am stupid"), leading to reduced self-esteem and self-efficacy (Corrigan and Watson 2002; Corrigan et al. 2011). Self-stigma has behavioral consequences when individuals with mental illness give up their life goals as a consequence of internalizing stigma; this is referred to as "why try effect" when someone does not feel worthy or able to pursue her or his goals (Corrigan et al. 2009). Self-stigma is also associated with shame, guilt, and secrecy or the tendency not to disclose one's mental illness to others (Link et al. 1991; Rüsch et al. 2006a).

Self-stigma is common among people with mental illness. In a large European survey of more than 1,000 participants with schizophrenia across 14 countries, nearly one in two reported moderate to high levels of self-stigma (Brohan et al. 2010). Among people with bipolar disorder or depression, about one in five had high self-stigma (Brohan et al. 2011). These numbers suggest that interventions to reduce self-stigma and its impact among people with mental illness are needed. We begin with an introduction of strategies to change self-stigma, followed by examples of intervention programs. We will conclude by discussing the efficacy of current interventions as well as problems and future directions.

Strategies

Psychoeducation

Psychoeducation for people with mental illness who suffer from self-stigma provides information about mental illness in order to reduce the agreement with prejudicial views and with discrimination against people with mental illness (Link et al. 2002). Psychoeducation informs about mental illness, including its etiology, prognosis, and available treatments; how self-stigma develops and affects individuals with mental illness; common myths about mental illness; and corresponding facts. It also presents examples of persons with severe mental illness who have successful careers and lead a happy life. The goal is to correct negative, distorted views about mental illness and provide a more balanced picture. Psychoeducation is the most frequently tested intervention so far (Mittal et al. 2012) and is also a strategy to reduce public stigma (see Table 24.1 in this chapter: education) (Jorm and Wright 2007).

Cognitive Restructuring

Cognitive restructuring is a core element of cognitive behavioral therapy (Beck et al. 1987). Participants learn about the links between events, thoughts, behaviors, and feelings. Cognitive behavioral therapy teaches how to identify and modify inaccurate thoughts. It helps to challenge dysfunctional thinking and to develop more adaptive thoughts. In this framework, self-stigma can be seen as a dysfunctional belief or self-concept. This approach can help counter self-stigmatizing beliefs. For example, a person with mental illness could think "I could never make things work because I am crazy," but he or she could then learn to address this self-defeating thought with contradictory evidence (e.g., "I have cleaned my room, I often cook for my family, I take care of my dog so well. These are all significant things to me. I do have a mental illness, but I can achieve important goals").

Disclosure

Disclosing one's mental illness may protect against stigma's negative effects (Rüsch et al. 2005; Corrigan et al. 2010). People who have disclosed aspects of their experience often report enhanced personal empowerment, self-esteem, and confidence in the pursuit of their life goals (Corrigan et al. 2013a). However, before people with mental illness share their experience with mental illness, they need to consider the risks and benefits of disclosure in different settings and to decide what to whom, and how to disclose. There are different levels of disclosure, from complete social avoidance and secrecy on the one end to indiscriminant disclosure and broadcasting on the other end (Corrigan 2004; Corrigan and Rao 2012). Many individuals choose selective disclosure as a middle path, disclosing their condition to some, but not all people in their environment. This choice may differ depending on the setting. Some individuals may find disclosure in their faith community or family easier than at their workplace.

Peer Support

The support of peers, that is, support by people with lived experience of mental illness for other individuals with mental illness, is an important resource in challenging self-stigma. It refers to more or less structured programs that are designed to enhance the sense of empowerment and self-determination. Peer support groups provide a range of services including emotional support, empathy, and care; help to feel connected and exchange experiences with others; and provide information on ways of recovery and coping skills. The act of sharing with or helping others gives people the opportunity to affirm their independence and sense of self-worth (Corrigan and Rao 2012). Participating in mutual-help groups promotes group identification or pride which may encourage people with mental illness to turn to peers for help and increase their sense of empowerment (Corrigan et al. 2013b; Rüsch et al. 2009).

Empowerment

Empowerment is a broad concept and involves power, control over one's treatment, activism, righteous indignation about unfair treatment, as well as optimism regarding one's future. Empowerment and self-stigma have been described as opposite poles of a continuum (Rüsch et al. 2006b). Enhancing personal empowerment is a main strategy to reduce self-stigma (Mittal et al. 2012). There are several ways to facilitate empowerment (Corrigan and Lundin 2001): (i) people with mental illness actively participate in treatment and get more satisfaction from services, giving them greater control over their lives; (ii) people with mental illness can act as mental health service providers, providing knowledge about mental illness, skills to deal with symptoms, and resources to meet personal goals; (iii) skills training can be provided by peer support groups, incl. specific coping skills, identifying solutions to problems by the group of peers, and validating solution lists and their suitability for real-life situations. Therefore the experience of mutual help can enhance a person's self-efficacy and well-being, and by enhanced empowerment, people with mental illness can develop more positive attitudes toward themselves.

Mindfulness

Mindfulness is a state of focusing one's attention to the present experience on a moment-to-moment basis nonjudgmentally (Kabat-Zinn 1994) (Marlatt and Kristeller 1999). It involves the training to maintain the awareness of one's present sensations, thoughts, or feelings, such as the breath or body sensations, to experience them as they arise and subside. People with mental illness are encouraged to nonjudgmentally notice self-stigmatizing evaluations and related emotions as passing events of their minds. Instead of struggling to get away from the stigmatizing beliefs or emotions, individuals practice to be with them, without agreeing with them (Hayes et al. 2004). This allows individuals to step back from their thoughts rather than to view them as necessarily accurate reflections of reality, reducing the risk of self-stigma. For example, every time a person noticed that in her mind she had the thought "I am a bad person, because I have a mental illness," she could reflect that "This is just one of my passing thoughts," observing it nonjudgmentally and not taking it for real.

Normalizing

Normalization is often used to target distressing psychotic symptoms and maladaptive understandings of mental illness in a collaborative empirical framework (Corrigan 2005). It is based on the notion that unusual experiences are common in the general population in a range of different circumstances (e.g., stressful events, trauma, hyperventilation, falling asleep, etc.). The aim of normalization here is to reduce the shame, anxiety, and self-stigma associated with mental illness. For example, in terms of the specific stressors on individuals, delusional ideation could be identified as "faulty cognition" with excessive self-reference, selective abstraction, or jumping to conclusions. As an intervention to reduce self-stigma, the goal of normalization is to destigmatize confusing and frightening experiences while not losing sight of the fact that something may be wrong (Kingdon and Turkington 1991).

Examples

Interventions may be delivered with one strategy only (e.g., psychoeducation) or a combination of different strategies as a multimodal treatment (e.g., psychoeducation with cognitive restructuring, self-acceptance with coping skills enhancement, or narrative enhancement with elements of CBT). Here are some examples of such structured intervention programs to reduce self-stigma (Table 24.2).

Narrative Enhancement and Cognitive Therapy (NECT)

This intervention has three central therapeutic approaches: psychoeducation, narrative strategies focusing on one's story, and cognitive restructuring (Yanos et al. 2011; Hasson-Ohayon et al. 2014; Yanos et al. 2012). The purpose of psychoeducation is to provide factual information and to correct stigmatizing beliefs. Narrative enhancement encourages participants to write or tell their personal story with mental illness, focusing on their achievements, hope, and recovery. Cognitive restructuring helps to identify and challenge dysfunctional beliefs (e.g., "I must be a weak person because I get depressed").

Cognitive Behavioral Therapy (CBT)

This program is based on Aaron Beck's cognitive theory (Beck et al. 1987) and includes cognitive and behavioral strategies for psychotic disorders (Kingdon and Turkington 1994). A strong therapeutic alliance is a key feature and CBT is always centered on the perspective of the person with mental illness. Stress-vulnerability

Table 24.2 Self-stigma reduction programs

Examples	Core strategies or approaches
Narrative Enhancement and Cognitive Therapy (NECT)	Psychoeducation, cognitive restructuring, narrative enhancement
Cognitive Behavioral Therapy (CBT)	Psychoeducation, normalization, cognitive restructuring, coping skills training
Coming Out Proud/Honest, Open, Proud (COP/HOP)	Support with disclosure decisions, peer support
Acceptance and Commitment Therapy (ACT)	Self-acceptance, mindfulness, value-directed behavioral intervention
Ending Self-Stigma (ESS)	Psychoeducation, cognitive restructuring, empowerment
Self-Stigma Reduction Program	Psychoeducation, motivational interviewing, cognitive restructuring, social skills training
Consumer-Operated Service Programs (COSPs)	Peer support, empowerment

models and normalization strategies are adapted to better understand the symptoms to combat stigma (Morrison et al. 2013). Besides challenging dysfunctional (self-) stigmatizing beliefs, self-acceptance is also encouraged. Social skills training is provided through behavioral rehearsal or role play; for example, people with mental illness can learn how to be assertive and to build a positive self-image in social situations. Other coping strategies such as relaxation techniques and emotional regulation skills are developed. At the end of such programs, plans for coping with future challenges are developed (Shimotsu et al. 2014).

Coming Out Proud/Honest, Open, Proud

Coming Out Proud (or now: Honest, Open, Proud) is a peer-led group program to support people with mental illness in their coping with stigma and disclosure-related distress. It was developed by Corrigan, other researchers as well as mental health service users based on a previous book by Corrigan and Lundin (2001) and informed by experiences with coming out among lesbian, gay, or bisexual individuals (Corrigan et al. 2013a). The goal of Coming Out Proud/Honest, Open, Proud is to support people with mental illness in their choices regarding disclosure versus nondisclosure. It is not the aim to make people disclose their mental illness but rather to help them find their way how to handle this choice in different settings. Coming Out Proud/ Honest, Open, Proud addresses three key issues related to disclosure, one in each session: (i) the costs and benefits of disclosure, (ii) different ways and levels of disclosure, and (iii) how to tell one's story (Rüsch et al. 2014a). The program includes suggestions and discussion points on how to present one's experience with mental illness. It is a group program that is run by peers with lived experience of mental illness.

Acceptance and Commitment Therapy (ACT)

ACT is a psychological intervention that uses acceptance and mindfulness strategies along with commitment and behavior change strategies to increase psychological flexibility (Hayes et al. 2006). It focuses on the relationship between thoughts, feelings, and overt behavior, rather than on attempts to modify the problematic stigmatizing thoughts and feelings themselves. ACT includes exercises that enable participants to notice how judgmental processes are related to stigmatizing attitudes. In the program, participants are trained to use psychological acceptance to increase self-understanding and empathy. The costs of self-stigma are discussed, and acceptance and nonjudgmental skills for stigma toward oneself and others are trained. Finally, it supports a behavioral commitment for change. Participants are encouraged to explore their life goals and values and to link the accomplishment of desired goals to values (Masuda 2014). This program has mainly been used to reduce self-stigma among people with substance use disorders (Luoma et al. 2012).

Ending Self-Stigma (ESS)

Ending Self-Stigma is a structured nine-session group intervention to reduce self-stigma among people with serious mental illnesses (Lucksted et al. 2011). The program includes lectures, discussions, sharing of personal experiences, teaching and practicing of skills, group support, and problem-solving exercises. Participants are asked to complete assignments between sessions.

Self-Stigma Reduction Program

This program aims to reduce self-stigma among people with schizophrenia. It contains 16 sessions, 12 group, and 4 individual follow-up sessions and includes five strategies: psychoeducation; motivational interviewing; cognitive behavioral therapy focused on combating beliefs of self-stigma; social skills training; and goal setting, action planning, and progress monitoring (Fung et al. 2011).

Consumer-Operated Service Programs (COSPs)

COSPs are self- and mutual-help programs managed by people with mental illness for people with mental illness. In these programs, individuals not only receive support and resources from peers but also support others. COSPs are a clear example that people with mental illness are able to take full responsibility of their care which increases their sense of empowerment (Segal et al. 2013; Corrigan 2006) .

Efficacy

Since few rigorous trials have evaluated the effects of interventions to reduce self-stigma, systematic reviews to date find little evidence for their efficacy. In a recent meta-analysis, only three intervention studies targeted self-stigma among people with mental illness. Two of them focused on people with mental illness in general, while a third focused on persons with schizophrenia. All interventions used multimodal psychotherapy, including psychoeducation, cognitive behavioral elements, acceptance, and commitment therapy, or narrative enhancement. The mean effect size was small and not statistically significant (Griffiths et al. 2014). In a recent narrative review, 8 out of 14 studies reported significant reductions of self-stigma (Mittal et al. 2012). Effect sizes were small to moderate. Psychoeducation was the most common intervention type. Booklets or information leaflets yielded small to medium effect sizes, and effect sizes of psychotherapy with cognitive behavioral elements ranged from 0.01 to 0.95. This suggests that cognitive behavioral methods can decrease self-stigma (Mittal et al. 2012). There is initial evidence from two randomized controlled trials in Europe and the USA that the peer-led Coming Out Proud/Honest, Open, Proud program reduces stigma-related stress, distress due to disclosure, as well as self-stigma (Rüsch et al. 2014a; Corrigan et al. 2015).

Future Directions

More randomized controlled trials with rigorous research methods and large sample sizes are needed. The fidelity of intervention delivery (e.g., professional training, manualization, and supervision) should be improved and self-stigma should be measured using appropriate outcome measures. For example, measures of perceived public stigma may very well capture the level of stigma a person perceives in society, but may be insufficient to capture self-stigma (Mittal et al. 2012). There is also a need for follow-up evaluations to test the sustainability of intervention effects.

The current literature has mainly focused on self-stigma among people with an established diagnosis of mental illness. It would be beneficial to design specialized interventions for young people at risk of psychosis (Rüsch et al. 2014b, c). Further research could explore the role of culture and ethnicity for interventions to reduce self-stigma as well as the cost-effectiveness of such programs. More research is needed to move from the question "Does it work?" to the question "Why and for whom does it work?" (Ehde et al. 2014). Answer this question can facilitate the future development of more effective interventions and their implementation for specific target groups. Finally, it will be relevant to examine the interactions between public stigma, structural discrimination, and self-stigma (Evans-Lacko et al. 2012) and the effects of interventions aimed at public or structural stigma on self-stigma levels. If societal attitudes became more positive, self-stigma is likely to decrease.

Interventions to Reduce Structural Discrimination

Strategies

Improving attitudes and behaviors of individuals is not sufficient to fight stigma, because discrimination can persist in long-lived social and cultural rules and regulations despite the best intentions of individuals (Hatzenbuehler and Link 2014). Comprehensive anti-stigma efforts can affect structural discrimination by specifically addressing legislation, mental health care funding, or health insurance policies which disadvantage people with mental illness. Some examples of these strategies are outlined below (Table 24.3). Differences between developing and developed countries should be taken into account (Rosen 2006), since structural discrimination and initiatives to fight it depend on legal and cultural local factors.

Table 24.3 Ways to reduce structural discrimination

Ways	Content
Education	Target individual-level and structural-level attitudes
Legislation	Anti-discrimination legislation (e.g., employment equity)
Media	Improve knowledge and attitudes of journalists in order to promote more balanced and recovery-oriented media coverage
Funding	Give equal resources to mental health care (as compared to physical health care), incl. access to outpatient psychotherapy and psychosocial interventions (e.g., supported employment)

Examples and Efficacy

There are two ways to reduce structural discrimination (Cook et al. 2014). First, individual-level interventions can over time change public attitudes, thus influencing legislative and other aspects of structural stigma. Second, interventions can specifically address the structural level, either in overall society or referring to institutions (e.g., within companies). Research showed that companies which actively stated ethnic diversity as an important goal were less threatening for individuals from ethnic minorities (Purdie-Vaughns et al. 2008). It may also be worthwhile to include education about structural aspects of healthcare and stigma in the curricula of future healthcare professionals (Metzl and Hansen 2014).

A second important avenue to reduce structural stigma is legislation. Recent US and European laws against discrimination of people with psychiatric or physical disabilities offer examples on how structural discrimination could be tackled, but also show limitations of this approach (Stuart 2007). Employment equity legislation aims to reduce discrimination against people with disabilities with respect to recruitment, retention, and promotion (Stuart 2006). However, the compliance of employers with the new legislation is often limited (Roulstone and Warren 2005), and for people with mental illness, it can be difficult to win anti-discrimination cases in court (Allbright 2005).

Finally, negative media portrayals of people with mental illness are often considered as structural stigma (Corrigan et al. 2005). Therefore interventions to improve the knowledge and attitudes of journalists toward people with mental illness are pertinent here (Stuart 2003; Campbell et al. 2009). There is also evidence that broad population campaigns can improve media reporting, thus potentially contributing to a virtual circle (Thornicroft et al. 2013).

Future Directions

To this date, there is very little empirical evidence on the efficacy of interventions to reduce the structural stigma associated with mental illness. This is a consequence of the relative neglect of structural aspects in this field until recently (Corrigan et al. 2004; Hatzenbuehler and Link 2014). Basic research is therefore needed on (i) structural-level interventions and their effects on members of the general public as well as on people with mental illness and (ii) on the interplay between individual- and structural-level interventions and their impact on structural stigma (Cook et al. 2014).

Conclusions

In summary, there is increasing evidence for the effectiveness of anti-stigma initiatives. On a more cautious note, individual discrimination, structural discrimination, and self-stigma lead to innumerable mechanisms of stigmatization. If one mechanism is blocked or diminished through successful initiatives, other ways to discriminate may emerge (Link and Phelan 2001). Therefore, to substantially reduce discrimination, stigmatizing attitudes and behaviors of influential stakeholders need to change fundamentally.

Future anti-stigma initiatives should tackle different aspects of stigma and discrimination simultaneously. In particular, they should measure success in terms of reduced discriminatory behavior as experienced by people with mental illness and the stability of these effects over time. Success will depend on the continuing collaboration of many groups in society, involving people with mental illness as well as key stakeholders such as teachers, mental health professionals, faith leaders, employers, police officers, and legislators. Judging from the history of the civil rights movement, a long-term collaborative effort is needed to achieve profound social change and substantially reduce mental illness stigma. Much more research and advocacy work is needed to understand, design, evaluate, and implement effective interventions. Therefore this seems to the beginning, rather than the end, of the story.

Information Box
- Contact and education are effective strategies to reduce public stigma.
- Cognitive as well as coping-focused approaches may reduce self-stigma.
- There is a lack of evidence on structural-level (e.g., legislative) interventions.
- Data on the medium- and long-term efficacy and on behavior changes are lacking.

References

Allbright AL (2005) 2004 employment decisions under the ADA title I – survey update. Ment Phys Disabil Law Report 29:513–516

Angermeyer MC, Holzinger A, Carta MG, Schomerus G (2011) Biogenetic explanations and public acceptance of mental illness: systematic review of population studies. Br J Psychiatry 199:367–372

Beck AT, Rush AJ, Shaw BF, Emery G (1987) Cognitive therapy of depression. Guilford Press, New York

Brohan E, Elgie R, Sartorius N, Thornicroft G (2010) Self-stigma, empowerment and perceived discrimination among people with schizophrenia in 14 European countries: the GAMIAN-Europe study. Schizophr Res 122:232–238

Brohan E, Gauci D, Sartorius N, Thornicroft G (2011) Self-stigma, empowerment and perceived discrimination among people with bipolar disorder or depression in 13 European countries: the GAMIAN-Europe study. J Affect Disord 129:56–63

Campbell NN, Heath J, Bouknight J, Rudd K, Pender J (2009) Speaking out for mental health: collaboration of future journalists and psychiatrists. Acad Psychiatry 33:166–168

Clement S, Lassman F, Barley E, Evans-Lacko SE, Williams P, Yamaguchi S, Slade M, Rüsch N, Thornicroft G (2013) Mass media interventions for reducing mental health-related stigma. Cochrane Database Syst Rev 7:CD009453

Cook JE, Purdie-Vaughns V, Meyer IH, Busch JT (2014) Intervening within and across levels: a multilevel approach to stigma and public health. Soc Sci Med 103:101–109

Corrigan PW (2004) Don't call me nuts: an international perspective on the stigma of mental illness. Acta Psychiatr Scand 109:403–404

Corrigan PW (2005) On the stigma of mental illness: practical strategies for research and social change. American Psychological Association, Washington, DC

Corrigan PW (2006) Impact of consumer-operated services on empowerment and recovery of people with psychiatric disabilities. Psychiatr Serv 57:1493–1496

Corrigan PW, Larson JE, Michaels PJ, Buchholz BA, Del Rossi R, Fontecchio M, Castro D, Gause M, Krzyżanowski R, Rüsch N (2015) Diminishing the self-stigma of mental illness by Coming Out Proud. Psychiatry Research 229:148–154

Corrigan PW, Lundin R (2001) Don't call me nuts! Coping with the stigma of mental illness. Recovery Press, Chicago

Corrigan PW, Penn DL (1999) Lessons from social psychology on discrediting psychiatric stigma. Am Psychol 54:765–776

Corrigan PW, Rao D (2012) On the self-stigma of mental illness: stages, disclosure, and strategies for change. Can J Psychiatr 57:464–469

Corrigan PW, Watson AC (2002) The paradox of self-stigma and mental illness. Clin Psychol Sci Pract 9:35–53

Corrigan PW, Markowitz FE, Watson AC (2004) Structural levels of mental illness stigma and discrimination. Schizophr Bull 30:481–491

Corrigan PW, Watson AC, Gracia G, Slopen N, Rasinski K, Hall LL (2005) Newspaper stories as measures of structural stigma. Psychiatr Serv 56:551–556

Corrigan PW, Larson JE, Rüsch N (2009) Self-stigma and the "why try" effect: impact on life goals and evidence-based practices. World Psychiatry 8:75–81

Corrigan PW, Morris S, Larson JE, Rafacz J, Wassel A, Michaels P, Wilkniss S, Batia K, Rüsch N (2010) Self-stigma and coming out about one's mental illness. J Community Psychol 38:1–17

Corrigan PW, Rafacz J, Rüsch N (2011) Examining a progressive model of self-stigma and its impact on people with serious mental illness. Psychiatry Res 189:339–343

Corrigan PW, Morris SB, Michaels PJ, Rafacz JE, Rüsch N (2012) Challenging the public stigma of mental illness: a meta-analysis of outcome studies. Psychiatr Serv 63:963–973

Corrigan PW, Kosyluk KA, Rüsch N (2013a) Reducing self-stigma by coming out proud. Am J Public Health 103:794–800

Corrigan PW, Sokol KA, Rüsch N (2013b) The impact of self-stigma and mutual-help programs on the quality of life of people with serious mental illnesses. Community Ment Health J 49:1–6

Dunion L, Gordon L (2005) Tackling the attitude problem. The achievements to date of Scotland's 'See Me' anti-stigma campaign. Ment Health Today March: 22–25

Ehde DM, Dillworth TM, Turner JA (2014) Cognitive-behavioral therapy for individuals with chronic pain: efficacy, innovations, and directions for research. Am Psychol 69:153

Evans-Lacko S, Brohan E, Mojtabai R, Thornicroft G (2012) Association between public views of mental illness and self-stigma among individuals with mental illness in 14 European countries. Psychol Med 42:1741–1752

Evans-Lacko S, Henderson C, Thornicroft G (2013a) Public knowledge, attitudes and behaviour regarding people with mental illness in England 2009–2012. Br J Psychiatry Suppl 55:s51–s57

Evans-Lacko S, Henderson C, Thornicroft G, McCrone P (2013b) Economic evaluation of the anti-stigma social marketing campaign in England 2009–2011. Br J Psychiatry Suppl 55:s95–s101

Evans-Lacko S, Malcolm E, West K, Rose D, London J, Rüsch N, Little K, Henderson C, Thornicroft G (2013c) Influence of Time to Change's social marketing interventions on stigma in England 2009–2011. Br J Psychiatry Suppl 55:s77–s88

Friedrich B, Evans-Lacko S, London J, Rhydderch D, Henderson C, Thornicroft G (2013) Anti-stigma training for medical students: the Education Not Discrimination project. Br J Psychiatry Suppl 55:s89–s94

Fung KM, Tsang HW, Cheung WM (2011) Randomized controlled trial of the self-stigma reduction program among individuals with schizophrenia. Psychiatry Res 189:208–214

Gawronski B, Bodenhausen GV (2006) Associative and propositional processes in evaluation: an integrative review of implicit and explicit attitude change. Psychol Bull 132:692–731

Greenwald AG, Poehlman TA, Uhlmann E, Banaji MR (2009) Understanding and using the Implicit Association Test: III. Meta-analysis of predictive validity. J Pers Soc Psychol 97:17–41

Griffiths KM, Carron-Arthur B, Parsons A, Reid R (2014) Effectiveness of programs for reducing the stigma associated with mental disorders. A meta-analysis of randomized controlled trials. World Psychiatry 13:161–175

Hadlaczky G, Hökby S, Mkrtchian A, Carli V, Wasserman D (2014) Mental Health First Aid is an effective public health intervention for improving knowledge, attitudes, and behaviour: a meta-analysis. Int Rev Psychiatry 26:467–475

Hasson-Ohayon I, Mashiach-Eizenberg M, Elhasid N, Yanos PT, Lysaker PH, Roe D (2014) Between self-clarity and recovery in schizophrenia: reducing the self-stigma and finding meaning. Compr Psychiatry 55:675–680

Hatzenbuehler ML, Link BG (2014) Introduction to the special issue on structural stigma and health. Soc Sci Med 103:1–6

Hayes SC, Bissett R, Roget N, Padilla M, Kohlenberg BS, Fisher G, Masuda A, Pistorello J, Rye AK, Berry K (2004) The impact of acceptance and commitment training and multicultural training on the stigmatizing attitudes and professional burnout of substance abuse counselors. Behav Ther 35:821–835

Hayes SC, Luoma JB, Bond FW, Masuda A, Lillis J (2006) Acceptance and commitment therapy: model, processes and outcomes. Behav Res Ther 44:1–25

Henderson C, Thornicroft G (2009) Stigma and discrimination in mental illness: time to change. Lancet 373:1930–1932

Henderson C, Thornicroft G (2013) Evaluation of the Time to Change programme in England 2008–2011. Br J Psychiatry Suppl 55:s45–s48

Jorm AF (2012) Mental health literacy: empowering the community to take action for better mental health. Am Psychol 67:231–243

Jorm AF, Wright A (2007) Beliefs of young people and their parents about the effectiveness of interventions for mental disorders. Aust N Z J Psychiatry 41:656–666

Jorm AF, Christensen H, Griffiths KM (2006) Changes in depression awareness and attitudes in Australia: the impact of beyondblue: the national depression initiative. Aust N Z J Psychiatry 40:42–46

Jorm AF, Kitchener BA, Sawyer MG, Scales H, Cvetkovski S (2010) Mental health first aid training for high school teachers: a cluster randomized trial. BMC Psychiatry 10:51

Kabat-Zinn J (1994) Wherever you go, there you are: mindfulness meditation in everyday life. Hyperion, New York

Kingdon DG, Turkington D (1991) The use of cognitive behavior therapy with a normalizing rationale in schizophrenia. Preliminary report. J Nerv Ment Dis 179:207–211

Kingdon DG, Turkington D (1994) Cognitive-behavioral therapy of schizophrenia. Guilford Press, New York

Kitchener BA, Jorm AF (2006) Mental health first aid training: review of evaluation studies. Aust N Z J Psychiatry 40:6–8

Kitchener BA, Jorm AF, Kelly CM (2010) Mental health first aid manual, 2nd edn. Orygen Youth Health Research Centre, Melbourne

Link BG, Phelan JC (2001) Conceptualizing stigma. Annu Rev Sociol 27:363–385

Link BG, Mirotznik J, Cullen FT (1991) The effectiveness of stigma coping orientations: can negative consequences of mental illness labeling be avoided? J Health Soc Behav 32:302–320

Link BG, Struening EL, Neese-Todd S, Asmussen S, Phelan JC (2002) On describing and seeking to change the experience of stigma. Psychiatr Rehabil Skills 6:201–231

Livingston JD, Milne T, Fang ML, Amari E (2012) The effectiveness of interventions for reducing stigma related to substance use disorders: a systematic review. Addiction 107:39–50

Lucksted A, Drapalski A, Calmes C, Forbes C, DeForge B, Boyd J (2011) Ending self-stigma: pilot evaluation of a new intervention to reduce internalized stigma among people with mental illnesses. Psychiatr Rehabil J 35:51–54

Luoma JB, Kohlenberg BS, Hayes SC, Fletcher L (2012) Slow and steady wins the race: a randomized clinical trial of acceptance and commitment therapy targeting shame in substance use disorders. J Consult Clin Psychol 80:43–53

Marlatt GA, Kristeller JL (1999) Mindfulness and meditation. In: Miller WR (ed) Integrating spirituality into treatment: resources for practitioners. American Psychological Association, Washington, DC, pp 67–84

Masuda A (2014) Mindfulness and acceptance in multicultural competency: a contextual approach to sociocultural diversity in theory and practice. New Harbinger Publications, Oakland

McCabe MP, Karantzas GC, Mrkic D, Mellor D, Davison TE (2013) A randomized control trial to evaluate the beyondblue depression training program: does it lead to better recognition of depression? Int J Geriatr Psychiatry 28:221–226

McCrone P, Knapp M, Henri M, McDaid D (2010) The economic impact of initiatives to reduce stigma: demonstration of a modelling approach. Epidemiol Psichiatr Soc 19:131–139

Mehta N, Clement S, Marcus E, Stona AC, Bezborodovs N, Evans-Lacko S, Palacios J, Docherty M, Barley E, Rose D, Koschorke M, Shidhaye R, Henderson C, Thornicroft G (2015) Evidence for effective interventions to reduce mental health-related stigma and discrimination in the medium and long term: systematic review. Br J Psychiatry 207:377–384

Mellor C (2014) School-based interventions targeting stigma of mental illness: systematic review. Psychiatr Bull 38:164–171

Metzl JM, Hansen H (2014) Structural competency: theorizing a new medical engagement with stigma and inequality. Soc Sci Med 103:126–133

Mittal D, Sullivan G, Chekuri L, Allee E, Corrigan PW (2012) Empirical studies of self-stigma reduction strategies: a critical review of the literature. Psychiatr Serv 63:974–981

Morrison AP, Birchwood M, Pyle M, Flach C, Stewart SL, Byrne R, Patterson P, Jones PB, Fowler D, Gumley AI, French P (2013) Impact of cognitive therapy on internalised stigma in people with at-risk mental states. Br J Psychiatry 203:140–145

Pettigrew TF, Tropp LR (2006) A meta-analytic test of intergroup contact theory. J Pers Soc Psychol 90:751–783

Phelan JC, Yang LH, Cruz-Rojas R (2006) Effects of attributing serious mental illnesses to genetic causes on orientations to treatment. Psychiatr Serv 57:382–387

Pinfold V, Toulmin H, Thornicroft G, Huxley P, Farmer P, Graham T (2003) Reducing psychiatric stigma and discrimination: evaluation of educational interventions in UK secondary schools. Br J Psychiatry 182:342–346

Purdie-Vaughns V, Steele CM, Davies PG, Ditlmann R, Crosby JR (2008) Social identity contingencies: how diversity cues signal threat or safety for African Americans in mainstream institutions. J Pers Soc Psychol 94:615–630

Rosen A (2006) Destigmatizing day-to-day practices: what developed countries can learn from developing countries. World Psychiatry 5:21–24

Roulstone A, Warren J (2005) Applying a barriers approach to monitoring disabled people's employment: implications for the Disability Discrimination Act 2005. Disabil Soc 21:115–131

Rudman LA, Ashmore RD, Gary ML (2001) "Unlearning" automatic biases: the malleability of implicit prejudice and stereotypes. J Pers Soc Psychol 81:856–868

Rüsch N, Corrigan PW (2012) Stigma, discrimination, and mental health. In: Knifton L, Quinn N (eds) Public mental health. McGraw Hill Europe/Open University Press, New York, pp. 94–100.

Rüsch N, Angermeyer MC, Corrigan PW (2005) Mental illness stigma: concepts, consequences, and initiatives to reduce stigma. Eur Psychiatry 20:529–539

Rüsch N, Hölzer A, Hermann C, Schramm E, Jacob GA, Bohus M, Lieb K, Corrigan PW (2006a) Self-stigma in women with borderline personality disorder and women with social phobia. J Nerv Ment Dis 194:766–773

Rüsch N, Lieb K, Bohus M, Corrigan PW (2006b) Self-stigma, empowerment, and perceived legitimacy of discrimination among women with mental illness. Psychiatr Serv 57:399–402

Rüsch N, Corrigan PW, Wassel A, Michaels P, Larson JE, Olschewski M, Wilkniss S, Batia K (2009) Self-stigma, group identification, perceived legitimacy of discrimination and mental health service use. Br J Psychiatry 195:551–552

Rüsch N, Todd AR, Bodenhausen GV, Corrigan PW (2010a) Biogenetic models of psychopathology, implicit guilt, and mental illness stigma. Psychiatry Res 179:328–332

Rüsch N, Todd AR, Bodenhausen GV, Corrigan PW (2010b) Do people with mental illness deserve what they get? Links between meritocratic worldviews and implicit versus explicit stigma. Eur Arch Psychiatry Clin Neurosci 260:617–625

Rüsch N, Evans-Lacko S, Clement S, Thornicroft G et al (2011) Stigma, discrimination, social exclusion, and mental health. In: Parker R, Sommer M (eds) Routledge handbook of global public health. Routledge, London, pp 394–401

Rüsch N, Abbruzzese E, Hagedorn E, Hartenhauer D, Kaufmann I, Curschellas J, Ventling S, Zuaboni G, Bridler R, Olschewski M, Kawohl W, Rössler W, Kleim B, Corrigan PW (2014a) The efficacy of Coming Out Proud to reduce stigma's impact among people with mental illness: pilot randomised controlled trial. Br J Psychiatry 204:391–397

Rüsch N, Corrigan PW, Heekeren K, Theodoridou A, Dvorsky D, Metzler S, Müller M, Walitza S, Rössler W (2014b) Well-being among persons at risk of psychosis: the role of self-labeling, shame and stigma stress. Psychiatr Serv 65:483–489

Rüsch N, Müller M, Heekeren K, Theodoridou A, Metzler S, Dvorsky D, Corrigan PW, Walitza S, Rössler W (2014c) Longitudinal course of self-labeling, stigma stress and well-being among young people at risk of psychosis. Schizophr Res 158:82–84

Sartorius N, Schulze H (2005) Reducing the stigma of mental illness: a report from a global association. Cambridge University Press, Cambridge

Sawyer MG, Pfeiffer S, Spence SH, Bond L, Graetz B, Kay D, Patton G, Sheffield J (2010) School-based prevention of depression: a randomised controlled study of the beyondblue schools research initiative. J Child Psychol Psychiatry 51:199–209

Schnittker J (2008) An uncertain revolution: why the rise of a genetic model of mental illness has not increased tolerance. Soc Sci Med 67:1370–1381

Schomerus G, Matschinger H, Angermeyer MC (2014) Causal beliefs of the public and social acceptance of persons with mental illness: a comparative analysis of schizophrenia, depression and alcohol dependence. Psychol Med 44:303–314.

Segal SP, Silverman CJ, Temkin TL (2013) Self-stigma and empowerment in combined-CMHA and consumer-run services: two controlled trials. Psychiatr Serv 64:990–996

Shimotsu S, Horikawa N, Emura R, Ishikawa SI, Nagao A, Ogata A, Hiejima S, Hosomi J (2014) Effectiveness of group cognitive-behavioral therapy in reducing self-stigma in Japanese psychiatric patients. Asian J Psychiatry 10:39–44

Stuart H (2003) Stigma and the daily news: evaluation of a newspaper intervention. Can J Psychiatr 48:651–656

Stuart H (2006) Mental illness and employment discrimination. Curr Opin Psychiatry 19:522–526

Stuart H (2007) Employment equity and mental disability. Curr Opin Psychiatry 20:486–490

Thornicroft G (2006) Shunned: discrimination against people with mental illness. Oxford University Press, Oxford

Thornicroft A, Goulden R, Shefer G, Rhydderch D, Rose D, Williams P, Thornicroft G, Henderson C (2013) Newspaper coverage of mental illness in England 2008–2011. Br J Psychiatry Suppl 55:s64–s69

Thornicroft G, Mehta N, Clement S, Evans-Lacko S, Doherty M, Rose D, Koschorke M, Shidhaye R, O'Reilly C, Henderson C (2016) Evidence for effective interventions to reduce mental health related stigma and discrimination. Lancet. doi:10.1016/S0140-6736(15)00298-6

Vaughan G, Hansen C (2004) 'Like Minds, Like Mine': a New Zealand project to counter the stigma and discrimination associated with mental illness. Australas Psychiatry 12:113–117

Wahl OF (1995) Media madness: public images of mental illness. Rutgers University Press, New Brunswick

Yamaguchi S, Wu SI, Biswas M, Yate M, Aoki Y, Barley EA, Thornicroft G (2013) Effects of short-term interventions to reduce mental health-related stigma in university or college students: a systematic review. J Nerv Ment Dis 201:490–503

Yanos PT, Roe D, Lysaker PH (2011) Narrative enhancement and cognitive therapy: a new group-based treatment for internalized stigma among persons with severe mental illness. Int J Group Psychother 61:576–595

Yanos PT, Roe D, West ML, Smith SM, Lysaker PH (2012) Group-based treatment for internalized stigma among persons with severe mental illness: findings from a randomized controlled trial. Psychol Serv 9:248–258

"Irre menschlich Hamburg" – An Example of a Bottom-Up Project

25

Thomas Bock, Angela Urban, Gwen Schulz,
Gyöngyver Sielaff, Amina Kuby, and Candelaria Mahlke

This chapter highlights the advantages and importance of bottom-up approaches in the fight against stigma. Where and how does stigmatization occur? Through uneducated neighbours, colleagues or psychiatric services itself? Does the diagnostic process unwillingly foster stigmatization by creating terminological barriers? Is it the case that today's prejudices against psychiatry reflect its failure of the past? Which concepts of mental health problems can strengthen or weaken prejudices, and which concepts can foster tolerance and sensitivity? What does successful work against stigma look like and what are the necessary prerequisites for such work? How should a field of psychiatry be constituted that allows for the natural transition between life crises and mental health problems that do not reject experiences with alienating terminology and concepts, but instead supports the assimilation of alienating experiences? Questions regarding stigmatization and in opposite regarding tolerance, sensitivity, prevention and hope

T. Bock (✉)
Center for Psychosocial Medicine, University Medical Center Hamburg Eppendorf, Martinistr. 52, 20249 Hamburg, Germany

Irre menschlich Hamburg e.V., Center for Psychosocial Medicine, University Medical Center Hamburg Eppendorf, Martinistr. 52, 20249 Hamburg, Germany
e-mail: bock@uke.de

A. Urban
Irre menschlich Hamburg e.V., Center for Psychosocial Medicine, University Medical Center Hamburg Eppendorf, Martinistr. 52, 20249 Hamburg, Germany
e-mail: info@irremenschlich.de

G. Schulz • G. Sielaff • A. Kuby • C. Mahlke
Center for Psychosocial Medicine, University Medical Center Hamburg Eppendorf, Martinistr. 52, 20249 Hamburg, Germany
e-mail: gwen.schulz@gmx.de; g.sielaff@uke.de; a.kuby@uke.de; c.mahlke@uke.de

© Springer International Publishing Switzerland 2017
W. Gaebel et al. (eds.), *The Stigma of Mental Illness - End of the Story?*,
DOI 10.1007/978-3-319-27839-1_25

are profoundly connected with the understanding of health and mental health problems, as well as the proposed concepts of support systems. Stigmatization due to mental health problems is judged as more distressing compared to stigmatization due to innate features or a minority status, given that the stigmatized person often held similar prejudices prior to their mental health problems. Whether people are stigmatized depends on the concept of human being, not merely on the idiosyncrasies of the individual. If a society propagates the picture of a successful, dynamic, eternally youthful person as the unquestioned standard, then any deviation from this can be stigmatized. A field of psychiatry that diagnoses every "deviation from the norm" and that endlessly extends its diagnostic categories is substantially responsible for the expansion of stigmatization.

Mental Health Problems and Prejudices

Prejudices against mental health problems are widespread, so the number of people suffering from prejudice is substantial. One-sided media reports, as well as former misjudgements made in psychiatry, serve to maintain negative stereotypes already disproved by scientific findings, e.g. that patients with mental health problems are "dangerous, incurable and unpredictable", that their personalities are "split" or that "their parents are responsible for the mental health problems". Patients with a diagnosis of schizophrenia and their families/relatives particularly experience stigmatization (Schulze and Angermeyer 2003). Fear and social withdrawal are possible consequences. Former studies revealed that fear of public stigma or self-stigma barrier mental health service use and relapse prevention (Clement et al. 2015). Prejudices endanger individual therapeutic progress, familial resources as well as ongoing structural developments in psychiatry. It is an excessive demand of the medical field alone to counteract prejudice. There is evidence shown in meta-analyses that medical illness models and analogies enhance rather than reduce fear and social distance towards people with mental health problems (Angermeyer and Schomerus 2012). Experiences within anti-stigma projects attest to these findings: The elimination of prejudices does not occur through reading about it or professional lectures, but through personal encounters and listening to someone's story. Therefore, to be credible and convincing, counteracting stigmatization has to be a joined effort of patients, relatives and those working in psychiatry. When targeting young people, anti-stigma works also have to have preventative aspects. For example, anti-stigma topics such as psychosis, mania and depression (bipolar disorder) have to be supplemented by topics such as eating disorders, self-harming behaviour and mental health problems through drug and alcohol consumption.

Stigmatization in Psychiatry?

Does stigmatization occur with discharge from a psychiatric institution? Or does it occur upon its initial diagnosis? What role do diagnostic labels and self-stigmatization play? When and where stigmatization occurs and who is responsible for it is debatable. Likewise are the models for how and where anti-stigma work needs to begin. According to sociologists, it is unquestioned that stigmatization occurs within psychiatry's diagnostic processes (Finzen 2001), not between classmates, colleagues or neighbours. Therefore, if psychiatry wants to counteract prejudices, it is only credible if this is done across all levels, publicly as well as internally. To do so, a common language is needed. To preserve and nurture this language was an essential reason for the establishment of the psychosis seminars. Psychosis seminars were established to foster a dialogue between three parties on eyelevel: people with experience of mental health problems, relatives and mental health professionals (Bock and Priebe 2005; Bock et al. 2013; Buck 2002). Furthermore, psychiatry in general and the diagnosing physician in particular are responsible for avoiding stigmatization wherever possible. The culture of trialogue provides the needed authenticity, whilst engaging in assessment sessions as well as public anti-stigma work (Alanen 2001).

If in psychiatric practice diagnoses are handled carefully, whilst efforts are made to achieve a common language and to understand and not only fight symptoms, self-understanding is fostered and thereby individual anti-stigma work delivered. This can be effectively complemented and enhanced through public relations activities. But if in today's psychiatric practice diagnoses and treatment standards are schematically allocated and symptoms are fought as a foreign matter, with disregard to underlying feelings and conflicts, the risk of distancing patients from their perceptions even further is high and is not in line with contemporary knowledge. Furthermore, a psychiatry which does not include relatives or includes them too late, and which does not offer treatment continuity, also contradicts contemporary best practice and participates in stigmatization by enhancing alienation on all levels instead of decreasing it.

Giving a mental health problem a name is not bad per se. Whilst it can frighten patients to name it, it can also allay their fears ("Rumpelstiltskin effect"). The diagnostic process alone does not determine weal and woe. Other determinants are the verbal context, the associated message and the simultaneously offered or denied relationship. Contrary to the generally limited understanding of illness insight and compliance, for example, Roessler et al. (1999) found that patients with an idiosyncratic illness concept have a higher quality of life. This derives the task for psychiatry: to conceptualize psycho-education more sensitively, more generously and in dialogue with the patient, to think of illness insight not as a one-sided requirement from the patient but as the responsibility of the therapist and to achieve compliance through cooperation, not subordination (Bock et al. 2007). This aim applies to children, adolescents and young "first-episode patients" in particular. Here, the diagnostic process needs to take place with particular caution. A sustainable therapeutic relationship and, as stated before, the use of a common language are prerequisites for the diagnostic process, not the result of such a process. To include parents, relatives and friends from the therapeutic process must be regarded as self-evident best practice.

Can an Anthropological Perspective Effectively Counteract Stigmatization?

It is important to regard mental health problems not only medically and pathologically, but also developmentally and anthropologically, meaning within their psychosocial and political context. The anthropological view shows that the transitions between health and mental health problems are fluent and that symptoms are not only alienating but of functional and/or protective relevance, as well as of profoundly human significance. We must not limit our thinking to the question of whether humanity is becoming increasingly psychologically ill. Instead, we must reflect on the fact that mental health problems are inherently human with just as much intensity. The following overview is meant to further elucidate the anthropological view, as well as potentially help with patient contact (Bock 2012a).

Anxiety: Ability or Disorder?

Without anxiety, people would be unable to protect themselves from danger. Humanity would be extinct. Anxiety as such does not need to be regarded as a disorder but, at least initially, as a necessary survival strategy. A persons' proximity to anxiety and his or her need for anxiety vary and are contingent upon that persons' biography and constitution. Only if anxiety spreads and takes on a life of its own, if it generalizes and uncouples itself from triggers, then it becomes the danger which it pretends to deter. If this happens, it can be helpful to reconstruct the story of one's anxiety, to reconnect it with precipitating conflicts, to remember possible triggers and moments of true potential danger, to make sense of the anxiety and to thereby tame it.

Compulsions: Prison or Grounding Ritual

Compulsive actions resemble superstitious rituals and religious rites; they are meant to stabilize an increasingly confused inner and outer world. Maybe, given the lack of religious/culturally accepted rites in our society, compulsive actions often take on an alienating character. The fact that compulsions are functional (i.e. that they create coherence) becomes apparent when contemplating the fact that people with psychosis potential sometimes decompensate after "successful" treatment of their compulsions. Similar to anxiety disorders, it is important to retrace the origination process of compulsions, to make sense of them, to stop their internal dynamic and to thereby to ease tension.

Depression: Protection Versus Harmful Dynamic

Initially, depression also appears to have a protective function: The psyche generates a feign death, comparable to an animal that hides until danger has passed. When something bad happens that exceeds our comprehensive faculties, when emotions are conflicting and cannot be sorted, when we feel overwhelmed and ask too much of ourselves and when decisions are pending that cannot be made, it can become necessary to let go. We develop depressive traits to protect ourselves. To emerge, we require time, silence, patience, reflection, consolation, support or encouragement etc. Problematically, depressive phases can develop own psychological, social and somatic dynamics. In other words, one's psyche, one's social environment and one's cerebral metabolism become increasingly sensitive. In a severe depressive episode, one's sense of time can get lost, to the extent that there seems to be no before or after. Also, one's black despair can become so insurmountable that death seems like salvation. Help is necessary. In severe depression, a balance between constructive and destructive forces can be found: The thought about dying can be all-encompassing, whilst the simultaneous paralysis can be a protection from its execution. Despair and self-protection balance each other. Suicide risk increases when antidepressants cause behavioural activation, whilst spirits are still low. Medication therefore requires a therapeutic relationship (Bock 2000).

Mania: Escape Forwards, But Where to?

Mania does not equate happiness. Whoever is truly happy and successful in life doesn't need to become manic. Whoever becomes manic is desperately happy – searching happiness far away from themselves. Mania and depression can promote each other: Whoever stays isolated during mania can drive himself to such profound exhaustion that a lapse into depression becomes ever more likely. Or depression can be experienced as so deep and boundless that only a flight forward into mania seems possible. Therapeutic support can offer other way of self-monitoring. After a while, however, serious (e.g. somatic) internal dynamics can develop. The above-mentioned loss of a sense of time does not cause bottomless despair but monumental recklessness, leading to the risk of self-harm (Koesler and Bock 2005).

Psychosis as Extreme Thin-Skinnedness

Looking at psychoses from an anthropological perspective – with a focus on it being a human continuum – they appear as an extremely permeable state: Inner conflicts and problems rise to the surface and take shape in hallucinations. Conversely, outside influences find their way inside without being filtered, without the chance to be weighed and ordered (paranoid perceptions). If a person becomes "paranoid", such a state is comparable to the perceptions of a toddler who sees everything in relation to himself or herself and, for example, feels guilty upon a parental argument. For children, this "egocentric" perception is a necessary developmental milestone. For adults, this perception seems inappropriate and out of touch with reality, therefore psychotic. Going through psychosis is comparable to dreaming – without the protection of sleep. In a dream it is safe to think of oneself as a bird; in a psychosis, it is not. There are dreams that bring pleasure and dreams that evoke fear. Similarly, a psychosis has aspects that may also bring pleasure or evoke fear. In a paranoid psychosis, these appear symbolically as a blend of meaningful significance and threat.

Throughout their lifetime, most people go through stable and unstable phases. Situations in which experiencing psychological distress is common include the process of individuation or attachment, the transition from school to work, loss of a job and birth of a child. In these situations, people with psychosis experience react more sensitively than others and therefore develop a psychosis. However, they do not react less humanely. It is therefore important not to declare relapse prevention the absolute goal. Such a stance implies stigmatization. It holds the danger that people not only avoid psychosis and its triggers but life altogether. In turn, this fosters negative symptoms and a post-schizophrenic depression. A detailed translation of psychotic symptoms according to the ICD-10 into a language for people with experience of mental health problems was created in the psychosis seminars and can serve as a basis for a narrative culture in psychiatry (Bock 2012b; Bock et al. 2007).

Borderline: In Between Closeness and Distance

People with a borderline personality disorder struggle through life crossing the borders between reality and dreaming; meanwhile wishes and fears appear irreconcilable or inseparable. The sense for nuances and synchronicities gets lost. Instead, certain needs or feelings are made absolute, whilst others are forcibly blocked out. It is a lifelong task of all human beings, not only of individuals with borderline personality disorders, to strike a balance between wishes and fears, between conflicting priorities such as closeness and distance, adaptation and resistance, attachment and autonomy. However, they experience them in an enhanced way and as existentially threatening. If self-harming behaviour occurs in this context, it is often an attempt to reduce tension, to affirm one's identity or to influence others. To escape the social, psychological and physical dynamics this ensues, therapeutic support is strongly advised. Anthropologically self-harming behaviour was and continues to be part of many cultures. It occurs, for example, in rituals and ceremonies whilst coming of age. In our culture, however, it has seemingly lost its cultural connection. With some restrictions, borderline personality disorder appears as a prolonged and enhanced adolescence, chronological linked to the transition into adulthood. Dependent on the level of gained internal dynamic, it can lose its impetus later in life.

Life Crises with Multidirectional Internal Dynamics

In contrast to all other living creatures, human beings must wrestle to achieve a sense of self. We can self-doubt – and despair as a result of that doubt; think beyond ourselves and loose ourselves in the process. Life crises present risk and opportunity. Mental health problems can be regarded as existential life crises of particularly thin-skinned people, with the risk of it developing multidirectional internal dynamics (i.e. psychological, social and somatic). These internal dynamics can strongly determine the onset and progress of mental health problems. This can be seen, for example, when cognitive patterns cause patients to spiral deeper into a depression or when the fear of stigmatization fosters social withdrawal and the resulting isolation fuels psychotic hallucinations. Such examples can be continued at will.

Uniting for Tolerance and Sensitivity: Project "Irre menschlich Hamburg"

The possibilities and difficulties of practical anti-stigma work shall be illustrated using the example of the association "Irre menschlich Hamburg e.V.". It was one of the first anti-stigma projects in Germany and arose from the trialogically organized Hamburg psychosis seminars. Working trialogically is the foundation for the continuing engagement of different target groups in varied contexts and topics, all revolving around psychological health and mental health problems (www.irremenschlich.de). Trialogue forums in general, of which there are now more than 100 in Germany, have proven to be a good training ground for anti-stigma work. Working through mutual prejudices creates a basis for combined efforts to reduce prejudices in the general public. This especially applies for the various advanced education opportunities. "Irre menschlich Hamburg" has a wide spectrum of tasks, and the topics and operating sites are conceptualized broadly. It began with anti-stigma work in the field of education delivering encounter projects in schools: First for the pupil and further on for the teachers as well. The field of anti-stigma campaigns and projects spread further to the university and most importantly to the education of mental health staff to fight stigma in the delivering of psychiatric services: encounter projects for nurses and students of medicine and psychology.

Also in administration, it seemed important to fight discrimination and raise awareness and tolerance, so encounter projects got established for social worker, youth supporters, pastors, probationary services and especially the police, having contact with mentally ill in extreme and acute situations. Also education and information projects in Hamburg businesses began, as well as regular education and training events for journalists and the housing industry. To raise public awareness, activities, e.g. various cultural events, like exhibitions, film screenings and theatre performances, are organized by "Irre menschlich Hamburg". The development, trial and execution of a curriculum to prepare people with experience of mental health problems for independent anti-stigma work and psychosocial care as peer support worker (EXperienced INvolvement, EX-IN) helped to deliver for all the rising fields and efforts.

Insights into the Work of "Err Human Hamburg"

To give some insight into the broad variety of anti-stigma projects, here a closer look into some activities of Irre menschlich. An overview is presented in (Fig. 25.1).

Anti-stigma in Education: School Projects and Further Development

Irre menschlich provides regular information sessions, materials, classes and prevention projects to Hamburg schools, tailored to all ages and subjects and annually open days for pupil and teachers. A variety of materials like "media suitcases" are developed.

Pioneer Work: Age-Appropriate Information and Personal Encounters

Youth facilities are not only designed to keep young people occupied, and the purpose of schools goes beyond increasing knowledge. Both aspire to provide problem-solving strategies that prepare young people for later life. Anti-stigma work can have direct preventative benefits, especially for young people who have experienced mental health problems directly or indirectly, as it allows teachers, educators and

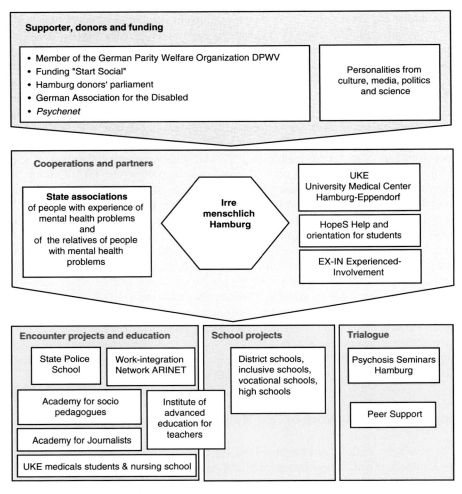

Fig. 25.1 Network of the project "Irre menschlich Hamburg e.V."

social pedagogues to engage students in discussions about life goals, life crises and personal/professional resources. "Irre menschlich Hamburg" began its anti-stigma work as a result of the strong positive response from schools following the release of the novel "The Begging Queen" ("Die Bettelkönigin"; Stratenwerth and Bock 2001). This urban fairy tale was based on the life of Hamburg artist Hildegard Wohlgemuth. In combination with her school visits, it laid the foundation for many anti-stigma projects. The youth novel "Pias lives…dangerously" (Bock and Kemme 2000) in conjunction with school visits by a former company leader of the German armed forces (role model for the book and now homeless) fulfilled a similar function for junior high students. Over the years a lot of authentic material for all ages and occasions was developed this way. The combination of authentic writing and direct personal encounters appears to best transport the idea of anti-stigma work.

A Lot of Experience and Varied Topics: Educational Policies and Health Policies

Over the past 10 years, "Irre menschlich Hamburg" has completed over 1,000 class projects with Hamburg school students. Core principles are the trialogue and direct personal encounters. Project topics have been continually extended, now including anxiety, psychosis, depression/burnout, self-harming behaviours/borderline personality disorder, eating disorders, psychosis and addiction. The topics gradually align with the experience of school students. Again, the trialogue/the authentic encounter with people with experience of mental health problems proves to be more convincing than conveying technical information or teaching from the moral high ground. The goal "More tolerance in dealing with others and more sensitivity in dealing with oneself" has rehabilitative and preventive aspects.

Experiences of the "Irre menschlich" School Projects

Participant observations, a systematic qualitative analysis of class sessions, and multiple surveys with students, teachers and other participants allow the following conclusions:

1. Students hold fewer prejudices than expected. Especially young students relate to people with experience of mental health problems with openness.
2. Within class sessions, encounters with psychiatry-experienced people exhibit considerable appeal. The "Irre menschlich Hamburg" material is used in preparation for and after these encounters. If encounters and material are reasonable linked, the project succeeds at its best. If the emphasis is on trialogical encounters, even short class sessions can have lasting effects.
3. Materials like the "media suitcases" can be flexibly assembled, dependent on the duration of the class, the students' ages as well as the qualifications and preferences of the consultant.
4. Class sessions over a period of 6 months may be conducted interdisciplinary (e.g. German/history, biology/philosophy/ethics, psychology/art). Teachers, whilst remaining responsible for structuring their classes, may be given advice on how to incorporate the material. This makes the projects economically viable and circumvents detrimental competition with teachers and consultants.
5. From a middle school level onwards, students are asked to think about their aspirations and goals in life, about their available resources and possible future conflicts. Discussing mental health problems in this way fosters self-confidence.
6. Learning effects are enhanced when students get a chance to organize their own activities. Students have visited an outpatient clinic, organized presents for consultants, written stories, drawn pictures, conducted interviews or discussed the lives of famous artists, scientists or politicians with mental health problems.

7. For consultants, being a crisis-experienced "life teacher" has an empowering effect ("It was like a second therapy").
8. The project fosters tolerance in dealing with others and sensitivity in dealing with oneself. Both are dependent on each other and strengthen one another. They are prerequisites for psychological health.
9. Within class sessions, worries and conflicts of students are not directly discussed (e.g. having parents with mental health problems). Instead, the sessions are designed to introduce students to the topics of mental health problems. Topics are not dealt with psychologically, but pedagogically, probably to the relief of students who are in distress.
10. Through direct personal encounters of people with experience of mental health problems and mental health professionals, students' awareness is enhanced and the threshold to seek professional help is lowered. This approach is likely to have a greater positive impact on mental health problem prevention than symptom-oriented early diagnoses.

"Life Coaches": Advanced Education for Teachers

The Institute of Advanced Education for Teachers offers regular courses on "psychological health/mental health problems as a class topic" and "psychological health/mental health problems in school students". At the yearly meeting of the UNESCO schools in Lübeck/Hamburg in the year 2005, the ideas of "Irre menschlich Hamburg" were well received. In the following year, these schools were encouraged to organize trialogical projects: topics such as inner peace and the protection of one's inner world were discussed alongside topics such as world peace and environmental protection.

Psychiatry Opens Its Door for Schools ("Psychiatrie Macht Schule"): Collaboration with the University Clinic

Between "Irre menschlich" and the University Medical Center Hamburg-Eppendorf (UKE), a constructive and mutually beneficial cooperation has emerged. "Psychiatrie macht Schule", an open day held at the UKE, has proven to be especially popular. Each year, more than 1.000 school students take part in approximately 60 trialogical workshops, readings and video lectures at the medical centre. The signature feature of these events is therapists, people with experience of mental health problems and relatives appearing together. Workshops include "Good times – bad times" (Bipolar disorders), "Extreme thin-skinned", "Hearing voices" (Psychoses) and "What's up?" (Eating disorders). An accompanying research project currently evaluates these workshops (Dorner et al 2014).

Perspectives on School Projects

In the future, "Irre menschlich Hamburg" and *Psychenet* intend to establish an ongoing presence at a number of exemplary schools. In particular, the projects aim to incorporate regular information sessions into school curricula, offer courses for teachers that can be tailored quickly upon demand and provide individualized support for students in need (e.g. one-on-one peer support). The projects have shown that trialogical work often makes young people realize that mental health problems can be dealt with in a non-stigmatizing appropriate way and that it can be discussed without having to put themselves in the centre of attention or being forced to take such a place. As such, the project fosters awareness of mental health problems, whilst avoiding the risk of stigmatization or of abusing the role of the teacher. In addition, speaking with consultants and listening to their stories can reduce patients' anxieties and open up new possibilities for help.

Shaping Attitudes: Fighting Stigma in Society, Work Life and Media

Fascinating Media: "First-Hand Information" for Journalists

"Irre menschlich Hamburg" conveys first-hand information to journalists. Reports about the project were televised on German channels such as ZDF and N3, and members of "Irre menschlich Hamburg" participated in various German talk shows, with the aim of conveying the human side of mental health problems. In addition, the newly designed website and a radio spot that was aired on several youth broadcasts have gotten positive feedback (www.irremenschlich.de).

Psychological Health and Mental Health Problems in the Working Environment: Specific Projects

Early on, "Irre menschlich Hamburg" began to organize trialogical projects for companies located within Hamburg. Again, the aim was to shape public perception of mental health problems towards a more human view and to foster the willingness of employers to recruit or continually employ people with mental health problems. Topics such as depression/burnout, as well as addiction and psychosis (e.g. in the advanced education course for teachers), were met with a particularly positive response. Together with the rehabilitation committee and the senator for town planning, "Irre menschlich Hamburg" participated in a large education campaign for the Hamburg housing industry. As with the other projects, the aim was to counteract prejudices and to develop new forms of cooperation, so people with mental health problems are able to find housing and sign their own housing contracts. Within the housing industry, more tolerance and sensitivity is also needed. Rare encounters occurred at a large opening event and at the regional advanced education courses.

Anti-stigma Work in Administration and Police Department

Youth Support: Raising Awareness Without Stigmatization

Since prejudices against mental health problems are common amongst young people, those who are at risk of developing mental health problems are quickly stigmatized and ostracized. Self-stigmatization is a frequently observed attempt to pre-empt social exclusion. Within the area of youth support, trialogical education courses with active participation of people with experience of mental health problems and their relatives have existed for many years. A 3-day basic course, which links anthropological understanding, support possibilities and a trialogue discourse, is regularly well attended. A long-term cooperation is planned as well and probationary services as well as unemployment/job-seeking services.

Supporting De-Escalation: Advanced Education for Police Officers

Within the Hamburg police, "Irre menschlich" has taken on a long-term responsibility to educate middle-level civil servants. Courses offer practical units on psychosis, mania and borderline personality disorder. The focus is on combining professional information with direct personal encounters, to correct one-sided views of mental health problems, reduce fears and search for de-escalation strategies. Rare encounters have occurred within this context. For example, at an advanced education course held in connection with the deaths of three people with mental health problems, a trialogical meeting occurred between the following parties: police executives, mental health professionals, people with experience of mental health problems, their relatives and a traumatized police woman, who, in distress, fired one of the fatal shots. Following an initial trial phase, police administration decided to anchor anti-stigma work within their curriculum by adding a training and encounter unit delivered by "Irre menschlich Hamburg". Its effect on the participants was assessed in 2014 measuring the social distance, causal attributions, emotional reactions, stereotyped attitudes, the assumed effect of different treatment and the prognosis for schizophrenia with questionnaires before and after the training. The results show the tendency of a positive effect of the training. The social distance is reduced, and less negative stereotypes and fear were observed. Besides that participants developed a more differentiated attitude towards effective treatment methods and considered more psychosocial causes of mental disorders, despite the agreement to biological causes, the expectation of anger and pro-social reactions did not change. Altogether a positive effect of the trialogical training could be shown.

Cooperation with *Psychenet*

For its proposed project *Psychenet* (Härter et al. 2012; Bock 2011), Hamburg was awarded "Health region of the future" in its subproject 1, and the encounter projects were intensified and extended. In addition, the trialogical education courses were enlarged. The media campaign (posters, film spots for cinemas) was successfully conceptualized trialogically; and people with experience of mental health problems modelled for the posters and wrote the accompanying text (rather than actors). Having gained confidence from this anti-stigma campaign, it was also decided to shoot film spots using people with experience of mental health problems. This project benefitted in particular from the photographer Thomas Rusch. Members of "Irre menschlich Hamburg" were able to influence the character of the anti-stigma campaign significantly.

The Future of "Irre menschlich Hamburg"

Recruitment and New Consultant Training

In the beginning – given its emergence from the psychosis seminars – "Irre menschlich Hamburg" focused on psychoses and bipolar disorders. For a few years now, the project has engaged consultants for many aspects of psychological health and mental health problems. Some of these consultants are recruited from the EX-IN programme. There has been an increasing amount of interest to participate in the project as a consultant. It has become apparent that the consultants benefit from their participation. Not only do they receive an income (for school projects only), they also receive a lot of personal encouragement.

Strengthening Preventative Project

Together with the professional "Ersterkrankten" project ("first-episode patients"), "Irre menschlich Hamburg" is aiming to support young people (and their relatives) in current crises. For example, dedicated (former) patients and their relatives might share personal experiences with young people who are searching for help. This can foster mindfulness and lower the threshold to seek professional help. This indirect trialogical approach is likely to have a greater effect on the prevention of mental health problems than early diagnoses.

Peer Support: EXperienced INvolvement (EX-IN), Achieving More Resistance to Stigmatization

"EX-IN" was an EU project set out to develop a curriculum for training people who had gone through psychological crises in order to help other people with similar psychological problems. By now, it has become a flourishing trialogical practice. An increasing number of clinical and subclinical institutions employ peer support worker as so-called recovery companions. The trialogical approach aims to strengthen patients' self-confidence, resources and quality of life. It aims to support patients during their recovery and offer relief and encouragement to relatives. According to the project experience, peer support has a threefold effect: (1) it strengthens self-efficacy and in result counteracts the risk for self-stigmatization, (2) it changes the perception of mental health problems amongst mental health staff, and (3) it reduces the risk for stigmatization against people with mental health problems in psychiatry. A number of international studies support the beneficial effects of this intervention (e.g. Davidson et al. 2012; Mahlke et al. 2014). As part of *Psychenet* Hamburg, "twofold peer support" was established in all psychiatric clinics in the Hamburg region, which entails people with experience of mental health problems supporting people in current crises as well as relatives supporting other relatives. A randomized study further evaluates its feasibility and effectiveness, as well as effects on the peer support worker themselves and attitudes of other mental health staff.

Information Box 25.1: Summary
1. Top-down anti-stigma campaigns run the risk of transmitting reductionist messages. Narrow medical illness concepts, as often propagated by pharmacological firms and still represented in mental health-care services, are not suited to decrease social distance or the risk of self-stigmatization.
2. A fluent transition between health and mental health problems counteracts the risk of (self-)stigmatization (Schomerus et al. 2012; Angermeyer and Schomerus 2012).
3. Encounters with individuals with mental health problems can reduce social distance and weaken prejudices.
4. Tolerance in dealing with others and oneself are worthwhile aims for prevention projects. Trialogical projects in schools and firms have rehabilitative effects as well as preventative effects.
5. Trialogical advanced education courses for journalists, teachers, the police, youth support services, health professions, housing associations, unemployment projects and probationary services reduce prejudices and mutual reservations. They strengthen the qualification of these professions and have an important political function towards inclusion (Bock and Priebe 2005).
6. In a clinical context, peer support can reduce the risk for self-stigmatization, whilst increasing self-efficacy and fostering self-help.
7. Peer support is likely to change perceptions of mental health problems within psychiatry, thereby minimizing the risk of stigmatization in and through this professional field.
8. The trialogical approach operates on multiple levels. Originating from the psychosis seminars/trialogue forums, it is effective for everyday work in psychiatry (e.g. open dialogue, treatment agreements), advanced education courses, congresses, organizations, complaints offices as well as psychiatry politics and immediate anti-stigma work. The ultimate aim is to achieve equitable cooperation between institutions and experts (people with experience of mental health problems, relatives, health professionals).
9. Success is more likely for local, long-term trialogical projects than top-down and exclusively medically oriented anti-stigma campaigns.
10. A trialogical citizen action committee is able to reach several groups: pupils, teacher journalists, police, pastors, health-care professionals, housing industry and others. With these projects Irre menschlich Hamburg has won a special award of the European unit as best practice model (*inno-serv.eu/de/content/irre-menschlich-ev-hamburg*).

Literature

Alanen, Y. O. (2001). Schizophrenie – Entstehung, Erscheinungsformen und bedürfnisangepaßte Behandlung. Stuttgart: Klett-Cotta

Angermeyer M, Schomerus G (2012) A stigma perspective on recovery. World Psychiatry 11:163–164

Bock T (2000) Gemeinsam gegen Vorurteile – zur Auseinandersetzung um eine Antistigmakampagne. Soziale Psychiatrie 24:16

Bock T (2011) Gesundheitsmetropole Hamburg, psychenet – aus der Perspektive von "Irre menschlich Hamburg" e.V. Kerbe Forum Sozialpsychiatrie 4:36–39

Bock T (2012a) Krankheitsverständnis – zwischen Stigmatisierung und Empowerment. Schweiz Arch Neurol Psychiatr 163:138–144

Bock T (2012b) Partizipation in Klinischer und Sozial-Psychiatrie – Impulse aus dem Trialog. In: Rosenbrock R, Hartung S (eds) Handbuch Partizipation im Gesundheitswesen. Vincentz-Verlag, Berlin

Bock T, Kemme G (2000) Pias lebt … gefährlich. Psychiatrie Verlag – Edition Balance, Bonn

Bock T, Priebe S (2005) Psychosis-seminars, an unconventional approach for how users, carers and professionals can learn from each other. Psychiatr Serv 56(11):1441–1443

Bock T, Buck D, Esterer I (2007) Stimmenreich. Psychiatrie Verlag, Bonn

Bock T, Meyer HJ, Rouhiainen T (2013) Trialog – eine Herausforderung mit Zukunft. In: Roessler W (ed) Handbuch Sozialpsychiatrie. Kohlhammer, Stuttgart

Buck D (2002) Laßt euch nicht entmutigen. Anne Fischer Verlag. Leipziger Universitätsverlag, Leipzig, Norderstedt

Clement S, Schauman O, Graham T et al (2015) What is the impact of mental health-related stigma on help-seeking? A systematic review of quantitative and qualitative studies. Psychol Med 45(1):11–27

Davidson L, Bellamy C, Guy K et al (2012) Peer support among persons with severe mental illnesses: a review of evidence and experience. World Psychiatry 11:123

Dorner R, Sander A, Bock T (2014) Psychiatrie macht Schule – ein Beitrag zur Prävention. Praxis. Wissen psychosozial. 18:46–49

Finzen A (2001) Psychose und Stigma – zum Umgang mit Vorurteilen und Schuldzuweisungen. Psychiatrie Verlag, Bonn

Härter M, Kentgens M, Brandes A (2012) Rationale and content of psychenet: the Hamburg network for mental health. Eur Arch Psychiatry Clin Neurosci 2:57–63

Koesler A, Bock T (2005) Gruppentherapie bipolarer Störungen, Psychotherapie im Dialog. Schwerpunktheft Psychotherapie in der Psychiatrie. Thiemeverlag, Stuttgart, pp 289–294

Mahlke CI, Krämer UM, Becker T et al (2014) Peer support in mental health services. Curr Opin Psychiatry 27(4):276–281

Roessler W, Salize HJ, Cucchiaro G et al (1999) Does the place of treatment influence the quality of life of schizophrenics? Acta Psychiatr Scand 100:142–148

Schomerus G, Schwahn C, Holzinger A, Corrigan PW, Grabe HJ, Carta MG, Angermeyer MC (2012) Evolution of public attitudes about mental illness: a systematic review and meta-analysis. Acta Psychiatr Scand 125:440–452

Schulze B, Angermeyer M (2003) Subjective experiences of stigma. A focus group study of schizophrenic patients, their relatives and mental health professionals. Soc Sci Med 56(2):299–312

Stratenwerth I, Bock T (2001) Die Bettelkönigin. (Kinderbuch) Koreverlag. Psychiatrie Verlag, Bonn

Illness Models and Stigma

26

Andreas Heinz

Introduction

So far, we have used different terms to talk about the problem at hand: In DSM-5 as well as in ICD-10, mental maladies are called "disorders"; other terms used include "illness", "disease" and "sickness" (Sartorius 2010). This variety of terms already indicates that there are different aspects of mental maladies. Some of them will be discussed below, mainly refer to the subjective experience of feeling impaired by the manifestation of the disease; others primarily refer to symptoms used to classify a disorder in medical terms or to the impairment of social participation. In somatic disorders, there is usually much less controversy whether to call a certain condition a disease or not. One reason for the rather controversial status of mental disorders in psychiatry and psychotherapy is a stigma associated with such problems and the inhuman history of psychiatric practices in several countries (Amnesty International 1977; Heinz 1998). Another reason for this controversy are problems associated with the concept of mental disorders per se. In somatic disorders, a disease is usually diagnosed if and only if a vital function of an organ is impaired. Hence, the inability to roll one's tongue is not a disease while the paralysis of a tongue is – the latter impairs the act of swallowing, which is necessary for survival, while the first is meaningless with respect to vital functions. The inability to roll one's tongue is a biologically explainable and heritable condition; however, neither heritability nor the existence of a biological explanation of the symptom is necessary or sufficient to call a certain dysfunction a symptom of a disease. Instead, whether a dysfunction is a symptom of a disease is decided upon its relevance for human life and survival (Boorse 1976). However, there is a problem when we try to transfer this approach to mental disorders: due to the variety of human behaviour, in association with age,

A. Heinz
Department of Psychiatry and Psychotherapy, Charité – Universitätsmedizin Berlin, Charitéplatz 1, 10117 Berlin, Germany
e-mail: andreas.heinz@charite.de

© Springer International Publishing Switzerland 2017
W. Gaebel et al. (eds.), *The Stigma of Mental Illness - End of the Story?*,
DOI 10.1007/978-3-319-27839-1_26

gender and culture as well as a variety of social effects, it can be substantially more difficult to identify mental functions necessary for human life and survival than in the case of e.g. motor functions and their impairment of neurology. In this essay, we will discuss different approaches towards defining mental disorders and suggest a definition that tries to reduce stigma but at the same time aims at the preservation of the protection that a disease classification can give to subjects within the health-care system.

Mental Disorders Do Not Depend on Abnormality

One straightforward approach to mental disorders could be to suggest that any cognitive motivational or emotional function is a symptom of a disease whenever it deviates from a norm. However, any such definition runs into the problem which is named above. There is a high diversity in human behaviour, and in several conditions, the functions are the norm and not normal functioning is the exception. A point in case is the existence of caries in Germany in the 1940s, when having problems with your teeth was the norm (Jaspers 1946). Accordingly, Jaspers insisted that the norm against which an abnormal symptom or function is defined is not a statistical norm (otherwise having caries would be the health condition and not having it would be the disease) but a certain "ideal norm", which has to be constructed upon assumptions about how a certain organ is supposed to function. However, can this be done within psychiatry and is it a useful approach even e.g. in neurology?

We suggest that this is not the case. No neurologist would try to diagnose e.g. paralyses according to a stroke by defining a norm of how a human body should move. Humans tend to move in all different directions, in various ways, with more or less speed etc. Instead, a paralysis is diagnosed by defining basic functions and aspects of a movement, so paralysis is diagnosed if the strength of a movement is reduced, if the muscular tone is altered and potentially also if there is muscular atrophy. Likewise, it appears absolutely impossible to define norms of normal "higher cognitive functions" at an abstract level. Rather, mental functions have to be broken down to basic functions, which are necessary for human life and survival and whose impairment then constitutes the symptom for a disease. Here, "disease" is the term to denote a malady in the medical context. This approach has for example been proposed by Boorse (1976). Boorse also suggested that beyond these functions that reduce the ability to survive also dysfunctions that reduce the ability to procreate constitute symptoms of a mental disorder. This, however, should be rejected, because it would allow to pathologize certain forms of sexual orientation among consenting adults. This would not only be inacceptable in any democratic society, it would also go profoundly against the aim of medicine, which is to serve the individual not to enforce social norms, whether they are disguised as biological demands or not, on the individual. On the other hand, the approach tested by Boorse functions well without burdening the individual with demands of biological procreation rates, as long as one focuses on functions necessary for survival. Those and only those functions that are necessary for survival are called symptoms when impaired. The definition of mental disorders would not deviate from the definition of somatic diseases. In both areas, a disease is then diagnosed if and only if a vital function is impaired.

However, here the question arises, which mental functions are necessary for survival. Again, given the diversity of human behaviour, it may be difficult to come up with a consensual definition of vital mental function. Indeed, in the introduction to DSM-5, no such definition is given, and instead, a number of partially overlapping terms (such as cognitive or motivational functions etc.) are presented. Here we suggest to focus on key symptoms of mental disorders as defined in traditional psychopathology. For example, there is little doubt that a delirium can be diagnosed worldwide as soon as vigilance, orientation and concentration are severely impaired. All of these symptoms have complex neurobiological correlates (as in the case of temporal and special orientation, which require for a person to locate himself or herself in his or her environment and to memorize certain aspects of recent activities); however, they can be diagnosed clinically rather easily. Likewise, a dementia can be diagnosed worldwide by assessing certain key memory functions (AMDP 1981; Heinz and Kluge 2010; Missmahl et al. 2012). Delirium and dementia have traditionally been called "exogenous psychosis" due to their association with organic brain dysfunction, either due to known pathological alterations in neuronal cell structure (as in Alzheimer's dementia) or external factors causing the syndrome (as in delirium tremens). We suggest that also the key symptoms what was previously called "endogenous psychosis", i.e. schizophrenia and major affective disorders, impair functions necessary for human life and survival. Indeed, effects have an intentional aspect and intimately link a subject with his or her environment. A severe impairment of the ability to experience various effects in changing environments, as in severe depression or mania, can threaten survival, e.g. because a person feels so desperate and hopeless that he or she stops eating and drinking. However, even if the survival of an individual is not directly threatened, a loss of the ability to experience different emotions in different contexts appears to profoundly impair a key aspect of human life, existential feelings that ground an individual in its surrounding (Ratcliff 2011; Slaby et al. 2011). Beyond major affective disorders, one can argue that ego disorders in schizophrenia, which are often called "passivity symptoms" in the Anglo-American context and include symptoms such as thought insertion or thought blockade, impair a key aspect of human life: the authorship and ownership of one's own thoughts, which is one of the prerequisites for human autonomy (Gallagher 2004; Souza and Swiney 2011; Vosgerau and Voss 2014). As can be seen in Table 26.1, key symptoms of exogenous and endogenous psychoses indeed appear to denote dysfunctions that impair the chance of the individual to survive and live in its environment.

The current controversy about illness models in psychiatry mainly arises from what has previously been called neurotic disorders and personality disorders (Table 26.2). In traditional psychopathology, such disorders were not labelled as

Table 26.1 Psychopathological assessment of key diagnostic symptoms

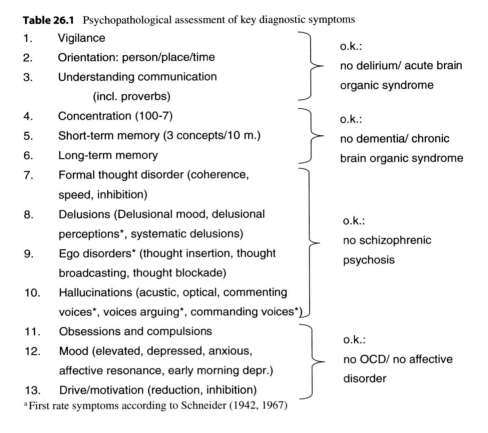

1.   Vigilance

2.   Orientation: person/place/time

3.   Understanding communication
        (incl. proverbs)

o.k.:
no delirium/ acute brain organic syndrome

4.   Concentration (100-7)

5.   Short-term memory (3 concepts/10 m.)

6.   Long-term memory

o.k.:
no dementia/ chronic brain organic syndrome

7.   Formal thought disorder (coherence, speed, inhibition)

8.   Delusions (Delusional mood, delusional perceptions*, systematic delusions)

9.   Ego disorders* (thought insertion, thought broadcasting, thought blockade)

10. Hallucinations (acustic, optical, commenting voices*, voices arguing*, commanding voices*)

o.k.:
no schizophrenic psychosis

11. Obsessions and compulsions

12. Mood (elevated, depressed, anxious, affective resonance, early morning depr.)

13. Drive/motivation (reduction, inhibition)

o.k.:
no OCD/ no affective disorder

ª First rate symptoms according to Schneider (1942, 1967)

Table 26.2 Mental disorders: diseases vs. variations

Exogenous psychoses (brain organic syndromes)	Endogenous psychoses	Variations
Acute e.g. delirium	The group of schizophrenias	Neuroses (trauma and conflict-related causes)
Chronic e.g. dementia	Major affective psychoses (unipolar and bipolar depression)	Personality disorders (traits)

diseases but rather as "normal" human variations. It is the status of these impairments that spark current debates: when should an anxiety be called a disorder? Which forms of suffering actually constitute a disease? How long should grief be allowed to exist before it can be labelled a depression and how long does a person have to suffer from grief following the loss of a loved one before he or she can receive therapeutic aid that is financed by the health insurance or maintenance organization? Here, questions of individual suffering and social participation appear to play a key role.

To Diagnose a Disease Is Not Enough: The Role of Illness and Sickness Aspects in Mental Disorder

If the term "disease" defines all medical aspects of a mental disorder and while its diagnosis depends on the impairment of vital functions, such impairments alone are not enough to justify a diagnosis of a mental disorder. A point in case are subjects hearing voices or experiencing some kind of thought insertion in their life – such symptoms appear to occur quite frequently without causing individual suffering or a relevant impairment of social participation (van Os et al. 2001). The existence of disease symptoms alone is thus not enough to diagnose a mental malady or disorder. Instead, Wakefield and others (Wakefield 2012 [1992]) have suggested that beyond the medical aspect of any disorder, the harm it causes for the individual needs to be specified. Here, we and others (Sartorius 2010) suggest to distinguish between the illness and the sickness aspect of any mental malady (see Fig. 26.1).

The illness aspect concerns the suffering it causes for the individual. The illness experience is at the root of our everyday understanding of a disease – we feel sick, ill and impaired, we suffer from pain, we experience fever or other unpleasant somatic symptoms and we can feel low or even depressed. As far as subjective impairments are concerned, all this suffering is subsumed under the concept of an "illness". However, there are certain mental disorders in which subjects display an impairment of certain mental functions, as in mania, the loss of the ability to feel grief or other negative feelings, which are not associated with any illness experiences. Instead, the subjects can feel great and powerful; they can be very creative and even want to stay in this elevated mood state. Here, a mental disorder can still be diagnosed but only if the disease symptoms (as in the ability to experience grief,

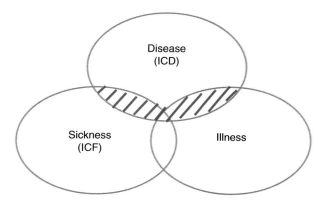

Fig. 26.1 The concept of a mental malady: disease plus illness or sickness. A mental malady should only be diagnosed if there are (1) symptoms of a disease, i.e. impairments of mental functions relevant for an individual's life and survival, and either (2) individual suffering due to these symptoms or some other form of subjective illness experience or (3) a substantial impairment of social participation due to the fact that activities of daily living are impaired by the mental dysfunctions

Table 26.3 Aspects of a mental malady

1.	*Disease*: this term aims at the medical aspect of any malady; a disease is defined by its core diagnostic symptoms, which reflect an impairment of functions that are relevant for an individual's life and survival (e.g. spatial disorientation)
2.	*Illness*: this term refers to the subjective experience of a malady including suffering and discomfort due to the disorder
3.	*Sickness*: the social aspect of a mental malady, defined by disabilities that impair social participation including activities of daily living (e.g. the inability to eat and drink in severe dementia)

the manic elevated mood) cause in other forms harm to the individual than described in the illness concept: an impairment of social participation. This aspect has often been termed the "sickness" aspect of any disorder. Indeed, persons showing manic symptoms can lose their social contacts and friends, they can alienate their loved ones by being unable to empathize with individual suffering of grief, they can endanger their own health by extremely incautious behaviour and they can lose all their financial resources and end up severely in debt, which they be profoundly regret when the manic episode is over. However, calling a social impairment a "sickness" requires extreme caution. The abuse of psychiatry in the Soviet Union teaches us that societies can demand a degree of conformity to social norms and label any forms of dissidence as indicators of a mental malady. Therefore, if a mental disorder causes an impairment of social participation, the aspects of this impairment should be limited to impairments in activities in daily living that are relevant for the wellbeing of person. For example, a demented person who is no longer able to acquire and prepare food and to keep up their personal level of hygiene indeed suffers from a profound reduction in social participation and hence clearly suffers from a mental malady, independent of whether the person feels ill at that moment or not. On the other hand, subjects with unusual belief systems, which may or not fulfil the disease criteria of a paranoia, should not be labelled mentally ill or diagnosed with a mental malady; they neither suffer from their symptoms nor are impaired in their activities of daily living. Otherwise, any deviation from a predominant worldview particularly if enforced in a dictatorship can be abused to label and stigmatize a person as being mentally ill. Therefore, we suggest a narrow concept of mental maladies (see Table 26.3) that requires the presence of an impairment of vital functions (the disease aspect) as well as either individual suffering (the illness aspect) or a severe impairment of social participation that interferes with activities of daily living (the sickness aspect).

How to Classify States of Suffering That Do Not Fulfil the Criteria of a Medical Disease?

Such a narrow classification of a mental malady has the advantage that it can hardly be abused in order to enforce social conformity by mislabelling political dissidents as a mental disorder or by enforcing certain sexual orientations as a norm. The recent introduction of the death penalty for homosexuality in certain countries worldwide warns us that there is an eminent danger of exclusion and stigmatization of diverse human behaviour and that psychiatry should be at the forefront of defending human rights. This struggle requires a cautious approach to mental maladies and a rather narrow disease concept that prevents political abuse. On the other hand, there are a substantial number of individuals suffering from mental disorders who do not receive appropriate treatment. For example, grief over the loss of a loved one can cause severe harm over the individual even if no vital functions are impaired, and therefore no medical disease in the narrow sense of the concept can be diagnosed. Here, we suggest that talking about mental disorders instead of "diseases" or "maladies" can be a useful approach. Shyness up to the degree of social phobia, depressed mood following personal losses, anxieties in situations of social discrimination or exclusion are not diseases, but subjects suffering from such impairments can substantially profit from psychotherapy, sometimes even medication. Should such illnesses and grievances be supported by the medical and psychotherapeutic health system, even if no disease in the narrow sense of the term can be diagnosed? The answer to this question depends on the resources that are given in any country. If the resources are very limited, it appears to be unfair to spread them out among all subjects with some kind of mental problem, and instead it seems to be necessary to focus them on those subjects suffering from mental diseases in the narrow sense. In richer countries, psychotherapeutic resources and even access to medications with low side effects can be provided for individuals suffering from everyday problems such as grief or common anxieties. The situation here is akin the decision whether to operate a nose that looks highly unusual and thus attracts unpleasant attention for the individual but does not impair breathing. In such cases, one may diagnose a mental disorder and provide health-care funds, and the degree of individual suffering and social exclusion appear to be the key aspects that should guide the decision whether an individual should be provided with therapy at the expense of insurances and health maintenance organizations. For any given society, it may even be wise to provide such medical and psychosocial services already for subjects who do not yet have the disease criteria, because early interventions can prevent the manifestation of a full-blown disease. One example would be interventions against substance use disorders already at the level when key symptoms of drug dependence such as tolerance development, withdrawal and loss of behavioural flexibility have not yet appeared. Again, this does not mean that it is useful to broaden concepts of substance use disorders too much: the current definition of alcohol use disorders in DSM-V allows to pathologize any kind of alcohol consumption in a country in which it is illegal. As long as the person wants to consume alcohol, spends a lot of time on its acquisition and exposes him- or herself to the legal consequences and the social problems associated with alcohol consumption, even moderate degrees of alcohol intake as common in many countries worldwide could be pathologized. This again warns against the danger of too broad disease categories and suggests to distinguish between mental maladies that fulfil criteria for the existence of a medical disease as well as for the presence of individual harm, either in the sense of suffering or impaired social participation and other forms of mental disorders in which suffering and impairments of social participation are the leading aspects of the state, but no vital functions are impaired.

However, any rational conceptionalization of mental maladies and disorders does not prevent that subjects suffering from such disorders or showing symptoms of such disorders are stigmatized. The fight against stigma is a must in any given society, no matter how broad or narrow a disease concept is articulated.

> **Information Box 26.1**
> 1. If the term "disease" defines all medical aspects of a mental disorder and while its diagnosis depends on the impairment of vital functions, such impairments alone are not enough to justify a diagnosis of a mental disorder.
> 2. Therefore, we suggest a narrow concept of mental maladies that requires the presence of an impairment in vital functions (the disease aspect) as well as either individual suffering (the illness aspect) or a severe impairment of social participation that interferes with activities of daily living (the sickness aspect).
> 3. Nevertheless, any rational conceptionalization of mental maladies and disorders does not prevent that subjects suffering from disorders or showing symptoms of such disorders are stigmatized. The fight against stigma is a must in any given society, no matter how broad or narrow a disease concept is articulated.

References

AMDP (Arbeitsgemeinschaft für Methodik und Dokumentation in der Psychiatrie) (1981) Das AMDP System. Manual zur Dokumentation psychiatrischer Befunde. Springer, Berlin/Heidelberg/New York

Amnesty International (1977) Bericht über die Folter. Fischer-Taschenbuch-Verlag, Frankfurt

Boorse C (1976) What a theory of mental health should be. J Theory Soc Behav 6:61–84

Gallagher S (2004) Neurocognitive models of schizophrenia: a neurophenomenological critique. Psychopathology 37:8–19

Heinz A (1998) Colonial perspectives in the construction of the psychotic patient as primitive man. Crit Anthropol 18(4):421–444

Heinz A, Kluge U (2010) Anthropological and evolutionary concepts of mental disorder. J Speculat Philos 24(3):292–307

Jaspers K (1946) Allgemeine Psychopathologie, Ein Leitfaden für Studierende, Ärzte und Psychologen. 1.Auflage 1913, 2. 1920, 3. 1923; 4. völlig neu bearbeitete Auflage. Springer, Berlin

Missmahl I, Kluge U, Bromand Z, Heinz A (2012) Teaching psychiatry and establishing psychosocial services – lessons from Afghanistan: migration and mental health. Eur Psychiatry 27(Supplement 2):S76–S80

Ratcliffe M (2011) Existentielle Gefühle. In: Slaby J, Stephan A, Walter H, Walter S (eds) Affektive Intentionalität, Beiträge zur welterschließenden Funktion der menschlichen Gefühle. Mentis, Paderborn, pp 144–169

Sartorius N (2010) Meta-effects of classifying mental disorders. In: Regier DA, Narrow WE, Kuhl GA, Kupfer DJ (eds) The conceptual evolution of DSM5. American Psychiatric Association, Airlington, pp 59–77

Schneider K (1942) Psychischer Befund und psychiatrische Diagnose. Thieme, Leipzig

Schneider K (1967) Psychopathologie, 8th edn. Thieme, Stuttgart

Slaby J, Stephan A, Walter H, Walter S (eds) (2011) Affektive Intentionalität. Beiträge zur welterschließenden Funktion der menschlichen Gefühle. Mentis, Paderborn, pp 170–205

Souza P, Swiney L (2011) Thought insertion: abnormal sense of thought agency or thought endorsement? Phenomenology and cognitive science. Springer, Berlin, published online 21. Sept 2011

van Os J, Hanssen M, Bijl RV, Vollebergh W (2001) Prevalence of psychotic disorder and community level of psychotic symptoms: an urban-rural comparison. Arch Gen Psychiatry 58:663–668

Vosgerau G, Voss M (2014) Authorship and control over thoughts. Mind Lang 29:534 (in print)

Wakefield JC (2012) [1992] Der Begriff der psychischen Störung: An der Grenze zwi.schen biologischen Tatsachen und gesellschaftlichen Werten. In: Schramme T (Hrsg). Krankheitstheorien. Frankfurt, Suhrkamp, pp 239–262

Part IV

"Fighting" Stigma
and Discrimination: Commentaries

Heather Stuart

There is increasing recognition that mental health-related stigma is a major public health problem that conveys a hidden burden of suffering on people who have a mental illness and their family members. In response, the number of countries and regions initiating anti-stigma programs is growing and, as international interest in anti-stigma programs has increased, so has the discourse surrounding what works, what does not, and why (Stuart et al. 2012). This chapter will provide a commentary on methods that have been shown to be effective and, in so doing, will selectively highlight some of the most promising practices in the field at macro (structural), meso (public), and micro (individual) levels.

What Constitutes Proof?

To answer the question what has proven effectiveness, it is first necessary to consider what constitutes proof. In medicine and the health sciences, evidence is rank ordered according to the methodological strength and rigor of scientific study designs used and their ability to provide unbiased estimates of underlying causal relationships. The gold standard for determining effectiveness is a high-quality review (or meta-analysis) of all relevant high-quality randomized controlled trials. Study designs that use nonrandomized, observational methods are deemed to be of lesser rank because they are more open to bias from unmeasured or confounding factors (something that randomization is supposed to avoid by balancing the groups) (Borgerson 2009).

H. Stuart
Centre for Health Services and Policy Research, Queen's University,
Abramsky Hall, 21 Arch Street, Room 324, Kingston, ON K7L 3N6, Canada
e-mail: heather.stuart@queensu.ca

© Springer International Publishing Switzerland 2017
W. Gaebel et al. (eds.), *The Stigma of Mental Illness - End of the Story?*,
DOI 10.1007/978-3-319-27839-1_27

This approach to evidence gathering has been criticized because of the large gap between the characteristics of individuals enrolled into clinical trials and the average day-to-day clients seen in clinical care settings. The meta-analyses of randomized trials can inform us as to what works under the best (most ideal) circumstances, where study subjects are handpicked, but not what works in day-to-day practice (Goldenberg 2009). In addition, in many public health situations, interventions are provided to entire nations or communities, making randomization difficult or impossible (Stuart 2008).

The nature of "proof" has important implications for the anti-stigma research field, where few randomized controlled trials have been conducted (and even fewer meta-analyses) and where much of our current knowledge comes from uncontrolled, observational study designs that would be considered fundamentally flawed by conventional evidence-based standards. As an illustration of this point, Griffiths and colleagues conducted a systematic search of randomized controlled trials focusing on the effectiveness of programs for reducing stigma (Griffiths et al. 2014). They identified 34 papers representing 33 trials, 26 of which contained sufficient data to conduct a meta-analysis. Because the trials examined different aspects of stigma, and results were heterogeneous across studies, it was difficult to make firm conclusions in many important aspects of stigma as they were underrepresented in the trial literature. For example, only one published study examined stigma reduction pertaining to generalized anxiety disorder and two focused on substance abuse. A range of conditions (e.g., bipolar disorder, panic disorder, post-traumatic stress disorder, and eating disorders) were not studied at all.

Findings from quasi-experimental and qualitative approaches, though more numerous, are often excluded from systematic reviews with the result that they never find their way into policy briefs. This situation significantly disadvantages anti-stigma strategies at the evidence and funding tables. Also, while it is difficult to argue with the importance of generating evidence to support action, the current paradigm largely ignores the social and cultural influences that govern the production of evidence. For example, it is now well recognized that mental illness-related stigma has slowed the production of evidence in the mental health field relative to other fields with equally disabling conditions. With fewer prospects for significant and sustained funding, researchers gravitate to other areas, leaving the field with a lack of capacity to produce high-quality evidence. Developing a strong evidence base to support best practices in anti-stigma programming remains an important challenge (Stuart 2008).

A more pragmatic approach would recognize that there is no simple formula for distinguishing what works from what does not. Such questions can only be answered with ongoing, extensive, and multifaceted evaluations designed to develop a bottom-up theory of truth (Goldenberg 2009). A pragmatic approach would also go beyond issues of efficacy and allow for an assessment of whether or not an intervention is appropriate (and/or valued) by the recipient and whether it is feasible to implement on a wide scale. Evans has argued that appropriateness and feasibility provide a sounder base for evaluating interventions acknowledging that many factors, other than the efficacy of an intervention under ideal conditions, can impact on its success (Evans 2003).

While scholarly interest in anti-stigma programming and evaluation is increasing, the evidence base to support anti-stigma initiatives remains underdeveloped. Prior to the 1990s, there was little evaluation evidence to draw upon, and current levels of work in this field continue to be meager when compared against evidence-based reports in other areas of mental health (Stuart 2008). Given that anti-stigma programming and evaluation are emerging fields, and given that interventions may not be amenable to the gold standard evidentiary practices, this review will adopt a broad understanding of effectiveness, including issues of appropriateness, feasibility, and scalability. Moreover, interventions that have been highlighted are those with the most plausible theories of change.

What Constitutes Stigma?

When considering the nature of anti-stigma interventions, it is important to first consider the nature of stigma. The Oxford online dictionary defines stigma as "a mark of disgrace associated with a particular circumstance, quality, or person" and gives as the main example, the stigma associated with mental disorders (Oxford Dictionaries 2014). This is consistent with Goffman's seminal work in which stigma was described as a mark of shame or infamy and where mental illnesses were identified as among the most deeply discrediting of all stigmatized conditions (Goffman 1963). Although Goffman understood stigma as deeply embedded in social relationships, his approach is now often criticized by advocates for placing too much emphasis on the attributes of the individual being stigmatized and insufficient emphasis on group behaviors. For example, Everett suggests that the term "discrimination" (rather than "stigma") better creates a dialogue that is rooted in a human rights paradigm that depicts prejudice and discrimination against people with a mental illness as forms of social oppression (Everett 2004).

Link and Phelan offer a contemporary definition of stigmatization that broadens the concept to include several interrelated components: identification and labeling of differences by the social group, cultural beliefs that link the label and the labeled individual to negative stereotypes, a categorical distinction between us and them, status loss and discrimination, and social structures that provide unequal access to social, economic, and political power (Link and Phelan 2001). This definition more clearly conceptualizes stigma as a multifaceted, multilevel social process that culminates in structural and power imbalances between groups. It is also more in keeping with the day-to-day experiences of people with a mental illness.

By moving away from explanatory models that focus on the social and cognitive elements of the stigmatizer who perceives a difference, endorses negative stereotypes, and behaves in a discriminatory manner (i.e., public stigma), it is possible to identify a broader range of structural factors that lead to discrimination against people with a mental illness (Corrigan et al. 2004). The recognition that social structures, through laws, policies, and institutional practices, can limit the rights and freedoms of people with a mental illness opens up new realms of possibilities for anti-stigma actions that could include such things as legal protest and social advocacy, which typically have not been included when considering anti-stigma activities (Arboleda-Florez and Stuart 2012).

The United Nations Declaration on the Rights of Persons with Disabilities adopts a similarly broad social-structural focus to promote the full inclusion of people with a disability. The Convention recognizes that disability is not the result of an individual's physical, emotional, or intellectual impairments but rather the result of the attitudinal and socio-environmental factors that may impede their full and effective participation in society on an equal footing with others. The Convention has forcefully shifted the paradigm away from the characteristics of individuals who have an impairment, to a human rights and social justice framework, one that recognizes that social inequities flow from social structures. Signatories to the Convention are challenged to remove economic, social, and political barriers that hinder social inclusion of people with disabilities (Stuart 2012).

In addition to public stigma and structural stigma, there is self-stigma. Self-stigma occurs when one internalizes the negative public beliefs about mental illnesses and applies them to oneself. It is a process of identity transformation that leads to a range of psychosocial consequences such as shame, secrecy, social withdrawal, depression, anxiety, reduction of hope and self-esteem, and poor quality of life (Sibitz et al. 2011). Brohan et al. (2010) surveyed 1,340 individuals with a psychotic disorder receiving treatment in 14 European countries (72 % response rate). Forty-two percent of the sample reported moderate or high levels of self-stigma, suggesting that self-stigma is a common and sometimes severe reaction to public and structural stigma.

The Importance of Multilevel Programs Targeting Behavioral Change

Link and Phelan (2001) have noted that the focus of much stigma research has been on public stigma and its consequences for those who are stigmatized. To address public stigma, many anti-stigma programs target changes in prejudicial attitudes using educational strategies. In *The Nature of Prejudice*, Allport defines prejudice as

> *an aversive or hostile attitude toward a person who belongs to a group, simply because he belongs to that group, and is therefore presumed to have the objectionable qualities ascribed to the group.* (Allport 2000, p. 20)

He makes an important distinction between misconceptions, where one organizes incorrect information, and prejudice. If individuals are capable of rectifying an erroneous judgment in light of new evidence, then they are not prejudiced. Prejudices are not reversible when exposed to new information. Unlike simple misconceptions, prejudices are resistant to all evidence to the contrary, and individuals tend to become emotional and hostile when their prejudices are threatened with a contradiction. Thus, it is not possible to rectify a prejudice without emotional resistance. Allport further makes the case that it is relatively ineffective to change prejudices by attempting to influence individuals because any lessons aimed at the individual will be smothered by cultural norms, expressed through the family, peers, media, and other social structures. He argues that it is easier to change cultural norms than it is to change individual attitudes. Once new norms are created, individual attitudes will follow. Thus, he would argue the importance of adopting a collectivist approach that targets behavioral (rather than attitudinal) change (Allport 2000).

The tendency has been to consider stigma in light of personal attributes rather than in light of the structural scaffolding that creates and perpetuates stigmatization. When powerful groups are motivated to stigmatize, social exclusion may be achieved in any number of ways. If, as Link and Phelan note, the stigmatized individual cannot be persuaded to voluntarily accept their lower status (as in the case of self-stigma), then direct discrimination may be used to accomplish the same outcome. If direct discrimination is ideologically difficult (i.e., viewed as socially undesirable), then sophisticated and covert forms of structural discrimination can achieve the same ends. Moreover, as long as the dominant group maintains a stigmatized view, decreasing one mechanism through which disadvantage is conferred creates the impetus to create another. Therefore, to be effective, anti-stigma interventions must recognize that approaches to change stigma must be multifaceted and multilevel. Not only must programs challenge the discriminating attitudes and behaviors of individuals operating within social groups, they must challenge and change the broader social structures in which these individuals operate (Link and Phelan 2001).

Promising Practices: Macro Level

Legislative Action and Advocacy

Though most would agree that legislation is not enough, legislative action is an indispensable tool in changing social structures and individual behaviors. This is because legislation has a significant symbolic and authoritative power, particularly when enforced and publicized. There have been many important strides taken to overturn legislation that explicitly discriminates or segregates people with a mental illness and in developing new legislation that better protects and promotes their rights (Callard et al. 2012).

Laws can govern actions even when they cannot change attitudes. Seat belt legislation stands as a good example of this principle. Prior to seat belt legislation, educational efforts were relatively ineffective in changing attitudes toward seat belts or increasing their use, even though the risk of a fatal injury for front seat occupants was widely known to drop by almost half if seat belts were worn. In a recent review of the literature, mandatory use legislation significantly increased seat belt use (to over 90 % in some countries), decreased fatalities to occupants, and decreased the rate of severe, nonfatal injuries (Rivara et al. 1999). In this case, the public health goal was achieved through legislation (and enforcement (Jonah et al. 1982)) in spite of individual beliefs. Today, it is likely that most people in countries with seat belt legislation are in favor of its use. A similar logic underlies mental health advocates' view that it does not matter what people think about those with a mental illness, as long as they are treated fairly and justly and have equal opportunities to become engaged in social and occupational activities (Sayce 2003).

While it may not be possible for the law to make people believe that those with a mental illness have human rights and social entitlements, it can prohibit discriminatory practices that make it difficult for those with a mental illness to get a job, obtain stable housing, or access treatment. In addition, law can establish protest mechanisms so that people who have had their rights violated have avenues of redress. Finally, law can impose duties on sectors and organizations to promote equality of opportunity and eliminate discrimination and harassment. In so doing, laws shift the emphasis away from the characteristics of the person who has been wronged and place the onus and responsibility on members of the social group (Callard et al. 2012).

The development of legislation to address discrimination on the basis of disability has gained importance over the last decades. By 2005, 40 out of the 189 United Nations member states have adopted some form of anti-discrimination legislation (Callard et al. 2012). Signatories to the United Nations Conventions on the Rights of Persons with Disabilities have an added impetus to promote legislative reform. The Convention is the first human rights instrument to offer comprehensive protections for persons with physical or mental impairments. It has reframed disability discourse from a focus on the individual to a rights-based model that emphasizes the social determinants of disability. The historical view of disabled people as the objects of charity, medical treatment, and social protection is firmly rejected. Instead the Convention strongly affirms that people with a disability have the right to be full and effective members of society. The substantive provisions are sweeping, covering both negative rights (e.g., freedom from any form of abuse or coercive treatment) and positive rights (e.g., rights to education, employment, and political participation). Signatories to the Convention are obliged to establish focal points for domestic implementation, a coordinating mechanism within government to facilitate intersectoral action, and a national reporting mechanism. An optional protocol (to which fewer countries have signed) empowers an international oversight committee to monitor and respond to individual and group allegations of violations. The Convention is a road map for structural transformation and will undoubtedly trigger a new generation of disability legislation and policies (Stuart 2012).

To be fully effective, however, legislation needs to be bolstered by social, structural, and political activities designed to eliminate economic, political, and social marginalization. It cannot stand alone. It needs strong advocacy to work. The World Health Organization describes mental health advocacy as a broad range of activities undertaken by a variety of players that are designed to promote the human rights of people with mental disorders under current law and ensure that mental health is on the agenda of policy makers and funders. Activities that often come under the broad umbrella of advocacy include awareness raising, dissemination of information, education, training, mutual help, counseling, mediating, defending, and denouncing. These activities are designed to remove barriers such as lack of mental health services, stigma, human rights violations, absence of mental health promotion, lack of housing, and unemployment. While systematic research quantifying the full effects of advocacy is lacking, the World Health Organization identifies positive outcomes including improvements in the policies and practices of governments and institutions, changes to laws and regulations, improvements in services, and improvements in human rights protections (The World Health Organization 2003).

Nowhere is the interaction between legislation and advocacy better demonstrated than in deinstitutionalization and its aftermath. Early reforms to mental health legislation, based on active civil rights advocacy, were an attempt to give greater emphasis to personal autonomy and eliminate coercive treatment practices. As a result, revisions to civil commitment legislation, which have occurred in many North American and European countries over the past 50–60 years, have removed the broad-based involuntary treatment criteria that kept people with mental illnesses segregated from mainstream society in large, geographically isolated and outdated institutions where they were subjected to harsh conditions and abuse (Stuart 2010).

During the 1960s in Canada, for example, psychiatric beds were at an all-time high of 66,000, having doubled over the preceding 30 years. Most of the buildings were obsolete, dating from the mid- to late 1800s, and overcrowded (up to 30 % over capacity) often housing up to 5,000 patients in deplorable conditions. Admission to a psychiatric institution was typically achieved using coercive legal means with the help of police. Once admitted, patients all but disappeared from social view and families broke off all ties (Reichman 1964). During the same time in the USA, numerous legal challenges arose to minimize civil commitment, the argument being that involuntary hospitalization was punitive with harmful outcomes. Beginning in the late 1960s, court cases and statutory reforms granted basic rights to people with a mental illness and placed significant restrictions on involuntary treatment. Subsequently, outpatient commitment legislation mandated treatment in the least restrictive alternative. Although the beds were emptied, the paucity of money and resources devoted to the community mental health system limited the efficacy of legislative reforms, resulting in poverty, homelessness, and disenfranchisement (Hiday and Wales 2013). Advocacy to protect negative rights must now give way to advocacy in the service of positive rights.

In Canada, successive waves of advocacy following bed closures have resulted in a fivefold per capita increase in expenditures on community-based psychiatric services from 6.97, in the late 1980s, to 35.90, in 1999 (Sealy and Whitehead 2004). Despite this investment, homelessness remains a serious problem signifying that important service and system failures persist and continued advocacy is necessary. The Mental Health Commission of Canada estimates that there are up to 300,000 people who are homeless across the country, costing Canadians 1.4 billion each year. Up to 67 % of those who are homeless report having had some mental health problem in their lifetime. In 2008, the Commission obtained a grant from the federal government for $110 million for a 5-year demonstration project to evaluate the effectiveness of a Housing First program. Based on the evidence provided by this project, and the resulting advocacy, the federal government's 2013 budget included $600 million for a homelessness partnering strategy to help address this problem (Goering et al. 2014).

Employment equity legislation provides another example of legislative action designed to remove discrimination that is in need of strong advocacy to make it work. The link between socioeconomic deprivation and mental disabilities has been widely acknowledged, prompting many governments to enact legislation to remove barriers to full economic participation. Such legislation typically imposes specific duties on employers to accommodate people with a disability. It prohibits employers from discriminating against qualified people in any aspect of employment, such as hiring, firing, return to work, or career advancement. Further, it requires employers to make reasonable accommodations for employees who are disabled so that they may fulfill their job requirements (Stuart 2007).

However, the impact of employment equity legislation on workplaces is the subject of considerable debate, especially as people with mental disabilities continue to experience significant employment discrimination. While most people with a mental health problem are willing and able to work, studies from various countries show that they are three to five times more likely to be unemployed compared to their nonmentally ill counterparts. In fact, people with mental illnesses report that employment discrimination is one of their most frequent stigma experiences. A weakness of employment equity legislation (and many other legislative approaches) is that it assumes that employers will adhere to the requirements and there is little active monitoring or enforcement to ensure that this is the case. In cases of wrongdoing, it is incumbent upon the individual who has been wronged to mount a legal protest. Individuals must know their rights and have the stamina and financial resources to put a claim forward and support an investigation. In some countries, a union may put forward a claim on the employee's behalf, and in many countries, human rights tribunals also exist to hear and settle claims (Callard et al. 2012).

To date there have been two reviews of the effectiveness of employment equity legislation in promoting employment for people with a mental illness—one in the USA (where employment equity legislation has the long history) and one in the UK. In both reviews, the legislation was described as a windfall for the employers, with the majority of claims (87 % in the UK and 63 % in the USA) being resolved in the employers' favor. This is because of the restricted understanding of disability with pronounced disadvantages for people with mental disorders (Stuart 2007).

As a result of strong advocacy, the Americans with Disabilities Act has since been amended to restore the original intent of the protections, broaden the definition of mental disability, and remove the strict standards that had been applied by Supreme Court decisions that required "severe" limitations to daily activities and excluded intermittent or episodic conditions (Callard et al. 2012). While similar problems exist in Britain, Sayce (2003) reports some improvement. For example, the proportion of British employers with disability policies went up from two-thirds in 2001 to 90 % in 2002, and the number stating that they employed people with disabilities rose from 87 % to 95 % during this time. Reasons included both a commitment to corporate social responsibility and compliance with Britain's Disability Discrimination Act.

It is clear from these examples that legislation can be an effective anti-stigma tool when there are procedural, organizational, policy, and financial supports, strong advocacy for social equity at each of these levels, and effective mechanisms of protest and redress.

Media Guidelines

News and entertainment media have created a vast storehouse of negative imagery surrounding the practice of psychiatry and people with a mental illness. Denigrating fictional images are some of the most potent portrayals of mental illnesses. Movies such as *The Snake Pit* or *One Flew Over the Cuckoo's Nest* have also provided dramatic images of the inhuman and oppressive effects of psychiatric treatments and institutions. Journalistic accounts of forced confinement and horrifying images of people living in the early psychiatric institutions have cast lasting doubts on the nature of psychiatric treatment and the motivation of psychiatric professionals. Indeed, investigative journalistic accounts of conditions in these facilities helped to spur the deinstitutionalization movement in North America (Stuart 2006).

News media, particularly newspapers, are among the most frequently identified sources of mental health (and health) information. However, standard story lines that focus on conflict, controversy, or public safety often place journalists in direct conflict with mental health advocates and professionals. As a result, there has been considerable interest in identifying recurrent themes used by news media to represent mental illnesses and the mentally ill. Reporters often emphasize the violent, delusional, and irrational behavior of people with a mental illness and may sensationalize headlines or story content (Stuart 2006).

In a recent Canadian study (Whitley and Berry 2013), for example, danger, violence, and criminality were direct themes in over 40 % of the 11,263 newspaper articles reviewed. The articles were from 20 of the best-selling English language Canadian newspapers. In many of these instances, journalists wrote sensationalist and titillating accounts of an event or person linking mental illness, as a general category, to unpredictable, shocking, or outlandish behavior. Often disease labels were assigned to people suspected of criminal behavior based on the reports of neighbors and police officers or even as a result of journalists' own speculations, without supporting evidence. Treatments for mental illnesses were discussed in 19 % of the articles, leaving the readers with the impression that mental illnesses are likely untreatable and incurable. Eighteen percent identified recovery or rehabilitation themes. Of most concern was the almost complete lack of voice from people with a mental illness. Eighty-three percent of the articles did not include a quotation or even a paraphrased statement from someone with a mental illness. In the 17 % where a quotation was included, less than half of the people were quoted positively. Similarly, 75 % of the articles did not include a quote from a psychiatric expert (psychiatrist, social worker, or spokesperson from a mental health advocacy organization). The voices of people with a mental illness and mental health experts were generally silenced. Moreover, no consistent improvements in media reporting between 2005 and 2010 were identified.

Despite the fact that the news and entertainment media have done little to convince the viewing public that people with a mental illness can recover and become productive members of society, journalists are an important and underused ally in anti-stigma work. Traditional approaches to media assume that the message will trigger the right behavior if the message is transmitted to the right person (a passive recipient) at the right time. However, media advocacy defines the problem more actively, as a power gap. By gaining access to the news media and framing public policy and health problems, community groups can apply pressure to change agendas and priorities. Often it requires greater emphasis on social dimensions of a problem such that personal troubles are translated into public issues. Working with community groups, journalists can shift emphasis away from victims to social and organizational structures that create and support inequities (Wallack and Dorfman 1996). Journalistic reports can help set the public agenda, set boundaries for the discussion, and amplify voices so that policy makers cannot ignore them. Journalists can also provide countervailing views of mental illnesses, model positive reactions to people with a mental illness, and illustrate the appropriate language to use when referring to people with a mental illness (Stuart 2006).

Toward this end, journalists in several countries have developed media guidelines for reporting on mental health-related events. In the foreword to the Canadian guide, Picard, a senior health columnist for *The Globe and Mail*, has indicated that, for meaningful change to occur, journalists need to be conscious of their failings and address them systematically, starting with language. An outdated and prejudicial turn of phrase, such as someone has "committed" suicide, or euphemisms like someone "died suddenly" need to be replaced with respectful, person-first language. Further, in his opinion, journalists also need to clean the slate of assumptions and misperceptions—the typical stereotypes that fuel notions that people with a mental illness are violent. In his opinion, they can do this by providing appropriate context when violent incidents occur. Finally, he points to equality in reporting. In his view, mental illnesses should be reported in the same way that physical illnesses are reported: "with curiosity, compassion, and a strong dose of righteous indignation when people are mistreated or wronged" (Canadian Journalism Forum on Violence and Trauma 2014, p. 4). In this way, journalism need not perpetuate stigma but provide opportunities to bring about meaningful change.

An Australian resource for media professionals provides up-to-date research relating to reporting of suicides and mental illnesses (National Media and Mental Health Group 2009). Advice includes considering whether a story about suicide needs to be run at all (as a succession of suicide stories may normalize this behavior), placing stories on the inside pages of a newspaper or other print media (as prominent placement of suicide stories may trigger copycats), considering the impact of the story on vulnerable audiences (as the impact may be higher when the reader, listener, or viewer identifies with the person in the report), avoiding detailed descriptions of the methods (as these may promote copycat suicides), not disclosing the location of a suicide (as it may become popularized for other suicides), and checking the language (avoiding words like "committed" or "failed suicide"). Interestingly, between 2001 and 2007, a large media-monitoring project reported a number of improvements in reporting following publication of this resource (Pirkis et al. 2008). For example, inappropriate language used by journalists to describe suicides dropped from 42 % to 6 % of stories. The majority of items on mental illness did not stereotype people as violent or untrustworthy. Stigmatizing reports dropped from 14 % in 2001 to 10 % in 2007.

Austria may have been one of the first countries to introduce media guidelines, in 1987, so it is in a unique position to assess the impacts on the subsequent frequency of suicides. Niederkrotenthaler and Sonneck (2007) statistically modeled suicide rates using an interrupted time-series design. Results showed a significant decline in suicides in the year following the introduction of the guidelines corresponding to a permanent annual decrease of 81 suicides. This drop corresponded to a significant improvement in the quality of media reporting in the 5 years after the introduction of the guidelines. Moreover, the improvement in the quality of the reporting was significantly correlated with the drop in the number of suicides, suggesting a causal link between media guidelines and dropping suicide numbers.

Pirkis and colleagues (2006) reviewed media guidelines from Australia, New Zealand, the USA, Canada, the UK, Hong Kong, Sri Lanka, and the World Health Organization, noting that they were all remarkably similar in their content. All recommended avoiding sensationalism, glamorizing, giving undue prominence, avoiding specific details, taking an educative role, and the importance of providing contact details for support services. However, the way in which the guidelines were developed differed markedly. Some guidelines had strong involvement from media professionals making them an active part of the process, ensuring that they felt some ownership for the result. Others did not. Both the Canadian and Australian media resources stand out because of the high involvement of media professionals in their production and dissemination. In Canada, for example, the Canadian Journalism Forum on Violence and Trauma developed *Mindset* with financial support from the Mental Health Commission of Canada but at arm's length (Canadian Journalism Forum on Violence and Trauma 2014). In Australia, a large task force including representatives from all major media outlets, consumer advocacy groups, and government representatives developed *reporting suicide and mental illness* (National Media and Mental Health Group 2009). These countries are also notable for the emphasis on reporting of suicide and mental illnesses (rather than focusing on suicide alone as many other countries have done).

Promising Practices: Meso Level

Contact-Based Education as Transformative Learning

People who hold prejudices selectively admit new information to their categorizations only if it confirms previous beliefs, making it possible to hold negative prejudgments in the face of considerable evidence to the contrary. One disarming device described by Allport (2000) is to admit an exception to the rule, keeping the negative structures intact for all other cases. This is called "re-fencing." When a fact cannot fit into a mental field, the exception is acknowledged and the field is hastily fenced in again. This is why traditional education, which conveys facts and explodes myths, is largely ineffective in reducing prejudices.

Moreover, there is a growing body of evidence to support the idea that factual knowledge about mental illnesses (i.e., good mental health literacy) can coexist with considerable amounts of stigma, suggesting that improved knowledge will not result in improved social acceptance. In the USA between 1950 and 1996, for example, pubic conceptions of mental illnesses had broadened and more closely approximated professional definitions. At the same time, stereotypes involving violence and other frightening characteristics linked to mental illnesses rose. In 1950, for example, 7 % of survey respondents mentioned violent incidents in relation to mental illnesses. This rose to 12 % by 1996. When considering violence related to psychotic illnesses, manifestations of violence increased from 13 % to 31 % (Phelan et al. 2000). Also, between 1996 and 2006, a greater proportion of the American public endorsed neurobiological explanations for major mental illnesses such as schizophrenia, depression, and alcohol dependence. Public endorsement for medical treatments for these disorders also increased. Despite improvements in knowledge, there was no corresponding decrease in any of the variables indicating public stigma, and levels of intolerance remained high. The majority of respondents continued to express an unwillingness to socialize with someone who had a mental illness. In some cases, neurobiological explanations actually increased the odds of a stigmatizing reaction (Pescosolido et al. 2010).

The contact hypothesis, originally articulated by Allport (1954), indicates that positive intergroup contact reduces prejudice and promotes better intergroup relations. He proposed that direct (face-to-face) intergroup contact would be more likely to reduce prejudice if it involved equal status between the groups, cooperation on common goals, and institutional support. Considerable research conducted across a host of different target groups has now demonstrated that intergroup contact can contribute to reductions in prejudice across a broad range of groups and contexts. A large meta-analytic study ($n = 515$ studies) reported that structured programs, especially those with institutional support, showed significantly stronger contact-prejudice effects (Pettigrew and Tropp 2006). The prejudice-reducing benefits of contact have also been shown to generalize beyond the immediate contact setting (or particular participants) to attitudes toward other settings and members of the larger group (Hewstone and Swart 2011).

Mezirow (1997) describes "habits of mind" as the frame of reference used to organize cognitive, conative, and emotional responses. They are broad, habitual ways of thinking, feeling, and acting that may be situated in cultural, social, educational, political, or psychological frames of reference. An example is the predisposition to regard people outside of one's social group prejudicially. In order to change a habit of mind, one must become critically reflective of the underlying assumptions, values, beliefs, and feelings. When done well, contact-based education has the potential to transform points of view by highlighting negative feelings and attitudes one may have about people with a mental illness, resulting in greater acceptance and transformative learning.

Contact-based education has been widely used to reduce prejudice and improve feelings of social distance toward people with a mental illness. Corrigan and colleagues (Corrigan et al. 2012) conducted a meta-analysis of 72 articles published between 1972 and 2010 that specifically focused on the ability of contact to reduce mental illness-related stigma. Results were based on 38,364 research participants from 14 countries in Europe, North America, South America, Asia, and Australia. College students, adolescents, and adults were the most frequently targeted. Children under the age of 12 and family members were rarely targeted. Contact yielded statistically significant improvements in attitudes and behavioral intentions (social distance). Both video contact and in-person contact showed statistically significant effects on attitudinal and behavioral intent measures, though in-person contact showed significantly greater effect sizes. The highest effect size (reflecting a moderate effect) was noted for in-person contact on behavioral intentions among adolescents. More recently, Griffiths and colleagues conducted a meta-analysis of randomized controlled trials and supported Corrigan's findings. The pooled effect of the five interventions employing contact with people who had a mental illness was moderate in magnitude ($d=0.29$, CI=0.16, 0.42, $p<0.001$) (Griffiths et al. 2014).

In addition to being provided to undifferentiated groups in the population, such as students, contact-based education can also be directed to subgroups who have particular influence in the lives of people with a mental illness. Recently, for example, Knaak and colleagues (2014) examined the key ingredients in 22 contact-based educational programs that targeted Canadian health providers. Using qualitative inquiry, they identified six ingredients that they considered were keys in reducing stigmatization. These included contact in the form of a personal testimony from a trained speaker who has lived experience of a mental illness, multiple forms or points of contact (e.g., live presentation and video presentations or multiple speakers), a focus on behavioral change through skill development, myth-busting, an enthusiastic facilitator who models a person-centered approach (as opposed to a pathology-first perspective), and a strong recovery theme. Each program was rated according to the presence or absence of these characteristics. Quantitative analysis showed that programs that included all six of the program elements performed significantly better than those that did not. Programs that used multiple forms of social contact and emphasized recovery were among the most effective. This is the first study to document key ingredients in contact-based education for health professionals, which is an important move toward establishing best practice standards for programs targeting this group.

Finally, in order for contact to change stigmatizing views and behaviors, it has to be repeated. Repeated interpersonal contact (rather than a one-off intervention) is necessary to disconfirm negative stereotypes. This is because any single piece of disconfirming information may elicit a minor or temporary change in the stereotype. Major change occurs gradually, only after an accumulation of many disconfirming instances (Hewstone 2000). Institutional support will be vital in ensuring that contact-based educational programs are maintained over time and become a routine part of orientation and development activities. This will require interactions between the social and organizational structures at the macro level, with programming aimed at changing public perceptions at the meso level.

Promising Practices: Microlevel

Stigma Management Strategies

To date, stigma research has predominantly focused on ways of reducing public stigma. However, given that public stigma will take many generations to erase, there has been a growing interest in self-stigma, particularly in stigma management strategies that could help individuals with a mental illness improve their sense of empowerment and self-esteem and promote recovery.

Goffman (1963) was the first to use the term "stigma management" to refer to coping strategies that a stigmatized individual uses to maintain a credible social identity. In the case of people who have a stigma that is not easily observable (such as in the case of a mental illness), one important strategy is to conceal one's stigmatized identify from others and then carefully manage the social information that is transacted in interpersonal situations. This would include such things as passing off the symptoms of one's mental illness as a more socially acceptable physical disorder or avoiding more intimate social relationships where a stigma may become known. However, such passing strategies can create considerable internal psychological strain and the worry that one will be found out.

Goffman (1963) also described revealing strategies, where individuals disclose their stigmatized status. This could range from strategic disclosure to a group of close supporters and friends, to a full-scale broadcast of everything to everybody. While there may be positive benefits to revealing, these can also lead to negative outcomes, in the case of selective disclosure, the worry that someone will divulge a confidence or in the case of broadcasting, the potential for discrimination and the need to manage uneasy social situations. Though Goffman did not rule out the possibility that, through disclosure, someone could be liberated from their internalized stigma, experience empowerment, and redefine their self-worth, most of the coping strategies he defined carried important negative psychosocial consequences.

Corrigan and Rao (2012) consider that disclosure may be an important first step in reducing self-stigmatization, one that has been linked to improved quality of life and a sense of control and power over their lives. Like Goffman (1963) they note that disclosure is not an all-or-nothing thing. There are levels. At one extreme, individuals avoid all situations where people may find out about their mental illness. They stay in the closet completely. Selective disclosure occurs when private information about one's mental illness is disclosed to a small group of friends or supporters who then keep this secret from others. Indiscriminant disclosure occurs when people make no active effort to conceal their mental illness. Finally, broadcasting one's experience means that one tells everyone in an effort to actively educate them.

Broadcasting can also improve one's sense of empowerment over the experience of a mental illness and the associated stigma.

An empowerment model (rather than a coping model) views stigmatized individuals as active participants who work to create positive outcomes and take control over their lives, rather than passive targets of stigma who try to conceal and avoid it. Further, it acknowledges that people can live successfully with a mental illness in spite of stigma. Within this context, Shih (2004) identifies three psychological mechanisms that are protective against self-stigma. The first is compensation, where stigmatized individuals develop skills to help them achieve their goals and overcome barriers associated with public stigma. Secondly, stigmatized individuals can selectively interpret their social environments to protect their self-worth, making comparisons to other similarly disadvantaged individuals. Self-efficacy is increased when one considers that one is doing as well or better than someone in similar circumstances. Finally, stigmatized individuals can protect their psychological well-being by emphasizing alternate social roles (other than someone with a mental illness) and actively overcome their illness identity.

In a similar vein, Thoits (2011) proposes five responses to stigma. At one extreme, one internalizes and agrees with the broad cultural stereotypes of mental illnesses and endorses these conceptions as self-descriptive. The other extreme is to challenge and confront stigma and overtly reject cultural images. In between, individuals may practice deflection by believing that cultural stereotypes do not apply to them or by recognizing that a mental illness is not the defining feature of their identity. Potential for harm is recognized but dismissed as a viable threat to the self. Avoidance is another strategy. Individuals anticipate public devaluation and avoid it by keeping their treatment history secret, by avoiding interacting with people who might be prejudiced, and by socializing primarily with others who share the same stigma. The final strategy is self-restoration. Individuals have been personally hurt by stigma and engage in self-esteem restoring strategies such as shifting their comparisons to other people with a mental disorder or disinvesting themselves from activities where they may fail. It is likely that individuals will use combinations of strategies and that strategies will change over the course of the illness and recovery process.

Mittal et al. (2012) systematically reviewed the literature published between 2000 and 2011 and identified 14 intervention studies designed to minimize self-stigma. Interventions ranged from psychoeducational interventions, sometimes accompanied with cognitive restructuring, to more complex multimodal interventions. Most targeted people with psychotic disorders. Eight of the studies reported a statistically significant decrease in self-stigma levels. Unfortunately, several studies used an outcome measure that did not directly assess self-stigma (but instead measured perceptions of public stigma) so it would not have been sensitive to individual-level change. These studies showed no effects. More recently, Rüsch and colleagues (2014) examined the efficacy of a three-module peer-based program (*Coming Out Proud*) designed to help people with a mental illness consider the applicability of various disclosure strategies to their own situations. Results of a randomized trial on 100 participants with a mental illness showed positive effects on the stigma stress-related variables and disclosure, but not on self-stigma or empowerment, which the authors thought may take more than three sessions to address.

Though stigma self-management interventions are in their early stages of research, they hold considerable promise for promoting empowerment and recovery.

Discussion

This chapter has examined approaches to stigma reduction at macro (structural), meso (public), and micro (individual) levels in an effort to identify combinations of practices that may be used to reduce the stigmatization of mental illnesses. A focus on social-structural approaches, such as legislation combined with advocacy along with the implementation of media guidelines to reduce ambient levels of negative stereotypes, holds promise as these have the potential to change behaviors directly. This chapter has also examined contact-based education as a promising method for improving social acceptance of people with a mental illness, typically aimed at specific target groups within the population, such as high school youth or health providers. In this context, contact occurs in person or indirectly when someone who has experienced a mental illness tells their recovery story and, ideally, engages members of the audience in dialogue in order to create a transformative learning experience. Finally, stigma self-management interventions have been identified as a promising new approach to support personal empowerment and recovery but one in need of more research. Given the entrenched nature of stigma, multiple approaches will be required at each of these levels to address this problem.

References

Allport G (1954) The nature of prejudice. Addison-Wesley Publishing Company, Reading
Allport G (2000) The nature of prejudice. In: Stereotypes and prejudice. Taylor and Francis, Philadelphia, pp 20–48
Arboleda-Florez J, Stuart H (2012) From sin to science: fighting the stigmatization of mental illnesses. Can J Psychiatr 57(8):457–463
Borgerson K (2009) Valuing evidence. Perspect Biol Med 52(2):218–233
Brohan E, Elgie R, Sartorius N, Thornicroft G (2010) Self-stigma, empowerment and perceived discrimination among people with schizophrenia in 14 European countries: the GAMIAN-Europe Study. Schizophr Res 122:232–238
Callard F, Sartorius N, Arboleda-Florez J, Bartlett P, Helmchen H, Stuart H et al (2012) Mental illness, discrimination and the law. Fighting for social justice. Wiley, Chinchester
Corrigan P, Rao D (2012) On the self-stigma of mental illness: stages, disclosure, and strategies for change. Can J Psychiatr 57(8):464–469
Corrigan P, Markowitz F, Watson A (2004) Structural levels of mental illness stigma and discrimination. Schizophr Bull 30(3):481–491
Corrigan P, Morris S, Michaels P, Rafacz J, Rusch N (2012) Challenging the public stigma of mental illness: a meta-analysis of outcome studies. Psychiatr Serv 63(10):963–973

Evans D (2003) Hierarchy of evidence: a framework for ranking evidence evaluating healthcare interventions. J Clin Nurs 12:77–84

Everett B (2004) Best practices in workplace mental health: an area for expanded research. Health Care Pap 5(2):114–116

Goering P, Veldhuizen S, Watson A, Adair C, Kopp B, Latimer E et al (2014) National final report cross-site at home/Chez Soi Project. Mental Health Commission of Canada, Calgary

Goffman E (1963) Stigma: notes on the management of spoiled identity. Prentice-Hall, Englewood Cliffs

Goldenberg M (2009) Objectivism, pragmatism, and the hierarchy of evidence. Perspect Biol Med 52(2):168–187

Griffiths K, Carron-Arthur B, Parsons A, Reid R (2014) Effectiveness of programs for reducing the stigma associated with mental disorders. A meta-analysis of randomized controlled trials. World Psychiatry 13:161–175

Hewstone M (2000) Contact and categorization: social psychological interventions to change intergroup relations. In: Stangor C (ed) Stereotypes and prejudice. Taylor and Francis, Philadelphia, pp 394–418

Hewstone M, Swart H (2011) Fifty-odd years of inter-group contact: from hypothesis to integrated theory. Br J Soc Psychol 50:374–386

Hiday V, Wales H (2013) Mental illness and the law. In: Aneshensel C, Phelan J, Bierman A (eds) Handbook of the sociology of mental health. Springer, New York, pp 563–584

Jonah B, Dawson N, Smith G (1982) Effects of a selective traffic enforcement program on seat belt usage. J Appl Psychol 67(1):89–96

Knaak S, Modgill G, Patten S (2014) Key ingredients of anti-stigma programs for health care providers: a data synthesis of evaluative studies. Can J Psychiatr 59(10 Suppl 1):S19–S26

Link BG, Phelan JC (2001) Conceptualizing stigma. Annu Rev Sociol 27:363–385

Mezirow J (1997) Transformative learning: from theory to practice. New Dir Adult Contin Educ Summer 74:5–11

Mittal D, Sullivan G, Chekuri L, Allee E, Corrigan P (2012) Empirical studies of self-stigma reduction strategies: a critical review of the literature. Psychiatr Serv 63(10):974–981

National Media and Mental Health Group (2009) Reporting suicide and mental illness. A mind-frame resource for media professionals. Commonwealth of Australia

Niederkrotenthaler T, Sonneck G (2007) Assessing the impact of media guidelines for reporting on suicide in Austria: interrupted time series analysis. Aust N Z J Psychiatry 41:419–428

Oxford Dictionaries (2014, 10 16). Retrieved 10 16, 2014, from www.oxforddictionaries.com: www.oxforddictionaries.com/definition/english/stigma

Pescosolido B, Martin J, Long J, Medina T, Phelan J, Link B (2010) "A Disease Like any Other?" A decade of change in public reactions to schizophrenia, depression, and alcohol dependence. Am J Psychiatry Adv 15:1–10

Pettigrew T, Tropp L (2006) A meta-analytic test of intergroup contact theory. J Pers Soc Psychol 90(5):751–783

Phelan J, Link B, Stueve A, Pescosolido B (2000) Public conceptions of mental illness in 1950 and 1996: what is mental illness and is it to be feared? J Health Soc Behav 41(2):188–207

Pirkis J, Blood W, Beautrais A, Burgess P, Skehan J (2006) Media guidelines on the reporting of suicides. Crisis 27(2):82–87

Pirkis J, Blood R, Dare A, Holland K, Rankin B, Williamson M, et al (2008) The media monitoring project. Changes in media reporting of suicide and mental health and illness in Australia 2001/2001-2006/2007. Commonwealth of Australia

Reichman A (1964) Royal Commission on Health Services. Psychiatric care in Canada: extent and results. Queen's Printer, Ottawa

Rivara F, Thompson D, Cummings P (1999) Effectiveness of primary and secondary enforced seat belt laws. Am J Prev Med 16:30–39

Rusch N, Abbruzzese E, Hagedorn E, Hartenhauer D, Kaufmann I, Curschellas J et al (2014) Efficacy of coming out proud to reduce stigma's impact among people with mental illness: pilot randomised controlled trial. Br J Psychiatry 204:391–397

Sayce L (2003) Beyond good intentions: making anti-discrimination strategies work. Disabil Soc 18(5):625–642

Sealy P, Whitehead P (2004) Forty years of deinstitutionalization of psychiatric services in Canada: an empirical assessment. Can J Psychiatr 49:249–257

Shih M (2004) Positive stigma: examining resilience and empowerment in overcoming stigma. Ann Am Acad 591:175–195

Sibitz I, Unger A, Woppmann A, Zidek T, Amering M (2011) Stigma resistance in patients with schizophrenia. Schizophr Bull 37(2):316–323

Stuart H (2006) Media portrayal of mental illness and its treatment. CNS Drugs 20(2):99–106

Stuart H (2007) Employment equity and mental disability. Curr Opin Psychiatry 20:486–490

Stuart H (2008) Building an evidence base for anti-stigma programming. In: Arboleda-Florez J, Sartorius N (eds) Understanding the stigma of mental illness: theory and interventions. Wiley, Chichester, pp 135–146

Stuart H (2010) Canadian perspectives on stigma because of mental illness. In: Streiner D, Cairney J (eds) Mental disorder in Canada: an epidemiologic perspective. University of Toronto Press, Toronto, pp 304–330

Stuart H (2012) United Nations convention on the rights of persons with disabilities: a roadmap for change. Curr Opin Psychiatry 25:365–369

Stuart H, Arboleda-Florez J, Sartorius N (2012) Paradigms lost: fighting stigma and the lessons learned. Oxford University Press, Oxford

The World Health Organization (2003) Advocacy for mental health. World Health Organization, Geneva

Thoits P (2011) Resisting the stigma of mental illness. Soc Psychol Q 74(6):6–28

Canadian Journalism Forum on Violence and Trauma (2014) Stigma and mental illness. In: Mindset: reporting on mental health. Canadian Journalism Forum on Violence and Trauma, London

Wallack L, Dorfman L (1996) Media advocacy: a strategy for advancing policy and promoting health. Health Educ Q 23(3):293–317

Whitley R, Berry S (2013) Trends in newspaper coverage of mental illness in Canada: 2005–2010. Can J Psychiatr 58(2):107–112

What Has Not Been Effective in Reducing Stigma

28

Julio Arboleda-Flórez

Persons with mental and emotional disabilities represent a significant proportion of the world's population. About one in four persons will suffer from a mental condition in their lifetime, and almost one million people die by suicide every year, with suicide being the third cause of death among the young. Depression is the most important cause of years lost to disability, and it is the third leading cause in the global burden of disease. Despite decades of mental health reform, in part aimed at the reduction of stigma, people with mental and psychosocial disabilities still experience significant economic, social and political inequities (Arboleda-Flórez 2001). This chapter will examine some of the current thinking related to stigma reduction and human rights that have acted as impediments to structural reforms designed to promote social inclusion of people with mental illnesses.

Historical Antecedents of Mental Illness Stigma

Few conditions in the history of medicine convey a sense of identity, as do tuberculosis, leprosy and mental illness. While a person could 'have' a touch of pneumonia, might 'suffer' from cirrhosis of the liver or 'have' a broken leg, *one is tubercular, a leper or mentally ill.* The first group is made up of medical conditions that people 'have', as one could have a jalopy or a leaking house. Those in the second group, however, are conditions that socially defined one's identity. These conditions are ways of being, as one might *be* Black, Oriental or European; short or tall; or fat or skinny. In addition, while there has been minimal stigma associated with those conditions in the first group, to be a leper or to be tubercular has, historically, incurred social banishment, such as being segregated in institutions and sanatoriums.

J. Arboleda-Flórez
Department of Psychiatry, Queen's University, Abramsky Hall,
Kingston, ON K7L 3N6, Canada
e-mail: julio.arboleda-florez@queensu.ca

© Springer International Publishing Switzerland 2017
W. Gaebel et al. (eds.), *The Stigma of Mental Illness - End of the Story?*,
DOI 10.1007/978-3-319-27839-1_28

Historically, people with a mental illness were banished by throwing them outside of the doors of the city or placed in ships with no port to disembark (Stuart et al.
2012).

Yet, for many medical conditions such as tuberculosis or leprosy, stigma has
been lessened, or even eliminated, once effective treatments have become widely
available. Not so with mental illness. For even when one is successfully treated and
the illness well managed, one is still schizophrenic, manic, depressed, or demented;
and the label itself conjures negative social reactions and discriminatory practices.
In addition, whereas other medical conditions with the exception of mutilating leprosy cases, could be hidden to a large extent, mental illnesses, by virtue of their
recurrent and/or acute symptoms or the disability they produce, are often difficult to
conceal. They are 'out there' for the world to see and to judge. In this respect, mental illnesses are not a private affair but a public identity requiring social judgement,
including legal determinations.

In regard to identity, this term usually refers to issues of culture, in recognition
that the individual is shaped by such things as race, ethnicity, gender, age, sexual
orientation, religious values, socio-economic status, migration, acculturation, language and nationality. Seldom it is considered that we are also shaped and identified
by our health status and our health conditions. Indeed, the hardest part of being
'mentally ill' might be confronting, de novo, a new and largely negative, social
identity.

'Mental illness identity' has deep historical roots as does stigma. The origin of
the word 'stigma' comes from ancient Greece. Among the ancient Greeks, *stizein*,
to tattoo or to brand, described a distinguishing mark burned or cut into the flesh of
slaves or criminals so that others would know who they were and that they were
less-valued members of society. Although branding of this sort was not applied to
people with a mental illness, stigmatizing attitudes about the mentally ill were
already apparent in Greek society. In Sophocles' *Ajax* or in Euripides' *The Madness
of Heracles*, mental illness was associated with concepts of shame, loss of face and
humiliation, and in his *Medea*, Euripides associated mental illness with criminality
in the form of multiple infanticide.

In the Christian world, the word *stigmata* applied to peculiar marks resembling
the wounds of Christ that some individuals develop on their palms and soles. Paul,
for example, proclaimed, 'I bear in my body the stigmata of Christ'. Although the
roots of the term are the same, the religious connotation of stigmata, as a mark of
grace, is not the same as current conceptualizations of social stigma as a mark of
disgrace (Arboleda-Flórez and Stuart 2012).

Hawthorne (2001) exemplified the mark of disgrace in *The Scarlet Letter*. In
this novel set in the puritanical New England town of Salem, Massachusetts, a
woman accused of being an adulteress is ordered to wear the scarlet letter 'A' to
signify her sin and shame. The town of Salem is also infamous for having been
the place of a mass execution of witches in 1662, a period in which the *Malleus
Maleficarum—the Witches' Hammer* (Kramer and Sprenger 1971)—was still a
highly regarded reference textbook for the management of witches. The inquisi-
torial approach to witches, many of whom had signs or symptoms of mental

illness, apart from being highly misogynous, also represented a negative and condemning attitude toward mental illnesses, and it may have been the origin of the stigmatizing attitudes toward those with mental illness that have existed in Christian cultures from the rise of rationalism in the seventeenth century to the present. Although present to some extent in other cultures, madness has long been stigmatized among Christians as a form of punishment on sinners inflicted by God.

The first European asylum for the insane was developed in 1409 by Father Gilabert Jofré, who observed one mentally ill individual being subjected to abuse in the streets of Valencia (Pinel 1988). While well motivated, this invention was later taken to the extreme in the wholesale banishment of the mentally ill who were locked up many times for life (Luis Vives 1980). And yet, banishment via institutionalization was only a continuation of a more pernicious social management style prevalent before the asylum in Valencia—the *Narrenschiff* or *Stultifera Navis*, the *Ship of Fools*, in which the mentally ill were condemned to navigate the waters of the rivers of Europe never finding a port but always banished from place to place (Brant 2005).

Sociopolitically, the asylums replaced the leprosaria. But whereas the latter were exclusive for lepers, the asylums became the place of what Foucault (1965) baptized as the 'Great Confinement'—places used to banish all sorts of undesirables, especially persons affected by mental conditions. In fact, the *lettres de cachet* contemplated in the 1838 Act on the Insane in France (Dômer 1974) gave the 'hospital archers' authority to round up and lock up, among others, 'beggars, vagabonds, the chronically unemployed, criminals, rebel politicians, heretics, prostitutes, syphilitics, alcoholics, madmen and idiots'. This became the blueprint for similar institutions all over the Western world. The characterization of the mentally ill as a 'wild beasts' left no other alternative but to put them away (Gracia and Lázaro 1992).

Social Dimensions of Health and Illness

The social dimensions of health and illness cover three main areas: the conceptualization of health and illness, the study of their measurement and social distribution and the explanation of patterns of health and illness, basically looked at from the point of view of society. Eisenberg (1977) and Kleinman et al. (1978) differentiated between *disease* (meaning the malfunctioning organ or the disturbance in a physiological function) and *illness* (the personal experience of being diseased). Talcott Parsons (1975), more perspicaciously, added *sickness* as a third element (to mean the reaction of society to the member who is diseased) in reference to the processes of social regulation and control that in his opinion also played an important part. However, Parsons had in mind persons who were physically ill, not the mentally ill. Society, as he described it, is prepared to make all sorts of accommodations for the physically ill in the context of the *sick role*. This role would specify that individuals must be genuinely sick with a demonstrable malady and that they must take care to recover, which would include the adherence to medical orders, taking the prescribed medications and changing unhealthy behaviours. Alas, society does not make such sick role accommodations for those with a mental illness. Since antiquity, the mentally ill have been the object of scorn, derision, abuse and discrimination and, in some eras, the objects of amusement and entertainment, as was common around the famous mental hospital of Bedlam in England (Stuart et al. 2012).

Stangor and Crandall (2000) hypothesized that stigma may develop via an original 'functional impetus' whose goal is to avoid a threat to the self either a *tangible* threat to a material or concrete good or a *symbolic* threat to the beliefs, values and ideologies upon which the group ordains its social, political or spiritual domains. The threat would be accentuated if a large number of individuals in the population agreed, whereupon the perceived threat would be consolidated through further social sharing of information. The sharing of stigma becomes an element of a society that creates, condones and maintains stigmatizing attitudes and behaviours. Thus, it may be that cultural perceptions of mental illness are associated with tangible threats to the health of society. In this respect, mental illnesses engender two kinds of fear: fear of physical attack and fear of contamination (i.e. that we may also lose our sanity). Further, to the extent that persons with mental illnesses are stereotyped as being lazy, unable to contribute and a burden to the system, mental illnesses also may be seen as posing a symbolic threat to the beliefs and values shared by members of the group.

Current Stigma Discourse

Colloquially, the term 'stigma' has been used to refer to the negative and prejudicial attitudes held by members of the public toward people with a mental illness, including their stigmatized attributes as well as the label of being mentally ill. Advocates for the mentally ill do not consider this conceptualization as entirely helpful. They have, therefore, proposed that the discussion about the challenges facing mentally ill persons in contemporary societies should be refocused. In their opinion, society should move away from the notion of stigma as a personal attribute, which they consider tends to bolster the view that mental illness is something that occurs to afflicted others, onto social structures that perpetuate oppression and inequity (Stuart et al. 2012).

In his seminal work, *Stigma: Notes on the Management of Spoiled Identity* (1963), Goffman, the renowned Canadian sociologist, conceptualized stigma as an attribute that is 'deeply discrediting' with the result that stigmatized persons are regarded as marked, tainted and of lesser social value. In his view, mental illness was among the most deeply discrediting of all conditions. Although Goffman has been criticized because of his emphasis on the attributes assigned to those who are stigmatized and his lack of emphasis on the complex power relationships that underlie the creation and maintenance of structural inequities, he did describe stigma as a *relational construct*, that is, something that the social group confers to some of its members.

From a social-psychological perspective, contemporary notions of stigma are rooted in psychological theory that examines the ways in which labels are connected to cultural stereotypes—how cognitive and attributional processes lead to the development and the maintenance of negative and erroneous stereotypes that provide the scaffolding for stigmatized worldviews. This perspective emphasizes the links between labelling, stereotyped attributions, emotional or prejudicial reactions and discriminatory behaviours. Although the process of stigmatization is not always as linear as attribution theory would suggest, research has demonstrated that people who hold moral models of mental illness—based on attributions that people who are mentally ill are blameworthy and in control of their illness, *could snap out of it if they wanted to* or are dangerous and unpredictable—are more likely to respond in negative and punitive ways. The important factor is that, once these types of stereotypical views develop, they may be followed by prejudicial attitudes and discriminatory practices, which, in turn, may lead to denial of legally recognized rights and entitlements (Stuart et al. 2012).

An unfortunate and unintended legacy of Goffman's work has been to deemphasize the widespread and systematic exclusion of people with a mental illness from economic and social life. The current paradigm has not provided the necessary rallying point for collective strategies to improve social inclusion. Increasingly advocates argue that the mark of shame should not reside with individuals who have a mental illness but with those who behave unjustly toward them. Thus, lately, stigma discourse has increasingly moved away from an attribute at the personal level and toward making it an issue of human rights. In fact, stigma is being reconceptualized as a form of social oppression that results from a complex sociopolitical process whereby the power imbalance between those who stigmatize and those who are stigmatized perpetuates and increases (Arboleda-Flórez and Stuart 2012). In this regard, Sayce (2000) identifies the thorny question of whether to talk about 'stigma' (meaning a negative attitude), 'discrimination' (an unfair behaviour) or 'social inclusion' (a structural characteristic). She notes that disabled people, in general, have not found the notion of stigma to be a useful concept because it supports an individualist approach to disability, with a focus on the discredited and the discreditable.

These different conceptual models are important because they point to different understandings of where the problem lies and different prescriptions for solutions. By focusing on discrimination and social oppression, it is possible to challenge power structures that create and maintain inequities, for example, by rendering discriminatory behaviours illegal or by using protest approaches, which aim to embarrass companies and organizations for discriminatory practices, including legal challenges when rights have been violated. In addition, the discrimination discourse is considered to offer a more useful approach as it resonates with other fields where it has already been established that discrimination is unethical and illegal (Sayce 2000).

Human Rights Discourse

In many developing countries, the mentally ill are expulsed from communities, where ordinarily they are expected to fend for themselves, or else, they are confined in small rooms or tied to trees or benches where they may be publicly humiliated and abused. Public knowledge of mental illness may have a detrimental effect on the entire family, such as in the case of potentially marriageable young people who may not find suitable partners for community fears that their descendants might be similarly tainted. In the developed world, the NIMBY (*not in my backyard*) syndrome has been described where communities refuse permission for supported housing or group homes to be developed in their neighbourhoods (Stuart et al. 2012). For example, a major newspaper in Canada, the *Toronto Star*, had in its edition of Sunday, May 18, 2014, second page, a piece titled 'Director of autism home upset with Ford remarks'. It appears that Toronto Councillor Doug Ford, brother of the city mayor, did chip in on a controversy in Etobicoke (a wealthy suburb of Toronto) by opining that a home for autistic teens has 'ruined the community', and he is further quoted as saying that 'if it comes down to it, I'll buy the house myself and resell it' (Ballingall 2014).

People with a mental illness also report experiencing unfair and negative treatment from their health professionals, whom they have rated as among the most stigmatizing of all groups. Recurrent themes in the literature in this regard include feeling punished, patronized, humiliated, spoken to as if they were children, being excluded from treatment decisions and being assumed to lack capacity to be responsible for their lives. Other problems include not being given sufficient information about their illness and treatment options, prognostic negativism and, at times, the unspoken threat of coercive treatment, which actually becomes overt in instances of mandated care through mental health legislation or through judicial treatment orders (Arboleda-Flórez and Stuart 2012).

People with a mental illness also face considerable employment discrimination (World Health Organization 2000). As well as experiencing higher than average unemployment, mental patients have problems finding suitable employment commensurate with their qualifications so often they tend to be underemployed. Once it is known that a young person has a mental illness, expectations of success in life are reduced. For example, if the person is a young student, it would not be surprising if he or she is advised not to proceed to higher educational achievements on the belief that the mental condition will eventually interfere with academic development and, certainly, with academic excellence. In fact, getting institutions to make necessary accommodations may be an ordeal in itself. Worse, in the workforce, mental patients oftentimes have difficulties collecting benefits because they are suspected of cheating or faking their conditions. Finally, many mentally ill persons suffer from *self-stigma* or the feeling that there must be something wrong with them, which is their fault. Many just give up the struggle, a situation dubbed the *why try effect* (Corrigan et al. 2009).

The growing realization of the extent and costs of mental conditions in many countries has accelerated a momentum for reform of mental health systems. Debate on the nature of such reform, however, has largely remained at the level of services and better financing and has excluded and exhaustive review of human rights issues. Ironically, even with the focus on improved service delivery, the plight of the mentally ill in the community does not seem to have improved and, in fact, may be getting worse as a result of neglect of national mental health systems and social marginalization and exclusion. Far from being a panacea, the mental health reforms culminating in the community mental health movement have not eliminated stigma as was hoped. Rather, they might have contributed to social inequities and human rights violations.

The WHO (2003, 2005) has listed the most common human rights violations experienced by people with mental disorders. First, it pertains to a lack of access to basic mental health care and treatment. Some countries lack adequate services, while in others, services are available only to certain segments of the population. For example, 32 % of countries reporting data to WHO have no community care facilities defined as 'any type of care, supervision and rehabilitation of mental patients outside the hospital by health and social workers based in the community', and 30 % don't have a specified budget for mental health. Of those that do, 20 % spend <1 % of their total health budget on mental health. There are also huge regional variations in the number of psychiatrists from more than 10 per 100,000 to <1 per 300,000. Worldwide, 68.6 % of psychiatric beds are in outmoded mental hospitals as opposed to general hospitals or other community settings. Second, the inappropriate and forced admission and/or treatment where informed consent is often not sought and people are forced to remain against their will for weeks, months or years. Third, there are violations within psychiatric institutions. People are restrained with rusting metal shackles, kept in caged beds and subjected to other inhumane treatment. They may be forced to live in filthy living conditions: lacking clothes, clean water, food, heating, proper bedding or hygiene facilities. Fourth, people are kept in seclusion for lengthy periods of time, often detained in large institutions, isolated from society far from families and loved ones. Finally, they may be deprived of their civil rights, such as the right to vote or the right to marry and have children and, as noted previously, may experience discrimination in all areas of life including employment, education and housing.

Human Rights and Reform

Human rights are inextricably linked to the degree of development of mental health systems, and, in all of these systems, abuses are perpetrated, from complete denial of such basic rights as liberty of the person in the custodial model to the loss of entitlements of citizenship in the deinstitutionalization model (Arboleda-Flórez 2004). Mental health reform, however, has continued apace in most countries in the world as a reaction to the abuses of previous models of care, to realizations of inequities in funding and to pressures of international agencies for change.

In a number of modules on mental health reform, the World Health Organization has spearheaded a multi-country mental health system reform project along different lines of action. One of those lines pertain to the promotion of human rights standards and principles in mental health legislation as emphasized in one of the modules of this initiative (World Health Organization 2003):

> All people with mental disorders have the right to receive high quality treatment and care delivered through responsive health care services. They should be protected against any form of inhuman treatment and discrimination.

The World Health Organization (WHO) emphasizes the need for protection of mentally ill persons when their mental conditions impact on their decision-making capacities and when they are in need of hospitalization against their will. In its approach, WHO articulates ten principles that are considered basic to proper mental health systems and for the protection of rights of the mentally ill:

- Promotion of mental health and prevention of mental disorders
- Access to basic mental health care
- Mental health assessment in accordance with internationally accepted principles
- Provision of the least restrictive type of mental health care
- Self-determination
- Right to be assisted in the exercise of self-determination
- Availability of review procedures
- Automatic period review mechanisms
- Qualified decision-makers
- Respect for the rule of law

In the module on mental health legislation and human rights (World Health Organization 2003), the WHO endorses the 25 principles contained in the United Nations General Assembly Resolution 46/119 (1991) that covers a gamut of areas that impact on the rights and care of the mentally ill such as:

- Protection of confidentiality
- Standards of care and treatment including involuntary admission and consent to treatment
- Rights of persons with mental disorders in mental health facilities
- Protection of minors
- Provision of resources for mental health facilities
- Role of community and culture
- Review mechanisms provided for the protection of the rights of offenders with mental disorders
- Procedural safeguards to protect the rights of persons with mental disorders
- Obligatory notification of rights

This effort of the WHO has been prompted by the realization of the extent and frequency of mental disorders worldwide and the dismal interest manifested by many countries in the provision of adequate services for this population, a fact that is easily measured in their national budgetary health allocations. The principles endorsed by the WHO and in declarations by scientific organizations such as the Declaration of Madrid of the World Psychiatric Association (1996) are framed with a sense of urgency and concern. The WPA document, for example, specifically, reminds psychiatrists that:

> The patient should be accepted as a partner by right in the therapeutic relationship [in order to] to allow the patient to make free and informed decisions.

More to the point on the matter of rights, in paragraph 4 of the Madrid Declaration, the WPA alerts psychiatrists that:

When the patient is incapacitated and/or unable to exercise proper judgment because of a mental disorder, or gravely disabled or incompetent, the psychiatrists should consult with the family and, if appropriate, seek legal counsel, to safeguard the human dignity and the legal rights of the patient.

Finally, on the matter of systems, the Declaration of the WPA (2005) emphasizes that:

As members of society, psychiatrists must advocate for fair and equal treatment of the mentally ill, for social justice and equity for all.

These concerns underline the close relationship between quality of mental health systems and treatment for mentally ill persons and the impact that systems and treatments could have on the human rights of mental patients. On the other hand, legal protections do not necessarily mean actual enforcement on the rights of individuals, especially when violations are entrenched in social beliefs that conspire to deny the rights and citizen entitlements that many other persons take for granted.

The entrenchment of protections and rights of mental patients in many declarations and official documents is an attempt to rectify the historical harms committed on them since asylums were developed and even before. Even gestures such as Pinel's, who imbued with the libertarian ideals of the French Revolution publicly cut the chains that, like prisoners, held the mentally ill to their posts at la Saltpêtrière in 1795 (Häfner 1991), have not been enough as old, and decrepit mental hospitals are still the preferred, and only, model of care in many countries. Sadly, removing the chains and allowing patients to return to the community have not liberated them from the yoke of yesteryears. In most countries, for example, even the most advanced and prosperous, people with a mental illness are no longer in asylums but in prisons, many of which having become de facto mental hospitals (Konrad 2002).

In an effort to protect basic rights to freedom, the path into criminalization has become overregulated and overseen by forensic psychiatrists who have become gatekeepers, or modern day superintendents, and courts of law (Arboleda-Flórez 2005). Indeed, the process of forensic evaluations has become another filter for treatment that keeps people with a mental illness (particularly those with a serious mental illness) in a limbo, ensconced among three seemingly inimical different systems: the health-care system, the justice system and the correctional system. At the end, however, the effect of a forensic evaluation may be the same—loss of liberty in a hospital for the criminally insane or deprivation of liberty in a jail pending legal dispositions. At this point, therefore, it would be appropriate to ask—what has been gained?

From Negative to Positive Human Rights

Human rights are customarily presented in terms of the obligations that the state has toward its citizens and whose violations could trigger individual or collective actions against the state. They are prohibitions on the state not to trespass, as they are part and parcel of individual freedoms. They include such things as protection against unlawful detentions, access to a lawyer, habeas corpus, inviolability of the person, privacy and protection of property. Despite their importance to individual freedoms, they have not promoted social inclusion for people who have a mental illness. The high levels of stigmatizing attitudes among the general public and even among clinicians are at the base of what Kelly calls 'structural violence' (Kelly 2005) or a pernicious and insidious form of discrimination and abuse not currently addressed by current human rights models aimed at protecting freedom and autonomy.

In society's efforts to protect individual freedoms, people with mental illnesses have gained the right to remain homeless in the streets where they could freeze to death on winter nights, be unemployed or be confined to a permanent existence of poverty and condemned to live on handouts. They also have the right to be robed, mugged, raped, beaten up or murdered in the streets, where they sleep for lack of proper accommodations or in high crime neighbourhoods where they live. Should they react violently, many times in self-defence, they are labelled as 'dangerous' and institutionalized or criminalized. Thus, they also have the right to be criminalized and to receive treatment, if any, in the anti-therapeutic environments of prisons and penitentiaries. The easy way in which people with mental illnesses are criminalized reinforces the stigmatizing attitudes in society by fuelling further fears that they are dangerous and unpredictable. In turn, this leads to further calls for expansion of controls via commitment legislation and a yearning for the good old mental institutions. The harshness of their existence has a negative impact on their illness as biological, psychological and social elements are in close interplay to reinforce etiological factors and to maintain disease status and disability. They do not have the right to social inclusion, full citizenship, financial means or places where they can enjoy some sense of privacy conducive to the development of intimate and emotionally rewarding relationships.

Unfortunately, people with a mental illness are largely powerless to modify their plight. Poverty, disenfranchisement, disability and championlessness are all partly to be blamed for this situation forming a circle from where there is little hope of escape. People with serious mental illnesses are usually at the lowest socio-economic levels, and many live in abject poverty. Their socio-economic status is related to the impacts of the illness, which often attacks before achieving their full development potential. Education may be truncated and, consequently, their economic marketability is significantly reduced. Many persons who develop mental illness when young cannot or do not access prompt treatment to help stem the illness and mitigate the impacts. Poor knowledge of the nature and presentation of mental conditions, fear of stigma among the family members, lack of financial resources and a health system that does not provide treatment facilities for the young unnecessarily prolong the period between appearance of the illness and first opportunity for treatment. For others, who became ill later in life, the problem is unemployment and underemployment. This leads to a catastrophic loss of income and a rapid fall in the socio-economic scale. Oftentimes, even claiming disability insurance, which had been paid for eventualities of this nature, becomes a nightmare. Insurance companies tend to see with suspicions any claims for mental disability, curtail the treatment options and cause the person to spend unnecessarily in legal costs and experts to redress the injustice.

Worldwide, people with a mental illness have little or no political voice. Many cannot even enter the electoral registries because they have no home address or live in institutional settings, so they cannot vote. Lobbying and political activism, as exercised by other disability groups in order to improve access to better health care including facilities and treatment options, are hard to organize when people are feared to be criminals, violent and unpredictable. Families may also live in poverty and be powerless to effect change. Politicians do not shake hands in mental hospitals or seek out the dispossessed in the streets to hand out leaflets. Disenfranchisement and lack of voice render social problems invisible so that the plight of the mentally ill and their families seldom enters the radar of politicians. This results in neglect of mental health systems, poor budgetary allocations, inadequate facilities and an utter disregard for their social situation. The mentally ill are not just disenfranchised, but they are totally alienated from the political system.

Powerless individuals who are unable to coalesce into social forces where numbers create political realities also lack political champions. Even when a champion surfaces and argues in favour of better services, the reason is often because of outrage out of a personal situation (usually a close relative has succumbed to a mental illness), and the champion has faced the reality of inadequate services. More often, however, fear of negative repercussions in political capital leads politicians to hide any mental illnesses among their relatives or themselves. A history of mental illness is a major roadblock to seek public office and a drawback to seek re-election. Clinicians who feel that they have to confront the social reality of their patients and who have a duty to advocate for them are often seen as self-serving or over controlling. If they gain political office, they move on to other issues, as they do not wish to be typecast as single-issue politician hammering at something for which there is no political resonance. Lack of voice, lack of social recognition and lack of political power have condemned people with serious mental illnesses to migrate into prison or to live their lives in mental health ghettos, jobless and dispossessed in the streets in utter poverty all the while enjoying their negative rights and freedoms (to be systematically abused, stigmatized and discriminated against). This is how the people with a mental illness have been celebrating their hard-gained rights and freedoms.

Redress

The point to be made is that, mere rhetoric about protection of basic rights to freedom and personal autonomy rings hollow as an empty exercise that harks back to old arguments appropriate to previous levels of development of mental health systems. Modern mental health systems do not depend on mental hospitals but on psychiatric units in general hospitals and on an array of community mental health agencies. These systems need a different level of discourse on human rights—one that addresses the economic discrimination, the disparities in access to health systems and the systemic, structural violence that people with mental illnesses are subjected to in the community. The human rights discourse has to evolve from an over-preoccupation on basic rights to freedom and autonomy (i.e. negative rights) toward a protection of citizen entitlements currently denied to people with a mental illness within the larger social system. In other words, it is time to consider how to implement positive rights—those that modern states provide to their citizens to help support their social and civic participation such as the right to health care, a job, basic income, housing and privacy. The struggle for those who care about human rights of people with a mental illness is to gain for them the same rights and entitlements that other citizens enjoy (Farmer 1999).

Finally, the serious consequences of stigmatization and the deleterious damages that it causes also include the belief among the victims that they must deserve it. *Self-stigma*, therefore, is another layer of reprobation that people with a mental illness have to carry on as they try to survive in a world that is hostile to them as a social class (Corrigan et al. 2009). There is no question, therefore, that fighting the stigma of mental illness is a worthwhile fight that should engage all those who care for those with a mental illness in our society. In that fight, there are many good strategies (as described in the previous chapter) and many that are unhelpful. Based on my experience, seven of these unhelpful strategies are presented below:

1. *The Sermon from the Mount*
   There are occasions when a very important person (often a celebrity) 'discovers' that people with a mental illness form a large portion of the population (perhaps because of a personal or family experience) and then decides to raise awareness or otherwise do 'something' about it. The 'do something' becomes a job with a passion, and the person becomes a crusader, giving inspirational speeches about the plight of those with a mental illness and what society ought to do to help. Such people may also charge for public appearances, sometimes-exorbitant sums. Given their status and position in the social hierarchy, mental health agencies are often prepared to pay large speaker fees in the desperate and vain hope of attracting even larger funds. However, the sermon from the mount may quickly become stale leaving little sustainable change.

2. *The Spokesperson*
   On another somewhat related situation, every now and then, an important political spokesperson does emerge, again often as a result of a personal or family experience with a mental illness. It is the search for mental health services that uncovers the dismal financial or staffing conductions under which mental health agencies operate. The 'how did this happen' or 'I had no idea'

spurs this individual to attempt to make difficult (and sometimes naïve) systemic changes. When change proves harder than expected, political speeches soon become diversified or watered down (lest business associates are antagonized or the public paints them as a single-issue politician) and enthusiasm fizzles.

3. *The Fathead Professor Grandiloquent Spuriousness*
   Together with those delivering the sermon from the mount and the important occasional self-interested spokesperson, it would be appropriate to place the professor who uses the lectern to give impassioned speeches about the need for healthy lifestyles away from alcohol, drugs, unbridled sexuality, consorting with prostitutes and becoming a spreader of sexually transmitted diseases. *Mens sana in corpore sano* is his motto, albeit he looks fat and flabby, smokes heavily, comes with a red nose and an alcoholic *tuphos* to deliver his classes, and rumours are heard among young male students that he has been seen frequenting houses of ill repute. 'Do as I say, not as I do'.

4. *Flash in the Pan Campaigns*
   Mental health agencies and governments are fond of 'campaigns'. These are showy and boisterous and garner much public attention. Pamphlets and posters are prepared and distributed nationally. Speeches are given by aforementioned very important persons and by mental health specialists. Messages are read in public radio stations, and info bytes and snippets on mental health issues appear on national television. Mental health gurus and agency officers may travel far and wide promoting strategies for better mental health in the population. Everyone is convinced that the campaign will work. However, military campaigns are known to be fast, aggressive and decisive, usually against a well-defined and circumscribed target. Alas, the target in mental health campaigns is large, not totally identified and often elusive. Also, many potential subjects to whom the campaign is directed would not like to be identified and so run the risk of being stigmatized. Because they are expensive, large-scale campaigns are often only a flash in the pan. Instead what is needed are mental health programmes that are well structured, well targeted, well financed and sustainable to bring about real improvements in the lives of people who have a mental illness and their family members.

5. *The Gurus of Salvation and Redemption*
   In classic times, mental illnesses were seen as belonging to individuals chosen by the gods, hence being enlightened. Sadly, in the Middle Ages, the notion of enlightenment gave soon way to idiocy (*mens captus*). More recently our understanding has centred on dangerousness, and unpredictability largely promulgated by selective presentations in the news and entertainment media (Steadman and Cocozza 1978; Stuart 2006). In some jurisdictions, dangerousness and unpredictability are more important in the decision to hospitalize (particularly involuntary hospitalization), than ensuring that the person has clear signs of a mental condition and is in need of treatment. For the gurus of salvation and redemption, treatment is not a decision to be made by the patient in consultation

with a physician and family but a state-made decision to be enforced by guards dressed in whites. Psychiatrists are agents of the state in charge of saving others from the mentally ill and, if per chance, to offer the hope of treatment for the few that have been clearly screened to be good treatment prospects.

6. *The Misguided Self-Actualization and In-Your-Face Patient Movements*
   As a counterculture, self-improvement and self-actualization are worthy goals that can be great motivators and extremely helpful to improve self-esteem for both the mentally healthy and those with mental health challenges. Those who are struggling to manage a mental illness should be encouraged to set goals and to strive to reach them, but a counterculture of antipsychiatry (e.g. Laing 1971) should not undermine more targeted treatment approaches for those who would benefit from them. Patient movements for self-governance should be encouraged especially as part of well-established mental health treatment and advocacy pro-grammes in hospitals and communities. However, in some circumstances, patient movements have become overly antagonistic—taking a hostile and vociferous stand against mental health professionals who are there to help them find those solutions. Making mental health professionals walk the gauntlet and harassing them with organized protests around places where they meet for their scientific congresses, menacing them with placards and shouting insults at them are hardly bases for improved dialogue and understanding.

7. *The Anti-therapeutic Zealots*
   Denying the existence of mental conditions or the effectiveness of modern treat-ments is an unscientific and harmful position. Mental illnesses are brain conditions whose neuroanatomy, pathological basis and symptomatology have been clearly demonstrated. Furthermore, their treatments, whether psychopharmacological, psychotherapeutic or both, are scientifically researched and developed under strict laboratory or clinical conditions, and their application protocols are the subject of constant study and refinement. Once improvement and remission are achieved, rehabilitation techniques, equally well established and tested, are utilized with great success. Denial of these realities is unhelpful to those who are managing their recovery process and who would benefit from these interventions.

Summary and Conclusions

This chapter has examined current conceptual models that support our understanding of stigma, mental illnesses and human rights. It has demonstrated that our current discourse is inadequate to promote full and effective participation of people with mental illnesses in society through civic, economic, political and social participation. We must move this rubric to one that focuses on solutions to entrenched structural inequities experienced by people with a mental illness, including conceptualizing anti-stigma interventions as those aimed at bringing about structural change. Greater emphasis on positive rights (rights that support social participation and inclusion) must now occur if we are to move beyond the current situation where people with mental illness are largely disenfranchised, powerless and championless.

References

Arboleda-Flórez J (2001) Stigmatization and human rights violations. In: Mental health: a call for action. World Health Organization, Geneva, pp 57–71

Arboleda-Flórez J (2004) Editorial – on the evolution of mental health systems. Curr Opin Psychiatry 17(5):377–380

Arboleda-Flórez J (2005) Forensic psychiatry: two masters, one ethics. Die Psychiatr 2:153–157

Arboleda-Flórez J, Stuart H (2012) From sin to science: fighting the stigmatization of mental illnesses. Can J Psychiatr 57(8):457–463

Ballingall A (2014) Autism home director 'Disappointed' by Doug Ford's opposition. rhestar.com, Sunday, 18 Jan (accessed at http://www.thestar.com/news/gta/2014/05/17/autism_home_director_disappointed_by_doug_fords_opposition.html. 18 Jan 2015)

Brant S (2005) Stultifera Navis: – 1497 – Internet, (Cited 2005, Dec 14]. Available from http://en.wikipedia.org/wiki/Ship_of_Fools_%28satire%29

Corrigan PW, Larson JE, Rüsch N (2009) Self-stigma and the "Why Try" effect: impact on life goals and evidence-based practices. World Psychiatry 8(2):75–81

Dômer K (1974) Ciudadanos y locos. Taurus, Madrid, p 29

Eisenberg L (1977) Disease and illness. Cult Med Psychiatry 1:9–23

Farmer P (1999) Pathologies of power: rethinking health and human rights. Am J Public Health 89(10):1486–1496

Foucault M (1965) Madness and civilization: a history of insanity in the age of reason. (Translated by R. Howard). Vintage Books, New York

Goffman E (1963) Stigma: notes on the management of spoiled identity. Prentice-Hall, Englewood Cliffs

Gracia D, Lázaro J (1992) Historia de la Psiquiatría. Chapter 2. In: Ayuso Gutierrez JL, Carulla LS (eds) Manual de Psiquiatría. Interamericana-McGraw-Hill, Bogotá

Häfner H (1991) The concept of mental illness. Chapter. In: Seva A (ed) The European handbook of psychiatry and mental health. Editorial Anthropos, Barcelona, p 20

Hawthorne N (2001) The scarlet letter: 1850. Infomotions, Chicago

Kelly BD (2005) Structural violence and schizophrenia. Social Science & Medicine 61(3);721–730

Kleinman A, Eisenberg L, Good B (1978) Culture, illness, and care: clinical lessons from anthropologic and cross-cultural research. Ann Intern Med 88(2):251–258

Konrad N (2002) Prisons as new hospitals. Curr Opin Psychiatry 15:583–587

Kramer H, Sprenger J (1971) The malleus maleficarum: 1487. Dover Publications, New York

Laing R (1971) Psychiatry and anti-psychiatry. Tavistock Publications, London

Parsons T (1975) The sick role and the role of the physician reconsidered. Millbank Memorial Fundam Q Health Soc 53(3):257–278

Pinel P (1988) Tratado médico-filosófico de la enajenación mental o mania: 1801. Editorial Nueva, Madrid

Sayce L (2000) From psychiatric patient to citizen. St. Martin's Press, New York

Stangor C, Crandall CS (2000) Threat and the social construction of stigma. In: Heatherton TF, Kleck RE, Hebl MR, Hull GJ (eds) The social psychology of stigma. The Guilford Press, New York, pp 62–87

Steadman H, Cocozza J (1978) Selective reporting and the public misconceptions of the criminally insane. Public Opin Q 41:523–533

Stuart H (2006) Media portrayal of mental illness and its treatments. CNS Drugs 10(2):99–106

Stuart H, Arboleda-Flórez J, Sartorius N (2012) Paradigms lost: lessons learned in the fight against stigma. Oxford University Press, Oxford

The World Health Organization (2000) Mental health and work: impact, issues, and good practices. World Health Organization, Geneva

The World Health Organization (2003) Mental health legislation and human rights. World Health Organization, Geneva

The World Health Organization (2005) Mental health atlas 2005, revised edition. World Health Organization, Geneva

United Nations (1991) Principles for the protection of persons with mental illness and for the improvement of mental health care (resolution 46/119). United Nations General Assembly, New York

Vives JL (1980) De Anima – Antología de Textos de Juan Luis Vives – 1538. (Translation by F. Tortosa). Universitat de Valencia, Valencia

World Psychiatric Association (1996) Madrid declaration on ethical standards for psychiatric practice. World Psychiatric Association, Madrid, http://www.wpanet.org. Accessed 19 Jan 2015)

World Psychiatric Association (2005) Madrid declaration on ethical standards for psychiatric practice—WPA informational folder 2002–2005. World Psychiatric Association General Secretariat, Geneva

Closing Mental Health Gaps Through Tackling Stigma and Discrimination

29

Sue Bailey

The Mental Health 'Gaps'

Mental health has historically been both a distant and poor relation to physical health (Bailey and Smith 2014). This is vividly illustrated by the four major 'gaps' that exist in England:

- *The mortality gap*
  The life expectancy for those with severe mental illness is on average 20 years less for men and 15 years less for women than for the population as a whole (Wahlbeck et al. 2011). Common mental health problems such as anxiety and depression also bring with them significant premature mortality (Russ et al. 2012).
- *The treatment gap*
  Across the lifespan and range of mental disorders, only a minority of people with mental health problems receive any intervention for their problem (McManus et al. 2009).
- *The funding gap*
  Although mental health accounted for 25 % of UK years' 'lost to disability' in 2010
  (Murray et al. 2013), it received approximately only 11.1 % of the NHS budget in 2010–2011 (Department of Health 2012).
- *The stigma gap*
  Stigma and discrimination significantly contribute to the treatment gap. Among people with a diagnosis of depression, eight out of ten report discrimination in at least one area of their lives (Lasalvia et al. 2013).

S. Bailey
Academy of Medical Royal Colleges, 10 Dallington Street, London EC1V 0DB, UK
e-mail: sue.bailey@aomrc.org.uk

© Springer International Publishing Switzerland 2017
W. Gaebel et al. (eds.), *The Stigma of Mental Illness - End of the Story?*,
DOI 10.1007/978-3-319-27839-1_29

This is not unfortunately limited to the public, but is a fundamental problem not only across the field of medicine itself but also for mental health services as well. The Time to Change campaign has demonstrated that the attitudes of mental health professionals have in fact shown the least improvement (Henderson et al. 2012).

Unfortunately there is often also a 'belief gap' on the part of fellow doctors and policy makers when the above facts, figures and failings are quoted.

Changing Attitudes of Targeted Groups

Mental Health Within Medicine

Mental health is every doctor's business (Bailey and Smith 2014). Comorbid mental health conditions exacerbate long-term physical health conditions – 8 billion pounds in additional costs to the English NHS every year. Mental health has a significant impact on many areas of physical health care. A fifth of patients with breast cancer are developing depression in the first year after their diagnosis. Forty-two percent of all tobacco use in England is by people with mental illness, but they are less likely to be offered smoking cessation programmes than those without mental illness (Bailey and Smith 2014).

Therefore, across medicine, we need to educate and support all doctors to watch out for diagnostic overshadowing where there is evidence that people with mental health problems do not receive either the same level of access, investigation or treatment for physical health complaints as people without them.

We need to give feedback to mental health colleagues about how we must and can improve the physical health of our patients. Improving lifelong training for psychiatrists on good physical health with regular monitoring of patients on antipsychotic medication.

Challenging stigma across the medical profession, where (e.g. liaison psychiatrists) work side by side with other doctors) they are well placed to gauge attitudes towards mental health.

We need to speak up for mental health services, where we can demonstrate better resourced mental health services can bring other savings to the wider NHS and improve physical health outcomes, but also more widely where early intervention for depression at work results in total returns of £ 5 for every £ 1 invested.

Doctors come into medicine to make peoples' lives better. The Cartesian view of the separate components of body and mind is being replaced with that of the whole person whose mental and physical health are codependent. This in itself will help tackle stigma and discrimination.

Mental Health Within Society

At a societal level, one in four adults and one in ten children are experiencing a diagnosed mental health problem at any one time (McManus et al. 2009). Stigma and discrimination against people with a mental illness have a substantial public health impact including poor access to physical and mental health care, reduced life expectancy and employment, increased risk of contact with the criminal justice system, victimisation, poverty and homelessness (Thornicroft et al. 2013).

From a recent review of stigma and discrimination (Thornicroft et al. [in Chapter 11 of the Annual Report of the Chief Medical Officer, England] 2013) on the subject of public mental health, the stark facts are that:

- Eighty-seven percent of mental health service users across England reported experiencing discrimination in at least one aspect of their life (English survey 2011).
- About 70 % of mental health service users feel the need to conceal their illness (Thornicroft et al. 2013).
- Still the most common newspaper articles on mental illness are those that contribute to stigma (Thornicroft et al. 2013).

In 2012 mental health service users described discrimination at all stages of the pathways into employment (Thornicroft et al. 2013). The Equality Act, England 2010, has opened the door to mental health users being able to take employers to employment tribunals on the basis of employers failing to make 'reasonable adjustments' in the case of those with mental illness. This is having some impact and also gives us valuable data with which to track what is happening.

Bringing About Change

In 1960 Goffman (1968) gave us this salutary definition of stigma: 'An attribute that is deeply discrediting and that reduces the bearer as a whole and usual person to a tainted, discounted one'. To bring about real change demands political will and funding to long-term scientifically evidenced campaigns. This is happening in England with Time to Change.

The key ingredients of this campaign:

- Have clearly defined the nature and degree of stigma and discrimination set in the context of what we know about other groups of people discriminated about.
- Work in true partnership with those with lived experience of mental health problems giving clear evidence on the severity and impact on the lives of people with mental illness.
- Have separated out and described population and target group level interventions and measured their effects: In phase 1 (2007–2011), targeting such groups as medical students, trainee teachers and employers; phase 2 (2011–current) has built on the learning from phase 1 with evidenced improvement in employer related attitudes, fewer discriminatory newspaper reporting and less self-reported discrimination experienced by service users.
- Have examined the particular detrimental effects of stigma and discrimination on health care, employment and citizenship.
- Have compared programmes in England with those in other countries.
- Have examined the relevant economic evidence.
- Have most importantly made clear evidence-supported recommendations for further stigma reduction in England.

They have also taken an important rights-based approach to this campaign using extant equality legislation to good effect embracing the key importance of patient self-empowerment by supporting and empowering mental health service users to respond to stigma and discrimination through addressing self-stigma, training in self-advocacy and peer support.

Legislation in England (The Health and Social Care Act; 2012) gave us parity between mental and physical health. A key component to having parity in practice is the eventual impact of campaigns such as Time to Change (Achieving Parity of outcomes, BMA Board of. Science may 2014).

To make real change in attitudes, we have to reach out early to children where we know attitudes across all aspects of their life take shape early and where we can support all children to respect difference and be supported to become emotionally resilient and support their peers to be the same including those of their peers with emerging mental health problems.

References

Bailey S, Smith G (2014) Why 'parity of esteem' for mental health is every hospital doctor's concern. Br J Hosp Med 75(5):277–280

British Medical Association (2014) Recognising the importance of physical health in mental health and intellectual disability: achieving parity of outcomes – May 2014. (http://bma.org. uk/-/media/files/pdfs/working%20for%20change/recognisingtheimportanceofphysicalhealth-inmentalhealthandintellectualdisability.pdf)

Department of Health (2012) 2003–04 to 2010–11 programme budgeting data. (http://www.gov. Uk/government/publications/2003-04-to-2010-11 programme-budgeting data. Accessed 2nd Apr 2014

Great Britain. Department of Health (2012). *Health and Social Care Act* 2012. The Stationery Office, Norwich

Goffman E (1968) Stigma: notes on the management of spoiled identity. Penguin, Harmondsworth

Henderson C, Corker E, Lewis-Holmes E, Hamilton S, Flach C, Rose D, … Thornicroft G (2012) England's time to change antistigma campaign: one-year outcomes of service user-rated experiences of discrimination. Psychiatr Serv 63(5):451–457

Lasalvia A, Zoppei S, Van Bortel T, Bonetto C, Cristofalo D, Wahlbeck K, … ASPEN/INDIGO Study Group (2013) Global pattern of experienced and anticipated discrimination reported by people with major depressive disorder: a cross-sectional survey. Lancet 381(9860):55–62

McManus S, Meltzer H, Brugha TS, Bebbington PE, Jenkins R (2009) Adult psychiatric morbidity in England, 2007: results of a household survey. The NHS Information Centre for for health and social care, Leeds

Murray CJ, Richards MA, Newton JN, Fenton KA, Anderson HR, Atkinson C, … Davis A (2013) UK health performance: findings of the Global Burden of Disease Study 2010. Lancet 381(9871):997–1020

Russ TC, Stamatakis E, Hamer M, Starr JM, Kivimäki M, Batty GD (2012) Association between psychological distress and mortality: individual participant pooled analysis of 10 prospective cohort studies. BMJ 345:e4933

The NHS Information Centre, Mental Health and Community (2011) Attitudes to Mental Illness – 2011 survey report. http://www.hscic.gov.uk/catalogue/PUB00292/atti-ment-illn-2011-sur-rep.pdf. Assessed 10 Aug 2015

Thornicroft G, Evans-Lacko S, Henderson C (2013) Stigma and discrimination. In: Davis SC (ed) Annual report of the chief medical officer 2013: public mental health priorities-investing in the evidence. Department of Health, London, pp 179–195, Chapter 11

Wahlbeck, K., Westman, J., Nordentoft, M., Gissler, M., & Laursen, T. M. (2011). Outcomes of Nordic mental health systems: life expectancy of patients with mental disorders. The British Journal of Psychiatry, 199(6), 453–458.

Part V

Overcoming Stigma and Discrimination: Recent Programmatic and Contextual Approaches

Improving Treatment, Prevention, and Rehabilitation

30

Wolfgang Gaebel, Mathias Riesbeck, Andrea Siegert,
Harald Zäske, and Jürgen Zielasek

Introduction

One of the major obstacles to seeking treatment for mental disorders is the stigmatization of mental disorders and the services of mental healthcare. This has been shown repeatedly, for example, for patients with alcohol addiction (Wallhed Finn et al. 2014). However, in some groups of mental disorders, perceived stigma only plays a small role when reasons for not seeking help are explored, for example, in persons with cannabis dependence (van der Pol et al. 2013). On the other hand, self-stigma is especially prevalent among those with mood disorders (Kelly and Jorm 2007). Early treatment of depression was shown to be associated with less stigmatization, but there was an intricate balance in attitudes toward depression treatment concerning issues of being not sick enough (stigma of "early treatment," when personal responsibility of those affected was perceived and thus illness invalidation stigma occurred) or of being too sick (stable dysfunction stigma; Henshaw 2014). Such stigmatizing attitudes are not only found in the general population but also in primary care physicians, who – as was shown in patients with depression – may underestimate the effects of stigma for help seeking and for treatment decisions (Keeley et al. 2014) and in families and other peer groups related to those affected by mental illnesses, with considerable detrimental effects on professional help seeking (Fernandez Y-Garcia et al. 2012). A lower level of social support is one of the negative consequences of stigmatization of those with alcohol addiction (Glass et al. 2013). Public health literacy and primary care specialist literacy regarding mental disorders, the stigmatization of mental disorders, and the treatability of mental disorders, appear central to lowering the perceived and the real stigma-related barriers to adequate access to mental healthcare services (Corrigan et al. 2012a;

W. Gaebel (✉) • M. Riesbeck • A. Siegert • H. Zäske • J. Zielasek
Department of Psychiatry and Psychotherapy, Medical Faculty, Heinrich-Heine-University,
LVR-Klinikum Düsseldorf, Bergische Landstr. 2, D-40629 Düsseldorf, Germany
e-mail: wolfgang.gaebel@uni-duesseldorf.de

© Springer International Publishing Switzerland 2017
W. Gaebel et al. (eds.), *The Stigma of Mental Illness - End of the Story?*,
DOI 10.1007/978-3-319-27839-1_30

Evans-Lacko et al. 2012; Wallhed Finn et al. 2014). Fostering help seeking is a key self-stigma reducing, empowering activity (Mittal et al. 2012). One of the areas in need of more studies is the stigmatization of persons with intellectual disabilities. A review showed that the evidence on the efficiency of anti-stigma interventions in this area was small, but changing awareness, attitudes and beliefs appear to be crucial components (Scior 2011). It is important to not only address individual stigmatizing experiences, but to also tackle public, institutional, and other societal types of stigmatization (Gaebel et al. 2004). Opening new avenues of therapy may increase the public perception of mental disorders as treatable health conditions. Promoting such a viewpoint, for example, increased the rate of diagnosis of schizophrenia (then relabeled) in Japan in the early 2000s (Umehara et al. 2011).

Prevention

Information Box 30.1
In the prevention of mental disorders, previous concepts of primary prevention (measures addressing those who never had a certain mental disorder) and secondary prevention (addressing those who had had a certain mental disorder) are increasingly superceded by a novel concept of universal prevention (addressing the whole population), selective prevention (addressing those without the mental disorder, but with certain risk factors), and indicated prevention (addressing those who already have mild symptoms of a mental disorder) (Saxena et al. 2006).

The stigmatization of mental disorders and of the institutions providing mental healthcare may be an important factor in limiting the effects of prevention programs, for example, by hindering people to use prevention programs dealing with mental disorders or by reducing the participation of people with mental disorders in programs aimed at reducing relapses (reviewed by Rüsch 2014). An important issue in the prevention of mental disorders is that in the case of mental disorders most primary preventive measures would need to target the population aged 18–25 years, and stigma research has shown that this age group may have special needs of how to reduce stigma and increase help seeking (Yap et al. 2011). For example, attributing mental illness to a personal weakness is a frequent misconception in this age group, and educational approaches to reduce stigma are more effective than in other age groups (Corrigan et al. 2012a). A recent meta-analysis investigated which childhood factors contribute to increased risks of adult mental disorders. These factors were psychological disturbances, genetic influences, neurological disorders, neuroticism, behavioral aspects, school performance, childhood adversity, child abuse or neglect, parenting and parent-child relationships, and disrupted and dysfunctional family structures. Evidence for the association with later mental ill-health was identified but with different degrees of magnitude (Fryers and Brugha 2013). While such research shows the multitude of factors involved in increasing the risk for mental disorders, it also indicates that prevention of all these factors already in childhood may be an insurmountable task. Therefore, preventive measures for adult mental disorders are usually developed in a disorder-specific way and address adolescents or adults.

Among the different types of prevention, universal prevention is mainly used to reduce the rate of alcohol consumption or drugs of addiction, but a recent health technology assessment report in Germany critically debated whether such measures are effective and whether they achieve sustained effects (http://portal.dimdi.de/de/hta/hta_berichte/hta309_bericht_de.pdf). A more recent meta-analysis showed that some programs were better than others and proposed a model including factors which may correspond with preventive efficacy (Sandler et al. 2014). Implementing such conceptual issues in future prevention programs may help to increase their efficacy. Novel anticraving substances like sodium oxybate (Skala et al. 2014) will need to be studied more extensively to show their efficacy in prevention, and novel concepts like addressing hyperglutamatergic neurotransmission in alcoholism may also open new avenues for prevention (Holmes et al. 2013). If such novel approaches are effective, the stigma of alcohol-related disorders may be reduced since their prevention will become more effective.

Better evidence for the efficacy of preventive measures exists for affective disorders, but these usually include complex psychological interventions over longer time periods. To cite one example, a study of indicated prevention in high-risk adolescents aged 13–17 years employed a cognitive behavioral method with eight weekly sessions followed by six monthly follow-up sessions. While the intervention showed preventive efficacy in adolescents whose parents did not develop depression during the study period, those adolescents who underwent the preventive intervention and whose parents became depressive during the study even had a worse outcome (Garber et al. 2009). This study shows that well-intended preventive measures may also have adverse effects, and similar to psychotherapy studies, the role of antidepressant medication in the secondary prevention of depression in children and adolescents is not conclusive given the diversity of methods used in prevention studies and adverse effects of medications in this age group (Cox et al. 2012). In adults, the situation is different and mood-stabilizing medication for bipolar disorder and long-term antidepressive maintenance therapy in unipolar depression are state of the art. Regarding psychological prevention programs, across all types of prevention (universal, selective, indicated), psychological interventions were effective in reducing the incidence of depression by 21 % and with a number needed to treat to spare one case of depression of 20 (van Zoonen et al. 2014). There is a trend to employ short, low-impact prevention interventions now for depression, and while they seem to be effective, their cost-effectiveness has yet to be shown especially in secondary prevention (Rodgers et al. 2012). As an alternative, increased physical activity has been consistently shown to prevent depression and could be used on the population level (Mammen and Faulkner 2013).

A more complicated situation has arisen in dementias. While previous studies on immunizing persons at risk have failed due to severe complications like meningoencephalitis, novel safe and efficient immunization schemes are currently being developed. Until these become available, preventive measures targeting vascular factors, which apparently play a major role in the pathogenesis of Alzheimer's disease, are the mainstay of effective dementia prevention, albeit with limited efficacy (Scarmeas et al. 2009; Defina et al. 2013). Another interesting approach employs novel secretase inhibitors, which may regulate amyloid protein processing and which is the way how nonsteroidal anti-inflammatory drugs exert their anti-dementia action. The latter, however, cannot be used for preventive therapies in Alzheimer's disease due to their side effects. Currently, therefore, prescribing regular physical activity and a Mediterranean diet accompanied by recommendations to keep up an enjoyable social lifestyle may be the best advice for dementia prevention. A major methodological challenge in studies on the prevention of dementias is the long observation periods necessary to show effects and the high propensities for side effects which may be expected in the elder target population. Also, the limited efficacy of the prevention measures makes large numbers of study participants necessary, increasing the costs and efforts of such studies.

A final part of this chapter deals with the prevention of schizophrenia. While it is now firmly established that the first onset of schizophrenia is usually preceded by a prodromal period of several years' duration, the prodromal symptoms are unspecific, and it is yet not clear which symptoms provide the best predictive value in individual cases and what would be the best treatment. In the current version of the American Association of Psychiatry *Diagnostic and Statistical Manual* (DSM-5, published in 2013), these reasons led to the addition of an "attenuated psychosis syndrome" only in the chapter on mental conditions deserving clinical attention and further research (Fusar-Poli et al. 2014), and we will discuss later in how far stigma questions came into play here. Currently, more research is needed in order to better identify those persons who have such prodromal symptoms and among these those who may profit from early psychological or medication interventions. Currently, it is advisable to identify such persons in specialized early recognition centers and closely monitor clinical progression with a view for inclusion in ongoing early treatment studies (Piras et al. 2014). Another important aspect is indicated prevention in those with incipient schizophrenia relapses. Interventions based on early warning signs are effective in preventing rehospitalization, although the cost-effectiveness of such prevention programs has not yet been established (Morriss et al. 2013). Targeted specialized interventions are less effective than maintenance antipsychotic therapy (Eisner et al. 2013), and although the optimal regimens still need to be determined, maintenance antipsychotic medication is state of the art in the secondary prevention of schizophrenia.

Treatment

Information Box 30.2
Treatment for mental disorders is usually multimodal, i.e., it is comprised of elements of psychosocial therapies and pharmacotherapy. Outcome measures for assessing the efficacy of treatment include symptom reduction, psychosocial functioning, and quality of life. Newer concepts like the "recovery" approach try to combine these outcome areas.

Over the last decades, various treatment strategies and interventions have been developed to improve the acute and long-term course of mental illnesses after the initial onset. In general, they aim at symptom reduction, preferably in all dimensions affected and below a subclinical level (i.e., remission), prevent symptom recurrence or relapse, and resume social and occupational functioning (i.e., recovery) to reach an adequate quality of life. Stigma, whether on the public or on the individual level, is highly associated with various aspects of treatment, e.g., treatment setting, treatment efficacy resulting in symptom reduction and benefits in long-term outcome, side effects, as well as treatment adherence (Gerlinger et al. 2013). In the following, treatment of schizophrenia as one of the most severe mental illnesses will be described in more detail and associations to stigma will be discussed.

Mainly over the last two decades, treatment options have been summarized in illness-specific clinical practice guidelines (CPGs) including evaluation of a broad range of interventions regarding efficacy (or effectiveness) and safety based on principles of evidence-based medicine to support clinicians and practitioners in their treatment decisions. As to schizophrenia, several CPGs were provided predominantly on a national level, however, many of them with limited quality (Gaebel et al. 2005). Nevertheless, also CPGs with high-quality levels are available (Gaebel et al. 2011), one of them the CPG of the UK National Institute for Health and Care Excellence (NICE 2009). Accordingly, description of treatment follows the NICE (2009) recommendations, which correspond to those of other high-quality CPGs in core treatment decisions (Gaebel et al. 2011). The NICE CPG was just re-updated (NICE 2014) with only minor revisions, which are considered here where appropriate.

The NICE CPG addresses stigma directly in the general introduction section: "Psychosis and schizophrenia are associated with considerable stigma, fear and limited public understanding" (NICE 2014, p. 5) together with the statement to "provide treatment and care in the least restrictive and stigmatising environment possible and in an atmosphere of hope and optimism" (NICE 2014, p. 28).

Regarding specific treatment options, antipsychotic drugs represent the mainstay in schizophrenia treatment and are recommended in oral formulation in the acute phase to reduce symptoms as well as in the stabilization or stable phase (after symptom remission) to prevent relapse and reach recovery. No single drug or drug group (in particular first- or second-generation antipsychotics; FGAs or SGAs) is preferred, given the similar efficacy in acute treatment or only slight advantages in relapse prevention for some (SGA) compounds (Kishimoto et al. 2013). Regarding safety or side effects, SGAs show advantages in extrapyramidal symptoms (Leucht et al. 2009); however, they have higher propensity for other side effects like weight gain or metabolic side effects. Thus, antipsychotic drug choice should be made in shared decision based on individual efficacy, side effects, and preference. Both efficacy and side effects of antipsychotic treatment are strongly related to stigma (Lysaker et al 2007; Seeman and Seeman 2012) and all three are in mutual interaction with treatment adherence (Tranulis et al 2011). Negative symptoms seem to play a major role in this regard, resulting in motivational and cognitive deficits and hamper "the power to resist" (Campellone et al 2014; Hill and Startup 2013). On the other side, antipsychotic drugs are less effective in reducing negative symptoms (as compared to positive symptoms), with some advantages of SGAs over FGAs (Leucht et al. 2009). Thus, negative symptoms are still an unmet need in schizophrenia (drug) treatment with impact on stigma experience and coping.

Another issue highly relevant for stigma are symptoms of aggressive behavior or violence (for a summary see Torrey 2011). Drug treatment likewise is an essential option in this regard, in the short-term management ("rapid tranquilization" with benzodiazepines or antipsychotics) as well as in the long-term course (antipsychotics). Since the latter is strongly associated with treatment adherence, the long-term drug strategy of depot or long-acting injectable antipsychotics (LAIs) is recommended as a feasible option. However, LAIs themselves have the image for patients, relatives, and clinicians to be related to stigma (Jaeger and Rossler 2010), so the pros and cons have to be weighted properly.

Psychological interventions represent another fundamental treatment strategy and should be offered routinely to all patients with schizophrenia (NICE 2009, 2014). Cognitive behavioral therapy (CBT) and family interventions are recommended explicitly. In addition, information regarding the illness and treatment should be provided in appropriate manner, so psychoeducation represents another treatment requisite. CBT is effective in reducing (persisting) positive as well as negative symptoms, and improves coping abilities, all related to stigma. A recent meta-analysis however failed to show a significant (direct) effect of CBT on stigma (Griffiths et al. 2014). On the other hand, psychoeducation for patients and relatives aims at improving insight, which is also related to stigma (Schrank et al. 2013).

Rehabilitation

Information Box 30.3

Definition

Rehabilitation includes all measures aimed at reducing the impact of disabling and handicapping conditions and at enabling the disabled and handicapped to achieve social integration. Rehabilitation aims not only at training disabled and handicapped persons to adapt to their environment but also at intervening in their immediate environment and society as a whole in order to facilitate social integration. The disabled and handicapped themselves, their families, and the communities they live in should be involved in the planning and implementation of services related to rehabilitation (WHO 1981).

Rehabilitation addresses both the disabilities produced by the mental disorder and the loss of opportunity that result from stigma and rehabilitation (Corrigan 2003). Beyond disabilities, rehabilitation now also takes the person's remaining resources into focus and is based on active participation and change management leading to increased "empowerment," which consists of the main elements autonomy, encouragement, and responsibility (reviewed by Lauber and Rössler 2004). Rehabilitation therapy is the mainstay of therapeutic interventions for those with chronic, severe mental illnesses. These patients mainly comprise patients with addiction disorders, schizophrenia, depression, or a comorbidity of these disorders. There is now clear evidence that several therapeutic measures used specifically in rehabilitation programs for the mentally ill have therapeutic efficacy. These studies were mainly performed with rehabilitation patients who had severe mental disorders like schizophrenia. Effective therapeutic measures include cognitive training and supported employment. Importantly, the relative therapeutic efficacy of such measures may heavily depend on the social services context in which the measures are applied. If rehabilitation therapy as usual already has substantial beneficial effects, any new therapeutic measures will have difficulties in demonstrating superior efficacy. This was shown for supported employment in a multinational study (Burns et al. 2007). Another point of interest is that combination therapies like those combining cognitive training and functional skills training are more effective when assessing "real-world" functioning than the individual programs (Bowie et al. 2012). A central question arises here in that the optimal timing and selection of therapeutic measures appropriate for the individual will need to be evidence based, but research and clear guidelines in this area are still lacking. Approaches to integrate cognitive remediation therapies with the whole psychosocial rehabilitation process are currently being developed (Penades et al. 2012). Another topic is the question whether more specific improvements of everyday functioning can be achieved with targeted social cognition therapies. Such therapies would address dysfunctions in emotion perception, attributional biases or "theory of mind"-related functions, and may include specialized neurocognitive training methods. Currently, issues of maintenance and generalization of therapeutic gains are considered including approaches based on social psychology (Roberts and Velligan 2012).

The success of vocational rehabilitation is dependent on patient variables like the presence of comorbid additional mental disorders or the degree of psychopathology. However, studies show that patient-related factors only account for approximately 10 % of the variance of long-term success of vocational therapy (Bond and Drake 2008). Environmental factors like the availability of rehabilitation services account for approximately 50 % of the variance, and the type of intervention (like cognitive training) may account for approximately 40 % of the variance (Bond and Drake 2008). Stigmatization leading to discrimination is a considerable problem in seeking employment for those with mental disorders in a competitive labor market, and this is a major factor in burdening the patient and the rehabilitative process (Stuart 2006). Measures to assess the effects of rehabilitation programs on self-stigma and related variables of depression, self esteem, and perceived devaluation and discrimination are currently being developed and validated (Boyd et al. 2014). While the reduction of acute symptoms will remain a mainstay of any rehabilitation intervention, environmental and social factors will need to be taken into account as significant modifiers of any treatment response in research aiming at developing novel rehabilitative strategies in the areas of the long-term rehabilitation of patients with mental disorders. This will include a lengthy process of reducing the stigmatization of those with mental disorders by those who are responsible for employing applicants with mental disorders, and any efforts to increase the likelihood of finding sustainable employment for those with mental disorders will have to address public stigmatizing attitudes and self-stigma (Corrigan et al. 2012b).

In the field of alcohol withdrawal and treatment of addiction, there are many effective interventions including those in specialized rehabilitation settings. A new and very necessary approach addresses persons with alcohol addiction in general hospital settings and primary care settings, in which brief interventions have been shown to reduce alcohol consumption and even death rates (the latter only for general hospital settings; Kaner et al. 2007; McQueen et al. 2011). From an anti-stigma point of view, implementing such therapies on a wider base in general hospitals may reduce stigmatization since it would show that even heavy drinking can be reduced and that therapeutic nihilism is not warranted. An important new area of research is the field of neurocognitive rehabilitation for those with alcohol-related chronic brain damage. A recent review came to the conclusion that there were only 16 studies in this important area, and most of these dealt with Korsakoff's syndrome (Svanberg and Evans 2013). Most studies focused on the rehabilitation of memory with only tentative conclusions possible due to variances in methodologies. More rigourous studies are needed to investigate the efficacy of specific treatment options, but a staged rehabilitation intervention process may offer the best practical approach to the multifaceted therapeutic challenges of this group of patients, including special home and social care services (Wilson et al. 2012).

The Relationship Between Stigma, Prevention, Treatment, and Rehabilitation of Mental Disorders

The stigma of mental illness interferes with mental healthcare, in particular with prevention, treatment, and rehabilitation of mental illness. Diverse kinds of relationships may exist between them, but there are no studies directly addressing in how far and to which extent these aspects are associated. Two recent aspects of the stigmatization of mental disorders have become very pertinent since they caused some debate and controversies, which reached into society as a whole, and since they are among the few instances in which some association between the diagnosis of a mental disorder and with stigmatization were addressed. These aspects are the prevention and early detection of schizophrenia promised by identifying persons with a specially high risk of developing schizophrenia and establishing a diagnostic entity of an "attenuated psychosis syndrome," and the Japanese example of renaming schizophrenia as a means to reduce the stigmatization associated with this term in Japan specifically.

DSM-5 and the Attenuated Psychotic Symptoms Syndrome

The stigma of mental illness, especially the stigma of psychiatric institutions and treatment, acts as a barrier to help seeking and to initiate treatment (Tanskanen et al. 2011). The stigma of being in need of psychiatric treatment was also a key issue in the recent debate about whether including the attenuated psychotic symptoms syndrome into the DSM-5 was warranted or not (Nelson and Yung 2011; Yung et al. 2010). It is remarkable that the risk of being stigmatized was used in argumentations of both perspectives.

Protagonists supporting the inclusion of the attenuated psychotic symptoms syndrome into DSM-5 assumed that adopting this diagnosis may improve early recognition and treatment of patients with this condition. They followed the rationale originating from the debate about the importance of early recognition and intervention measures for psychosis: Both measures reduce the burden of stigma in the long run, since people at an early stage of psychosis would otherwise suffer from the consequences of longer prodromal periods and worsened illness courses, which both are associated with increased burden due to stigma (McGorry et al. 2001).

The risk of labeling people with a psychiatric diagnosis who would not have developed a psychosis (the "false-positive" cases) stood against this. These "false-positive" persons would be prone to suffer from stigma due to the fact that a mental disorder label was used to characterize their situation or the fact that they were in contact with the psychiatric healthcare system (see Nelson and Yung 2011 for a detailed discussion of these points).

One cannot decide whether one of these stigma issues outweighs the other, because empirical evidence of the relevance for either of them is lacking, despite the vast existing body of mental illness stigma research (Yung et al. 2012). In particular, there is a dearth of research addressing stigma experiences and perceptions of people suffering from mental illness regarding specific stages of illness (Gerlinger et al. 2013). The attenuated psychosis symptom syndrome was finally not introduced into DSM-5 as a novel mental disorder, but the defining clinical characteristics were listed in a separate chapter of DSM-5 about mental health conditions warranting further clinical studies. The main reason for this decision was that the predictive value of identifying such a syndrome was not considered sufficiently high enough and that the best treatment for such conditions was still under investigation.

The following chapters give some examples on the field of schizophrenia.

Renaming Schizophrenia: The Japanese Example

The question of renaming schizophrenia is a further interesting stigma-related issue, since the term "schizophrenia" by itself has become connected with negative connotations in some languages. Generally, the improvement and further development of illness concepts (and as a consequence thereof, of treatment methods) should reduce the stigmatizing potential of an illness. Nevertheless, it is questionable whether the change of a diagnostic label alone reduces stigma (Lieberman and First 2007). Along with such a change in name, a new appraisal of the whole illness concept is needed, as the example from Japan has shown (cf. for the following: Zäske et al. 2010; Umehara et al. 2011).

In the year 2002, the Japanese Society of Psychiatry and Neurology (JSPN) changed the Japanese name for "schizophrenia" ("seishin-bunretsubo"; literally "split-mind disorder") into togoshitcho-sho ("integration disorder"). The original Japanese term "seishin-bunretsubo" derives from the original definition of schizophrenia by Bleuler implicating the splitting of mental functions (German: "Spaltungsirresein"). As Sato (2006) discusses, the Japanese culture perceives the body and mind as a unity, meaning that a person suffering from "seishin-bunretsubo" was being perceived as being abnormal in his/her whole essence ("seihsin"). This leads to the false prejudice that schizophrenia causes a decay of personality (Sato 2006). In contrast to this, the new Japanese term "togoshitcho-sho" implicates a biopsychosocial illness concept relying on the vulnerability-stress model; it emphasizes the treatability of the illness and the patients' chances for recovery.

Since 2005, the new name for schizophrenia has been officially acknowledged through the Japanese Ministry for Health, Labor, and Welfare. Further studies showed that positive effects prevail, e.g., the rate of patients who were being informed about their diagnosis increased from 36.7 to 69.7 % (Sato 2006). Also, the new term seems to be lesser associated with criminality than the old one (Takahashi et al. 2009). Nevertheless, as Umehara et al. (2011) argue, a significant percentage of the patients with schizophrenia (up to 40 %) are still not able to name their correct diagnosis.

Conclusions

As both examples show, issues of the relation of the stigma of mental illness with issues of early detection and prevention or the general concept of the disorder are complex, dependent on the historical and cultural context of the respective societies, and sometimes opposing. Despite the large body of stigma research in the last 10–20 years, many specific questions about the relation of mental healthcare, prevention, and treatment with stigma and discrimination are not yet answered sufficiently. Besides the conceptual and terminological issues discussed above, personal factors may play a significant role as well; as some authors have stated (Tanskanen et al. 2011; Anderson et al. 2013), the "fear of being stigmatized" was one cause for not seeking help in case of mental health problems. Are there specific personal sources of stigmatization that are more important than others hindering the person to seek help? Which role does the availability and the public perception of mental health services play? How do people in need of mental healthcare deal with the two aspects of the treatment of mental disorders – in that treatment adds to stigmatization by providing clues for others that one has a mental disorder but at the same time preventing or alleviating stigmatization because of reductions of visible or otherwise notable symptoms of mental disorders? Examining such questions might be promising to find new individually tailored and differentiated strategies to reduce the "fear of being stigmatized" and hence to improve the acceptance of seeking mental healthcare if needed.

References

Anderson KK, Fuhrer R, Malla AK (2013) "There are too many steps before you get to where you need to be": help-seeking by patients with first-episode psychosis. J Ment Health 22:384–395

Bond GR, Drake RE (2008) Predictors of competitive employment among patients with schizophrenia. Curr Opin Psychiatry 21:362–369

Bowie CR, McGurk SR, Mausbach B et al (2012) Combined cognitive remediation and functional skills training for schizophrenia: effects on cognition, functional competence, and real-world behavior. Am J Psychiatry 169:710–718

Boyd JE, Otilingam PG, Deforge BR (2014) Brief version of the Internalized Stigma of Mental Illness (ISMI) scale: psychometric properties and relationship to depression, self esteem, recovery orientation, empowerment, and perceived devaluation and discrimination. Psychiatr Rehabil J 37:17–23

Burns T, Catty J, Becker T et al (2007) The effectiveness of supported employment for people with severe mental illness: a randomised controlled trial. Lancet 370:1146–1152

Campellone TR, Caponigro JM, Kring AM (2014) The power to resist: the relationship between power, stigma, and negative symptoms in schizophrenia. Psychiatry Res 215:280–285

Corrigan PW (2003) Towards an integrated, structural model of psychiatric rehabilitation. Psychiatr Rehabil J 26:346–358

Corrigan PW, Morris SB, Michaels PJ et al (2012a) Challenging the public stigma of mental illness: a meta-analysis of outcome studies. Psychiatr Serv 63:963–973

Corrigan PW, Powell KJ, Rüsch N (2012b) How does stigma affect work in people with serious mental illnesses? Psychiatr Rehabil J 35:381–384

Cox GR, Fisher CA, De Silva S et al (2012) Interventions for preventing relapse and recurrence of a depressive disorder in children and adolescents. Cochrane Database Syst Rev 11:CD007504

Defina LF, Willis BL, Radford NB et al (2013) The association between midlife cardiorespiratory fitness levels and later-life dementia: a cohort study. Ann Intern Med 158:162–168

Eisner E, Drake R, Barrowclough C (2013) Assessing early signs of relapse in psychosis: review and future directions. Clin Psychol Rev 33:637–653

Evans-Lacko S, Brohan E, Mojtabai R et al (2012) Association between public views of mental illness and self-stigma among individuals with mental illness in 14 European countries. Psychol Med 42:1741–1752

Fernandez Y-Garcia E, Duberstein P, Paterniti DA et al (2012) Feeling labeled, judged, lectured, and rejected by family and friends over depression: cautionary results for primary care clinicians from a multi-centered, qualitative study. BMC Fam Pract 13:64

Fryers T, Brugha T (2013) Childhood determinants of adult psychiatric disorder. Clin Psychol Rev 33:637–653

Fusar-Poli P, Carpenter WT, Woods SW et al (2014) Attenuated psychosis syndrome: ready for DSM-5.1? Annu Rev Clin Psychol 10:155–192

Gaebel W, Baumann A, Zäske H (2004) Gesellschaftsrelevante Ansätze zur Überwindung von Stigma und Diskriminierung. In: Rössler W (ed) Psychiatrische rehabilitation. Springer, Berlin, pp 875–886 [Article in German]

Gaebel W, Weinmann S, Sartorius N et al (2005) Schizophrenia practice guidelines: international survey and comparison. Br J Psychiatry 187:248–255

Gaebel W, Riesbeck M, Wobrock T (2011) Schizophrenia guidelines across the world: a selective review and comparison. Int Rev Psychiatry 23:379–387

Garber J, Clarke GN, Weersing VR et al (2009) Prevention of depression in at-risk adolescents: a randomized controlled trial. JAMA 301:2215–2224

Gerlinger G, Hauser M, De Hert M et al (2013) Personal stigma in schizophrenia spectrum disorders: a systematic review of prevalence rates, correlates, impact and interventions. World Psychiatry 12:155–164

Glass JE, Mowbray OP, Link BG et al (2013) Alcohol stigma and persistence of alcohol and other psychiatric disorders: a modified labeling theory approach. Drug Alcohol Depend 133:685–692

Griffiths KM, Carron-Arthur B et al (2014) Effectiveness of programs for reducing the stigma associated with mental disorders. A meta-analysis of randomized controlled trials. World Psychiatry 13:161–175

Henshaw EJ (2014) Too sick, not sick enough?: effects of treatment type and timing on depression stigma. J Nerv Ment Dis 202:269–292

Hill K, Startup M (2013) The relationship between internalized stigma, negative symptoms and social functioning in schizophrenia: the mediating role of self-efficacy. Psychiatry Res 206:151–157

Holmes A, Spanagel R, Krystal JH (2013) Glutamatergic targets for new alcohol medications. Psychopharmacol (Berl) 229:539–554

Jaeger M, Rössler W (2010) Attitudes towards long-acting depot antipsychotics: a survey of patients, relatives and psychiatrists. Psychiatry Res 175:58–62

Kaner EF, Beyer F, Dickinson HO et al (2007) Effectiveness of brief alcohol interventions in primary care populations. Cochrane Database Syst Rev 2:CD004148

Keeley RD, West DR, Tutt B et al (2014) A qualitative comparison of primary care clinicians' and their patients' perspectives on achieving depression care: implications for improving outcomes. BMC Fam Pract 15:13

Kelly CM, Jorm AF (2007) Stigma and mood disorders. Curr Opin Psychiatry 20:13–16

Kishimoto T, Agarwal V, Kishi T et al (2013) Relapse prevention in schizophrenia: a systematic review and meta-analysis of second-generation antipsychotics versus first-generation antipsychotics. Mol Psychiatry 18:53–66

Lauber C, Rössler W (2004) Empowerment: Selbstbestimmung oder Hilfe zur Selbsthilfe. In: Rössler W (ed) Psychiatrische rehabilitation. Springer, Berlin, pp 146–156 [Article in German]

Leucht S, Corves C, Arbter D et al (2009) Second-generation versus first-generation antipsychotic drugs for schizophrenia: a meta-analysis. Lancet 373:31–41

Lieberman JA, First MB (2007) Renaming schizophrenia. BMJ 334:108

Lysaker PH, Davis LW, Warman DM et al (2007) Stigma, social function and symptoms in schizophrenia and schizoaffective disorder: associations across 6 months. Psychiatry Res 149:89–95

Mammen G, Faulkner G (2013) Physical activity and the prevention of depression: a systematic review of prospective studies. Am J Prev Med 45:649–657

McGorry PD, Yung A, Phillips L. (2001) Ethics and early interventions in psychosis: keeping up the pace and staying in step. Schizophr Res. 51:17–29

McQueen J, Howe TE, Allan L et al (2011) Brief interventions for heavy alcohol users admitted to general hospital wards. Cochrane Database Syst Rev 8:CD005191

Mittal D, Sullivan G, Chekuri L et al (2012) Empirical studies of self-stigma reduction strategies: a critical review of the literature. Psychiatr Serv 63:974–981

Morriss R, Vinjamuri I, Faizal MA et al (2013) Training to recognise the early signs of recurrence in schizophrenia. Cochrane Database Syst Rev 2:CD005147

Nelson B, Yung AR (2011) Should a risk syndrome for first episode psychosis be included in the DSM-5? Curr Opin Psychiatry 24:128–133

NICE National Institute for Health and Care Excellence (2014) Psychosis and schizophrenia in adults NICE clinical guideline 178; http://guidance.nice.org.uk/cg178. Accessed 29 Aug 2014

NICE National Institute for Health and Clinical Excellence (2009) Schizophrenia. Core interventions in the treatment and management of schizophrenia in adults in primary and secondary care (update). http://guidance.nice.org.uk/CG82 Accessed 29 Aug 2014

Penadés R, Catalán R, Pujol N et al (2012) The integration of cognitive remediation therapy into the whole psychosocial rehabilitation process: an evidence-based and person-centered approach. Rehabil Res Pract 2012:386895

Piras S, Casu G, Casu MA et al (2014) Prediction and prevention of the first psychotic episode: new directions and opportunities. Ther Clin Risk Manag 10:241–253

Roberts DL, Velligan DI (2012) Can social functioning in schizophrenia be improved through targeted social cognitive intervention? Rehabil Res Pract 2012:742106

Rodgers M, Asaria M, Walker S et al (2012) The clinical effectiveness and cost-effectiveness of low-intensity psychological interventions for the secondary prevention of relapse after depression: a systematic review. Health Technol Assess 16:1–130

Rüsch N (2014) Prävention und das Stigma psychischer Erkrankungen. In: Rössler W, Ajdacic-Gross V (eds) Prävention psychischer Störungen. Kohlhammer, Stuttgart, pp 19–28

Sandler I, Wolchik SA, Cruden G et al (2014) Overview of meta-analyses of the prevention of mental health, substance use, and conduct problems. Annu Rev Clin Psychol 10:243–273

Sato M (2006) Renaming schizophrenia: a Japanese perspective. World Psychiatry 5:53–55

Saxena S, Jané Llopis E, Hosman CMH (2006) Prevention of mental and behavioral disorders: implications for policy and practice. World Psychiatry 5:1

Scarmeas N, Stern Y, Mayeux R et al (2009) Mediterranean diet and mild cognitive impairment. Arch Neurol 66:216–225

Schrank B, Amering M, Hay AG et al (2013) Insight, positive and negative symptoms, hope, depression and self-stigma: a comprehensive model of mutual influences in schizophrenia spectrum disorders. Epidemiol Psychiatr Sci. doi:10.1017/S2045796013000322

Scior K (2011) Public awareness, attitudes and beliefs regarding intellectual disability: a systematic review. Res Dev Disabil 32:2164–2182

Seeman MV, Seeman N (2012) The meaning of antipsychotic medication to patients with schizophrenia. J Psychiatr Pract 18:338–348

Skala K, Caputo F, Mirijello A et al (2014) Sodium oxybate in the treatment of alcohol dependence: from the alcohol withdrawal syndrome to the alcohol relapse prevention. Expert Opin Pharmacother 15:245–257

Svanberg J, Evans JJ (2013) Neuropsychological rehabilitation in alcohol-related brain damage: a systematic review. Alcohol Alcohol 48:704–711

Stuart H (2006) Mental illness and employment discrimination. Curr Opin Psychiatry. 19:522–526

Takahashi H, Ideno T, Okubo S et al (2009) Impact of changing the Japanese term for "schizophrenia" for reasons of stereotypical beliefs of schizophrenia in Japanese youth. Schizophr Res 112:149–152

Tanskanen S, Morant N, Hinton M et al (2011) Service user and carer experiences of seeking help for a first episode of psychosis: a UK qualitative study. BMC Psychiatry 11:157

Torrey EF (2011) Stigma and violence: isn't it time to connect the dots? Schizophr Bull 37:892–896

Tranulis C, Goff D, Henderson DC et al (2011) Becoming adherent to antipsychotics: a qualitative study of treatment-experienced schizophrenia patients. Psychiatr Serv 62:888–892

Umehara H, Fangerau H, Gaebel W et al (2011) [From "schizophrenia" to "disturbance of the integrity of the self": causes and consequences of renaming schizophrenia in Japan in 2002]. Nervenarzt 82:1160–1168 [Article in German]

Van der Pol P, Liebregts N, de Graaf R et al (2013) Facilitators and barriers in treatment seeking for cannabis dependence. Drug Alcohol Depend 133:776–780

Van Zoonen K, Buntrock C, Ebert DD et al (2014) Preventing the onset of major depressive disorder: a meta-analytic review of psychological interventions. Int J Epidemiol 43:318–329

Wallhed Finn S, Bakshi AS, Andréasson S (2014) Alcohol consumption, dependence, and treatment barriers: perceptions among nontreatment seekers with alcohol dependence. Subst Use Misuse 49:762–769

WHO (1981) Disability prevention and rehabilitation. Report of the WHO Expert Committee on Disability Prevention and Rehabilitation, WHO Technical Report Series 668. WHO, Geneva, http://whqlibdoc.who.int/trs/WHO_TRS_668.pdf

Wilson K, Halsey A, Macpherson H (2012) The psycho-social rehabilitation of patients with alcohol-related brain damage in the community. Alcohol Alcohol 47:304–311

Yap MB, Wright A, Jorm AF (2011) The influence of stigma on young people's help-seeking intentions and beliefs about the helpfulness of various sources of help. Soc Psychiatry Psychiatr Epidemiol 46:1257–1265

Yung AR, Nelson B, Thompson AD et al (2010) Should a "Risk Syndrome for Psychosis" be included in the DSMV? Schizophr Res 120:7–15

Yung AR, Woods SW, Ruhrmann S et al (2012) Whither the attenuated psychosis syndrome? Schizophr Bull 38:1130–1144

Zäske H, Cleveland HR, Gaebel W (2010) Die Semantik des Begriffs "Schizophrenie" und das damit verbundene Stigma. Was lässt sich von der japanischen Umbenennung lernen? Kerbe Forum Sozialpsychiatrie 28:26–28 [Article in German]

Stigma and Recovery

31

Elizabeth Flanagan, Anthony Pavlo, and Larry Davidson

"The best antidote to stigma is recovery" – American policy maker.

The statement quoted above has many possible meanings. It could be taken, for example, to refer to the body of research reviewed in this volume that suggests that exposure over time to people in recovery who are occupying valued social roles is the most effective way to reduce stigma. Or, it could be taken to mean that recovering from a serious mental illness is the best way to disprove and dispel the stigma, shame, and self-blame that many people unfortunately have internalized from the society in which they live. Within the context in which the statement was made, though, the speaker's intent was rather that governments and private philanthropies would be better advised to spend the resources they were considering to allocate to fighting stigma (e.g., though community education campaigns) on funding psychiatric treatment, thereby (presumably) enabling people to recover *despite* stigma. While there may be some merit to this sentiment—insofar as mental health care remains vastly underfunded in virtually all societies around the globe—the speaker appeared to be making at least two problematic assumptions. First, she assumed that receiving psychiatric treatment was sufficient to ensure recovery regardless of stigma and other social and environmental factors (e.g., social determinants of health). Second, she was assuming that the psychiatric treatment that would be provided would not itself be perpetuating the same stigmatizing attitudes and beliefs that she was interested in dispelling.

The following chapter will be concerned primarily with the second of these two assumptions. A growing body of literature addresses many of the factors and forces

E. Flanagan (✉) • A. Pavlo • L. Davidson
Department of Psychiatry, Yale University School of Medicine,
319 Peck Street, Bldg. One, New Haven, CT 06513, USA
e-mail: elizabeth.flanagan@yale.edu; larry.davidson@yale.edu

© Springer International Publishing Switzerland 2017   551
W. Gaebel et al. (eds.), *The Stigma of Mental Illness - End of the Story?*,
DOI 10.1007/978-3-319-27839-1_31

that lie beyond the scope of mental health care that influence recovery, and this literature falls outside of the scope of this volume as well. What has received less attention in the research thus far is the degree to which mental health services and systems may actively contribute to, rather than work to reduce and eliminate, stigma—at least as much as, if not more than, the broader community itself. What little research that has been conducted thus far suggests, though, that mental health practitioners hold many stigmatizing attitudes and beliefs toward people with mental illness (Corrigan et al. 2014; Schulze 2007). Should this be the case, simply funding more of the same services as those already being provided will do little to dispel stigma. This chapter therefore focuses on identifying some of the ways in which mental health staff and settings serve, albeit unwittingly, as agents of stigma, thereby impeding rather than promoting recovery.

We believe that it is important to address stigma within the mental health system, not only in order to honor the Hippocratic oath of "first, do no harm" but also because we recognize that these stigmatizing beliefs, attitudes—and we will now add, practices—are largely inherited from earlier eras and do not reflect mal-intent on the part of present-day staff. Like other forms of discrimination, stigma manifests itself in mental health settings both in obvious, blatant ways (e.g., telling a client that he or she will never return to school, never work, or never fall in love) and in subtle, but at times even more destructive, ways (e.g., through the same type of "micro-aggressions" experienced by persons who are the object of other forms of discrimination; Deegan 2007; Gonzales et al. 2014; Sue et al. 2007).

We draw on both quantitative and qualitative research to identify ways in which stigma may be communicated within mental health settings. These data were collected over the last 5 years through a series of studies aimed at understanding and reducing stigma in mental health settings. In conducting this research, we proposed a model of the mechanisms of stigma in mental health settings. Our model was based on the stigma models of three prominent stigma theorists: Bruce Link, Jo Phelan, and Pat Corrigan. Link and Phelan (2001) defined stigma as occurring "when elements of labeling, stereotyping, separation, status loss and discrimination co-occur in a power situation that allows them to unfold" (p. 367). Later they added that emotional reactions from both the stigmatizer and the stigmatized also need to be represented in this definition (Link et al. 2004). Corrigan and colleagues (2003) included other factors in the occurrence of stigma in the general public including perceptions about the controllability of the cause of the disorder, personal responsibility, and dangerousness as well as familiarity (i.e., knowledge and experience) with mental illness.

Based on these two definitions of how stigma works in the general public, we proposed a model of how stigma might work in mental health settings (see Fig. 31.1).

Our model starts with a cognitive-emotional response in a clinician, activated by the presence of a diagnostic label. This cognitive-emotional response includes: stereotypes, attributions about the causes of mental illness, perceptions of dangerousness, emotional reactions, and behavioral reactions in the clinician. This cognitive-emotional response occurs within a power differential between the clinician and consumer and through separation of the clinician from the consumer. The outcomes of our model are internalized stigma in mental health consumers

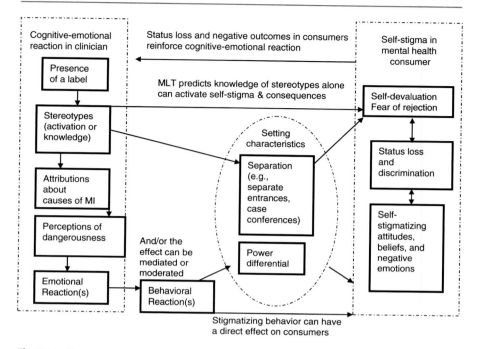

Fig. 31.1 Conceptual mode for the mechanisms of stigma within mental health settings. Note: These factors combine modified labeling theory as used by Link, Phelan, and Corrigan in previous studies (i.e., Link and Phelan 2001; Link et al. 2004; Corrigan 2000; Corrigan and Calabrese 2005)

including: self-devaluation, fear of rejection, status loss, discrimination, and self-stigmatizing attitudes, beliefs, and negative emotions. Our discussion of stigma in mental health settings in this chapter will focus on the cognitive-emotional experience in the clinician and the structural aspects of the setting (i.e., separation, power differential) that result in negative outcomes in the consumer. Given space limitations, we will not discuss in-depth negative outcomes in the consumer.

The first of these studies was a comprehensive assessment of stigma in the statewide system of care in the State of Connecticut through its Department of Mental Health and Addiction Services (CT DMHAS) Local Mental Health Authorities. There are 18 community mental health centers in CT DMHAS, seven of which are operated by the state and 11 are private nonprofit agencies. A total of 445 clinicians completed surveys that assessed their negative stereotypes, negative emotions, negative attributions, and negative behaviors toward people with mental illness as well as demographic factors. A total of 394 service users completed surveys that assessed their perception of negative stereotypes, emotions, attributions, and behaviors from the staff at their agency and its subsequent effect on their experiences of discrimination, status loss, low self-efficacy, and negative coping behaviors. Finally, a total of 334 community members in Connecticut completed a similar set of surveys as the clinicians as a comparison group for the clinicians' responses. The full report of the analysis of these data is available elsewhere (Flanagan et al. 2016a).

The goal of the second study was to examine in depth the experience of stigma in a single community mental health center in the CT DMHAS system, using qualitative research methods. Interviews were conducted with 14 mental health clinicians and 12 consumers by a person with similar experiences (i.e., clinician interviews were conducted by an experienced mental health clinician; consumer interviews were conducted by a mental health consumer; neither of the interviewers were active in the CT DMHAS mental health system). Consumers were asked about what it was like to come to the mental health center, what it was like working with their clinician (e.g., a time the clinician was helpful and not helpful, what their relationship was like), how the policies and procedures of the place affected their treatment, and what they thought about the issue of stigma in mental health settings. Clinicians were asked what it was like coming to the mental health center, what it is like working with their clients, what it was like doing their job in the mental health center, and what they think about stigma in mental health settings. Data analyses were conducted by a team of seven experienced qualitative researchers who reviewed the transcripts. The clinician and consumer transcripts were analyzed separately. Each transcript was reviewed by at least three researchers in addition to the principal investigator. The research team met over a series of weeks to come to a consensus about themes in the interviews and identify potential quotes to illustrate the themes. The full report of the analyses of these data also is available elsewhere (Flanagan et al. 2016b).

Theoretical Model of Stigma Within Mental Health Settings

Presence of a Label

Our model starts with the presence of a label. In mental health settings, labeling consumers with a diagnostic category may happen immediately upon entry to the system, and a person's labels may then follow him or her around the system. In Link and Phelan's (2001) definition, the label is the signal that sparks the stigma. The issue of labeling was studied in depth in Flanagan et al. (2009), which was a qualitative study of the diagnostic process in the Connecticut Mental Health Center. Our research suggests there are several ways the presence of label initiates stigma in mental health settings.

First, the possibility of stigma occurring is greatly increased by the diagnostic process being foreshortened because of the need to give a diagnosis quickly for reimbursement purposes. As a result, clients are often diagnosed in a rush and based on the criteria needed for disability or service eligibility rather than as a comprehensive diagnostic understanding. As one clinician described:

> You got to get them going, you got to get a diagnosis, we can't get paid without a diagnosis... We focus on that because of system constraints and we don't treat the client. As my supervisor says, "unfortunately, we treat the chart." The chart has to be x, y, and z. We can't get [entitlements] for this guy without a strong Axis I, but we need something to base it on … the frustration is trying to rush through and get your best guess in order to try to satisfy the system and not necessarily treating the client. (cited in Flanagan et al. 2009)

Second, some people receive diagnoses as a result of negative behavior that upsets the staff rather than because the diagnostic criteria were properly applied. Again, it may be due to rushing to make a diagnosis. As two clinicians described:

> As soon as they come in and have a conflict or they're splitting staff, everybody's Borderline … what you often see in young African-American males is sociopathic personality disorder … I do think it does a disservice to label people before you have a clear assessment of what's going on. I think you need a length of time to do that, and I … think our system doesn't allow us the time to do that. We need to get people in the system, diagnosed, treated, and moved on. (cited in Flanagan et al. 2009)
>
> In this field, if you are so inclined, and someone challenges something you say, you can give them another diagnosis. If you're telling me that you don't want a certain medication and you'd rather have such and such, I might call you "drug seeking"… If you get angry with me because I answer a phone call while you're in my office, during an appointment, I might say you have some kind of personality problem … If you happen to think my treatment approach is not working and you let me know that, I might label you in some other way. So, basically, it's the power of the pen. The practitioner has the power to make these diagnoses. Once you put these diagnoses in someone's chart, they can follow them for their whole lives. (cited in Flanagan et al. 2009)

Third, people's diagnoses may be used against them, as a reason to discontinue treatment or withhold services.

> Many people I've worked with came to me with diagnoses of Borderline Personality Disorder, partly because they were challenging, partly because they didn't agree with their therapists, and the therapists felt they could no longer work with the client, the client no longer wanted to work with them either, so they get transferred. But they get transferred with labels. (Flanagan et al. 2009)

A fourth important role of labeling in the development of stigma in mental health settings is that it serves to distance the client from the clinician, helping the clinician to manage his or her negative emotions and thoughts:

> I think the idea of "mental disorder"… is a desire to take something that is frightening or something which is inexplicable or not conventional and make it a foreign entity to be objectified, analyzed, reviewed, and cured … because it's hard to deal with being in situations which are disempowering and which are confusing. (cited in Flanagan et al. 2009)

Thus, our research shows that diagnostic labels play an important part in many of the factors involved in the model. Labels produce stereotyping, negative emotions, and negative behaviors in clinicians.

Stereotypes

Stereotypes are a central aspect of prejudice and discrimination in many settings, and mental health settings appear to be no exception. Historically, there have been numerous stereotypes about people with mental illness. The most prominent ones are that they are dangerous, unpredictable, and/or childlike. People with mental illness may also be depicted as cruel, as in the American television show "Criminal Minds." Clinical settings are no different. Clients are often seen as dangerous: at our local mental health center there is a metal detector to enter the building operated by a public safety officer and "panic" buttons are included in each room and in the hallways. This is in stark contrast to the cancer center just across the street where anyone can enter with no search procedures (and there is a piano in the lobby). Clients are often seen as unpredictable as well. Not keeping appointments is seen as par for the course, and clients are often expected to have difficulty in housing and in managing symptoms and addictions. Clients are also viewed as childlike, dependent on the system, and helpless to take care of themselves or pursue any goals.

In the survey study described previously, stereotypes were assessed with Penn's characteristics scale (Penn et al. 1994). These characteristics include: weak, boring, insensitive, naive, shy, unsociable, emotional, cruel, awkward, unintelligent, sad, unsuccessful, unenthusiastic, insecure, defensive, cold, untrustworthy, and ineffective. Clinicians were asked to rate the extent to which their clients embody these characteristics. Consumers were asked to rate how the staff at the mental health setting viewed them in relation to these characteristics. Community members were asked to rate the characteristics of people with mental illness. The top five characteristics that clinicians ascribed to their clients were: emotional, insecure, awkward, sad, and unsuccessful.

Another stereotype of people with mental illness that came across in the clinician interviews was that consumers were viewed as extremely needy. As one clinician said: "Our patients are very, very needy. I mean I may often describe them as ... huge Hoover vacuums which kind of want to get in to you and that's it, but they just want to suck the life right out of you."

The survey data allowed us to analyze the variables in our model that were related to negatives stereotypes toward people with mental illness (e.g., negative emotions, negative behaviors). Stepwise regression, putting all of the model variables in a regression model, showed that for clinicians, negative stereotypes were predicted by desire for social distance, negative emotions, and how much pity they feel for the person.

Attributions About the Causes of Mental Illness (i.e., Controllability, Responsibility)

Attributions about controllability and responsibility of mental illness are extremely important in mental health settings. Clients are penalized when clinicians think that the illness is controllable or the person is seen as responsible for his/her illness. A prime example of this is blaming people with substance use disorders for "just not stopping" or returning to neighborhoods or friends who are still using substances, despite the research evidence that addictions are chronic disorders (e.g., Dennis and Scott 2007; McLellan et al. 2000). Another example of this is people who engage in self-harming behaviors, who are often viewed as in control of their behavior and responsible for the aftereffects of the interpersonal difficulties or the physical damage as a result of their self-harming behaviors. Anger about returning to substance use or self-harming behavior can be used as a reason for withholding services, health care, housing, money, transportation, and social activities. Consumers with mental illnesses also report medical professionals in emergency departments expressing anger to them about how their physical damage as a result of self-harm that is their "own fault" and that medical procedures such as stitches or stomach tubes have been given roughly or even without anesthetic by medical staff who were angry about their self-harm.

In our survey study, clinicians gave low ratings of controllability over illness and responsibility for illness to a case description of person with schizophrenia or depression. Community members indicated that they thought the person with schizophrenia or depression had significantly more control and was more responsible for his/her illness than clinicians indicated ($d = 0.26$, $p < 0.001$). However, when clients were asked how the staff at their mental health center felt about how in control and responsible a person with schizophrenia or depression was, consumers gave significantly higher ratings than clinicians ($d = 1.05$, $p < 0.001$). These results suggest that although clinicians report holding people less responsible for and in control of a mental illness than community members do, clients perceive that clinicians hold people responsible for their illness and view the person as more in control than the clinicians indicate.

Perceptions of Dangerousness

Dangerousness is one of the most prevalent and common perceptions of people with serious mental illness by the general public (e.g., Corrigan et al. 2002; Link et al. 1999). This perception appears to be no different in mental health settings (Stuber et al. 2014). As stated previously, the mental health center studied in the qualitative study has a metal detector at the door and public safety officers as guards. Clients are asked to empty their pockets and are searched for weapons upon entry to the building while staffs are not. Perceptions of dangerousness have serious implications in mental health settings as they can result in hospitalization, placement in a group home, partial hospitalization, mandatory inpatient or outpatient treatment, and even incarceration.

In our survey study, clinicians rated a case of a person with schizophrenia or depression as significantly less dangerous than community members did. But consumers' ratings indicated that they thought clinicians perceived a person with schizophrenia or depression as much more dangerous than clinicians reported. On a separate question, clinicians also rated a person with schizophrenia or depression as less likely to be harmful to others than community members and consumers rated when describing their own beliefs. Clinicians and consumers also gave lower ratings to the likelihood that the person would be violent to self than community members did. When asked about going through the metal detector, some consumers reported liking the metal detector and feeling more comfortable since other people with mental illness were not going to be allowed to be dangerous. Our data thus suggest that the attribution that people with mental illness are dangerous is just as prevalent, if not more so, in mental health settings, even among clients. In the words of one consumer participant:

> I think some of the workers, like the maintenance and the cafeteria, they should be a little bit more schooled. Because they act like they're scared to look at you or if they brush against you, like it's going to rub off on them or something like that. You know, sometimes even the guard downstairs can be a little … like, you know, we're not mass murderers that are medicated. You know, it's a feeling that you get…when you come in the door. I think that there are workers here [who] need to be more educated, as far as the mental health. It doesn't mean that the person will pull out a knife and cut your throat or something. You know, it ain't like you see on TV … It's nothing like that.

Thus, both the quantitative and qualitative research in our study suggest that consumers are seen as dangerous within mental health settings as well as in the general public.

Emotional Reactions

Emotional reactions are not typically parts of stigma models, but Link et al. (2004) made a very important addition to their definition of stigma when they added that variable. Emotional reactions are particularly important for stigma in mental health settings. Clinicians are in close contact with people with mental illness, often for many years and spanning many different treatment services. The process of clinicians monitoring and changing their emotional reactions had been an important part of clinical work in the past, such as with the concept of countertransference, but this has not been emphasized in clinical work more recently. Nevertheless, clinicians have many emotional reactions to clients, and these emotions need to be recognized, understood, and their effect on clinical care needs to be monitored.

We used several measures of emotions in our survey study. Penn's affective reactions scale (Penn et al. 1994) asks people to rate their feelings on ten bipolar adjectives (e.g., calm vs. anxious). The AQ-27 (Corrigan 2003) measured anger, pity, and fear felt toward a person diagnosed with schizophrenia or depression. Clinicians and community members were asked to rate their own feelings, while consumers were asked to rate how the staff at their mental health center feel. In the measure of a variety of negative emotions (i.e., pessimistic, anxious, resentful, fearful, angry, disgusted, apprehensive, irritable, tense, nervous), clinicians reported feeling more negative emotions than did community members ($d=-0.35$, $p<0.001$), and service users reported perceiving more negative emotions from clinicians than clinicians reported ($d=0.35$, $p<0.001$). In the AQ-27, clinicians and community members reported similar levels of anger toward someone with schizophrenia or depression, and consumers reported perceiving significantly more anger from clinicians than clinicians reported ($d=0.79$, $p<0.001$). Clinicians reported significantly less fear toward someone with schizophrenia or depression than community members ($d=0.25$, $p<0.001$), and consumers perceived more fear from clinicians than clinicians reported. With regard to pity, clinician report and consumers' perception of clinician stigma were similar, but community members reported less pity for someone with schizophrenia or depression than clinicians' report and consumers' perceptions of clinicians.

Perceptions of clinicians' negative emotions were very important, as regression analysis showed that perception of negative emotions from clinicians predicted low self-esteem/self-efficacy (stdB = 0.38, $p<0.001$), powerlessness (stdB = 0.12, $p<0.05$), low activism/autonomy (stdB = 0.20, $p<0.001$), and low optimism/control over the future (stdB = 0.23, $p<0.001$ in consumers). Our research also investigated what predicted negative emotions in clinicians. When stepwise regression was conducted, results showed the following variables predicted negative emotions: (1) negative stereotypes, (2) anger, (3) the desire not to help, (4) male gender of the clinician, (5) having previous inpatient experience, (6) and endorsing the view that a person with schizophrenia or depression should be segregated from the community. Given the importance of negative emotions in clinical work, the prediction of negative emotions by variables in the model, and the finding that perceiving negative emotions from clinical staff predicted a range of negative outcomes in consumers, our research suggests that negative emotions may be central to the function of stigma in mental health settings.

Behavioral Reactions

Behavioral reactions are where the rubber meets the road with regard to stigma. This is where the internal cognitive-emotional experience becomes translated into actions that are discriminatory. In the community, many different actions may be considered discriminatory, including exclusion and discriminatory practices in hiring, housing, health care, etc. In clinical settings, discriminatory behavioral reactions can take many forms including avoiding clients, coercing them into treatment (e.g., inpatient, crisis, partial hospitalization), segregating them from society (e.g., mental hospitals, group homes), preventing them from receiving needed services, and discharging them from care.

In the survey, we measured wanting to avoid, help, coerce into treatment, and segregate a person from society who has schizophrenia or depression. The avoidance measure was essentially a social distance measure that did not translate well to a clinical setting. It asked how comfortable the person would be interviewing for a job, sharing a car pool, and renting an apartment to a person with schizophrenia or depression. Clinicians' report and consumers' perceptions of clinicians' willingness to engage in such experiences were similar, while community members were significantly less willing than clinicians to have these kinds of interactions with someone with schizophrenia or depression ($d=0.51$, $p<0.001$). When asked about helping, clinicians' report was significantly higher than consumers' perceptions of clinicians' desire to help, and community members had significantly lower desire to help than both groups (clinicians vs. community members, $d=-1.87$, $p<0.001$).

When asked about coercion into treatment, clinicians' reported desire to coerce someone with schizophrenia or depression into treatment was lowest, followed by consumers' perceptions of clinicians' desire for coercive treatment ($d=0.66$, $p<001$), and then community members endorsed the most desire to force someone into treatment ($d=1.47$, $p<0.001$). Similarly, clinicians reported the lowest desire to segregate someone with schizophrenia or depression from society, followed by community members ($d=0.31$, $p<0.001$), and then consumers' perceptions of clinicians' ($d=1.31$, $p<0.001$) desire to segregate someone into treatment was highest.

Because coercion into treatment is such an important aspect of discrimination in mental health settings, we used stepwise linear regression to see which factors in clinicians were most strongly related to deciding to coerce someone into treatment. In this study, coercing someone into treatment included the items: (1) "[Client] should be forced into treatment with his doctor, even if he doesn't want to"; (2) "If I were in charge of the person in the description's treatment, I would require him/her to take medication"; and (3) "If I were in charge of the person's treatment, I would force him/her to live in a group home." Agreeing that a person with schizophrenia or depression should be forced into treatment was predicted by: (1) how much you think the person is a risk to his neighbors and it is best for him/her and the community if she/he is hospitalized; (2) thinking the person is not able to make his own decisions about treatment; (3) The extent to which your own views are not recovery-oriented; (4) thinking it is not likely that the person's mental illness will improve on its own; (5) the extent to which agency policies are not recovery oriented; (6) thinking that client is dangerous; and (7) having pity for the client.

These findings are quite illuminating. People are forced into treatment and/or segregated from society when clinicians perceive them to be at risk of grave disability or imminent harm to self or others. This perception seems to be more common in settings and among practitioners that are not as recovery oriented and seems to involve viewing the consumer as relatively powerless in the face of the illness. It therefore is reasonable to expect such clinicians to rely more heavily on coercion in their work, as they do not see much of a role for the consumer other than to take the medications being prescribed. Similarly, while pity is seen as a pro-social emotion that inspires people to help, the only kind of help some clinicians were able to identify was help that was given against the person's will.

Separation

Separation of the stigmatizer from the stigmatized group is essential for stigma to occur (Link and Phelan 2001). In most stigma models, the stigmatizers have little personal experience with the stigmatized group, so it is easy to apply stereotypes, to be afraid of, and to avoid a group of people you are separated from. The variable of separation plays an interesting role in mental health settings. In many ways clinicians and consumers are not separated. They spend multiple hours together in the very intimate act of therapy through which the clinician comes to know many private details about the client. In a community mental health center, they might be together in group therapy, in medication management meetings, and in center events such as speakers, performances, and holiday parties.

But clients and clinicians are also separated in very important ways, ways that often point to the power differential that is discussed next. Clients and clinicians often use separate bathrooms, separate entrances to buildings, and separate cafeterias in manners that are reminiscent of historic segregation practices in the Southern United States. Clinicians also have keys to the building while clients have to enter through the metal detector and be searched. In our local mental health facility, clients are not allowed to have or use cameras, while staff have no such restrictions. Clients are also excluded from treatment team meetings and medication management meetings where their own treatment is being discussed. Through these, and other related structures, even clinicians who are firm in their belief in the personhood of persons with mental illnesses may find it hard to hold onto their sense of common humanity with the people they serve.

Power Differential

The other setting characteristic that Link and Phelan (2001) argue needs to be present in order for stigma to occur is a power differential. In the community, power differentials often occur because of differences in affluence and social capital between people with mental illness and the general public. In clinical settings, there are many elements used to maintain a power differential between clients and clinicians. There are power differentials in the relationship between clinicians and consumers in that the clinician is perceived as the expert while the client is seeking treatment. The clinician has the power to make treatment decisions with or without the clients' consent. There are structural power differentials embedded in the entrances, security, keys, cafeterias, and bathrooms of mental health settings as described in the previous section. Power differentials are also communicated by race ethnicity (i.e., the staff are mostly White, the clients are mostly African-American and Hispanic), socioeconomic status (i.e., staff receive a paycheck for their services while clients receive disability entitlements), and education (i.e., most staff have higher education while many clients have high school or less education).

In the survey, the only measure of power was from the consumers' perspective. Rogers et al.'s (1997) empowerment scale was used to measure the amount of power mental health consumers felt "at this mental health center." Stepwise regression with all variables in this study was conducted to determine the factors most strongly related to client empowerment. Results showed that the following variables are predictive of consumers' sense of a lack of power at the mental health center (in rank order of importance in predicting empowerment): (1) perceived devaluation/discrimination of consumers, (2) perceived negative emotions from clinicians, (3) stigmatizing experiences, and (4) decrements in self-esteem as a result of having a mental illness.

The Context of Stigma in Mental Health Settings

In the following section, we will summarize the results from the qualitative study of the context of stigma in mental health settings that was conducted after the quantitative assessment. The goal of this research was to examine the experience of stigma in mental health settings from the perspectives of consumers and clinicians. The methods for this study were described earlier in this chapter. The following presents an analysis of the clinician and consumer data.

Overall, clinicians tended to believe that stigma is less prevalent (or, in some cases, nonexistent) in mental health care than in the general community. They tended to believe that they did not convey stigma toward their clients but often were able to identify sources of stigma outside of themselves, such as systemic issues, other colleagues, the community, and self-stigma among clients. Despite their belief that they did not convey stigma to their clients, some clinicians often unintentionally expressed stigmatizing beliefs and attitudes juxtaposed with instances of approaching clients in a more respectful way. Consumers, on the other hand, often were able to identify instances of stigma with staff. They also felt respected and safe, especially in the context of satisfying relationships with clinicians.

Clinicians

Relationships. Clinicians tended to focus on two aspects of the relationships they had with consumers: (1) experiencing intimacy with some consumers and (2) the centrality of relationships to care. With few exceptions, clinicians described feeling fulfilled as a result of their work with clients. They described a commitment and dedication to their work and, at times, described their relationships with consumers in familiar, even friendly, rather than clinical ways. Furthermore, they described reciprocity in their relationships with clients. For example, one provider described how consumers felt like "family" and had her best interests in mind when she was pregnant:

> I mean just when I sit there and I can complain like, "Oh, this person … wants too much and blah, blah, blah." But there's other people that are so warm and so generous and give so much of themselves and are just like I feel like they're, you know, family practically. You know, I have a group that I run … [a]nd last year I was pregnant and they were … all about my pregnancy and making sure I was doing the right thing and eating healthy … as involved as they can possibly be. And it was just really sweet to see and then they're constantly like checking up on me and that type of thing which [is] nice … I mean I see my work as being reciprocal. I probably usually get more from them than I could ever give to them.

Another clinician described what her work meant to her. She expressed warm, close relationships with clients and highlighted the role of these relationships in facilitating client safety:

> I really like what I'm doing. It's not that I am doing it because it pays well. I'm doing it because I know that somebody out there is going to benefit from it and may be a better person ... It gives me a heart full of gratitude to come in and work with my clients. I'm going to be honest here. I really love my clients, I do. I look forward to seeing them coming here. I think the reason why I don't have so many people getting into crisis with me is my relationship with them, so I don't have a lot of crisis.

Another participant described how she did not experience stigma in the community and continued by describing how she had a preference for those diagnosed with serious mental illnesses:

> And so you know I don't necessarily say, I'm walking down the street and I see someone who's walking down the street and kind of fidgety with his hands and talking to himself. I don't necessarily cross that street or get nervous or clutch my purse or move my child from one side to the other. I don't do that because like I said, I have a high tolerance for people who are presenting differently ... [I]t's really about educating people and trying to dispel some of those myths. Because some of the people with the most severe illness have been like just the greatest, warmest, kindest, genuine people that I've ever met and sometimes much nicer than some people who are quote unquote sane.

Similarly, a few clinicians described how they liked the consumers better than their fellow staff. One provider described how it was a "nice feeling" when consumers went out of their way to greet him in the hallways of the mental health clinic. He continued by describing how "the clients really, in my mind, have a lot more in the way of, you know, social skills, a lot more in the way of an ability to appreciate somebody making an effort to help them than some of the people that are paid to be here."

Other clinicians described facets of the therapeutic relationship they thought were most helpful. For example, one participant described the importance of being genuine and consistent within the therapeutic relationship. He said:

> Intrinsically you have to bring who you are to the table ... you need your engagement with people and your relationships that you establish with people or it's really what the work is. It's not the paperwork; it's not even the phone call or the thing you do with the patient. It's really you just being you and consistently being there ... Just genuine ... that's what people respond to.

When asked what is helpful, another clinician described fostering hope within the relationships: "Give them hope. I think hope is not something that a doctor can dispense or prescribe. It's something that people can give to people. Other clinicians emphasized seeing clients as people rather than diagnoses: "My clients are some people that I am very close with. I say close with not in a sense of being close, but people that I respect and really want to help. I see them as individuals. I don't see them as bipolar, schizophrenic, or personal[ity] disorders." When another participant was asked what she thought she could do to make consumers happy, she responded:

> I listened to someone speak here … She was talking about what it was like to be a person with mental health problems. The thing she said, over and over again in different ways, was what made a difference was kindness. She just wanted people to be nice to her. I think that's it. I think that's a big part of it.

The system. Clinicians described how policy, procedures, paperwork, and a lack of resources tended to get in the way of their work with consumers. These issues resulted in their experiencing higher levels of stress and frustration, resulting in feeling less effective. For example, one clinician said:

> That, you know, there just simply aren't the resources out there and it's beyond their, the client's control and beyond my control … You know most of the real frustrations I get around here are not with the clients, they are with … the policies and with, with just the basic management in the building.

A common concern was extremely high caseloads and clinicians often felt a lack of safety as a result:

> I think we're experiencing, at least on this team, we're experiencing huge case loads that are a little scary, unsafe. You know, as a licensed clinician I feel that … my license is at risk because of the nature of the work that we do … we're seeing more and more severe, persistent mental illness coupled with the needs of what these people with these issues have. Then coupled with … not having the resources.

Another said, "It's extremely stressful right now due to the high caseloads. It's—I have to say—I love what I do. I love the population that I work with and I wouldn't want a different job. I just wish it were a little less stressful." These systemic issues posed difficulties for clinicians leading to feeling less effective and more frustrated. As we will discuss in the next section, these systemic issues provide a context for clinicians engaging in stereotyping.

Burnout—giant Hoover vacuums. Clinicians described feeling overwhelmed by their work at times. They described feeling overworked, overwhelmed, and had trouble "put[ting] down … work at the end of the day." They often described feeling overworked but also expressed enjoying their work. For example, one participant said, "Draining, exhausting, but it's a job I love." A few clinicians described feeling conflicted about coming to work due to this kind of stress. One participant described how she was kept up at night due to her worries about consumers and her day-to-day work. Another one said:

> I'm usually happy to come here, energetic. I love my patients. I like to work with the population that I work with. There are some days that yes, I don't want to get out of bed and say, I just don't want to go to work, or it's—I don't know—I guess we all have those days when I [we?] feel frustrated. Not with the patients but mostly with the system.

These systemic issues appeared to affect clinicians' sense of satisfaction with their work, resulting both in feeling overwhelmed and frustrated and, at times, behaving in avoidant ways. For example, one clinician (who tended to describe clients in mostly positive and person-centered ways) commented: "Our patients are very, very needy. I mean I may often describe them as ... huge Hoover vacuums which kind of want to get in to you and that's it, but they just want to suck the life right out of you." We suggest that it was this clinician's experiences of feeling overwhelmed and "burned out" that led her to characterize her clients in such a more detached and demeaning manner.

Symptoms versus persons. Another major theme in the clinician data was the narrow focus on pathology, symptoms, and limitations rather than viewing the whole person. For example, clinicians often discussed the importance of controlling symptoms to the exclusion of other issues in consumers' lives. Furthermore, clinicians often expressed low expectations for consumers with serious mental illness. For example, one participant said:

> Most often they go back to their residence [when they are not here]. They ... might just watch TV or some go to social club, some just go home and stay in their apartments without TV, some live in group homes. I mean it's different for just about everyone of them ... I think for the most part those that have housing and are happy with that housing are pretty much status quo; they're pretty happy with their life. I mean they all wish they could have more money. But other than that, I think they're pretty content.

This participant did not have much hope for her clients beyond a very restricted and empty life. Furthermore, her belief that people were "pretty content" communicated that she did not feel they could do (or could want) more. Later in the interview, in response to being asked what was helpful for clients, she continued:

> Just sometimes just coming in and they just, there's nothing going on, they're just coming in to kind of check in, that's helpful. Just they got out of the house a little bit, you know, got to sit in talk with someone. So that I think is helpful. Just meeting with the doctor, getting their meds renewed, that's helpful ... I don't know if I've ever really felt that I haven't [been helpful]...

This notion that patients did not need very much because they would not benefit from more intensive treatment appeared often in these interviews. Clinicians tended to focus on medication to the exclusion of other treatments or engagement in any meaningful activities that might promote recovery.

Other clinicians invalidated consumers' experiences and reduced their emotions to symptoms. For example, one participant attributed her client's anger to a symptom of her mental illness. She said:

> "Oh, well, you know, like if a patient is "pissed off" at me because, you know, they want X, Y and Z, and, you know, unfortunately they're not entitled to it [because of] the guidelines of a program." Another participant described the effects of a client discontinuing his medication. She said:
> One of his symptoms was paranoia. And he would think that people in his apartment building were out to get him or something like that. So, he would do things like bang on

people's doors at late hours of the night. Or leave his door open and sit in a chair right in front of his door to see who was passing by his door, because he thought people were coming by and sending rays or waves or something through his door.

Rather than attempting to understand this person's fears and their impact on his ability to live alone, the clinician reduced his emotional experience to a symptom of severe mental illness ("paranoia"). She continued by expressing frustration that her patient could not "see the relationship between not taking his medicine and losing his apartments ... The frustration was coming from the fact that myself—and like I said, the rest of my team—would try to help him understand, you know, why he was constantly losing his apartment or his housing." While losing housing is significant and frustrating for clinicians, participants did not describe trying to understand their clients' fears about medication or difficulties in living independently (among other issues). Instead, they focused on insisting that people remain on their medication as the only possible solution, without exploring the consumer's preferences. Other times, clinicians expressed a fatalistic attitude about recovery. For example, one participant said: "[F]or my clients, I want them to be as independent as they were deemed—as their destiny deemed them to be."

Examples of provider stigma. With few exceptions, clinicians often expressed stigmatizing beliefs or language despite their beliefs that (1) stigma was less prevalent in mental health settings than in the past and/or (2) they did not behave in stigmatizing ways. This conflict was most striking in clinician narratives that were marked by flexibility and acceptance. In other words, participants who appeared to behave in non-stigmatizing ways or saw themselves as anti-stigma agents also expressed stigmatizing beliefs at the same time. Whether participants were aware of this conflict was unclear from the interviews. One participant put this conflict well:

> I think we're caught in a time and place where mental health providers are aware of the stigma of mental health conditions and aware of how we discriminate against people with mental health conditions and an awareness that we really probably shouldn't that—that that's not really a good thing, that's not really a healthy thing—but we still do.

When asked about staff's use of derogatory or stigmatizing language, one participant described how he "developed a reputation as the guy who you have to watch out what you say around." However, he also set fairly low expectations for individuals diagnosed with serious mental illness in terms of their possible recovery. Another participant, whose interview was marked by commitment to his work and views of consumers as not just patients, labeled some consumers as having "character disorder agendas" when they did not agree with him. Another clinician described this tension between treating persons with serious mental illness in discriminatory ways despite working closely and alongside them. First, she described her unhappiness with how co-workers with "mental health issues" were treated by other staff:

> There are clinicians here that have mental health issues. Even amongst the clinical department, some of those people have been clearly ostracized from others. It's like, "Don't talk to her," "Don't talk to that person because …" To me, that's really sad because at least in my belief, I'm trying to fight against stigma, and that promotes stigma and keeps us stuck in it.

Later, she described how she thought the hiring of peers was characterized by a similar tension:

> The other thing is we have peer mentors, and with the peer mentors, they're technically hired staff but they don't have the privileges of staff. They don't have keys and they're not really treated like staff; they're treated like clients. I think that reinforces the idea of "us" and "them," and that's something I fight against. I have a struggle with that.

Consumers

The findings from the consumer interviews were analogous to the provider data in that relationships, expectations, and systemic issues were most prominent. When discussing either specific relationships with staff or particular staff members with which they had particularly meaningful relationships, consumers tended to discuss their experiences of the mental health center in ways that did not indicate stigma. However, when discussing systemic issues, the staff at large, or the "clinic," they described feeling stigmatized.

Relationships. Significant relationships with clinicians appeared to be important in their care. In general, consumers felt less stigmatized when describing specific or particularly beneficial relationships. For example, one participant said:

> For me personally, my clinician has been pretty, pretty reasonable, willing to listen to what I really have to say. She wasn't very opinionated which I found to be really good. You know, she just sat and listened and then when I would finish saying what's on my mind, she would gladly you know, give a response. But it was just that, just a response. It wasn't being judgmental, it wasn't saying this is what I should do and she just did, I think for the most part, pretty much helped set my mind at ease to the things I did talked to her about.

Participants indicated wanting to be understood and accepted by clinicians. One participant described how it was important for him to have a collaborative relationship with his clinician in which both parties were responsible for making decisions. In response to being asked how staff could be helpful, he responded:

> That's a tough question. I will say to help me you have to understand me. So to understand me, you have to be me. So you can't be me and understand me. But to understand me is to know your soul. And then you could probably know me. So if I know me and I know what's going on with me, to help me you have to know me and then you can help me.

Another participant described a staff training that she thought would help staff be less stigmatizing:

> The training would involve role playing … I would have the client play as a provider, and I would have the provider play as the client, and talking about ways of kind of being accepting, and knowing that you know, the way you speak, the way you talk, the way you walk, and the way you look, somebody can pick up on that.

Consumers' comments tended to describe wanting to feel safe and respected within their relationships with clinicians. In some respects, both consumers and clinicians valued the potential role positive relationships could play in recovery. However, consumers also described how these relationships could be stigmatizing in ways that may not be apparent to clinicians but feel hurtful and damaging nonetheless.

Experiences of stigma in mental health settings. Participants described feeling stigmatized when they perceived that staff had little hope for them or other consumers. Similarly, they felt stigmatized when providers had low expectations for them. These experiences made them feel invalidated and less motivated for treatment. For example, one participant said:

> I even overheard clinicians talk about a client in the elevator, and they didn't have any hope for him. They said, "Oh, that's what he does. Oh, well." It's just really sad. Because if you don't have hope for us, and you were feeling that way, it's going to come out in the meeting when you meet with the person, and so we can pick up on stuff like that, and it makes it where, you know, we don't really want to be there, we don't really want to talk to them. So it's not therapeutic or anything. Just kind of like we just go to show up to try to get help for ourselves, but … In some ways … I go there to help myself, but I don't enjoy going there because it's almost like it makes me just feel bad.

Another participant described how it felt to be stereotyped as weak and, as a result, feeling like change or recovery was impossible: "This is just my personal feelings…if you have someone who can't get it, and who has been struggling for years and years and years, I think that person is looked at as weak, and not being able to be helped. So I think I see a lot of frustration with a lot of the clinicians around that." Rather than suggest way clinicians may have failed to help this person or ways they might try to help differently, this participant described how there are people "who can't get it," placing blame solely on the consumer.

Consumers described feeling as though their clinicians did not view them as people but rather as static labels:

> It's labels versus people, and the sad part is, a lot of clinicians, I believe, even though they went to school, you know, they have all this knowledge, they don't have hope for some of us. And I think that that's really sad, because I think that they just go for a paycheck, it's not really about helping us. And so I do, I think that the stigma is not even like in the population of our people outside, it's actually in the mental health system itself, through the clinicians and all that.

Other consumers described invalidation when their emotions were treated as symptoms of mental illness. One participant said:

You know, it's like you can't be too happy and you can't be too sad because you never know who's looking at you. Before you know it, they be putting you in this group or putting you in this facility or that facility. You know what I'm saying? They're not really ... don't look at you or ask what's going on to get that reaction ... you become accustomed to ... like I'm sitting here talking to you. Now, you'd think I'd have a PhD or something or whatever, based on my mental health issues, but I can talk. I can, you know, say what I got to say. But there are times when ... days happen in my life and I just get lip locked. You know.

Systemic issues. Participants described how systemic issues affected their perceptions of care, often resulting in feeling unsafe and having negative feelings about themselves. For example, one participant described the difficulties he experienced having to trust a new therapist every year. He said:

Yeah, for me it's not usually the same person, and I find it very difficult, because it's like you get used to one person, and you share all of this story with that person, or about yourself, and then boom, you're thrown to somebody else to do it all over again, and it feels like you know, I just repeat my story over and over again to a whole bunch of people, and it kind of makes me feel like, naked and vulnerable.

Participants also described how they did not feel welcome at times. They also felt stigmatized in that staff perceived clients as dangerous. These issues made pursuing treatment more difficult. One participant said: "It does feel a little scary when you have to walk through the doors where the guards are, and they're not as friendly, and they search you, and it sort of makes you feel like you kind of did something wrong when you go there for an appointment when you're trying to get help."

In summary, when taken together, the results of the qualitative analysis of the clinician and consumer interviews provide a way of understanding how stigma manifests in mental health care. Because clinicians did not see themselves as stigmatizing, they did not discuss ways in which they held stereotypes and behaved in discriminatory ways. They could describe how broader, systemic factors could result in consumers experiencing stigma. However, consumers were able to describe instances in which clinicians behaved in stigmatizing ways, often in the form of subtle yet painful communications about their capacities and potential for recovery. The qualitative interviews describe the context in which many of the findings of the quantitative data could be understood. Participants described a context that could easily lead to stigma despite clinicians' inability to identify stigma within themselves. However, the results also indicate that providers often hold positive beliefs and opinions about their clients, potentially signaling ways that stigma can be combated in these settings.

Conclusions

This chapter presented a model of stigma in mental health settings that describes a cognitive-emotional reaction in a clinician within a setting of separation and power differential from mental health consumers, and we described our quantitative findings testing that model. Because of space limitations, we did not discuss the negative outcomes of self-stigma and discrimination that occurs in the consumer as a result of this form of stigma. Then we presented our findings from a follow-up study that examined the context of stigma in mental health settings. We hope that this chapter has served to identify and discuss the factors related to stigma in mental health settings that are part of the clinician's cognitive-emotional reaction and structural aspects of mental health settings in ways that can generate new and effective interventions. We also look forward to future research and discussion on this important topic.

References

Corrigan, P. W. (2000). Mental health stigma as social attribution: Implications for research methods and attitude change. Clinical Psychology: Science and Practice, 7(1):48–67.
Corrigan PW (2003) An attribution model of public discrimination toward people with mental illness. J Health Soc Behav 44:162–179
Corrigan PW, Rowan D, Green A., Lundin R, River P, Uphoff-Wasowski K, … Kubiak MA (2002) Challenging two mental illness stigmas: personal responsibility and dangerousness. Schizophr Bull 28(2):293
Corrigan P, Markowitz FE, Watson A, Rowan D, Kubiak MA (2003) An attribution model of public discrimination towards persons with mental illness. J Health Soc Behav 44:162–179
Corrigan, Patrick W. & Calabrese, Joseph D. In Patrick W. Corrigan, (Ed), (2005). On the stigma of mental illness: Practical strategies for research and social change. Washington, DC, US: American Psychological Association pp.239–256.
Corrigan PW, Druss BG, Perlick DA (2014) The impact of mental illness stigma on seeking and participating in mental health care. Psychol Sci Public Interest 15(2):37–70
Deegan P (2007) Mentalism, microaggressions, and the peer professional. Posted at: http://www.patdeegan.com/blog/archives/000014.php
Dennis M, Scott CK (2007) Managing addiction as a chronic condition. Addict Sci Clin Pract 4(1):45
Flanagan EH, Miller R, Davidson L (2009) "Unfortunately, We Treat the Chart:" sources of stigma in mental health settings. Psychiatry Q 80(1):55–64
Flanagan EH, Pavlo A, Corrigan PW, Link BL, Davidson L (2016a) Understanding clinician stigma: clinician, service user, and community member perspectives. In preparation
Flanagan EH, Pavlo A, Davidson L (2016b) The experience of stigma in a community mental health center: consumer and clinician perspectives. In preparation
Gonzales L, Davidoff KC, Nadal KL, Yanos PT (2014) Microaggressions experienced by persons with mental illnesses: an exploratory study. Psychiatr Rehabil J 38:234–41
Link BG, Phelan JC (2001) Conceptualizing stigma. Annu Rev Soc 27:363–385
Link BG, Phelan JC, Bresnahan M, Stueve A, Pescosolido BA (1999) Public conceptions of mental illness: labels, causes, dangerousness, and social distance. Am J Public Health 89(9):1328–1333
Link BG, Yang LH, Phelan JC, Collins PY (2004) Measuring mental illness stigma. Schizophr Bull 30(3):511–541
McLellan AT, Lewis DC, O'Brien CP, Kleber HD (2000) Drug dependence, a chronic medical illness: implications for treatment, insurance, and outcomes evaluation. JAMA 284(13):1689–1695
Penn DL, Guynan K, Daily T, Spaulding WD, Garbin CP, Sullivan M (1994) Dispelling the stigma of schizophrenia: what sort of information is best? Schizophr Bull 20(3):567–574
Rogers ES, Chamberlin J, Ellison ML, Crean T (1997) A consumer-constructed scale to measure empowerment among users of mental health services. Psychiatr Serv 48(8):1042–1047
Schulze B (2007) Stigma and mental health professionals: a review of the evidence on an intricate relationship. Int Rev Psychiatry 19:137–155. doi:10.1080/09540260701278929
Stuber JP, Rocha A, Christian A, Link BG (2014) Conceptions of mental illness: attitudes of mental health professionals and the general public. Psychiatr Serv 65:490–7
Sue DW, Capodilupo CM, Torino GC, Bucceri JM, Holder A, Nadal KL, Esquilin M (2007) Racial microaggressions in everyday life: implications for clinical practice. Am Psychol 62(4):271

Stigma and the Renaming of Schizophrenia

32

Toshimasa Maruta and Chihiro Matsumoto

Introduction

Schizophrenia is a common disease with a prevalence rate of 1 %. Worldwide, roughly 24 million people suffer from it. The condition, initially coined "dementia praecox" by Kraepelin, was later termed "schizophrenie (schizophrenia)" by Bleuler, and the name has been used for over a century. In recent years, however, there has been a discussion whether schizophrenia, the disorder label, should be reconsidered.

This movement has supposedly been influenced by a situation in Japan, where in 2002, the Japanese Society of Psychiatry and Neurology (JSPN) changed the name for the condition from "seishin-bunretsu-byo (mind-split disease)" to "togo-shitcho-sho (integration disorder)." This also impacted on its surrounding countries, where Chinese characters are similarly used in their languages. The renaming movement in Japan was favorably received by the patients and their families, which supposedly is also an encouraging factor. As we are witnessing the revision of the two international classifications of mental disorders in the current decade, the USA and Europe are likely to take account of the situation in Japan.

In this article, an overview of the situation concerning renaming will be provided, and expectations will be discussed.

The original version of this chapter was revised.
An erratum to this chapter can be found at DOI 10.1007/978-3-319-27839-1_38

T. Maruta (✉)
Health Management Center, Seitoku University,
Iwase 550, Matsudo City, Chiba Prefecture, 271-8555, Japan
e-mail: maruta@seitoku.ac.jp

C. Matsumoto
Department of Psychology, Rikkyo University,
1-2-26 Kitano, Niiza-shi, Saitama, 352-8558, Japan

© Springer International Publishing Switzerland 2017
W. Gaebel et al. (eds.), *The Stigma of Mental Illness - End of the Story?*,
DOI 10.1007/978-3-319-27839-1_32

The Renaming Movement in Japan

In Japan, the term "seishin-bunretsu-byo (mind-split disease)" was accepted as an official translation for schizophrenia by the terminology committee formed within the JSPN in 1937, and it has been used ever since. In 1993, the National Federation of Families with Mentally Ill in Japan (NFFMIJ) submitted a petition to the JSPN to request the renaming for the following reasons: The term "seishin-bunretsu-byo" (1) gives an impression of an incurable disease, depriving the patients and their families of hope; (2) is socially burdened with stigma; and (3) after renaming, the disorder is becoming more treatable, including improved treatment outcomes (Sato 2006). Upon receiving this request, the terminology committee took the petition into consideration. Of note, in 1997, before the renaming was officially approved, Koishikawa et al. (4) reported that "only 16.6 % of the patients and 33.9 % of their families were able to report the diagnosis accurately" (Koishikawa et al. 1997).

In 1999, Ono et al. (1999) reported that "52 % of JSPN Council members informed their patients only occasionally on a case-by-case basis of the diagnosis of schizophrenia, and only 7 % of them informed all their patients of the diagnosis". Thirty-seven percent of the members informed only the patients' families.

In 1996, the terminology committee decided on the following principles upon discussing the new disorder name: the new term should (1) not result in any social disadvantage to the patients; (2) reflect the concept of schizophrenia; (3) not intend to represent the disease entity, but its syndrome; (4) be easy to understand; and (5) be distinguished from other disorders. The committee frequently held face-to-face meetings, and ultimately, the following three terms became the final candidates: "togo-shitcho-sho (integration disorder)," "sukizofurenia (a form of a loan word)," and "Bleuler Disease." Members of the JSPN were requested to comment on those three candidates, and at the JSPN General Assembly, "togo-shitcho-sho (integration disorder)" was voted as the new term to replace the old one. The new term was publicly promoted at the 12th International Congress of the World Psychiatric Association, and a month later, the approval by the Japanese government followed.

While it is widely known that the renaming took place in Japan, what is less known is the fact that the renaming was intended to coincide with an introduction of a new conceptualization of the illness. According to Sato (2002, 2015), following the renaming from "seishin-bunretsu-byo (mind-split disease)" to "togo-shitcho-sho (integration disorder)", the following changes were promoted: the concept from "dementia praecox (disease)" to "clinical entity (syndrome)", etiology from "endogenous" to "vulnerability to schizophrenic episode", pathophysiology from "unknown to "neurotransmitter dysfunction", axis I and II from "same dimension" to "different dimensions", diagnosis from "psychopathology" to "a theoretical in etiology", outcome from "untreatable" to "treatable", psychoeducation from "difficult" to "easy", and treatment from "somatic treatment" to "comprehensive treatment".

The Situation in Asian Countries

Some countries, besides Japan, that use Chinese characters also seem to be moving toward renaming.

In Korea in 2012, the Korean Psychiatric Association changed the term of schizophrenia from "jeongshin-bunyeol-byung (mind-splitted disorder)" to "johyun-byung (attunement disorder)" (Kim et al. 2012). The old term was heavily loaded with prejudice against the patients and their caregivers, as well as mental health professionals. Also, the old term was often confused with dissociative identity disorder. Commenting on the new term, Lee et al. reported that "Johyeon literally means 'to tune a stringed musical instrument'. In the context of schizophrenia, attunement is a metaphor for tuning the strings of the mind" (Lee et al. 2013).

In China, the corresponding term for schizophrenia is "jing shen fen lie zheng (mind-split disease)", which is seen as highly stigmatizing and as yet is still in use. In order to approve a new medical term in China, the decision would have to go through various channels such as associations and committees in a hierarchical manner, which could hinder the renaming movement (Sartorius et al. 2014).

In Hong Kong, "jing shen fen lie (splitting of mind)" still remains in use, but also a new term "si jue shi tiao" has been introduced. This new term denotes "dysfunction of thought and perception" and also indicates an increased treatability. While it has not been empirically shown that the new term will reduce stigma, the new one is likely to gain awareness (Sartorius et al. 2014; Ouyang and Yang 2014).

In Taiwan, the Taiwanese Society of Psychiatry changed the term form "jing shen fen lie zheng (mind-split disease)" to "si jue shi tiao zheng (dysfunction of thought and perception)" in 2014.

At the moment, no similar renaming movement is observed in Singapore (Sartorius et al. 2014).

The Situation in the USA and Europe

There are researchers and organizations that advocate for renaming in the US and Europe as well. Table 32.1 shows the terms that have been proposed to replace schizophrenia, showing the increasing interest in renaming in mainly the US and Europe.

This trend may be partially due to the *Diagnostic and Statistical Manual of Mental Disorders, Fifth Edition* (DSM-5), recently published by the American Psychiatric Association, and the soon-to-be completed International Classification of Diseases and Related Health Problems, 11th Revision (ICD-11) by the World Health Organization. The DSM-5 is a classification system intended to be used primarily within the USA, published in May 2013, and naturally it largely reflects the scientific findings and opinions from the USA. In contrast, the implementation of the ICD-11 is to be preceded by the approval of the World Health Assembly in 2017, allowing for further discussion on the topic. Also, by nature, the ICD-11 is expected to reflect more international perspectives.

Table 32.1 Proposed alternatives for the term "schizophrenia"

Proposed names	Author(s)
Kraepelin-Bleuler disease	Kim and Berrios (2001)
Dopamine dysregulation disorder	Sugiura et al. (2001)
Neuro-emotional integration disorder (NEID)	Levin (2006)
Salience (dysregulation) syndrome	van Os (2009a, b)
Youth onset conative, cognitive, and reality distortion syndromes (CONCORD)	Keshavan et al. (2011)
Dysfunction perception syndrome (DPS)	George (2012)
Bleuler's syndrome	George (2012), Henderson and Malhi (2014), and Lasalvia et al. (2015)
Psychosis susceptibility syndrome (PSS)	George and Klijn (2013a, b)

Modified table, originally extracted from Lasalvia et al. (2015)
Gathered from literature published in European and North American countries

Lasalvia et al. (2015), having reviewed existing literature, summarize the pros and cons of renaming schizophrenia. The pros include that the new term will (1) be more acceptable for users, (2) be more acceptable for professionals, (3) improve the public image of the disorder and of people suffering from it, and (4) give a more realistic picture of the condition, providing hope and promoting recovery. On the other hand, the cons include that renaming would (1) lead to disagreement among professionals and hinder diagnostic communication, (2) give rise to confusion in the public, (3) wrongly suggest that some fundamental truth about schizophrenia has been newly discovered, (4) be only semantics, and (5) have the effort to blame the person rather than the illness. Thus, renaming schizophrenia is a complex issue.

In the Netherlands, "Anoiksis," a completely consumer-run association of people with chronic psychoses or schizophrenia, not a group of researchers, has been actively advocating renaming (George 2012; George and Klijn 2013a, b). Their activities resemble those taken by the NFFMIJ in Japan, which eventually brought around the renaming. Unfortunately, no activities of similar nature and size have been reported from the US or other parts of Europe.

Two Surveys Conducted by the Authors

The authors have conducted two surveys concerning renaming of schizophrenia (Maruta et al. 2008, 2014). The results of the surveys are briefly described below.

Study 1 was carried out in 2006. In addition to sociodemographic information, our questionnaire included other questions and space for comments. This questionnaire was sent to 80 members of the Section on Classification, Diagnostic Assessment, and Nomenclature of the World Psychiatric Association, using the 2006 member list. We sent a questionnaire by e-mail or, if an e-mail address was not identified, by hard copy. Twenty-one (26.3 %) responded, from Kenya, Nigeria, Egypt, the UK, Switzerland, Germany, the Czech Republic, Italy, South Korea,

Japan, the US, Canada, Nicaragua, Cuba, Brazil, and Argentina. The mean length of careers of the respondents as a psychiatrist was 32 years (SD = 14 years).

Study 2 was carried out in 2013, using a modified version of the questionnaire used in the first study. We surveyed the members of the Section on Schizophrenia of the World Psychiatric Association ($N=35$) and those of the European Psychiatric Association ($N=44$). The memberships of 13 individuals were found to overlap, and their response was treated as that of one respondent. The questionnaire was sent via e-mail to 66 members, of which 38 members (57 %) responded. The mean length of their career as a psychiatrist was 25 years (SD = 11 years).

On the results of Study 1, the most remarkable finding was that 45 % answered "no" to the question (appropriateness of the term "schizophrenia"). In addition, half of the respondents considered that the term "schizophrenia" had a stigmatizing meaning. Among them, 60 % agreed on the need for a name that would reduce stigma.

As alternative terms for schizophrenia, the following suggestions were proposed: integration disorder, integrative disorder, disintegrative disorder, schizophrenic syndrome, non-affective psychotic disorder, detachment syndrome with dissociative features, "flat" psychosis, monoamine dysregulation disorder, connecting disorder, chronic detachment syndrome, multi-symptomatic psychosis, and processing disorder. On the other hand, as alternative terms for schizoid, they suggested introvert, isolation, or pseudo-dissociative, while for schizotypal they suggested odd or eccentric or post-detachment.

In Study 2, the idea of renaming seemed somewhat supported, with 57 % of the respondents expressing their opinion that the term "schizophrenia" was not appropriate. A total of 84 % of such individuals thought schizophrenia denoted stigma, 72 % of whom explicitly supported renaming schizophrenia. Concerning the timing of renaming, 57 % of the respondents thought that it would be desirable to bring about the change by the publication of the 11th revision of the ICD (ICD-11) (Table 32.2).

In addition to appropriateness of the term and possible timing for renaming, respondents were asked about possible alternatives. They were divided into five categories (Table 32.3).

In addition, Table 32.4 shows possible alternatives for schizoid and schizotypal.

When asked about the rational to support renaming, the respondents mainly provided the following reasons: The term schizophrenia is extremely stigmatizing and imposes a great deal of psychological burden on the patients and their families, and it does not represent the fundamental nature of the condition. In contrast, those who were against renaming mentioned that a premature renaming before successfully elucidating the nature of the condition would cause confusion, that renaming alone would not eliminate stigma, that the stigma does not come from the name itself, and that the English term, namely, schizophrenia, is not causing as much stigma as the Chinese character-based ones, which happened to be bad translations to begin with.

Furthermore, when asked whether the new term should convey an acceptable scientific concept, the respondents stated that treatment outcomes of the illness have improved recently, and it is no longer an untreatable disorder as commonly perceived. The concepts promoted by Kraepelin, Bleuler, and their followers are to blame for stigma, and that the stigma can be removed by improving the treatment outcomes, not just a renaming.

Table 32.2 Questionnaire as used in Study 2

	Yes	No
1. How long have you been working as a psychiatrist?		
2. Do you use the term "schizophrenia" or its equivalent in your language when you explain the diagnosis to the patient?	28	10
3. If you do not use the word "schizophrenia", please write the term you use and which language it is		
4. Do you think that the term "schizophrenia" is an appropriate term for the disorder?	16	21
5. Do you think that the term "schizophrenia" denotes stigma?	31	6
6. *If you answered "yes" to No. 5*, should "schizophrenia" be changed to another term, to reduce stigma?	21	8
7. In your language, is the term "schizophrenia" concordant with the meaning of "split-mind disease"?	28	5
If you answered "no" to No. 7, what does it mean in English?		
8. In your country or in your main psychiatric society, is there any action or movement to change the term "schizophrenia"?	4	34
9. *If you answered "yes" to No. 6*, please mark when it should be changed		
(a) As soon as possible	5	–
(b) By the publication of ICD-11	12	–
(c) Later	3	–
(d) Did not answer "yes" to Q.6	1	–
10. *If you answered "yes" to No. 6*, what term do you think is more appropriate than the current term, i.e., "schizophrenia"? Please provide your suggestions below		
11. Should the new name convey an acceptable scientific concept or concepts?	27	4
12. *If you answered "yes" to No. 11*, what scientific concept(s) should be reflected?		
13. *If you answered "no" to No. 11*, why do you not think so?		
14. Do you think that the terms "schizoid" and "schizotypal" should also be changed?	17	20
15. For question 14, if you answered "yes", what terms do you think are more appropriate instead of the terms "schizoid" and "schizotypal"? Please write your suggestions below		

This questionnaire is a modified version of the first study's questionnaire and includes the distribution of responses, regarding the term "schizophrenia". Participants were 38 members of the section "schizophrenia" from both the World Psychiatric Association (WPA) and the European Psychiatric Association (EPA)

Study 2 was conducted seven years after Study 1. In Study 1, to the question "Do you think that the term 'schizophrenia' is an appropriate term for the disease," less than half of the respondents answered negatively; in contrast, more than half did so in Study 2. The participants of Study 1 were primarily classification experts, whereas those of Study 2 were primarily schizophrenia experts, which discourages a simple comparison. Even so, the sheer increase in the response rate (from 26 % to 57 %) seems to indicate a heightened awareness of the issue.

Table 32.3 Terms for schizophrenia as recommended by the participants of Study 2

Proposals
I. After a person's name
Bleuler's syndrome
Eugen Bleuler's syndrome
Schneider's syndrome
Kraepelin disease
John Nash's syndrome
II. Referring to
1. An integration failure
Disintegration disorder
Disintegration disorder of brain
Brain disintegration disorder
Integration disorder
Integrative mental disorder
Mind integration failure disorder
Salience dysregulation syndrome
2. An organization failure
Brain tuning disorder
Discoordination disorder
Dysfunctional thought disorder
Disorganized disorder
Disorganized thinking disorder
Thought disorder
3. A neurodevelopmental process
Developmental psychosis
Neurodevelopmental psychosis
Neurodevelopmental vulnerability disorder
Vulnerability based psychosis
Social brain disorder
III. Others
Idiopathic psychosis
Idiopathic (or primary) psychosis
Endogenous psychosis
Psychosis
Psychosis spectrum disorder
Non-affective (enduring) psychosis
Dopamine dysregulation disorder

See Table 32.2 – question 10

Table 32.4 Terms for schizoid and schizotypal as recommended by the participants of Study 2

Associated to both (schizoid and schizotypal)	Associated to one in particular
Alienated	Kretschmer's disorder (personality)
Dys-social	Social anhedonia (schizoid)
With restricted affect	Introversive (schizoid)
With eccentric thinking	Psychotic personality disorder (schizotypal)
Anhedonic	Distinctive (schizotypal)
Psychotic spectrum personality disorders	
Minor psychotic disorders	
Psycho-introverted	
Unbalanced	
Disintegrated	

See Table 32.2 – question 15

Summary

The movement of renaming schizophrenia, which largely originated from Japan and Southeast Asia, is now drawing international attention. As described above, one can infer that it has much to do with the upcoming publication of the ICD-11. Schizophrenia is among the cardinal mental disorders, which explains the high interest.

Renaming has drawn various opinions. The utmost significance of renaming resides in reducing stigma that is associated with the condition and removing obstacles for those trying to reach mental health care. Perhaps the translation of schizophrenia in Chinese character-based languages, including Japanese, was not appropriate. At that time, the translation was done without a perspective of or for the patients and their families, thereby lacking an insight into how the disorder label might impact them, and with very scarce scientific knowledge about the pathology. While the etiology of schizophrenia still remains largely unknown, today we know much more, which seems to encourage revisiting the term for the condition in question. It is most likely that renaming per se will do very little to remove stigma, but it will certainly serve as a first step. Very recently, upon the Ebola outbreak, the WHO issued a statement to discourage use of names of animals, locations, or persons in the terms for newly identified diseases, highlighting the impact that disease labels can carry.

The choice of a new name should be made in consultation with the patients and their families, not just with mental health professionals, as it was done in Japan. In Study 2, described above, when asked whether the new name should convey an acceptable scientific concept, many experts felt so. While larger-scaled studies are needed to say anything conclusive, it is apparent that a new name, if and when renaming does take place, needs to be accompanied by a new concept. To help reduce stigma, public education will also be imperative.

The ICD-11 is expected to receive the WHO's approval in 2017. With less than 2 years until the completion of the ICD-11, it is unclear whether we can reach a consensus about the renaming of schizophrenia in time. While the revision of the

ICD has fueled the discussion, even if the ICD-11 ends up adopting schizophrenia as its predecessors did, renaming of schizophrenia should be continuously debated, so that the stigma associated with the name and the condition will be reduced and the patients and their families will feel more hopeful.

References

George B (2012) What's in a name? Stigma Res Action 2:119–122

George B, Klijn A (2013a) A modern name for schizophrenia (PSS) would diminish self-stigma. Psychol Med 43:1555–1557

George B, Klijn A (2013b) A sweeter smelling rose: a reply to our commentators. Psychol Med 43:2015–2016

Henderson S, Malhi GS (2014) Swan song for schizophrenia? Aust N Z J Psychiatry 48:302–305

Keshavan MS, Nasrallah HA, Tandon R (2011) Schizophrenia, "Just the Facts" 6. Moving ahead with the schizophrenia concept: from the elephant to the mouse. Schizophr Res 127:3–13

Kim Y, Berrios GE (2001) Impact of the term schizophrenia on the culture of ideograph: the Japanese experience. Schizophr Bull 27:181–185

Kim, SW, Jang, JE, Kim, JM et al. (2012) Comparison of stigma according to the term used for schizophrenia: split-mind disorder vs attunement disorder. J Korean Neuropsychiatr Assoc. 51: 210–217

Koishikawa H, Kim Y, Yuzawa C et al (1997) Investigation of the consciousness of the patients and families about the given information of the disease. In: Uchimura H (ed) Studies on clinical features, treatment, and rehabilitation of schizophrenia. Ministry of Health and Welfare, Tokyo (in Japanese)

Lasalvia A, Penta E, Sartorius N, Henderson S (2015) Should the label "schizophrenia" be abandoned? Schizophr Res 162(1–3):276–284

Lee YS, Kwon JS (2011) Renaming schizophrenia. J Kor Neuropsychiatr Assoc 50:16–19

Lee YS, Kim JJ, Kwon JS (2013) Renaming schizophrenia in South Korea. Lancet 382(9893):683–684

Levin T (2006) Schizophrenia should be renamed to help educate patients and the public. Int J Soc Psychiatry 52:324–331

Maruta T, Iimori M (2008) Schizo-nomenclature: a new condition? Psychiatry Clin Neurosci 62:741–743

Maruta T, Volpe U, Gaebel W, Matsumoto C, Iimori M (2014) Should schizophrenia still be named so? Schizophr Res 52:305–306

Ono Y, Satsumi Y, Kim Y, Iwadate T, Moriyama K, Nakane Y, Nakata T, Okagami K, Sakai T, Sato M, Someya T, Takagi S, Ushijima S, Yamauchi K, Yoshimura K (1999) Schizophrenia: is it time to replace the term? Psychiatry Clin Neurosci 53(3):335–341

Ouyang WC, Yang YK (2014) Renaming schizophrenia in far east Asian countries. Taiwan J Psychiatry 28:63–64

Sartorius N, Chiu H, Heok KE, Lee MS, Ouyang WC, Sato M, Yang YK, Yu X (2014) Name change for schizophrenia. Schizophr Bull 40(2):255–258

Sato M (2006) Renaming schizophrenia: a Japanese perspective. World Psychiatry 5(1):53–55

Sato M (2015) www.jspn.or.jp/modules/activity/index.php?content_id=77. (Cited on 2nd of June, 2015, in Japanese)

Sato M (2002) Togo-Shitcho-Sho. What is changed from split-mind-disease. Special committee report. Jpn Soc Neurol Psychiatry (in Japanese)

Sugiura T, Sakamoto S, Tanaka E, Tomoda A, Kitamura T (2001) Labeling effect of Seishin-bunretsu-byou, the Japanese translation for schizophrenia: an argument for relabeling. Int J Soc Psychiatry 47:43–51

van Os J (2009a) A salience dysregulation syndrome. Br J Psychiatry 194:101–103

van Os J (2009b) 'Salience syndrome' replaces 'schizophrenia' in DSM-V and ICD-11: psychiatry's evidence-based entry into the 21st century? Acta Psychiatr Scand 120:363–372

Trialogue: An Exercise in Communication Between Users, Carers, and Professional Mental Health Workers Beyond Role Stereotypes

33

M. Amering

"Nothing About Us Without Us"

The reality of "Nothing About Us Without Us" seems to have arrived and is irreversibly here to stay: no policy development, no amendment of legislation, or elaboration of new regulations shall be undertaken without including experts in their own right, persons with a lived experience of mental health problems and services. Whether the Mental Health Action Plan for Europe, the WHO Global Mental Health Action Plan, or the recommendations of the first trialogic task force of the World Psychiatric Association (WPA) providing for a partnership with users of services and their families and friends (Wallcraft et al. 2011), the call for "user involvement," a "partnership approach," or participatory approach is evidence that henceforth no significant development can be advanced without the meaningful involvement of experts in their own right.

In many ways the first human rights treaty of the twenty-first century epitomizes the essentials of recovery orientation. Forged between diplomats and a throng of civil society representatives – many of them persons with disabilities as experts in their own right, including those with psychosocial disabilities (Sabatello and Schulze 2014) – the treaty is the product of a truly participatory process. In a corresponding logic, it makes the consultation of its constituency – persons with disabilities and their representative organizations, respectively – an obligation: "In the development and implementation of legislation and policies to implement the present Convention, and in other decision-making processes concerning issues relating to persons with disabilities, States Parties shall closely consult with and actively

M. Amering
Department of Psychiatry and Psychotherapy, Medical University of Vienna,
Waehringer Guertel 18-20, 1090, Vienna, Austria
e-mail: michaela.amering@meduniwien.ac.at

© Springer International Publishing Switzerland 2017
W. Gaebel et al. (eds.), *The Stigma of Mental Illness - End of the Story?*,
DOI 10.1007/978-3-319-27839-1_33

involve persons with disabilities, including children with disabilities, through their representative organizations" (Article 4 Para 3 CRPD).

Such participation is a response to the growing understanding of the impact of decades of societal and therewith structural exclusion. It is, however, also a key method to enable genuine autonomy for a societal group that has been largely ostracized from mainstream society and frequently been subject to various forms of paternalism, neglect, and oftentimes violence in different forms. Ensuring equality for persons with disabilities thus necessitates an intervention into the composition and structures of debates and decision-making processes. Interactions have to be re-tooled based on the understanding that disablement is importantly a result of social and attitudinal barriers of the mainstream. Stereotypes, prejudices, and imagery of disability are the main hurdles that need to be overcome.

"Fix Society, Not People"

"Fix society, not people," captures the core of the Convention (Schulze 2014). The focus on the perceived deficits of a person has to be replaced by an understanding that impairment is "an evolving concept" and, importantly, one that is far more defined by the attitudes of society than the impairment as such. New forms of interaction and negotiation strategies emerged from the process toward the UN Convention for the Rights of Persons with Disabilities. Maya Sabatello and Marianne Schulze's book (2014) on how the CRPD came to be gathers exciting accounts about new strategies and forms of communication and negotiation. Two aspects stand out in relation to the topic of Trialogue. Firstly, the notion that *everyone* ultimately has an intimate interest in upholding disability rights" as disability is viewed as "an integral part of common human experience" (Sabatello 2014). Based on the prevalence rates for disabilities across the life span, clearly, almost everybody will have either personal lived experience or experience within the group of family and friends. Secondly, the acknowledgment of the fact that many diplomatic delegations and civil rights organizations "simply lacked the expertise, knowledge, and understanding to properly address the needs of persons with disabilities" and the willingness to learn from organizations and people with a lived experience background highlights an urgent need for change with regard to communication skills. Despite difficult circumstances from financial to organizational matters, the inclusion of persons with disabilities into the negotiation process was furthered by their great engagement as well as welcomed by different United Nations bodies. These historical developments lead to new and essential opportunities of impact and were successful in breaking down existing barriers: "the proportion of delegates with disabilities at the AHC (*Ad Hoc Committee*) simply made the phenomenon impossible to ignore" (Sabatello 2014). Among the resulting "new diplomacy" strategies, abstract legal terminology was importantly amended by communications that were able "to challenge their imagination, as if it all happens to them" (Grandia 2014) and "providing first-hand testimonies of persons with disabilities who experienced discrimination and who could point to what should have been done differently": "With hundreds of persons with disabilities in the UN corridors, in the negotiating room, in the various meetings, and in the cafeteria" ... "it became impossible to avoid a dialogue" (Sabatello 2014).

Never again letting the dialogue breakdown had been an essential goal of the creators of Trialogue and the Trialogue movement. The experience of the worst forms of human rights violations, including forced sterilization and the murder of people with disabilities, especially also people with mental health problems, at the time of the Nazi regime in Germany had motivated the survivor Dorothea Buck. She talks about how she *experienced the psychiatric system as so inhumane, because nobody spoke with us. A person cannot be more devalued than to be considered unworthy or incapable of conversation.* This very notion brought it about that in the 1980s Mrs. Buck shared her ideas about the need to prevent such inhumane conditions with Thomas Bock and Ingeborg Esterer and as a consequence the Trialogue was born (Bock et al. 2000). "Trialogue" stands for communication among and between the three main groups of individuals who deal with psychiatric problems and disorders and with the mental health system – people with experiences of severe mental distress, family members/friends, and mental health professionals. Trialogue encounters occur under special conditions – outside familial, institutional and therapeutical hierarchies, and clinches. Trialogue group participants meet on neutral ground and communicate on equal footing.

An illustration of the historical context and the difficulties of speaking to each other openly and on eye level is the fact that for the first time only decades after the atrocities, in the year 2010, during its annual congress in November, did the German Association for Psychiatry and Psychotherapy ask the victims and relatives of the victims for forgiveness (www.dgppn.de/english-version/history/psychiatry-under-national-socialism.html). In his speech the president of the association Frank Schneider said among many other things:

> *I stand before you today as President of an association that has taken nearly 70 years to end this silence and recall the tradition of enlightenment through science in which it stands.*
> *...... At this point I would like to express my admiration for Dorothea Buck. The sculptor and author, who was herself one of the victims, co-founded the "Federal Organisation of (Ex-) Users of Psychiatry" in Germany. She has tirelessly dedicated herself to raising awareness of the issues and to ensuring that they are not forgotten.*
> *..... In the name of the German Association for Psychiatry and Psychotherapy, I ask you, the victims and relatives of the victims, for forgiveness for the pain and injustice you suffered in the name of German psychiatry and at the hands of German psychiatrists under National Socialism, and for the silence, trivialisation and denial that for far too long characterised psychiatry in post-war Germany.*

In Austria the similarly difficult process of ending the silence following the same atrocities was greatly enhanced by the efforts of Harald Hofer, a prominent user/survivor activist. He focused in a commemorative speech 1995 on a *conspiracy of indifference* as the obstacle to recognizing victims of discrimination and exclusion not only historically but also today (Hofer 1997). He also was a founding member of the First Vienna Trialogue in 1994 (Amering et al. 2002).

The Trialogue Experience: An Exercise in Communication Between Service Users, Families, and Friends and Mental Health Workers on Equal Footing

What is true for the hope-inspiring historical firsts of the negotiation processes and the "new diplomacy" in the context of the UN Convention on the Rights of Persons with Disabilities (Sabatello 2014) as well as for trying to overcome the silence after a history of horrific crimes and discrimination against persons with disabilities is of course strongly related to the communication between the Trialogue partners everywhere: we need to learn new forms of communications, a language that allows us to interact in a context of nondiscrimination.

Trialogue groups are training grounds for working together on an equal basis. It is a new and exciting form of communication, a chance to interact beyond role stereotypes, and an opportunity to gain new insights and knowledge. Participants learn to accept each other as "experts by experience" and "experts by training." In other words Trialogue participants acquire skills that are well suited to recovery-oriented and rights-based work as well as to participatory approaches in therapeutic and service development decisions as well as policy developments (Amering and Schmolke 2009).

"Trialogue" stands for the encounter of the three main groups of individuals who deal with psychiatric problems and disorders and with the mental health system – people with experiences of severe mental distress, family members/friends, and mental health professionals – on equal footing (Amering et al 2012). This encounter occurs under special conditions – outside the family, outside psychiatric institutions, and outside a therapeutic setting. Trialogue facilitates communication about the personal experiences in dealing with psychiatric problems and disorders and their consequences. Participants of diverse experience backgrounds – lived experience as users and carers as well as professional working experience in mental health services – strive toward giving up their isolation and lack of common language. Mutual understanding and necessary delimitation from the vast variety of the participants' different backgrounds concerning experience and knowledge are to be established. Trying to understand and share the complex and very heterogeneous subjective experiences leads toward establishing a common language, in which different forms of expertise and experience of participants of the three groups can be exchanged. For any particular topic of discussion, a wealth of knowledge and experience is brought to exchange and provides a comprehensive resource for problem solving. Every participant has the chance to observe different interpretations of similar roles in participants of his or her own groups as well as of the other two groups. Subjective views can be complemented by objective knowledge and put into perspective of different interpretations and handling of similar experiences. Thus a skill base for effective forms of collaborations can be acquired, which then extends its value into other situations, like clinical encounters or problem solving within family life as well as working together on different levels of policy development and decisions.

The "First Vienna Trialogue" was established after the World Conference for Social Psychiatry in Hamburg in 1994 by a small group of people representing users, relatives, and professionals. Since then, Trialogue meetings are being held twice a month with 10–40 people in attendance. In the beginning, the meetings were only publicized verbally, followed by newspaper ads and announcements within user- and professional organizations. Trialogue is an *open group* – everyone interested in participating is welcome. It was our experience from the start that users formed the largest share of regular participants, followed by family members and friends and professionals (social workers, psychologists, nurses, patient's advocates, guardians, psychiatrists). As an open group, the number of attendants and the compositions of members from the three groups vary each time, and there is a mix of regulars and of those who drop by to see what the group is like. During the time of the group's existence, the venue of meetings has changed a couple of times. For many years now, the Trialogue groups in Vienna enjoy the hospitality of a highly reputed adult education facility. Besides financial considerations, we strived toward finding a place outside psychiatric institutions, unaffiliated with a particular self-help organization and apart from therapeutic or family relations thus offering a *neutral ground* that does not offer an advantage or a privilege for any of the participating groups. For the same reason, we prefer a rotating system of different members in the role of moderator to a model of professional moderation.

Psychosis Seminars

The role model for the "First Vienna Trialogue" was the psychosis seminar in Hamburg. Currently, over 150 of these seminars can be found in Germany, some of them using different names such as "exchange of experiences with psychosis" or "from dialogue to trialogue" and some in Switzerland and Austria. As a result of a meeting of many different members of such groups, a team of people began to evaluate the results of the psychosis seminars and published a guideline (Bock et al. 2000).

The published accounts of our experience of the first years of Trialogue (Amering et al. 2002), which we reported in a trialogic format, were meant to demonstrate how new, different, extraordinary, and unusual this type of encounter is. We emphasize the unique personal and professional learning opportunities it engenders as well as highlight the difficulties that can arise when you engage in a Trialogue as a whole person, start to accept the different members of the group as equally entitled experts, and try not to avoid relevant conflicts of interest. However, when we encourage taking Trialogue seriously, we also point out all the fun that it brings. *There is much laughter within the Trialogue, which is seen as a powerful remedy* is one important conclusion by a mother talking about her experiences as a Trialogue group member.

Trialogues and psychosis seminars usually take place weekly, biweekly, or monthly and last between 90 and 120 min (often including a short break). Attendees vary between 10 and 60 people. Ideally there should be an about equal number of participants from the groups of professionals, users, and carers. Community, education, or communication centers are well-suited locations. Trialogue groups are moderated. Moderators can be recruited from all three attending groups. They can rotate or stay stable for some agreed time. Rules concern mainly that only one person should be speaking at a time and that personal information disclosed should not be spread outside the group. Participants may introduce themselves with their full name and identify themselves as belonging to one of the groups. However, this is not necessary if anonymity is desired.

A few years ago, a woman and a man attended a Trialogue by mistake of entering the wrong room. They had nothing to do with mental health issues, but during the group exchange about a specific psychotic experience of one of the participants, the woman, who used the chance to talk about her hurtful experiences with her sister, got very emotional and was supported by the group. At the end of this particular Trialogue group, she and her husband thanked the group and expressed that they had not yet encountered a social environment that granted them such freedom of expression and thus, was such a relief for a big problem that had been waiting to be formulated and shared for a long time.

The above example illustrates the exceptional nature of the communication possible within the Trialogue framework and its opportunities to reach out to people outside the psychiatric subculture in the wider community. More specifically, the experience gained in Trialogue groups is also extremely useful for people who want or need to engage into policy activities that need the participation of all three groups represented in Trialogue, like serving on quality control boards of psychiatric services, in advisory groups for planning and evaluating psychiatric services, in anti-stigma and anti-discrimination initiatives, and in all sorts of other much-needed advocacy activities.

Research

One may conclude that Trialogue groups have been widely established with a wealth of practical experiences and anecdotal evidence for positive effects in all three participating groups and on their efforts to collaborate more successfully. Yet, the effects have only rarely been systematically studied. One reason might be that they represent an unconventional setting, which is in line with neither the didactic approaches of psychoeducation nor the usual rules of group psychotherapy. However, there are strong indications that all participants do gain in knowledge and that language and communication style develops and therapeutic effects can be documented.

Bock und Priebe describe in their 2005 publication characteristics, history, and possible benefits of psychosis-seminars and trialogue groups (Bock and Priebe, 2005). From a lot of experience and from the few data on psychosis seminars, in Germany it looks like:

- Many participants are characterized by a lot of experience, often over many years.
- Main benefits for carers stem from gaining knowledge, sharing experience, and being able to discuss concrete issues they struggle with within their family with persons, who know similar situations from their own experience, but with whom they are not intimately entangled through emotional and biographical bonds.

- Consumers benefit from respect for their psychotic experiences and a chance to make sense of these and other experiences in their personal social and biographical context.
- Professionals value not only the opportunity to gain new insights into the experience of psychiatric problems but also review their role and their practices in new and comprehensive perspectives.
- Many attendants share the wish to improve current psychiatric practices and advance the concepts of mental illness and health.

The European Families Organization (EUFAMI 2003) recommend Trialogue groups also for those outside German-speaking countries. Looking at example of topics covered by Trialogue groups does lend credit to the idea that people all over the world might benefit from such exchanges:

- Stigma and discrimination
- Work and social integration
- Power, powerlessness, and empowerment
- The family doctor as a Trialogue partner
- From dialogue to trialogue – where are the professionals?
- The "good" psychiatrist – users' and relatives' perspectives
- When help has more unwanted than wanted effects
- Diagnosis as a trap – being put in a box
- Religion and psychosis
- False hopes for recovery and healing
- Day clinics – why so few?
- Clinical and field trials – experimenting with patients
- Silent users – who is helping them?
- From aftercare to prevention – easy access to early help

A recent mixed method study of a newly emerging Trialogue in Berlin (von Peter et al. 2015) clearly showed that communication in Trialogue groups is considerably different from communication in clinical encounters. All three groups cherish and aspire to interest for each other, goodwill, and openness. Daily clinical routine with role prescriptions, power balance, and constant pressure to act is experienced as an obstacle. Sadly, professionals feel that they cannot be the persons they want to be in their working environments. And that they are not empowered to change this situation, which certainly is a source of disappointment when realized by family carers and users of these services. Users and ex-users describe the healing effect of creating a narrative in a public environment and are willing to allow insights into their lived experience thus enabling family carers, friends, and mental health workers to better understand and cope with difficult situations. Family carers worry that their own family member with a psychiatric diagnosis might have more serious problems than the users or ex-users attending the Trialogue. They appreciate the chance to pose their questions to somebody with a lived experience, who is not their own relative, and they do feel empowered to keep up the hope also after long times of great difficulties through the stories of their Trialogue partners with similar experiences.

Trialogue is found to facilitate a discrete and independent form of communication and acquisition and production of knowledge. Trialogue groups seem to be experimental grounds, teaching participants how to develop equal relationships.

The group around Thomas Bock in Hamburg has developed an instrument to measure subjective experience and meaning of psychoses: the German Subjective Sense in Psychosis Questionnaire (SUSE) involving user and professional experience (Klapheck et al. 2012). They used this instrument as well as measurements of coping and recovery to assess quite large groups of Trialogue participants with user, family carer, and psychiatric professional backgrounds. Results show a positive effect on Trialogue participants with experience of psychosis either themselves or as carers with regard to a more positive attitude toward symptoms, less anxiety and better sense of coherence, as well as wider mutual understanding, and more empowerment for everybody (Ruppelt et al. 2014).

International Developments

Trialogue experiences in other parts of the world have shown impressively how the Trialogue setting has very similar effects in different cultures. Trialogue meetings at WPA Congresses in recent years in Istanbul, Buenos Aires, and Beijing (Amering 2010) invariably resulted in animated discussions that were characterized by an openness and mutual appreciation of diverse experiences and positions. Considerable interest and energy toward implementing and sustaining a setting that regularly allows such moving and richly informative exchanges were expressed.

This is in line with WPA's work in its first trialogic working group within the framework of the WPA Action Plan 2008–2011. The Task Force on Best Practice in Working with Service Users and Carers under the leadership of Helen Herrman published its recommendations to the international mental health community in 2011 (Wallcraft et al. 2011). The ten recommendations call for a partnership approach on all levels of mental health policy and care and *promote shared work worldwide to identify best practice examples and create a resource to assist others to begin successful collaboration*. In consultation with the task force, the WPA Committee on Ethics drafted a paragraph based on these recommendations that has been unanimously endorsed as an amendment to its Madrid Declaration on Ethical Standards for Psychiatric Practice by the WPA General Assembly in 2011.

Trialogue meetings in North America have in the past often been difficult due to long-standing conflicts between the user and survivor movement geared toward alternatives to the biomedical model and families looking for best practice in professional help for their relatives. A commitment to trauma-informed language and communication styles for Trialogues has been identified as an important prerequisite for talking openly to each other, especially in the face of the growing database on the association of different diagnoses from the psychosis spectrum and traumatic life histories of people affected (e.g., Schaefer and Fisher 2011).

Growing international interest has led to the recent establishment of Trialogue groups in Poland, French-speaking Switzerland, France, Greece, and Ireland. The

Mental Health Trialogue Network Ireland (MHTNI) is an exciting new community development initiative in Irish mental health and will also serve as a web base for international exchange on Trialogue in the future (www.trialogue.co). The aim of the Irish Network was to *empower communities in Ireland to become proactive in communicating about mental health through a powerful open dialogue and participatory process called Trialogue.* Project leaders talk about how *in the past mental health was often seen as the domain of service providers, carers, and the people who used the mental health services. However, within communities there is a huge diversity of knowledge and experience that can be used to transform our services.*

This aspect highlights the possible effects of Trialogues on the wider communities over time. Trialogue groups can serve large part of communities. Reaching out to everybody with a firsthand lived experience – that is a lot of people as we know from epidemiological research – friends and family – is there anybody who is not at some point during their life? – and people working in mental health and mental health-related fields, Trialogue really does not leave nobody out. Consequently, if a community can use the learning opportunities that Trialogue provides, expertise with successful interventions with regard to secondary and tertiary prevention for persons with mental health problems could grow. Such growing capacity is likely to profit also in terms of primary prevention for the wider community. Learning about mental health and illness and helping community members with mental health problems can strengthen communities' mental health capacities and improve mental health literacy for everybody. The currently often hidden knowledge of a large part of the community – namely, that of families and friends of people with mental health problems as well as the expertise of those who are dealing with or have overcome such problems in their own lives – can be validated and shared for the benefit of all.

References

Amering M (2010) Trialogue in Beijing – meeting of Chinese and international users, carers and mental health workers beyond role stereotype. WPA NEWS, Sept 2010, p 15 http://www.wpanet.org/uploads/Newsletters/WPA_Newsletter/Past_Issues/news3-2010.pdf

Amering M, Schmolke M (2009) Recovery in mental health. Reshaping scientific and clinical responsibilities. Wiley-Blackwell, London

Amering M, Hofer H, Rath I (2002) The "First Vienna Trialogue" – experiences with a new form of communication between users, relatives and mental health professionals. In: Lefley HP, Johnson DL (eds) Family interventions in mental illness: international perspectives. Praeger. S, Westport, pp 105–124

Amering M, Mikus M, Steffen S (2012) Recovery in Austria: mental health trialogue. Int Rev Psychiatry 24(1):11–18

Bock T, Priebe S (2005) Psychosis seminars: an unconventional approach. Psychiatr Serv 56(11):1441–1443

Bock T, Buck D, Esterer I (2000) Es ist normal, verschieden zu sein. Psychose-Seminare & Hilfen zum Dialog. Arbeitshilfe 10. Psychiatrie Verlag, Bonn

EUFAMI (2003) Trialogue: the benefits of three-way communication. www.eufami.org

Grandia L (2014) Imagine: to be part of this. In: Sabatello M, Schulze M (eds) Human rights & disability advocacy. University of Pennsylvania Press, Philadelphia, Pennsylvania

Hofer H (1997) Die Verschwörung der Gleichgültigkeit. In: Smekal C, Hinterhuber H, Meise U (eds) Wider das Vergessen. VIP-Verlag, Innsbruck

Klapheck K, Nordmeyer S, Cronjäger H, Naber D, Bock T (2012) Subjective experience and meaning of psychoses: the German Subjective Sense in Psychosis Questionnaire (SUSE). Psychol Med 42(1):61–71

Mental Health Trialogue Network, Ireland (retrieved on 090216) www.trialogue.co

Psychiatry under National Socialism – Remembrance and Responsibility (retrieved on 090216) www.dgppn.de/english-version/history/psychiatry-under-national-socialism.html

Ruppelt F, Klapheck K, Bock T (2014) Erfolgreiche Evaluation: Psychoseseminare stärken Sinnsuche und Genesung. Soziale Psychiatrie 145:28–31

Sabatello M, Schulze M (eds) (2014) Human Rights & Disability Advocacy. University of Pennsylvania Press, Philadelphia, Pennsylvania

Schulze M (2014) The Human Rights of Persons with Disabilities. In: Mihr A, Gibney M (eds) The SAGE Handbook of Human Rights Volume 1. SAGE, Thousand Oaks, CA

Schäfer I, Fisher HL (2011) Childhood trauma and posttraumatic stress disorder in patients with psychosis: clinical challenges and emerging treatments. Curr Opin Psychiatry 24(6):514–8

von Peter S, Schwedler H_J, Amering M, Munk I (2015) This Openness Must Continue – Changes Through Trialogue Identified by Users, Carers, and Mental Health Professionals. Psychiatr Prax 42(7):384–91

Wallcraft J, Schrank B, Amering M (2009) Handbook of service user involvement in mental health research. Wiley-Blackwell, London

Wallcraft J, Amering M, Freidin J, Davar B, Froggatt D, Jafri H, Javed A, Katontoka S, Raja S, Rataemane S, Steffen S, Tyano S, Underhill C, Wahlberg H, Warner R, Herrman H (2011) Partnerships for better mental health worldwide: WPA recommendations on best practices in working with service users and family carers. World Psychiatry 10(3):229–236

Empowerment and Inclusion: The Introduction of Peer Workers into the Workforce

34

Geoff Shepherd and Julie Repper

History and Background

The idea that people with mental health problems may receive support from others who share their experiences has a long history in mental health services (Davidson et al. 2012). For example, Davidson notes how Pinel and his colleagues, working in the Bicetre hospital in Paris at the end of the eighteenth century, were convinced that a major factor in the reform of mental health care must be the employment of people with '*lived experience*'. '*As much as possible, all servants are chosen from the category of mental patients. They are at any rate better suited to this demanding work because they are usually more gentle, honest and humane*' (Jean Baptiste Pussin in a letter to Pinel, 1793, quoted in Davidson et al., p. 123). With the advent of more medical models of mental illness, the use of peer support in hospitals declined in the later part of the nineteenth century as the mental health professionals – medical, nursing, psychology, social work – established themselves. It made a reappearance in the 1960s and 1970s in the therapeutic community movement, with a renewed emphasis on the potential of peers to help one another (Campling 2001). Now peer support is popular again, with more than half of the US states making it billable under Medicaid and trained peer workers being employed in many countries all over the world (Repper 2013a; Slade 2009).

G. Shepherd (✉)
ImROC Programme, Centre for Mental Health,
134-138 Borough High Street, London SE1 1LB, UK

Department of Health Services and Population Research,
Institute of Psychiatry, University of London, London, UK
e-mail: geoff.shepherd@centreformentalhealth.org.uk

J. Repper
ImROC Programme, Centre for Mental Health,
134-138 Borough High Street, London SE1 1LB, UK

© Springer International Publishing Switzerland 2017
W. Gaebel et al. (eds.), *The Stigma of Mental Illness - End of the Story?*,
DOI 10.1007/978-3-319-27839-1_34

In the UK, peer support has long played a central role in voluntary sector and user-led services/groups (Basset et al. 2010; Mental Health Foundation 2012; Scottish Recovery Network 2011, 2012) but peer worker roles in statutory services have been slower to develop (Rinaldi and Hardisty 2010). Nevertheless, the English Department of Health has recognised that peer support can play an important role in providing individualised support, facilitating self-management, aiding prevention and reducing health inequalities (Department of Health 2010, 2011). It also recommends peer support as a potentially important route whereby people with mental health problems can participate in paid employment. The recent Schizophrenia Commission report (2012) specifically recommends that, '*all mental health providers should review opportunities to develop specific roles for peer workers*' (p. 35).

What Is Peer Support?

Before going any further, we should define what we mean by '*peer support*' and review the different types of peer support that have been developed. Peer support may be defined simply as, "offering and receiving help, based on shared understanding, respect and mutual empowerment between people in similar situations" (Mead et al. 2001). Thus, it occurs when people share common concerns and draw on their own experiences to offer emotional and practical support to help each other move forwards. Peer support encompasses a personal understanding of the frustrations sometimes experienced with the mental health system and serves to reframe recovery as making sense of what has happened and moving on, rather than identifying and eradicating symptoms and dysfunctions (Adams and Leitner 2008; Bradstreet 2006). It is through this trusting relationship, which offers companionship, empathy and empowerment, that feelings of isolation and rejection can be replaced with hope, a sense of agency and belief in personal control. '*I wanted to be able to show people that however low you go down, there is a way up, and there is a way out…. The thing I try to install is, no matter where you are, if you want to get somewhere else you can, there's always a route to get to where you want to be*' (*Peer support worker, Nottingham Healthcare*).

The shared experiences of peers in mental health settings are most commonly their mutual experiences of distress and of surviving trauma. However, it is not always enough for them simply to tell their stories. Support is often most helpful if both parties have other things in common such as cultural background, religion, age, gender and personal values (Faulkner and Kalathil 2012). The peers from user-led groups interviewed by Faulkner and Kalathil also found that relationships were more supportive if both people were willing both to provide *and* receive support and had gained some distance from their own situation so that they were able to help each other think through solutions, rather than simply give advice based on their own experiences. For these reasons, training, supervision and support are essential for peer workers employed in services (see section "Characteristics of effective peer support" below).

There are several different ways in which peer workers can be employed within mental health services. For example, they may work in *dedicated peer support teams*, responding to referrals for peer support from clinical teams (Repper and Watson 2012). In this arrangement they are likely to be used as a source of specialist advice for the local mental health service regarding recovery-focused practices such as WRAP, or other forms of personal recovery planning. They may also contribute to service-wide functions, e.g. speaking at staff induction, reviewing policy documents, undertaking quality assurance exercises, providing mentorship for staff, etc.

Alternatively, they may be employed *alongside traditional staff in existing teams* (inpatient or community) to bring a specific focus on the needs of service users. In inpatient settings they may facilitate early discharge, using their experiences to help the person identify and prioritise goals and develop their own control and self-management strategies. Working closely with the professional staff team can help ensure that the person does not spend any longer in hospital than they need to and is best prepared for managing their own condition on discharge. Peer workers are also in a good position to work flexibly across boundaries, liaising with staff in community teams, to help the person engage with follow-up supports. For example, they may improve the benefits of outpatient appointments by helping the service user think through their questions and concerns prior to the appointment and how best to convey these to the professional thus facilitating a '*shared decision making*' approach (SAMSHA 2010; Torrey and Drake 2009). One of the most important roles for peer workers in community teams is to facilitate social inclusion by using their personal knowledge of the local community to identify resources and activities which might help the person and then supporting them to engage by accompanying them until they are confident to attend alone (Repper and Watson 2012).

Whatever the form of peer support or the nature of the role, there are a number of core principles that peer support workers should aim to maintain. These are summarised in Box 34.1. These principles can be used to guide training and supervision and to maintain the integrity of the peer role wherever they are located and whoever employs them.

Effectiveness and Cost-Effectiveness

Despite considerable interest in introducing peer workers into the workforce in recent years, the evidence for their effectiveness is limited. There have been few randomised controlled trials those which have been performed often evaluate very different forms of peer support. Not surprisingly, meta-analytic reviews which restrict themselves to randomised controlled trials tend to come up with rather negative results (Pitt et al. 2013; Evans et al. 2014). However, other reviewers who have also considered non-RCT evidence, including '*grey*' as well as published literature, present a more positive picture (Davidson et al. 2012; Repper and Carter 2011; Trachtenberg et al. 2013; Warner 2009). Not surprisingly, because of the variable quality of the evidence and the use of different samples, different

Box 34.1: The Core Principles of Peer Support (From Repper 2013a, Reproduced with Permission)

Mutual	The experience of peers who give and gain support is never identical. However, peer workers in mental health settings share some of the experiences of the people they work with. They have an understanding of common mental health challenges, the meaning of being defined as a '*mental patient*' in our society and the confusion, loneliness, fear and hopelessness that can ensue.
Reciprocal	Traditional relationships between mental health professionals and the people they support are founded on the assumption of an expert (professional) and a nonexpert (patient/client). Peer relationships involve no claims to such special expertise, but a sharing and exploration of different world views and the generation of solutions together.
Non-directive	Because of their claims to special knowledge, mental health professionals often prescribe the '*best*' course of action for those whom they serve. Peer support is not about introducing another set of experts to offer prescriptions based on their experience, e.g. "You should try this because it worked for me". Instead, they help people to recognise their own resources and seek their own solutions. "Peer support is about being an expert in not being an expert and that takes a lot of expertise" (Recovery Innovations, 2007)
Recovery focused	Peer support engages in recovery-focused relationships by: Inspiring *HOPE*: they are in a position to say '*I know you can do it*' and to help generate personal belief, energy and commitment with the person they are supporting Supporting people to take back *CONTROL* of their personal challenges and define their own destiny Facilitating access to *OPPORTUNITIES* that the person values, enabling them to participate in roles, relationships and activities in the communities of their choice.
Strengths based	Peer support involves a relationship where the person providing support is not afraid of being with someone in their distress. But it is also about seeing within that distress the seeds of possibility and creating a fertile ground for those seeds to flourish. It explores what a person has gained from their experience, seeks out their qualities and assets, identifies hidden achievements and celebrates what may seem like the smallest steps forward.
Inclusive	Being '*peer*' is not just about having experienced mental health challenges, it is also about understanding the meaning of such experiences within the communities of which the person is a part. This can be critical among those who feel marginalised and misunderstood by traditional services. Someone who knows the language, values and nuances of those communities obviously has a better understanding of the resources and the possibilities. This equips them to be more effective in helping others become a valued member of their community.
Progressive	Peer support is not a static friendship, but progressive mutual support in a shared journey of discovery. The peer is not just a '*buddy*', but a travelling companion, with both travellers learning new skills, developing new resources and reframing challenges as opportunities for finding new solutions.
Safe	Supportive peer relationships involve the negotiation of what emotional safety means to both parties. This can be achieved by discovering what makes each other feel unsafe, sharing rules of confidentiality, demonstrating compassion, authenticity and a nonjudgemental attitude and acknowledging that neither has all the answers.

reviewers come to slightly different conclusions. Nevertheless, a number of consistent findings do emerge.

- In no study has the employment of peer support workers been found to result in worse health outcomes compared with those not receiving the service. Most commonly the inclusion of peers in the workforce produces the same or better results across a range of outcomes.
- The inclusion of peer support workers tends to produce specific improvements in patients' feelings of empowerment, self-esteem and confidence. This is usually associated with increased service satisfaction.
- In both cross-sectional and longitudinal studies, patients receiving peer support have shown improvements in community integration and social functioning. In some studies they also bring about improvements in self-reported quality of life measures, although here the findings are mixed.
- In a number of studies when patients are in frequent contact with peer support workers, their stability in employment, education and training has also been shown to increase.

As indicated, some of these findings are not replicated across all studies and the overall methodological quality of the evidence is limited. Nevertheless, the general findings of an increased sense of empowerment and positive benefits in terms of social inclusion are consistent.

Regarding cost effectiveness, Trachtenberg et al. (2013) examined a sample of outcome studies ($n=6$) which aimed to evaluate whether the introduction of peer support workers into community crisis teams or acute inpatient wards reduced the use of hospital beds either by preventing or delaying admissions to a hospital, or by shortening the length of inpatient stays. Across the studies, the average benefit/cost ratio (taking into account sample size) was more than 4:1. Thus, the estimated financial value of cost savings in terms of reduced inpatient bed days consequent upon introducing peer workers was very significant. This was a small study, but the results provide preliminary support for the proposition that adding peer support workers to existing mental health teams result in cost savings. This conclusion is echoed in a recent review commissioned by the UK charity Rethink (2014) from the Personal Social Services Research Unit, led by Professor Martin Knapp, at the London School of Economics. They suggest, '*An approach which may also in time offer the biggest scope for cost savings in mental health care is to promote and expand co-production, drawing on the resources of people who are currently using mental health services, for example in peer support roles*' (p. 6).

In addition to these benefits for people receiving this kind of support, there is also evidence of benefits for the peer workers themselves. They feel more empowered in their own recovery journey and have greater confidence and self-esteem and feel more valued (Mowbray et al. 1998; Repper and Carter 2011; Salzer and Shear 2002). They also acquire a much more positive sense of identity. As one of the peer workers in the ImROC programme said, '*I work hard to keep myself well now, I've got a reason to look after myself better…. It's made a real big difference to me you know, just contributing something, to them. You know and hopefully changing their lives for the better'.*

Finally, our recent experience with the ImROC (Implementing Recovery through Organisational Change) programme is that the introduction of peer workers is a powerful way of driving a more recovery-focused approach within the whole organisation (Shepherd et al. 2010). Just as peer workers provide hope and inspiration for service users, so they challenge negative attitudes of staff and provide an inspiration for all members of the team. They provide a living example that people with mental health problems can make a valued contribution to their own and others' recovery if they are given the opportunity (Repper and Watson 2012). As this team leader said, *'The values and leadership of consumers are driving the shift from a system focused on symptom reduction and custodial care to self-directed recovery built on individual strengths'.* This specific impact on organisations is common among services where peer workers are introduced but, to our knowledge, it has not been formally investigated. We shall return to this theme later.

To summarise, there is reasonably good evidence to support the idea that the introduction of peer workers, alongside other traditional mental health staff in the workforce, may have significant benefits in terms of increasing feelings of empowerment and social inclusion both for those receiving the service and for those delivering it. Furthermore, there is some evidence that the introduction of peers into the workforce may be highly cost-effective. There is also evidence that there are benefits for the organisations in which they operate in terms of inspiring a more positive, *'recovery-oriented'* approach. Of course, these kinds of benefits do not happen automatically. They requires a high quality implementation of the intervention and there is still considerable variability in what kind of support is provided. This lack of standardisation of the *'independent variable'* undoubtedly accounts for some of the variability in outcomes. So, can we specify in more detail the nature of effective peer support?

Characteristics of Effective Peer Support

As part of the ImROC programme, we now have experience in supporting the development of more than 300 peer posts (Shepherd in press). On the basis of this experience we can begin to identify some the key characteristics of effective peer support. (This section is based on one of the ImROC Briefing papers, Repper (2013b) and this text is reproduced with permission).

When developing peer worker posts, it is useful to think of four sequential phases. The first involves *preparation* – of the organisation as a whole, of the teams in which peers will be placed and, obviously, of the peers themselves. The second involves *recruitment* of trained peers to the posts that have been created. Given the likelihood that peer applicants may have not worked for some time, nor been through an interview process with all of the formalities and checks that this brings, this whole process needs careful support. Thirdly, there is the safe and effective *employment* of peer workers in mental health organisations. Finally, the *ongoing development* of peer worker opportunities and contributions needs to be considered in the context of the wider healthcare system and the changing culture of services. These different phases are summarised in Box 34.2 below.

Box 34.2: Developing Peer Worker Posts: 4 Phases (Reproduced from Repper 2013b, with Permission)

1. Preparation
   - Preparing the organisation
   - Preparing the teams
   - Defining roles
   - Common myths and misperceptions
   - Preparing the peer workers (training)
   - Developing job descriptions and person specifications
2. Recruitment
   - Advertising
   - Benefits advice
   - Applications
   - Interviews
   - Occupational health
   - CRB checks
   - Supporting people who are not offered posts
3. Employing peer workers
   - Selecting placements
   - Induction/orientation
   - Supervision and support
   - Staff myths
4. Ongoing development of the role
   - Career pathways
   - Training opportunities
   - Wider system change

Preparation

The development of peer worker posts must begin with consideration of the context in which they will be employed. A local project/steering group therefore needs to be established and its membership should include representatives from the various parts of the organisation that will be affected – e.g. HR, management, professional groups, communications, etc. It is also important to include people who use the services, their family and friends and members from relevant local partner organisations.

This group then needs to work through a number of critical issues, beginning with the fundamental questions, '*Why do we want to employ peers?*' and '*What differences do we hope they will make?*' In the current climate, it is particularly important to be aware of the danger of creating peer support roles for the sole purpose of saving money, or simply to carry out tasks that other staff are unwilling to do. The vision for peer workers needs to be communicated to all relevant departments and teams with an invitation to find out more, or to get involved for those who are interested. A variety of communication methods will be necessary to achieve this, including workshops, information days, staff briefings, newsletters, etc. Potential peer workers should be involved directly in all these initiatives. Once committed, the organisation then needs to address a number of key organisational processes.

(a) *Human Resources (HR)* – At the heart of establishing successful peer support worker programmes will always be the support of HR departments (indeed, some of the most successful schemes have been led by HR professionals). Ensuring that HR colleagues understand the aims and philosophy of peer support workers and are in a position to offer their guidance regarding recruitment, job descriptions, interviewing, supervision, etc. is therefore essential. If people are to be employed in '*proper*' jobs, then they will need '*proper*' job descriptions and person specifications. These should be developed locally.

(b) *Workforce Planning* – Predicting the future balance of traditional professionals and peer workers is a key problem. No one believes that peers could – or should – replace *all* professionals, but there is an issue of balance to be resolved. What should this be? Local services need to agree local targets and prepare to work towards them. In Nottinghamshire Healthcare Trust (England) the aim has been expressed in terms of at least two peer workers (not necessarily full-time) in every clinical team. This may require a process of consultation with local trade unions to help them see the benefits for staff inherent in these new developments.

(c) *Occupational Health (OH)* – Occupational health services have a critical role to play in providing advice regarding appointments of new staff (peers) and return-to-work plans for peers who have periods of absence due to recurrence of illness. Although the same rules should apply to peer workers as to other staff, OH clinicians may be particularly anxious regarding fitness and '*return-to-work*' issues when the person is known to have had mental health problems and is returning to work in a mental health service setting. They may also be unfamiliar with the concept of '*reasonable adjustments*' to the workplace as applied to people with mental health issues (*see* Perkins et al. 2009). Members of the project team will therefore have to ensure that OH colleagues are fully involved in the project from the outset and that their continuing input is secured.

(d) *Facilities* – Peer support workers will need their own base for meeting, peer supervision, informal support and to complete records. This should be close to their workplace but not necessarily based in the clinical teams.

(e) *Finances/Management* – If new posts are to be created, or existing posts redefined, this may have financial and other management implications. Funding needs to be identified to cover basic salary and '*on-costs*', recruitment, training, peer-led advice/supervision, relief cover, travel, administration and equipment costs. If comprehensive costs are not identified at the beginning of the project they will inevitably return to haunt the project team at a later date.

(f) *Involving Staff 'Learning and Development Units'* – The employment of peer workers may create new opportunities for learning and development departments to work collaboratively with peers in developing and delivering training to a variety of staff groups (and groups outside the organisation, e.g. police, GPs, etc.).

(g) *Developing Relationships with Local Social Services Departments and Non-statutory Partners* – Peers' roles may usefully cross over boundaries between services, so any steering group is likely to need to include relevant partner organisations. For example, social services departments may provide funding for joint training; local peer-led or voluntary sector organisations might be involved in the preparation, training and supervision of peers. This is particularly important in the early stages of the project as user-run organisations may have considerable existing experience relating to the topic and may be able to provide advice, support and active collaboration regarding training and supervision. However, if not handled sensitively, it may also give rise to conflicts.

Once established the Project Group then needs to develop a clear plan, within the identified financial envelope, with specific actions, accountabilities and timescales. Of course, this will change as the project evolves, but clear planning at this stage is essential to keep the project '*on track*'. It may be assisted by having some external monitoring of progress.

If the introduction of peer workers is to be successful then the teams where they are to be placed have to be prepared. The whole team must understand and (hopefully) own the process and in several pilot studies it has been reported that they are less likely to be successful or effective in teams that are not already working in a recovery-focused manner and not committed to engaging with peers as team members (Repper and Watson 2012; Scottish Recovery Network 2011). Therefore, it is strongly recommended that teams in which peer workers are placed have already accessed training in recovery-focused practice and have a commitment to making the service more recovery focused (e.g. have used the '*Team Recovery Action Plan*', Repper and Perkins 2013).

In practical terms, it is most helpful if the team is given an opportunity to try out working together. This can be done in a training day in which everyone meets and considers the role of peer support and how it differs from other roles in the team. Team members also need the opportunity to hear the experience of peer workers and mental health practitioners from other teams where they have been successfully introduced. They should be encouraged to discuss their hopes and concerns honestly and to develop a sense of collective ownership of the relative roles and responsibilities of peer workers in their own, specific, team context. In these meetings it is helpful if senior managers can also attend (at least partly) to provide reassurance, answer questions and confirm that there is a commitment to these developments from the '*top*'.

Next we must consider the training of workers. '*The Peer Support Training took me on a massive journey of discovery about myself and gave me an appreciation for my strengths. Through it came to realise that all those scary places I had been during my time of being unwell, were going to allow me to hold up a torch for others during their dark times and help them on their road to recovery – it wasn't wasted time*' (cited in Pollitt et al. 2012). Although peer worker training has been developed and delivered in several different countries and settings, there is a reasonably high degree of consistency across the content of the course the style of teaching and intended learning outcomes. The core skills required are active listening and problem solving, clarity about how to facilitate recovery and the role and relationships of the peer worker. Courses therefore generally cover communication skills (particularly active listening), mutual problem solving/solution focused skills, WRAP, managing challenging situations, valuing difference, code of conduct and ethical considerations, team working and managing personal information/telling your own story. Most courses are very much '*strengths based*' and also place emphasis on students learning from one another how to support recovery using an interactive format. Marked differences exist in the intensity ('*depth*') of the teaching and length of courses (from a few days to several weeks). Some courses are linked to formal accreditation with local Colleges of Further Education, some are not. With such a wide range of training it is not surprising that the outcomes of peer workers have often been highly variable. However, at the moment, there are no empirical grounds for deciding between different training options.

Recruitment

Recruitment begins with advertising. There is no simple answer regarding how best this is done. Prospective peer workers who are not in active contact with specialist mental health services are unlikely to read professional journals and may not access newspapers, so other options for local publicity may need to be considered (e.g. direct communication with local user groups). But simply contacting local user groups may exclude many people who have experience of mental health problems, who have not chosen to join a local group. These processes of how and where to advertise therefore needs careful consideration and a relevant local strategy developed accordingly. Whatever the advertising strategy decided upon, local '*orientation sessions*' for prospective candidates are a useful way of providing information. They can also be used as part of a '*preselection*' process.

Whatever the recruitment process it is important to provide financial advice for potential applicants in terms of the possible effects of employment on their social security pensions. The benefits system is usually complicated and highly individual, so it is important for applicants to get an expert, personal '*back to work*' calculation. If this is not provided, many good candidates may be significantly deterred from applying.

Because of the nature of the likely applicants, it is also necessary to consider how best to support them in the recruitment process. Some applicants may have been out of employment for some time and will lack the confidence and skills to apply. Applications can be particularly challenging for people who have spent time in the hospital, homeless, or in prison. The process usually assumes familiarity with IT, an ability to explain interruptions in employment and housing, and to answer questions about criminal history. All of these can be very off-putting and may constitute a real barrier to the very people who could be most helpful peers – those having most in common with the average person using services. Support for prospective applicants can be provided either within the organisation or delivered by a partner agency specialising in employment support.

Given the complex and sensitive nature of the role, applicants need to be interviewed to assess their baseline communication skills, their understanding of recovery and their ability to share constructively their own journey and what helps them to stay well. These interviews can be conducted on an individual or group basis. They can take the form of role play interviews which allow relationship and communication skills to be observed.

In most countries peer support workers – like any other new employee – will need to complete some kind of check regarding possible criminal record (CRB). Criminal record checks can be very stressful for peer applicants and they may need help to complete the relevant forms. In England the NHS is clear that it cannot employ people who have a serious criminal history, but it is not unusual for applicants to peer posts to have a record of minor crime and some discretion is given to the appointing authority. The challenge for the service is therefore to assess the risk involved in employing this particular person and to make judgments about the likelihood of criminal acts being repeated. This has to be undertaken on a case-by-case basis and the decision needs to take into account the seriousness of the offence, when it occurred, and its potential relevance to the role. Some decisions will be easy, some will not. Where the incidents are clearly related to periods of mental ill-health, it is easier to put safeguards in place to prevent reoccurrence. However, where the incidents are more serious, more frequent, or unrelated to periods of mental instability, then it may be more difficult to identify triggers and develop effective safety plans. The employing organisation therefore needs to be clear at the outset how these decisions will be taken and by whom.

If the person is then offered a position in a local service then, in England, occupational health colleagues need to come back into the process to ascertain if the successful applicant requires any *'reasonable adjustments'* under the provisions of the *'Disability and Discrimination Act'* (HMG 1995, 2005). In this context, *'reasonable adjustments'* might include:

- Specifying work hours to take account of particular problems with early mornings, rush hour traffic, or side effects of medication
- Offering support with aspects of the role that are particularly difficult due to nature of mental health challenges (e.g. sealing envelopes may be difficult for people who feel compelled to check)
- Increasing feedback to people who tend to repeatedly worry over possible mistakes ensuring that they are thoroughly debriefed at the end of each shift.

These kinds of simple changes may be crucial to helping people with psychiatric disabilities function in these new roles.

Finally, we need to consider how best to support unsuccessful candidates. Following an intensive training programme, people will naturally feel despondent and their confidence will drop if they are unsuccessful in their job interview. It is therefore very important to discuss thoroughly with the person the reasons for not appointing and to explore alternative options. For some this will take the form of further interview practice, for others a period working as a peer volunteer, or doing some courses in the recovery college might be more appropriate.

Employment

So, we come to the phase of actual employment, again a number of elements need to be considered. First, the choice of initial placement: where there is a choice, peers can be allocated according to their personal attributes, experiences and preferences. Certainly, at least in the beginning, it is sensible to place peers in teams that already actively support recovery and are keen to welcome these new colleagues. It is not a good idea to choose the most difficult place to start.

It is also worth thinking more broadly than simply matching people in terms of the peer's mental health problems with the peers to be worked with. By placing a peer with a specific diagnosis on a unit that specialises in this particular set of difficulties, there is a danger of perpetuating a narrow diagnostic categorisation. Of at least as much value is the placement of a peer in a team that has identified a gap in certain skills or interests that the peer can fill (e.g. membership of a particular age or ethnic group). Wherever possible peers should be placed in groups of at least two per team, with some overlapping working hours. This will help prevent isolation, provide support and help create a greater impact on the team culture.

There are specific issues if the peer is placed in a team that is currently providing her mental health support or has done so in the recent past. There are advantages (e.g. she/he can be an inspirational role model for other peers and staff) and disadvantages (e.g. she/he is seen as '*special*' and not like other patients). These issues need to be discussed with the peer worker and the staff together and a joint decision reached.

In terms of induction for new peer workers, it is helpful to allocate a staff mentor to each peer (possibly the team recovery champion) to provide information, support and to give informal tips about routines and informal procedures ('*how we do things around here*'). The mentor is also then in a good position to help set up an induction plan. Many peer workers – just like other staff – find adjusting to the demands of a new and complex organisation quite stressful. '*Returning to work was a daunting issue in itself and it became clear that peers need tailored support during this period. Even though I described processes such as sickness reporting, how to apply for annual leave, using information systems, whereabouts sheets, client records, etc.*

many times; for some peers embedding this into their everyday working life proved very difficult. Even basic tasks like organising telephones and computer access and how to obtain diaries, keys, 'pigeon holes', etc. was time consuming and the team would have benefitted from a slow induction period to ensure that each peer was fully confident and familiar with these processes before they started working' (Peer support team coordinator, Nottingham).

Once they have begun to settle in, the questions of supervision and support then need to be addressed. Supervision and support is vital for peers – just as it is for other staff – and, ideally, this should be provided through a combination of *'managerial'* supervision (from the team leader or a care coordinator) and *'professional'* supervision (from a senior peer or through contact with a group of peer workers). Individual and group supervision offer opportunities to model and practice the principles of mutuality: sharing strategies, challenges and successes, developing skills, knowledge and expertise in the group and creating confidence that difficulties are not unique and can be overcome.

The value of bringing all peer workers together for group supervision and mutual support cannot be overestimated. Once together, peers become more confident about sharing their hopes, fears, their personal stories and challenges. As a group they gain strength and solidarity, they can support each other effectively and solve problems together. Even when peers are working in separate parts of the service, it is a good idea to bring them together from time to time so that they can continue to develop their identity and retain clarity about their distinctive contribution.

There are some aspects of peer working that need particular attention. These are specific to the role and do not lend themselves to clear rules or *'black and white'* solutions. First, there is a big difference between telling your own story in the classroom setting and using your experience to build a relationship with someone who you are supporting. Peer workers often need additional support in the early days to clarify their own boundaries and develop a personal account or narrative that feels safe. The second challenge lies in their double role and identity as both a *'practitioner'* (staff) and a *'patient'* (service user). Peers may be accustomed to relating to mental health workers as *'the expert'* (sometimes the *'enemy'*) but not as a colleague with whom they can work as equals, in a relationship based on mutual respect. Similarly, they are more used to relating to service users as friends, rather than peers, so it can be challenging for them to maintain professional boundaries.

While peer workers can find it difficult to separate their role as practitioner from their role as *'patient'*, staff seem to find this even more difficult. Too often the challenges reported by peer workers focus on their problems gaining the respect of staff. In some instances staff are reluctant to refer to peers, unclear about what peer workers offer, lacking in confidence that peer workers can cope with people who might present complex challenges. Staff will have many said and unsaid fears and anxieties about the introduction of peers and these have to be addressed. Some of the common myths and misinterpretations are shown in Box 34.3.

Box 34.3: Common Myths and Misperceptions About Peer Workers (From Repper 2013b)

Myth #1 – Peer support is just a way of saving money.

Myth #2 – Peers will be too fragile, they are likely to *break down* at work.

Myth #3 – Peers cannot be expected to conform to usual standards of confidentiality.

Myth #4 – There is no difference between Peer support workers and other staff who have personal experience of mental health problems.

Myth #5 – The presence of peer support workers will make staff worried about *saying the wrong thing*.

Myth #6 – The only way to be sure of getting a job these days is to say you have a mental health problem.

Myth #7 – Peers get to do all the nice things – talking to patients, taking them out, going home with them – the rest of us have to do the boring admin and medication, handing out meals, making beds etc.

Myth #8 – Peers don't know the difference between friendships and working relationships.

Myth #9 – Peers will be subversive, they will be *anti-psychiatry* and *anti-medication*.

Myth #10 – Peers will take up so much time that traditional staff roles will be made much harder, not easier.

Myth #1 – Peer support is just a way of saving money. As indicated earlier, this is where many of the debates about peer support workers generally begin. We have argued elsewhere that promoting recovery requires a great deal more than traditional therapeutic approaches (Repper and Perkins 2003: Shepherd et al. 2008). Providing hope, helping people make sense of their lives, finding meaning in what has happened, helping people take control over their destinies and manage the challenges of everyday life: these do not require professional expertise. Those who have faced similar challenges are often far better equipped to support these endeavours. To extend the domain of professionals to span all facets of life both deskills everyone else – friends, families, carers – it is also wasteful of the considerable resources involved in training and employing specialist professionals. The use of peer support workers is simply an attempt to complement these *'professional'* skills with *'life experience'* so as to ensure that both are provided (hopefully in at least equal measure) in the most cost-efficient way. It is clearly *not* simply a case of *'saving money'*.

Myth #2 – Peers will be too fragile, they are likely to 'break down' at work. People with lived experience of mental health challenges have long been employed in mental health services in a variety of positions from clinicians to managers, it is just that they seldom disclose this fact. Does this mean that all these workers are *'too fragile'* and *'likely to break down'*? The evidence actually suggests that, if provided with appropriate support, employees with mental health challenges may take *less* time off sick than those without (Perkins et al. 2000).

Myth #3 – Peers cannot be expected to conform to usual standards of confidentiality. Anyone working in a mental health service – from statutory to voluntary to peer-led will be required to observe formal rules relating to confidentiality. Peer workers are no different. Indeed, because of their lived experience, peer workers are often particularly sensitive to issues relating to confidentiality. Indeed, our experience is that issues of confidentiality have been more frequently raised by peer workers complaining about other staff breaching confidentiality by chatting about the clients with whom they work outside the workplace.

Myth #4 – There is no difference between employing peer support workers and employing other staff who have personal experience of mental health problems. Peer workers are employed *because of* their personal experience of mental health issues in the belief that with proper training and support they can use these experiences to help others. A psychologist, or a psychiatrist or a nurse with their own lived experience is primarily employed because of their professional qualifications and experience – although their personal experience will, hopefully, help to improve their professional role. Introducing peer workers into the workforce does, of course, raise the issue of how best to support people in traditional professions who have their own lived experience. They often fear discrimination and exclusion if they disclose their history. However, acknowledging their additional experience is not only *'healthy'* in terms of recognising the reality of human experience for both staff and service users, it can also enhance the quality of the service by encouraging traditional mental health staff to use this experience to inform their work.

Myth #5 – The presence of peer support workers will make staff worried about 'saying the wrong thing'. Everyone, peer or professional, has, at some time, said or done something that they later regret. Without the capacity for humility – and the courage to accept and accommodate feedback to reflect on our behaviour – any relationship, whether it is between partners, friends or the providers of services, is likely to break down. Thus, the willingness to reflect and learn from our behaviour is a key process for improving the quality of interactions and most groups have some mechanisms (formal or informal) for reflecting on these problems as they arise. As indicated, opportunities for supervision and reflection on practice are therefore an essential and necessary aspect of good practice.

Myth #6 – The only way to be sure of getting a job these days is to say you have a mental health problem. Within mental health services many types of expertise are required: professional expertise, expertise resulting from experience outside the mental health arena, and the expertise of lived experience of mental health challenges, trauma and recovery. To date, pride of place in mental health services has been accorded to professional expertise at the expense of the other two. Therefore there is a continued need to break down barriers and actively value the expertise and insights that experience of mental distress brings. It is not the case that this is the only thing that is important, but it should be valued and not be a source of stigma and discrimination.

Myth #7 – Peers get to do all the nice things – talking to patients, taking them out, going home with them – the rest of us have to do the boring admin and medication, handing out meals, making beds etc. In any relationship, group or service there are tasks that have to be done. What distinguishes peer relationships is not what is done but the nature of the relationship: *'peer to peer'* rather than *'expert to non-expert'*. Peer support can thus occur in the course of any activity whether it is making a bed, going for a walk or just sitting and talking. Thus, it is not the case of peers getting to do all the *'nice things'*, it is simply that peers may have greater opportunities to use their relationships productively. The key question this raises for staff is actually how to engage in the *'nasty things'*, while preserving positive relationships.

Myth #8 – Peers don't know the difference between friendships and working relationships. There are many differences in the relationships between peer support workers and peers and those of friends, particularly in terms of self-disclosure, the degree of choice involved and the explicitness of *'rules'* (conventions of behaviour). But formal rules don't obviate the need for judgement and sensitivity. Peer support worker relationships therefore do involve more judgements than friendships – when and what to disclose, when and what *'rules'* to obey, etc. These judgements need to be considered as part of the training of peer support workers and reinforced by careful reflection and supervision.

Myth #9 – Peers will be subversive, they will be 'anti-psychiatry' and 'anti-medication'. The essence of peer support is not to prescribe what others should think, feel or do. Thus, peers should not be telling people whether or not to take medication, or to use conventional services, complementary therapies, etc. Rather, peers should be aiming to help people explore different ways of understanding, ways of coping and growing that make sense to them. Such exploration may involve challenges to orthodox views, but orthodox views are nearly always limited by the attempt to generalise from the performance of a group to the experience of an individual (e.g. in large scale treatment trials). Individual exploration is facilitated by the diverse narratives of others who have faced similar challenges.

Myth #10 – Peers will take up so much time that traditional staff roles will be made much harder, not easier. As indicated earlier, peer support workers may require additional employment support, particularly when the roles are being established. But these should not be different from any other worker. Peer workers may then make the jobs of other practitioners easier by relieving them of aspects of support that do not require their specialist professional expertise. This potential is clearly there if the problems are properly addressed at the outset. If peer workers are simply *'thrown into the mix'* then they will save neither time nor money.

Development of Peer Worker Roles

Once in post, just like other staff, peers should be given regular opportunities to review their role and consider if they wish to pursue avenues for career development. As they gain experience they will become clearer about the sort of training they might need to qualify for more specialist peer roles (e.g. in supervision and/or peer management, peer training or peer research). These positions are likely to attract higher remuneration. Peer workers may even decide to apply for training to equip them to enter traditional professional roles (e.g. counselling).

Regarding the development of new peer worker positions, given appropriate training, support and supervision, they will be their own best advocates. As indicated earlier, staff soon come to value peer posts and recognise the unique and complementary skills that they can bring to a service. There is therefore a demand for new posts to be created or converted and numbers grow. For example, in Nottinghamshire Healthcare the service chose to review all suitable vacancies as they arose and consider the possibility of converting them into peer posts (for example, converting a healthcare assistant posts into peer/healthcare assistant post – doing the same things in a different way).

The employment of peer workers also drives forward positive changes across the whole organisation. As already described, it becomes necessary to review recruitment, occupational health, management and supervision and career progression for *all* staff. Once in post, the peers themselves will begin to challenge policies, procedures and familiar assumptions about the work performance of people with mental health problems. This may have significant implications for members of staff who are employed in traditional professional roles, but also have their own '*lived experience*' of mental health problems. These challenges to existing practices are part of the cultural change that having peers employed inside services can bring.

But, they may also have other effects on the organisation. Let us begin to explore these as we try to understand the processes which underpin the effects of peer workers on individuals.

A Theory of Change Based on Stigma Reduction

We have seen already that support from peer workers is consistently associated with feelings of increased empowerment and improvements in various aspects of social inclusion (employment, education, community involvement, etc.) for those receiving this kind of support. But, how do these changes occur? What are the underlying mechanisms? We believe that they are specifically linked to reductions in self-stigma and stigmatising attitudes in staff in the organisations in which the peer workers are located.

The stigma associated with mental illness is pervasive. It is perhaps the most important social consequence of mental illness and may persist long after symptoms have subsided. Stigma takes two forms, '*external*', where the focus is on the effects of stigmatising attitudes on the part of neighbours, workmates, employers, etc., and '*internal*', where the focus is on processes of '*self-stigmatisation*'. Most of the research has concentrated on attempts to measure – and to change – external stigmatising attitudes (Thornicroft 2006), relatively less attention has been paid to the alleviation of '*self-stigma*'.

Self-stigma refers to '*an internalisation of negative beliefs about the self, which are largely based on shame, the acceptance of mental illness stereotypes, a sense of alienation from others, and consequent low mood*' (Henderson et al. 2014). These authors note that self-stigma is usually negatively correlated with empowerment, i.e. it is a state *dis*empowerment. Corrigan and his colleagues have developed a progressive model for the effects of self-stigma in people with serious mental illness (Corrigan et al. 2009, 2011; Rusch et al. 2010). They suggest that it arises from three related processes: (i) an *awareness* of the stereotypes regarding mental illness, (ii) an *acceptance* that these stereotypes are largely '*true*' and (c) a subsequent *application* of these ideas to the self (internalisation), together with an assumption of personal responsibility. These beliefs lead to feelings of disempowerment, reductions in self-esteem and loss of hope, which in turn lead to a reluctance to engage in positive activities which might help the person pursue their life goals. Corrigan et al. call this the "why try?" effect. Hence, the person asks themselves, '*Why should I even try to get a job? Someone like me – someone who is incompetent because of mental illness – could never successfully meet work demands …. Why should I even try to live independently? Someone like me is just not worth the investment to be successful…. Why should I pursue education?*' (etc.).

In an earlier paper (Corrigan and Watson 2002) also note that some people with serious mental illness may be aware of the stereotypes but reject their '*truth*' and reject the notion that these stereotypes apply to them. These people may then become justifiably angry ('*righteous anger*') at what they see as simple, unwarranted prejudice. They are most likely to be active in pushing for change in mental health system and, indeed, in society more generally. Thus, what might sometimes seem to be militant, irrational rhetoric may, in fact, be more accurately viewed as a perfectly rational response to an unfair situation.

Is it possible to change these processes of self-stigmatisation? The research cited earlier on effective methods to reduce external stigma (e.g. Thornicroft 2006) suggests that effective anti-stigma programs need to contain three key components:

1. Attempts to *combat ignorance* through the provision of accurate information about mental health problems, their prevalence, what is known about causes and precipitating factors, effective treatments, etc.
2. *Addressing prejudice* (negative emotional reactions) through engineering direct contact between members of the group who hold the prejudiced attitudes and those they are prejudiced about which is of sufficient duration, and is managed in such a way, that the groups can explore their prejudices and (hopefully) conclude that, faced with the evidence of real people, they are not possible to maintain.
3. *Reducing discrimination* by continually monitoring and challenging discriminatory behaviour.

Applying these conclusions to the context of peer support, this implies that:

(a) If people are provided with *information* about what can be achieved by peers (for example, through the use of personal narratives and stories) then this may help them question negative stereotypes. It may help inspire hope as they realise that it may be possible to pursue their personal recovery goals after all.

(b) If they then have the opportunity to meet with others with whom they can identify, who are coping in positive ways, then they may be helped to *re-examine their negative emotional reactions to themselves* (i.e. their prejudice towards self) and, in this way, improve self-esteem and confidence. Specifically, the person can begin to see that what they felt most ashamed of in themselves (the stigma of mental illness) is actually an experience which might be extremely valuable and might be used to help others. Thus, the negative effects of self-stigma are *'turned on their head'*.

(c) Finally, if they are given *ongoing support to monitor and challenge 'self-discriminatory behaviour'* this might overcome the *"why try?"* effect. Their negative cognitions are challenged and they should feel more willing to take up opportunities which will help them purse their personal recovery goals. This combination of exposure to contradictory beliefs and emotional support from others it is possible to identify with, seem a potentially powerful combination to increase feelings of empowerment and move people towards a state where they can begin to engage with their own recovery.

This formulation is consistent with the findings of a recent study by Corrigan and Sokol (2013) which showed that self-stigma was directly reduced through participation in mutual help programmes, particularly where the person identified with other members of the group. This model needs much further work and testing but, if correct, it highlights a number of ways in which peer support might be made even more effective and might have even more far-reaching benefits.

The same model can also be applied to the processes of organisational and cultural change that we noted earlier in relation to the effects of peers. Thus, it has already been shown that stigmatising attitudes are common *within* mental health services as well as outside (Henderson et al. 2014). They are more common in younger, less experienced staff and are undoubtedly reinforced by the biased sample of service users which staff tend to see (i.e. *'sick'* people, rather than those that are doing well). Hence, the presence of peers in the workforce who can talk about positive personal stories provides staff with living examples which challenge negative stereotypes. They can also get to know these people, over extended periods of time, in formal and informal settings, and (hopefully) this will reduce prejudiced attitudes and increase expectations. Finally, the provision of this counter-attitudinal information, and a chance to address prejudice, should challenge discriminatory behaviour. Staff should then think twice before saying things like, *'You will just have to accept it..... I am afraid that you are stuck with your condition for life.....You will never get completely better......You will always have to take medication .....I wouldn't think of trying to live on your own / get a job / maintain a relationship (etc.)'*.

This explains why the introduction of peer workers can have a powerful effect on changing the culture of mental health organisations and driving forward a recovery-oriented approach by challenging stigmatising attitudes among staff. As this team leader said, '*Peer workers have significantly changed the recovery focus of our team, they challenge the way we talk about people from a problem and diagnosis focus to one of strengths and possibilities........ I just stand back and watch him work his magic. Not just with the patients who come in here so frightened and hopeless, but with staff too. He can help them see things in a completely different way*' (Pollitt et al. 2012).

Conclusions and Future Directions

We have seen how the provision of support from suitably trained and managed peer workers is consistently associated with increases in feelings of empowerment, self-efficacy and hope for the future. There is also evidence that this leads to positive behavioural changes in the direction of increased social inclusion. These changes can be achieved in ways that are cost-effective and seem best understood in terms of the reduced self-stigma and contact with living examples of people who contradict low expectations and stigmatising attitudes in the workforce. We have argued that, in a similar way by challenging stigmatising attitudes, the presence of peer workers in mental health organisations may be a powerful mechanism for increasing hope and expectations among staff, making it more likely that they will support peoples' recovery.

However, much remains to be done. As indicated earlier, most of the available outcome data on the effectiveness of peer support is based on simple, prospective follow-up studies or matched control designs; there are few randomised controlled trials. To conduct meaningful randomised controlled trials we need to know more about the key ingredients of effective peer support and be able to '*standardise*' – at least make replicable – the intervention itself (the '*independent variable*'). We have made some suggestions about what we consider to be some of the essential ingredients based on our experience, but these ideas need to be empirically investigated. In addition, the theoretical model proposed here, based on stigma reduction, particularly the reduction of self-stigma, needs much more rigorous testing. This could be done in conjunction with further outcome trials.

We believe that this research is important. If peer support can be shown to be effective in the ways described above and if it works for the reasons suggested, then we might have a highly cost-effective intervention, with far-reaching effects, which is both cheaper and better. This would be a very exciting prospect for the future.

References

Adams AL, Leitner LM (2008) Breaking out of the mainstream: the evolution of peer support alternatives to the Mental Health System. Ethical Human Psychol Psychiatr 10:146–162

Basset T, Faulkner A, Repper J, Stamou E (2010) Lived experience leading the way peer support in mental health. Available from: http://www.together-uk.org/wp-content/uploads/downloads/2011/11/livedexperiencereport.pdf

Bradstreet S (2006) Harnessing the 'lived experience'. Formalising peer support approaches to promote recovery. Ment Health Rev 11:2–6

Campling P (2001) Therapeutic communities. Adv Psychiatr Treat 7:365–372

Corrigan PW, Sokol KA (2013) The impact of self-stigma and mutual help programs on the quality of life of people with serious mental illnesses. Community Ment Health J 49:1–6

Corrigan PW, Watson A (2002) Understanding the impact of stigma on people with mental illness. World Psychiatr 1:16–20

Corrigan PW, Larson JE, Rusch N (2009) Self-stigma and the "why try" effect: impact on life goals and evidence-based practices. World Psychiatr 8:75–81

Corrigan PW, Rafacz J, Rusch N (2011) Examining a progressive model of self-stigma and its impact on people with serious mental illness. Psychiatry Res 189:339–343

Davidson L, Bellamy C, Guy K, Miller R (2012) Peer support among persons with severe mental illnesses: a review of evidence and experience. World Psychiatr 11:123–128

Department of Health (2010) Putting people first: planning together – peer support and self directed support. Department of Health, London

Department of Health (2011) No health without mental health: a cross-government mental health outcomes strategy for people of all ages. Department of Health, London

Faulkner A, Kalathil K (2012) The freedom to be, the chance to dream: preserving user-led peer support in mental health. Together, London, Available from: www.together-uk.org

Henderson C, Noblett J, Parke H, Clement S, Caffrey A, Gale-Grant O, Schulze B, Druss B, Thornicroft G (2014) Mental health-related stigma in health care and mental health-care settings. Lancet 1:467–482

HMG (1995) Disability Discrimination Act. Available from: www.legislation.gov.uk/ukpga/1995/50/pdfs/ukpga_19950050_en.pdf

HMG (2005) Disability Discrimination Act 2005. London: legislation.gov.uk. Available from http://www.legislation.gov.uk/ukpga/1995/50/contents

Lloyd-Evans B, Mayo-Wilson E, Harrison B, Istead H, Brown E, Pilling S, Johnson S, Kendall T (2014) A systematic review and meta-analysis of randomised controlled trials of peer support for people with severe mental illness. BMC Psychiatry 14:39, http://www.biomedcentral.com/1471-244X/14/39

Mead S, Hilton D, Curtis L (2001) Peer support: a theoretical perspective. Psychiatr Rehabil J 25:134–141

Mental Health Foundation (2012) Peer support in mental health and learning disability. Mental Health Foundation/Need 2Know Publications, London

Mowbray CT, Moxley DP, Colllins ME (1998) Consumer as mental health providers: first person accounts of benefits and limitations. J Behav Health Serv Res 25:97–411

Perkins, R., Evenson, E. and Davidson, B. (2000) The pathfinder user employment programme. Southwest London & St. George's Mental Health NHS Trust, Trust Headquarters, Springfield University Hospital, 61 Glenburnie Road, London SW17 7DJ, London

Perkins R, Farmer P, Litchfield P (2009) Realising ambitions: better employment support for people with a mental health condition. Department of Work and Pensions CM 7742, London, Available from: www.gov.uk/government/uploads/system/uploads/attachment_data/file/228818/7742.pdf

Pitt V, Lowe D, Hill S et al. (2013) Consumer providers of care for adult clients of statutory mental health services. Cochrane Database Syst Rev 3:CD004807. doi:10.1002/14651858.CD004807.pub2.

Pollitt A, Winpenney E, Newbould J, Celia C, Ling T, Scraggs E (2012) Evaluation of the peer worker programme of Cambridge and Peterborough NHS Foundation Trust. RAND Europe, Cambridge, UK, Available from: www.rand/org/pubs/documented_briefings/DB651.html

Repper J (2013a) Peer support workers: theory and practice, ImROC Briefing Paper 5. Centre for Mental Health and Mental Health Network, NHS Confederation, London, Available from www.ImROC.org

Repper J (2013b) Peer support workers: a practical guide to implementation, ImROC briefing paper 7. Centre for Mental Health and Mental Health Network, NHS Confederation, London, Available from www.ImROC.org

Repper J, Carter T (2011) A review of the literature on peer support in mental health services. J Ment Health 20:392–411

Repper J, Perkins R (2003) Social inclusion and recovery: a model for mental health practice. Bailliere Tindall, London

Repper J, Perkins R (2013) The team recovery implementation plan: a framework for creating recovery focussed services, ImROC Briefing No. 6. Centre for Mental Health and Mental Health Network, NHS Confederation, London, Available from www.ImROC.org

Repper J, Watson E (2012) A year of peer support in Nottingham: lessons learned. J Ment Health Train Educ Pract 7:70–78

Rethink (2014) Investing in recovery – making the business case for effective interventions for people with schizophrenia and psychosis. Available from www.rethink.org/?gclid=CJyCsMm mjcYCFYnJtAodHnsAbg

Rinaldi M, Hardisty J (2010) Harnessing the expertise of experience: increasing access to employment within mental health services for people who have themselves experienced mental health problems. Divers Health Care 7:13–21

Rusch N, Corrigan PW, Todd AR, Bodenausen GV (2010) Implicit self-stigma in people with mental illness. J Nerv Ment Dis 198:150–153

Salzer M, Shear S (2002) Identifying consumer-provider benefits in evaluations of consumer-delivered services. Psychiatr Rehab J 25:281–288

SAMSHA (2010) Shared decision-making in mental health care: practice. Research and future directions, HHS Publication No. SMA-09-4371. Centre for Mental Health Services, Substance Abuse and Mental Health Services Administration, Rockville, Available from http://store.samhsa.gov/product/Shared-Decision-Making-in-Mental-Health-Care/SMA09-4371

Schizophrenia Commission (2012) The abandoned illness. The Schizophrenia Commission, London

Scottish Recovery Network (2011) Experts by experience: guidelines to support the development of Peer Worker roles in the mental health sector. Available from www.scottishrecovery.net

Scottish Recovery Network (2012) Experts by experience: values framework for peer working. Available from www.scottishrecovery.net

Shepherd G (in press) Recovery-focussed interventions in psychosis. In: Pradhan B, Pinninti N and Rathod S. (eds) To appear in 'Brief interventions for psychosis: a clinical compendium'. Springer Publications

Shepherd G, Boardman J, Slade M (2008) Making recovery a reality. Centre for Mental Health, London, Available from www.ImROC.org

Shepherd G, Boardman J, Burns M (2010) Implementing recovery: a methodology for organisational change. Centre for Mental Health, London, Available from www.ImROC.org

Slade M (2009) Personal recovery and mental illness. Cambridge University Press, Cambridge

Thornicroft G (2006) Shunned: discrimination against people with mental illness. Oxford University Press, Oxford

Torrey W, Drake R (2009) Practicing shared decision making in the outpatient psychiatric care of adults with severe mental illnesses: redesigning care in the future. Community Ment Health J. doi:10.1007/s10597-009-9265-9, Published online: 08 November 2009

Trachtenberg M, Parsonage M, Shepherd G, Boardman J (2013) Peer support in mental health care: is it good value for money? Centre for Mental Health, London, Available from: www.centreformentalhealth.org.uk/peer-support-value-for-money

Warner (2009) Recovery from schizophrenia and the recovery model. Curr Opin Psychiatr 22:374–380

Targeting the Stigma of Psychiatry and Psychiatrists

35

Ahmed Hankir, Antonio Ventriglio, and Dinesh Bhugra

Introduction

The phenomenon of a group of people or communities (across the different cultures) treating an individual who has a mental health problem as 'the other' can be traced as far back as antiquity. Superstition held that these people were deemed to have consorted with the occult in some way or another and as such were possessed by a malevolent entity. The only 'treatment', therefore, was to exorcise or expunge the nefarious spirit by consulting some necromancer who would invariably, among other things, whisper incantations, trephine holes in skulls and resort to other forms of witchcraft and quackery.

Although psychiatry is a medical specialty, its scientific basis has been ridiculed ever since its inception. Indeed psychiatry, psychiatric patients and psychiatrists have often been at the receiving end of the cruel and harmful effects of stigma. For example, patients with mental illnesses were once referred to as *aliens* and their doctors as *alienists* as if these people were not even human. Such disparaging terms clearly indicated the lack of recognition and respect that psychiatry, psychiatric patients and mental health practitioners received. This discrimination, prejudice and stigma have survived the ravages of time and have persisted throughout the centuries although, as we will show later on in this book chapter, rays of hope are starting to glimmer as the trend is beginning to change in some parts of the world.

A. Hankir
Department of Psychiatry, Carrick Institute for Graduate Studies, Cape Canaveral, Florida, USA

A. Ventriglio
Department of Clinical and Experimental Medicine, University of Foggia, Foggia, Italy

D. Bhugra (✉)
Institute of Psychiatry, King's College London, De Crespigny Park, Box P025, London SE5 8AF, UK
e-mail: dinesh.bhugra@kcl.ac.uk

© Springer International Publishing Switzerland 2017
W. Gaebel et al. (eds.), *The Stigma of Mental Illness - End of the Story?*,
DOI 10.1007/978-3-319-27839-1_35

The ramifications of mental health stigma are serious. For psychiatric patients, fear of exposure to stigmatization can contribute to secrecy and symptom concealment, and many people continue to suffer in silence despite the availability of effective treatment. Indeed, people with mental health problems have low levels of help-seeking behaviour which may, for example, deprive them of receiving the benefits of early intervention. Moreover, many people with a mental health problem never make it as far as the mental health services at all (and those who are *fortunate* enough to make it that far often present by the time the disease has developed into a full blown crisis (i.e. suicidal behaviour). Even doctors are not *immune* to the stigma attached to mental illness and its fatal consequences. For example, in recent times Dr. Daksha Emson, a brilliant British psychiatrist based in London, tragically killed herself and her baby daughter during a psychotic episode. An independent inquiry into Dr. Emson's death concluded that she was the victim of stigma in the National Health Service (NHS). Succinctly put: stigma is killing people. Thus, at every stage of a patient's journey – from the onset of symptoms to recovery – stigma and discrimination rear their ugly faces.

Stigma plays the dual role of affecting mental health patients on the one hand and mental health practitioners on the other. In relation to the former and its implications, the Global Burden of Disease (GBD) study has revealed that not only is there a burgeoning rise in the prevalence of mental illnesses but by 2020 depression is likely to become the most common disorder overtaking physical diseases such as cardiac pathology and cancer. Thus, in order to relieve the globe of the tremendous burden that mental diseases will place on it, the stigma attached to these conditions must be challenged. In relation to the latter, this has had an unfortunate effect on recruitment and retention into psychiatry so much so that the World Health Organization (WHO) has identified a chronic shortage of psychiatrists worldwide (albeit there are variations in recruitment and retention rates between countries).

The stigma associated with a person having a mental health problem combined with the stigma associated with being a psychiatrist means that many people with psychopathology continue to suffer needlessly and unnecessarily. It can only be with a sense of urgency then that we, the global community from grassroots to governmental level, collectively address the challenges that psychiatric diseases place on humanity. In this book chapter we discuss and describe the salient findings and implications of initiatives launched to combat stigma by individuals, groups and organizations. We start off by defining the term stigma itself.

Defining Stigma

Although the term stigma has ancient origins, it was only in the twentieth century that the term was introduced into the psychological and sociological lexicons. Evans-Lacko et al. conducted a systematic mapping of the literature on the state of the art in European research on reducing social exclusion and stigma related to mental health. As part of their research, they investigated whether published papers included a formal definition of the social issue being examined in order to gain a better understand of the theoretical underpinnings of the studies (Evans-Lacko et al. 2014). When explicitly defined, Goffman's seminal definition of stigma as *'an attribute that is deeply discrediting and that reduces the bearer from a whole and usual person to a tainted, discounted one* (Goffman 1963)' was often quoted. In recent years, Link, Phelan and colleagues have revisited this definition to reflect advances in stigma research. Their definition distinguishes between five main components of stigma: labelling, stereotyping, separation, status loss and discrimination and was used in the majority of the studies that included a definition (Link et al. 2004).

Stigma Against Psychiatric Patients

Fear, prejudice and discrimination towards those who experience mental health problems can be a result of ignorance (i.e. lack of knowledge), misinformation and the plethora of myths that abound. However, prejudice runs deep and attitudes may be difficult to change in spite of education and training. Moreover, people with a mental illness may also hold stigmatizing views towards themselves (Henderson et al. 2013), and this can have an effect on the perception of the treatment available for psychiatric disorders and whether patients decide to comply with therapy or not (Lewer et al. 2015).

   The country that a person with a mental health problem is from can influence the attitude that he or she may have towards psychiatric treatment. For example, a recent multinational study revealed that respondents from Germany, Slovak Republic and Russia had a general propensity towards psychotherapy as potential treatment in comparison with pharmacotherapy (Angermeyer et al. 2005) (indeed, a separate study revealed that an increased tendency to prescribe psychotropic medication was seen as a negative aspect of psychiatry (Shore 1979)). Thus, a degree of cultural variation in the type of help-seeking behaviour that a person demonstrates may exist (Bhugra 2014), reflecting differing attitudes and the explanatory models that a person may formulate in an attempt to fathom the psychological phenomena that he or she is experiencing.

Stigma Towards Psychiatrists

Psychiatry is lambasted by antipsychiatrists who are perhaps the most vehement and vociferous group who campaign against the existence and practice of a particular medical specialty. Trainees in psychiatry often have to confront and cope with questions like: 'Am I a real doctor?', and this can lower morale and result in a reduction in the self-confidence of its practitioners.

   In the NHS in the UK and in other healthcare systems elsewhere in the world, there has been a separation between mental healthcare from physical healthcare, inevitably resulting in fewer medical colleagues understanding the role of psychiatry particularly so if they have not had adequate exposure to psychiatry during their undergraduate or postgraduate training (Carney and Bhugra 2013) (over recent years, the disparity of esteem between mental illness and physical illness in the UK has resulted in the closure of many psychiatric inpatient wards. There have been reports of people with a mental health problem who are in a crisis having to travel hundreds of miles from where they reside in order to receive emergency inpatient mental health treatment (http://www.theguardian.com/profile/alex-langford).

The reality is that psychiatry, unrivalled by any other medical specialty, deals with the spectrum of human emotion and considers all aspects of the human experience: exuberance, despair, flights of fancy and notions of romanticism, confusion, perception and memory and its devastating fragmentation. In perinatal psychiatry, the psychiatric practitioner may be consulted to assess a mother who is perplexed and terrified by her unbidden thoughts of harming her child. In general adult psychiatry, doctors see the family of a young man who have watched him become a complete stranger, muttering wild accusations about conspiracies and attending to unseen and inaudible stimuli. Psychiatrists aim to be the doctors who know what the best recourse is in these circumstances. They also strive to be the doctors who purvey empathy and comfort to the next of kin as well as instil optimism in them (and most importantly the patient) that effective treatment exists and that recovery is not just possible but a reality for many who have been through similar experiences (Hankir et al. 2014a).

There are numerous reasons as to why being a psychiatrist is deemed undesirable; foremost among them is the pivotal role that popular culture plays (Stuart et al. 2015). Indeed, portrayals of psychiatrists (and indeed of psychiatric patients) in literature, film and the media are powerful influences in shaping individual and collective perceptions and the decision-making process in terms of career choices that medical graduates make (Farooq et al. 2013a).

The Role That Film Plays in the Perceptions of Mental Illness

Films are extremely popular across the different cultures. India is the country that produces the largest number of films every year. In 2009 alone the Hindi film industry Bollywood contributed to producing a staggering 1,288 Indian feature films (Annual Report 2009). The USA, Hong Kong and Nigeria are examples of other countries where film industries are booming.

One could argue that as long as human beings continue to seek entertainment and escapism – for, as the twentieth-century Nobel Laureate T.S. Eliot said, '*mankind cannot bear very much reality*' – cinema will remain deeply embedded in our societies.

The storylines of films are influenced by the society we live in. Given that one in four of us has a mental illness at some point in our lives (*The World Health Report 2001 – Mental Health: New Understanding, New Hope*), mental illness and the psychiatrists who treat these illnesses play huge roles in our societies and on our screens. In view of this, Bhugra et al. examined Bollywood films produced since the early 1960s as a means to analyse the changes in Indian society's attitudes towards mental health issues (Deakin and Bhugra 2012).

Bhugra's analyses revealed how in post-colonial India in the 1950s and 1960s there were many films featuring people with mental illness who were subjected to ridicule but there were also some films that had sympathetic portrayals of sufferers of mental illness. In the 1970s and 1980s when the country was going through major economic, social and political upheavals, the portrayal of mental illness in film was very much of psychopaths who could not rely on the system to provide for the vulnerable so they were vigilantes taking the law into their own hands. This image of mental illness sufferers transformed in the 1990s when there were many motion pictures that portrayed the theme of morbid jealousy. These films typically involved men who were trying to control women and who viewed them as a kind of commodity. This period overlapped with the economic liberalization that was taking place in India at the time which gave people the power and freedom to own property and other objects. Many men extended this to include women (i.e. they viewed the sociopolitical changes in India at the time as a means to justify the 'objectification' of women) and viewed them as property that they could (and should) rightfully own (Deakin and Bhugra 2012).

Recruitment into Psychiatry

Lydall et al. conducted a review on a number of studies from around the world that analysed the factors that influenced the recruitment of medical graduates into psychiatry. The main issue with recruitment and retention that Lydall et al. found was that psychiatry continues to be considered by many as unscientific and this remains the major reason as to why graduates do not specialize in this branch of medicine (Farooq et al. 2013b).

The worldwide picture in terms of recruitment into psychiatry is heavily influenced by the wealthier countries' ability to recruit to shortage specialties from International Medical Graduates (IMG) (Farooq et al. 2013b). Goldacre et al. found that IMGs from black minority ethnic (BME) groups were significantly over-represented in general adult psychiatry, learning disability and old age psychiatry (Goldacre et al. 2009). Fazel and Ebmeier looked at UK centralized recruitment data and noted that for UK graduates psychiatry was the sixth most popular choice, whereas it was the fourth most popular choice for IMGs (Fazel and Ebmeier 2009).

The first review on recruitment was conducted by Eagle and Marcos. The authors described two distinct groups of people who opt for a career in psychiatry. The first group is composed of people who decided that they wanted to specialize in psychiatry prior to starting medical school. The second (larger) group is comprised of people who decide that they want to specialize in psychiatry during medical school or after they qualify. Eagle and Marcos broadly describe the latter as having a 'general practitioner, humanitarian orientation', with the potential for being 'pulled' towards either primary care or psychiatry depending on economic and social factors. Eagle and Marcos also identified the characteristics of people who chose psychiatry as a career (Eagle and Marcos 1980) (see Table 35.1).

Sierles and Taylor conducted a review of over 200 English language publications on the causes of the plummeting rate of recruitment into psychiatry (see Table 35.2).

The authors summarized historical trends of recruitment into psychiatry in the USA in the context of changing sociopolitical and economic circumstances. They discovered that recruitment into psychiatry in the USA improved significantly after World War II (with the realization of the magnitude of mental health challenges affecting fitness for conscription for military service as well as the impact that conflict had on a veteran's mental health) and in the 1960s which coincided with a shift in the provision of mental health services from hospitals into the community and the

Table 35.1 Eagle and Marcos factors (Eagle and Marcos 1980)

Eagle and Marcos characteristics of students choosing psychiatry as a career (Eagle and Marcos 1980)
More likely to be single
From large metropolitan areas
Politically liberal
Uninterested in religion
Interested in humanitarian ideas
More likely to have majored in arts, humanities and social sciences before medical school
Score low on measures of authoritarianism and self esteem
High capacity to tolerate ambiguity
Score highly on anxiety and fear of death
Express positive attitudes to psychiatry and psychiatrists
Exposure to, and taking responsibility for, psychiatric patients, especially those with a good prognosis

Table 35.2 Sierles and Taylor's hypotheses on the causes of falling psychiatric recruitment (Sierles and Taylor 1995)

1. Messianic failure: this refers to the enthusiasm that swept psychiatry in the mid twentieth century as a means of producing social change, represented by the community mental health movement. The authors comment on the perceived failure of this movement
2. Conventionality and competition: this refers to the gradual shift in the field from psychodynamic to a biological paradigm, so becoming more 'conventional' or more similar to other fields of medicine. Alternative training pathways have opened for those interested in psychotherapy training for non-medical graduates, thus increasing the competition for medical graduates
3. Money: graduates with high indebtedness (i.e. graduates who have attended private medical schools in the USA) have been shown to opt for high-income specialties on graduation. Psychiatry is among the lowest-paid specialty, and it has been argued that this influences recruitment of medical graduates into the specialty
4. Demographic change: in the USA there has been a huge increase in the number of women in medicine (from 9.1 % in 1969–1970 to 41.9 % in 1993–1994). Women were twice as likely as men to choose psychiatry in the 1970s, but this ratio had dropped to 1.57 times as likely in the 1990s
5. Generalist competition: some authors have proposed a link between choosing psychiatry and generalist specialties, suggesting interested graduates are more likely to have these in their top preferences, with competition between the two for graduates (this hypothesis, however, has conflicting evidence)

manufacturing of effective psychotropic medication. The authors report a fall of medical graduates who were recruited into psychiatry in the 1970s which was subsequent to cuts in the allocation of resources to the US National Institute Mental Health (NIMH) training budget (this was due to a 'shifting' of the provision of healthcare from specialists to generalists in response to escalating healthcare costs) (Sierles and Taylor 1995).

Case Study: Recommendations to Increase Recruitment into Psychiatry in the UK

Halder et al. conducted a quantitative, cross-sectional online survey to understand the factors that contributed to recruitment into psychiatry in the UK. A total of 484 students from 18 medical schools throughout the UK responded. Halder et al. revealed that there was little difference in the quality ratings of lectures and small

Table 35.3 'Pull factors': recommendations to improve recruitment into psychiatry in the UK (Halder et al. 2013)

Lectures about mental health earlier in the medical school curriculum
Recruit consultant psychiatrists and psychiatry trainees as medical student tutors (e.g. for communication skills)
Encourage students to adopt an active role in decision-making (in discussions with doctors) during their psychiatry placement
Ensure good quality teaching within psychiatry placements for students by involving teaching-oriented psychiatrists
Greater exposure of students to sub-specialties of psychiatry to enhance understanding of the variety of in psychiatry
Encourage and support the development of enrichment activities including social psychiatry clubs, special study modules and research in psychiatry within each medical school
Cultivate more role models in teaching, leadership and research
Challenge misconceptions of patients (e.g. being 'difficult, dangerous or untreatable') – this applies to students and other doctors
Work with medical colleagues to eliminate stigmatizing attitudes that subsequently influence students

group teaching between those interested in psychiatry and those who were not. Experience of 'enrichment activities' (i.e. psychiatry special study modules, university psychiatry clubs) was significantly more likely to take up psychiatry. The authors do, however, report that caution should be taken when interpreting these results and that causality cannot be determined by their study. The authors formulated recommendations to improve recruitment into psychiatry in the UK (see Table 35.3) and concluded that addressing psychiatry teaching and exposure may improve recruitment into the specialty (Halder et al. 2013).

Case Study: 'The Wounded Healer': An Effective 'Double-Pronged' Approach to Increasing Recruitment into Psychiatry and Reducing the Stigma Associated with Mental Illness?

Despite the perception that medical students and doctors should be 'invincible', mental health problems are common in this population (Harvey et al. 2009). Medical students and doctors, thus, have the capacity to become treatment seeking patients. In Canada, for example, a study using an objective measure of emotional exhaustion revealed that 80 % of doctors were suffering from burnout (Thommasen et al. 2001). Suicide rates are also high with 400 doctors dying from this cause of death every year in the USA alone (www.afsp.org). The use of cannabis and illicit drugs among medical students is also reported to be on the rise: UK studies in Leeds (Ashton and Kamali 1995) and Newcastle upon Tyne (Pickard et al. 2000) have demonstrated high levels of alcohol consumption and illicit drug use, and high anxiety and depression scores.

Like other people who have mental health problems, medical students and doctors who have these experiences also have low levels of help-seeking behaviour. The results of a recent study, for example, identified stigma as an explicit barrier to the use of mental health services by 30 % of first- and second-year medical students experiencing depression (Givens and Tjia 2002).

The 2008 Stigma Shout Survey of almost 4,000 people using mental health services and carers revealed that healthcare professionals are a common source of stigma reported by people with mental illness (http://www.time-to-change.org.uk/news/stigma-shout-survey-shows-real-impact-stigma-and-discrimination-peoples-lives). In order to address the pernicious issue of stigma in healthcare professionals, a starting point would be for each and every healthcare provider to be honest with himself or herself in order to develop an insight and to challenge any preconceptions and prejudice that they may have. Another way to change negative attitudes towards healthcare professionals with psychopathology is to realize that those kinds of experiences may actually be beneficial as opposed to being disadvantageous. A motif in the narratives of doctors who have first-hand experience of psychiatric illness is that they have become more insightful and empathetic (Hankir 2013).

Carl Jung used the term the Wounded Healer as an archetypal dynamic to describe a phenomenon that may take place in the relationship between analyst and analysand. Jung discovered the Wounded Healer archetype in relation to himself, for Jung, '…it is his own hurt that gives a measure of his power to heal…' (Jung 1994).

We felt that there was a need to develop a novel anti-stigma intervention targeted at healthcare professionals and professional trainees. Corrigan et al. conducted a meta-analysis of outcome studies challenging the public stigma of mental illness and concluded that social contact was more effective than education at reducing the discrimination towards mental illness in adults (Corrigan et al. 2012). In view of this we designed and developed the Wounded Healer which is a 1-h contact-based anti-stigma intervention. The Wounded Healer has been described as an innovative method of pedagogy that blends the humanities with science (Hankir and Zaman 2013).

The intervention incorporates an autobiographical narrative from the primary author, a trainee in academic psychiatry in the UK who has first-hand experience of profound oscillations in mood. The aims of the intervention are to engage, enthuse, enthral and educate by making reference to film, literature and poetry in order to convey the subjective experience of bipolar disorder (and thus illustrate its association with the artistic temperament). It also contains factual information on mental health challenges in order to dispel the many myths on mental illness that abound (Hankir et al. 2014b).

The Wounded Healer has been delivered to 5,000 medical students and doctors in 14 medical schools throughout the UK and in countries all over the world including the USA, Canada, Portugal, Slovenia, Lebanon and Italy. We created and hand distributed paper questionnaires to participants in six cohorts who attended the Wounded Healer: Manchester Medical School ($n=36$), Cambridge University ($n=97$), Sheffield Medical School ($n=21$), Southampton Medical School ($n=23$), Foundation Doctors in the North West of England ($n=51$) and Manchester University International Society ($n=25$) (total sample size $n=256$, response rate 219/256 (85.5 %)). The questionnaire contained stigma constructs and answers were on a Likert-type scale. There was also space for free-text comments which were subjected to thematic analyses (Hankir et al. 2014b).

The feedback that we have received has been exceptionally positive (Table 35.4). Thematic analyses of free-text comments revealed eight broad themes, three of which are included below:

Theme 1: Inspirational

> Superb. Inspirational story, excellent view into psychiatry. Foundation Doctor (Hankir et al. 2014b)

Theme 2: Positivity towards the health humanities

> Excellent talk. Really enjoyable, fantastic use of literature, poetry and film. The best lecture I have had in medical school so far. Manchester Medical Student (Hankir et al. 2014b)

Theme 3: Stigma

> Drawing from personal experiences and dismantling the stigma surrounding mental illness especially in medical professionals was inspiring. Leeds Medical Student (Hankir et al. 2014b)
>   Lectures like these should be given to all medical students to help reduce stigma and to encourage anyone struggling to get help.... Sheffield Medical Student (Hankir et al. 2014b)

Moreover, an unintended but positive effect of the Wounded Healer is that respondents (medical students and junior doctors) reported that they developed an interest in specializing in psychiatry as evidenced by the following free text comment from a respondent who attended the Wounded Healer in Liverpool Medical School (Hankir et al. 2014b):

> Unbelievable. This guy had charisma in spades. It was so reassuring to know that a doctor with mental health challenges can overcome them and be so successful. Quite possibly the poster boy for my future career decision. (Hankir et al. 2014b)

Table 35.4 Summary of immediate postintervention evaluation responses by item (Hankir et al. 2014b)

	Strongly disagree	Disagree	Neither agree nor disagree	Agree	Strongly agree
	Frequency (%)	Frequency (%)	Frequency (%)	Frequency (%)	Frequency (%)
The talk was interesting (n=219)	2 (1 %)	0 (0 %)	1 (1 %)	79 (36 %)	137 (63 %)
My views towards mental health issues are more positive after the talk (n=219)	1 (1 %)	1 (1 %)	43 (20 %)	122 (56 %)	52 (24 %)
The talk dispelled some common myths about mental illness and zand to think more rationally about psychiatry (n=219)	1 (1 %)	1 (1 %)	32 (15 %)	125 (57 %)	27 (24 %)
A talk on the mental health of doctors and medical students given by a doctor with personal experiences of mental illness is preferable than from someone who has not had those experiences (n=219)	0 (0 %)	1 (1 %)	22 (10 %)	76 (35 %)	120 (55 %)
The talk made me more understanding and accepting of medical students and doctors who suffer from mental illness (n=219)	1 (1 %)	4 (2 %)	42 (19 %)	108 (49 %)	64 (29 %)
I am more aware of the importance of registering with a GP and consulting him/her if I feel I am under mental distress (n=219)	0 (0 %)	6 (3 %)	57 (26 %)	100 (46 %)	56 (26 %)
The talk made me realize that medical students and doctors who suffer from mental illness can recover and achieve their goals (n=219)	1 (1 %)	0 (0 %)	11 (5 %)	83 (38 %)	124 (57 %)

	Definitely not	No	Neither yes or no	Yes	Definitely yes
	Frequency (%)	Frequency (%)	Frequency (%)	Frequency (%)	Frequency (%)
I would recommend the talk to a friend of colleague (n=219)	0 (0 %)	0 (0 %)	8 (4 %)	90 (41 %)	121 (55 %)

Interestingly, recent research has revealed that first-hand experience of mental health challenges is a factor that can influence why medical graduates decide to specialize in psychiatry (Farooq et al. 2014) and since mental health challenges are common in medical students and doctors this might be why the Wounded Healer has such an appeal to this population.

The Wounded Healer anti-stigma intervention appears to have influenced participants to view psychiatric disorders in healthcare professionals in a more positive way. The Wounded Healer has successfully been introduced into the medical school curricula of King's College London, Dundee University, Cambridge University and University of East Anglia. Moreover, filmmakers from the London College of Communication have successfully obtained funding from the Institute of Inner Vision to commission the production of a film on the Wounded Healer so we can reach out to an even larger audience nationally and internationally.

Having received invitations to lecture in the Portuguese Medical Student Association and the Spanish Medical Student Congresses in 2015 (which is forecasted to be attended by more than 1,000 European medical students), the Wounded Healer and similar initiatives might offer opportunities for international organizations such as World Psychiatry Association and European Psychiatry Association to conduct future research to assess if such an intervention can cause a sustained reduction in the stigma associated with psychopathology in the medical profession and if the Wounded Healer can indeed increase recruitment into the specialty (Fig. 35.1).

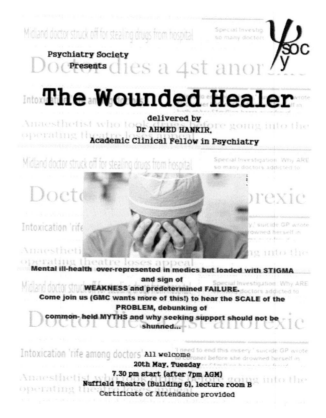

Fig. 35.1 Leaflet designed by the Southampton Medical School – Psychiatry Society on the Wounded Healer. This leaflet was used as promotional material to publicize the event and recruit participants (Hankir et al. 2014b)

Conclusion

Stigma and discrimination are pervasive phenomena which exert a negative influence, through a multitude of ways, on the lives of many individuals affected by mental illness. Anti-stigma work targeting specific groups, such as healthcare staff, or strategies which empower individuals facing discrimination are likely to play a key role in reducing the impact of stigma. Interventions building on the principle of contact frequently show promise at reducing the stigma associated with mental health challenges, and we need to continue to incorporate personal stories and narratives into interventions in order to build awareness at local and national levels. We have not reached the end of stigma. However, there are positive signs on the horizon indicating that at last the society is aware and beginning to talk about mental illness, mentally ill and those who care for them – whether lay or professional.

References

Angermeyer MC, Breier P, Dietrich S, Kenzine D, Matschinger H (2005) Public attitudes towards psychiatric treatment. Soc Psychiatry Psychiatr Epidemiol 40:855–64
Annual report 2009 (PDF) Central Board of Film Certification, Ministry of Information and Broadcasting, GOVERNMENT OF INDIA. Cited 2015
Ashton CH, Kamali F (1995) Personality, lifestyles, alcohol and drug consumption in a sample of British medical students. Med Educ 29(3):187–192
Bhugra D (2014) Globalization, culture and mental health. Int Rev Psychiatry 26(5):615–616. doi:10.3109/09540261.2014.955084
Carney S, Bhugra D (2013) Education and training in psychiatry in the U.K. Acad Psychiatry 37(4):243–247. doi:10.1176/appi.ap.12060109
Corrigan PW, Morris SB, Michaels PJ, Rafacz JD, Rüsch N (2012) Challenging the public stigma of mental illness: a meta-analysis of outcome studies. Psychiatr Serv 63(10):963–973. doi:10.1176/appi.ps.201100529
Deakin N, Bhugra D (2012) Families in Bollywood cinema: changes and context. Int Rev Psychiatry 24(2):166–172. doi:10.3109/09540261.2012.656307
Eagle PF, Marcos LR (1980) Factors in medical students' choice of psychiatry. Am J Psychiatr 137:5
Evans-Lacko S, Courtin E, Fiorillo A (2014) The state of the art in European research on reducing social exclusion and stigma related to mental health: a systematic mapping of the literature. Eur Psychiatry 29(6):381–389. doi:10.1016/j.eurpsy.2014.02.007
Farooq K, Lydall GJ, Bhugra D (2013a) Research into recruitment: critical gaps in the literature. Int Rev Psychiatry 25(4):366–370. doi:10.3109/09540261.2013.822853
Farooq K, Lydall GJ, Bhugra D (2013b) What attracts medical students towards psychiatry? A review of factors before and during medical school. Int Rev Psychiatry 25(4):371–377. doi:10 .3109/09540261.2013.823855
Farooq K, Lydall GJ, Malik A, Ndetei DM, ISOSCCIP Group, Bhugra D (2014) Why medical students choose psychiatry – a 20 country cross-sectional survey. BMC Med Educ 14:12. doi:10.1186/1472-6920-14-12
Fazel S, Ebmeier KP (2009) Specialty choice in UK junior doctors: is psychiatry the least popular specialty for UK and international medical graduates? BMC Med Educ 9:77
Givens JL, Tjia J (2002) Depressed medical students' use of mental health services and barriers to use. Acad Med 77(9):918–921
Goffman E (1963) Stigma: notes on the management of spoiled identity. Prentice-Hall, Englewood Cliffs

Goldacre MJ, Fazel S, Smith F, Lambert T (2009) Choice and rejection of psychiatry as a career: surveys of UK medical graduates from 1974 to 2009. Br J Psychiatry 202:228–234

Halder N, Hadjidemetriou C, Pearson R, Farooq K, Lydall GJ, Malik A, Bhugra D (2013) Student career choice in psychiatry: findings from 18 UK medical schools. Int Rev Psychiatry 25(4):438–444. doi:10.3109/09540261.2013.824414

Hankir A (2013) Review and overview: autobiographical narrative and psychopathology. CEPiP 1:254–260

Hankir A, Zaman R (2013) Jung's archetype, 'The Wounded Healer', mental illness in the medical profession and the role of the health humanities in psychiatry. BMJ Case Rep. doi:10.1136/bcr-2013-009990, pii: bcr2013009990

Hankir AK, Northall A, Zaman R (2014a) Stigma and mental health challenges in medical students. BMJ Case Rep. doi:10.1136/bcr-2014-205226, pii: bcr2014205226

Hankir A, Zaman R, Evans-Lacko S (2014b) The wounded healer: an effective anti-stigma intervention targeted at the medical profession? Psychiatr Danub 26(Suppl 1):89–96

Harvey S, Laird B, Henderson M et al (2009) The mental health of healthcare professionals. Department of Health, London

Henderson C, Evans-Lacko S, Thornicroft G (2013) Mental illness stigma, help seeking, and public health programs. Am J Public Health 103(5):777–780. doi:10.2105/AJPH.2012.301056, Epub 2013 Mar 14

Langford A (2013) Why mental health bed cuts make me ashamed to work for the NHS. http://www.theguardian.com/society/2013/oct/23/mental-health-bed-cuts-ashamed-nhs. Accessed 18 Mar 2015

Time to Change (2008) Stigma Shout survey shows the real impact of stigma and discrimination on people's lives. http://www.time-to-change.org.uk/news/stigma-shout-survey-shows-real-impact-stigma-and-discrimination-peoples-lives. Accessed 20 Mar 2015

Jung SA (1994) quoted in Anthony Stevens. Jung. Oxford, 110

Lewer D, O'Reilly C, Mojtabai R, Evans-Lacko S (2015). Antidepressant use in 27 European countries: associations with sociodemographic, cultural and economic factors. Br J Psychiatry 207(3):221–226. pii: bjp.bp.114.156786

Link BG, Yang LH, Phelan JC, Collins PY (2004) Measuring mental illness stigma. Schizophr Bull 30(3):511–541

Pickard M, Bates L, Dorian M et al (2000) Alcohol and drug use in second year medical students at the University of Leeds. Med Educ 34(2):86–87

Shore MF (1979) Public psychiatry: the public's view. Psychiatr Serv 30:768–771

Sierles FS, Taylor MA (1995) Decline of U.S. medical student career choice of psychiatry and what to do about it. Am J Psychiatr 152:11

Stuart H, Sartorius N, Liinamaa T, Images Study Group (2015) Images of psychiatry and psychiatrists. Acta Psychiatr Scand 131(1):21–28. doi:10.1111/acps.12368

The world health report 2001 – mental health: new understanding, new hope. The World Health Organization website. Published 2001. Updated 2001. Cited 2015. http://www.who.int/whr/2001/en/

Thommasen HV, Lavancy M, Connelly I et al (2001) Mental health, job satisfaction, and intention to relocate. Opinions of physicians in rural British Columbia. Can Fam Physician 47:737–744

American Foundation for Suicide Prevention (2014) Physician and Medical Student Depression and Suicide Prevention. http://afsp.org/our-work/education/physician-medical-student-depression-suicide-prevention. Accessed 20 Mar 2015

Exemplary Contribution of Professional Scientific Organizations: The European Psychiatric Association

36

Marianne Kastrup, Andreas Heinz, and Danuta Wasserman

Stigma affects psychiatry and psychiatrists in two ways: firstly, through its negative effects on the patients' illness course, help-seeking behavior, treatment adherence, and social inclusion; secondly, negative views about psychiatry and psychiatrists are also common in the medical profession itself (Gaebel et al. 2015). The negative image of psychiatry and psychiatrists may keep medical graduates from choosing psychiatry as their professional career.

Thus, stigma is an issue that links patients and therapists, as the stigma that mentally ill frequently experience may be a reason why psychiatrists also become subject to stigma as a profession. As a consequence, the fight against stigma should be fought from many angles and using many vehicles to reach the goal.

One such tool may be international professional organizations, and the present chapter will outline some of the ways that an international professional organization – in casu the European Psychiatric Association (EPA) – may contribute to the abolishment of stigma.

M. Kastrup (✉)
Centre for Transcultural Psychiatry,
Psychiatric Centre Copenhagen, Copenhagen, Denmark
e-mail: d121304@dadlnet.dk

A. Heinz
Department of Psychiatry and Psychotherapy,
Charité – Universitätsmedizin Berlin,
Charitéplatz 1, 10117 Berlin, Germany
e-mail: andreas.heinz@charite.de

D. Wasserman
Department of Public Health Sciences, NASP, Karolinska Institutet,
Stockholm, Sweden
e-mail: danuta.wasserman@ki.se

© Springer International Publishing Switzerland 2017
W. Gaebel et al. (eds.), *The Stigma of Mental Illness - End of the Story?*,
DOI 10.1007/978-3-319-27839-1_36

European Psychiatric Association

The organization was founded in 1983 and has its origin in Strasbourg, but its members represent all parts of Europe. The objective of the EPA (then AEP, Association of European Psychiatrists) founding members was to establish an Association of French and German Psychiatrists, which would promote European Psychiatry in the fields of research, treatment, and teaching, three axes considered to be unequivocally complementary.

Another objective was to establish an association of psychiatrists that would act as a privileged mediator between practitioners, official councils, and public authorities on matters relating to mental health policies. Besides, in the mind of its founding members, this Franco-German Association was to be the first step towards the creation of an association gathering psychiatrists from all European countries.

In order to reach these goals, EPA gradually set up the organization of the annual European Congress of Psychiatry, as well as other regular scientific meetings, the publication of a scientific international journal, the awarding of research grants, and the creation of sections as working groups corresponding to subdisciplines in psychiatry.

Since its foundation and the inaugural symposium held in May 1984, the number of EPA members has been growing steadily, representing many countries in Europe and abroad. With active individual members in as many as 81 countries and meanwhile 39 National Society/Association Members who represent almost 80,000 European psychiatrists, the EPA is the main association representing psychiatry in Europe.

EPA's activities address the interests of psychiatrists in academia, research, and practice throughout all stages of career development. It deals with psychiatry and its related disciplines, and it focuses on the improvement of care for the mentally ill, the reduction of stigma towards mentally ill, as well as on the development of professional excellence.

EPA is the most visible psychiatric association in Europe, basing its growth on the development of collaborative projects with other major psychiatric organizations, as well as organizations of families and relatives. What joins all members together is that they all work or are qualified to work within psychiatry in Europe. There is thus a close link to psychiatric practice, and members have an extensive insight in all aspects of psychiatric care and knowledge about the stigma they are encountering. Consequently fighting this stigma is high on the agenda, and the association is involved in a number of activities that directly or indirectly are having an impact on stigma.

Council of Europe

Having its headquarters in Strasbourg, it is natural that the EPA since years has close contact with the Council of Europe, Europe's oldest international organization aiming at defending human rights. The EPA was granted in February 1989 a consultant status at the Council of Europe followed by a participatory status in 2003. This position allows the EPA continuously to have insight knowledge of issues that are being debated at the Council and interact in matters of concern for the EPA. As part of this collaboration, the EPA has jointly with the Council of Europe organized symposia at some of the annual EPA Congresses covering topics of mutual concern. Thus, e.g., in 2005, the EPA confirmed its cooperation with the Council by organizing a Human Rights Workshop held during the 13th EPA Congress in Munich (under the Auspices of the Secretary General of the Council of Europe), titled "The role of psychiatrists in ensuring the respect of the rights of persons deprived of their liberty" with a particular focus on the need for European psychiatrists to actively participate in the supervision of the human rights of psychiatric patients deprived of their liberty. The EPA Human Rights Workshop involved the European Committee for the Prevention of Torture and Inhuman or Degrading Treatment or Punishment (CPT), and the legal standards introduced by the CPT in the domain of psychiatry to prevent abuses were discussed as well as concrete results obtained in the field (e.g., in psychiatric hospitals) following the visits of the CPT – a clear example of the synergy of a joint effort.

EPA Congresses

The EPA organizes every year a scientific congress that attracts about 3,000 participants from all over Europe as well as from outside Europe. The objective of the congresses is to have the highest possible scientific standards and to provide high-quality educational courses.

Of particular interest in the present context is the high profile given to ethical topics related to the care of the mentally ill. As an example there have been several Presidential Symposia covering this topic, e.g., in 2006 where the Presidential Symposium was dealing with ethical issues concerning the treatment of mental disorders. In 2007 there was a Presidential Forum on "European Union Strategy for Mental Health" with the involvement of representatives of the EU, the Council of Europe, and the WHO/Europe.

The annual EPA Congresses are increasing in importance and visibility and gather thousands of researchers, clinicians, and teachers who in a collegial atmosphere discuss the latest and clinically most relevant findings. There is a particular focus on young scholars that are encouraged to network but also to interact with more senior colleagues to progress in their scientific endeavors. This interaction could be a fruitful means to discuss ethical behavior, communication with patients, etc., and in this way seen as yet another step towards diminishing stigma. But also the opening ceremonies of several EPA Congresses excellently have an anti-stigma impact by showing how famous artists despite mental problems have been able to produce wonderful artistic work.

European Round Table

In 2008 the Presidential Forum was entitled "Ethical Issues Related to Diagnosis and Classification of Psychiatric Disorders" [with, e.g., topics such as "The Differential Diagnosis Between Depression and 'Normal Sadness'" and "Ethical Issues Relevant to the Definition of Mental Disorders"].

By placing such topics directly as Presidential symposia, EPA shows its concern for the provision of care for the mentally ill and the need to fight for breaking the stigma these may encounter.

The fight for better care and a step towards reduction of stigma was not only one of the aims of the Presidential symposia. EPA took the initiative in 2007 to organize its first European Round Table with National Psychiatric Societies in Europe on the theme "Identity and Harmonisation of European Psychiatry". Here the opportunity was provided to identify areas of shared interests and to provide inputs on activities and challenges and aiming to harmonize standards within Europe. This step towards a European Platform of Psychiatrists could be seen as a long-term project for the association but also an opening towards further collaboration with consumer organizations for the promotion of standards of quality care across Europe.

At the 23rd European Congress of Psychiatry in 2015, the EPA initiated an annual Forum on "Improving Mental Health and Mental Health Care across Europe". Its aim was to foster a dialogue between the EPA and other European and international stakeholders in the field of mental health and mental health care (participants were, e.g., the EPA Council of National Psychiatric Association, the WHO, the World Psychiatric Association, the World Federation for Mental Health, the UN, the Union of European Medical Specialists, the European Brain Council, the European Association of Neurology, the European College of Neuropsychopharmacology, the ROAMER project, EUFAMI, and GAMIAN-Europe). Following up on the 2015 Forum, the theme of the next Forum at the 24th European Congress of Psychiatry in 2016 is "A Common Language in European Psychiatry – can it be achieved?" and again brings together a variety of organizations in the field of mental health.

The intention behind the format of EPA Forums is to cover a broad range of perspectives. Therefore, representatives from a variety of organizations have been invited to present their view on mental health in Europe. The provision of a platform for the exchange of opinions, ideas, and intentions of a diversity of interest groups helps to foster discussions in a trialogue manner contributing to de-stigmatization.

The EPA 30th Anniversary Symposium

In order to celebrate the EPA 30th Anniversary, a symposium "Are People with Mental Illness Truly Citizens of Europe?" led by EPA's Committee on ethical issues took place on 15 November, 2013.

The aim of this specific symposium was to promote awareness regarding the importance of appropriate legislative actions and provisions in order to protect people affected from a mental illness throughout Europe. Such anti-stigma efforts are highly relevant as they – in the long term – may help affected individuals to gradually and equally become recognized as European citizens. The symposium comprised political, ethical, and cultural aspects of the problem (European Psychiatric Association 2013). The venue of the symposium was the Council of Europe in

Strasbourg, and it was held under the auspices of the Secretary General of the Council of Europe and in the framework of the European Year of Citizens.

This anniversary event had a significant symbolic importance by manifesting how seriously EPA takes the rights of mentally ill and how high this is on the EPA agenda for the future.

As a result of this event and as guidance for future action, a declaration on the quality of psychiatry and mental health care in Europe was formulated (see Box 36.1).

Box 36.1: Selected Statements of the Declaration on Quality of Psychiatry and Mental Health Care in Europe of the European Psychiatric Association on the Occasion of Its 30th Anniversary, Strasburg, 2013

- To promote and advocate the respect for people with mental illness and the development and implementation of laws and other regulations that aim to ensure that the human rights and civil rights of people with mental illness, their families and other carers are respected
- To fight against discrimination and for the provision of equitable and quality care for people with mental illness regardless of their gender, age, sexuality, nationality, religion, or ethnic origin
- To act as individuals and psychiatric societies against all discrimination on the grounds of mental illness or impairment and do whatever is in their power to prevent and overcome the stigmatization by mental illness
- To protect the confidentiality of information about people with mental illness handled by health-care personnel and by any other person or institutions/organizations/bodies involved in the provision of mental health care and related tasks, never allowing that the concern for confidentiality is used as an excuse for deprivation of people with mental illness

(European Psychiatric Association 2014)

EPA Ethics Committee

The EPA decided to establish an Ethics Committee in 2010 with the aim among other things to promote ethical standards of psychiatric research and care in Europe. The Committee should initiate and disseminate EPA positions statements on ethical subjects, advise the EPA Board about actions concerning ethical transgressions brought to the EPA, and collaborate with European National Psychiatric Associations, the Council of Europe, and other international organizations in matters concerning ethics and human rights. Furthermore, the Committee is making surveys on how ethics in psychiatry is being managed in Europe and assembles information concerning ethical challenges facing European psychiatry. It is important to reach out to collaborate with other medical professions and develop activities based on a multidisciplinary approach to ethics.

The Committee receives regular requests from mentally ill from different countries who feel that their treatment is mal-managed or that they are subject to medical abuse and discrimination. Trying to disentangle such complicated situations and provide advice to the claimant is paving the way to a reduction of the stigma that they clearly feel subjected to.

The Committee sees it as one of its most valuable tasks to contribute to a greater understanding of how an awareness of the ethical dimension may have an impact on the degree of stigma.

The EPA Committee on Ethics has contributed with symposia at several of the EPA Congresses on topics such as Ethical Challenges and Perspectives for the European Psychiatrist, Research Ethical Questions, Coercive Treatment, and Ethics in European Psychiatry.

EPA Educational Activity

It has been said that the best way to overcome stigma is through research activities. Thanks to research findings it may be demonstrated that mental illness to a very large extent is curable and that there are close links between physical and mental disorders.

The EPA Summer Schools that were established a few years ago have proven a great success for junior colleagues. Till now they have had a focus on the link between somatic illness and mental illness thereby contributing to the objective that there should be equal access to care for mentally ill with a somatic illness like there is for non-mentally ill. A second topic/subject is that mental illness ranks as high as somatic illness, and so there should be equity in the amount of resources allocated to the two, but also showing that there is much communality between the two disorders.

By focusing on the interaction between somatic and mental illnesses, the EPA Summer Schools pay their part in the reduction of any taboos linked to psychiatric disorders.

In addition to the summer school events, the EPA also organizes two types of Continuing Medical Education (CME) courses. These were launched in 2002 during the 11th European Congress of Psychiatry in Stockholm and are designed to match the demands of professionals working in mental health care. The courses are open to all members seeking continuing medical training and international education programs. Ever since, the courses were of particular success, especially the courses on "How to Develop a Program against Stigma and Discrimination because of Schizophrenia" and "Fighting Stigma and Discrimination on a Limited Budget".

EPA Guidance

The EPA has produced a number of guidance documents that have been developed by top researchers in the respective fields. Of major interest for the topic of stigma is firstly the article published in European Psychiatry titled "EPA Guidance on how to Improve the Image of Psychiatry and of the Psychiatrist" (Bhugra et al. 2015a). In this paper potential causes and explanations regarding negative attitudes towards psychiatry and psychiatrists were explored and some counter-strategies proposed. A second EPA guidance document on "The Role and Responsibilities of Psychiatrists" (Bhugra et al. 2015b) declared the role and responsibilities of psychiatrists towards planning and delivering high-quality services and their responsibility to advocate for the patients and the clinical services. The aim of this guidance document was to define the values and competencies necessary to deliver the best care for the patients – care that is patient-centered, safe, and effective. Concerning the fight against stigma, national psychiatric societies and psychiatrists themselves – as professionals – are asked to take on a leading role and become advocates for patients and their families.

Guidance recommendations may contribute to the better understanding of mental illness, its etiology, and treatment. As such they provide a significant input to the fight against stigma. One of their aims is to contribute to a more rational approach to mental illness and to demonstrate how solid, scientific work has resulted in greater insight and knowledge about mental illness and how it may be treated and overcome. By such efforts irrational approaches towards psychiatric disorders may be reduced, and the stigma towards the illness consequently diminished.

References

Bhugra D, Sartorius N, Fiorillo A, Evans-Lacko S, Ventriglio A, Hermans MM, Gaebel W (2015a) EPA guidance on how to improve the image of psychiatry and of the psychiatrist. Eur Psychiatry 30(3):423–430

Bhugra D, Ventriglio A, Kuzman MR, Ikkos G, Hermans MM, Falkai P, Gaebel W (2015b) EPA guidance on the role and responsibilities of psychiatrists. Eur Psychiatry 30(3):417–422

European Psychiatric Association (2013) Are people with mental illness truly citizens of Europe. http://www.europsy.net/wp-content/uploads/2013/11/epa-strasbourg-symposium-programme.pdf. Assessed 07 Oct 2015

European Psychiatric Association (2014) Declaration on Quality of Psychiatry and Mental Health Care in Europe of the European Psychiatric Association on the occasion of its 30th Anniversary. http://www.europsy.net/wp-content/uploads/2014/07/Declaration_for-publication.pdf. Assessed 05 Oct 2015

Gaebel W, Zäske H, Zielasek J, Cleveland HR, Samjeske K, Stuart H, Arboleda-Florez J, Akiyama T, Baumann AE, Gureje O, Jorge MR, Kastrup M, Suzuki Y, Tasman A, Fidalgo TM, Jarema M, Johnson SB, Kola L, Krupchanka D, Larach V, Matthews L, Mellsop G, Ndetei DM, Okasha TA, Padalko E, Spurgeon JA, Tyszkowska M, Sartorius N (2015) Stigmatization of psychiatrists and general practitioners: results of an international survey. Eur Arch Psychiatry Clin Neurosci 265(3):189–197

Addressing Stigma: The WHO Comprehensive Mental Health Action Plan 2013–2020

37

Shekhar Saxena

Introduction

The awareness of mental disorders as being common and a major public health issue has increased substantially in the last few decades. In 1995, a book was published entitled *World Mental Health*: *problems and priorities in low-income countries* (Desjarlais et al. 1995). A few years later in 2001, WHO devoted its World Health Report to *Mental Health*: *New Understanding, New Hope*, and the US Institute of Medicine brought out *Neurological, Psychiatric, and Developmental Disorders*: *Meeting the challenge in the Developing World* (WHO 2001; Institute of Medicine 2001). These publications were amongst the first to build a case for mental health starting from the finding that, due to their chronic course and disabling nature, MNS (mental, neurological and substance use) disorders contribute very significantly to the Global Burden of Disease. Each report also drew strong attention to the extremely unsatisfactory situation in most low- and middle-income countries regarding the availability, quality and range of treatment services and produced a series of recommendations for research and training, service provision and policy.

In a number of respects, much progress has been made since then. Awareness and acceptance of the value of mental health and the challenge posed by mental ill health has continued to grow, both at the international level and in an increasing number of countries. New alliances and partnerships have been formed, including civil society organisations advocating for better rights and service access for persons with mental disorders and their families. In addition, the evidence base around what resources are available in countries and which interventions are effective,

S. Saxena
Department of Mental Health and Substance Abuse, World Health Organization,
Geneva CH-1211, Switzerland
e-mail: saxenas@who.int

© Springer International Publishing Switzerland 2017
W. Gaebel et al. (eds.), *The Stigma of Mental Illness - End of the Story?*,
DOI 10.1007/978-3-319-27839-1_37

feasible and affordable to implement in the context of low- and middle-income countries (LMICs) has improved dramatically (WHO 2010, 2011; Prince et al. 2007; Patel and Thornicroft 2009).

In other respects, however, the situation now is not greatly different to how it was 20 years ago. There continues to be widespread stigma, discrimination and human rights violations against persons with mental disorders and psychosocial disabilities (Drew et al. 2011). Resources allocated to mental health remain extremely modest; the treatment gap is as large as ever (WHO 2011; Lora et al. 2012).

World Health Organization (WHO) is the lead United Nations agency to advise and assist its 194 member states, virtually covering the entire world, on all matters related to health. Since the WHO concept of health includes physical, mental and social wellbeing, mental health is an essential and integral part of WHO's efforts, right from its inception. With increasing availability of scientific evidence on the epidemiology, burden, phenomenology, effective interventions and human rights aspects of mental disorders, the case for a political commitment by countries was ready. In May 2013, all member states of WHO endorsed the *Comprehensive Mental Health Action Plan 2013–2020* (WHO 2013; Saxena et al. 2013). This new effort now commits governments, as well as WHO and other partners, to taking defined actions across a number of areas of implementation. This article briefly sets out what these actions are, whose responsibility they are and how they support the important agenda of decreasing stigma against mental illness.

Development of the Plan

The process for the action plan started with a proposal by a number of Member States to include an agenda item on mental health at the Executive Board meeting of the WHO in January 2012; this was accepted and led to a Resolution, first at the Executive Board and subsequently at the World Health Assembly (WHA) of that year, on the global burden of mental disorders and the need for a comprehensive, coordinated response from health and social sectors at the country level. The WHA Resolution requested the Director-General, inter alia, to develop a comprehensive mental health action plan, in consultation with Member States, covering services, policies, legislation, plans, strategies and programmes.

So began an intensive period of drafting and consultation, not only with WHO Member States but also with non-governmental organisations, WHO Collaborating Centres and other academic institutions. A 'zero' draft prepared by the WHO Secretariat in the summer of 2012 was made available for comment to all interested parties via a web consultation and was used for global and regional consultation meetings.

Following revision and its approval by the Executive Board in January 2013, the final draft was submitted to and adopted by the WHA in May 2013.

Key Elements of the Plan

The *Comprehensive Mental Health Action Plan 2013–2020* is centred around four objectives, all of which are designed to serve the overall goal to 'promote mental well-being, prevent mental disorders, provide care, enhance recovery, promote human rights and reduce the mortality, morbidity and disability for persons with mental disorders' (WHO 2010). The objectives are:

1. To strengthen effective leadership and governance for mental health
2. To provide comprehensive, integrated and responsive mental health and social care services in community-based settings
3. To implement strategies for promotion and prevention in mental health
4. To strengthen information systems, evidence and research for mental health

For each objective, a series of defined actions are identified for Member States, for international and national partners and for WHO Secretariat (see Table 37.1). Relating to governance and leadership, for example, proposed actions for Member States cover the development, strengthening and implementation of mental health policies, strategies, programmes, laws and regulations; resource planning; engagement and involvement with all relevant stakeholders; and empowerment of people with mental disorders and psychosocial disabilities.

For each action area, a set of implementation options are also provided, which reflects not only the diversity of current resources and opportunities amongst countries, but also the different ways by which key actions can be effectively accomplished. Looking across the Member States, there are enormous differences with respect to national income, resource availability and the state of the healthcare system, which are expected to have an important influence on the precise set of actions that actually can be undertaken.

Monitoring Implementation of the Plan

Each of the four objectives is accompanied by one or two specific targets, which provide the basis for measurable collective action and achievement by Member States towards global goals (see Table). Since these six targets and associated indicators represent only a subset of the information and reporting needs that Member States require to be able to adequately monitor their mental health policies and programmes, the WHO Secretariat was requested to prepare and propose a more complete set of indicators for Member States to use as the basis for routine data collection and reporting to WHO. Additional indicators include:

- Government health expenditure on mental health
- Number of mental health workers
- Number and proportion of primary care staff trained in mental health

- Extent of participation of associations of persons with mental disorders and family members in service planning and development
- Number of mental healthcare facilities at different levels of service delivery
- Number and proportion of admissions for severe mental disorders to inpatient mental health facilities that (a) exceed 1 year and (b) are involuntary
- Number of persons with a severe mental disorder discharged from a mental or general hospital in the last year who were followed up within 1 month by community-based health services
- Number of persons with a severe mental disorder who receive disability payments or income support

Table 37.1 Comprehensive mental health action plan 2013–2020: objectives and global targets

Objective	Action areas	Key indicators	2020 target
Leadership and governance for mental health	Policy and law	Existence of a national policy/plan for mental health that is in line with international human rights instruments	80 % of countries
	Resource planning		
	Stakeholder collaboration		
	Empowerment of persons with mental disorders and psychosocial disabilities	Existence of a national law covering mental health that is in line with international human rights instruments	50 % of countries
Comprehensive, integrated and responsive services	Service reorganisation and expanded coverage	Proportion of persons with a severe mental disorder who are using services	20 % increase
	Integrated and responsive care		
	Mental health in emergencies		
	Human resource development		
	Address disparities		
Mental health promotion and prevention	Mental health promotion and prevention	Functioning programmes of multisectoral mental health promotion and prevention in existence	80 % of countries
	Suicide prevention		
		Number of suicide deaths per year per 100,000 population	10 % decrease
Information, evidence and research	Information systems	Core set of identified and agreed mental health indicators routinely collected and reported every 2 years	80 % of countries
	Evidence and research		

Baseline data collection for this set of core mental health indicators has been undertaken via a revised 2014 version of the Mental Health ATLAS (WHO 2014). It is anticipated that this ATLAS exercise will be repeated every 3 years, which will enable progress towards implementation of the plan as well as global targets to be monitored.

Regional and National Adaptation of the Plan

Agreement on the overall structure and content of a global plan of action, with strong buy-in and consensus across stakeholders, is a vital step towards more coordinated and unified action towards improving mental health system access, quality and outcomes globally. Ultimately, however, policies are determined, resources are allocated and services are developed at the national level. It is therefore equally vital that such a global action plan be subject to a process of adaptation to prevailing local circumstances, standards and priorities.

This process has been facilitated by WHO through the development of regional action plans and implementation frameworks, which has enabled groupings of countries with shared cultural values to better reflect their own needs and preferences. Thus, in the Eastern Mediterranean Region, the initial consultation held at the drafting stage of development has been followed by a technical intercountry meeting at which regionally focussed objectives, implementation strategies and performance indicators could be reviewed, discussed and approved by national counterparts. A similar process has been undertaken in the Western Pacific and the American regions of WHO.

Addressing Stigma

The action plan clearly recognises the importance of stigma against mental disorders. It notes that because of stigmatisation and discrimination, persons with mental disorders often have their human rights violated and many are denied economic, social and cultural rights, with restrictions on the rights to work and education, as well as reproductive rights and the right to the highest attainable standard of health. The vision of the action plan also addresses stigma. The vision is a world in which mental health is valued and promoted, mental disorders are prevented and persons affected by these disorders are able to exercise the full range of human rights and to access high-quality, culturally appropriate health and social care in a timely way to promote recovery, all in order to attain the highest possible level of health and participate fully in society and at work free from stigmatisation and discrimination. The action plan also includes actions to combat stigmatisation, discrimination and other human rights violations towards people with mental disorders and psychosocial disabilities including in the workplace. The action plan clearly recognises that efforts will be needed by the governments but also by the civil society partners, including persons and families with mental disorders to reduce stigma.Conclusion

Adoption of the *Comprehensive Mental Health Action Plan 2013–2020* by the World Health Assembly in May 2013 provides the clearest example to date of an increasing commitment by governments to enhance the priority given to mental health within their health and public policy. The agreement by all countries – large and small, rich and poor and from all regions of the world – on a common vision for mental health along with objectives to reach defined targets within a specified time period represents an important step in a longer process to improve mental health across the world. This new commitment is likely to result in a larger proportion of persons with mental disorders to access care and treatment and also to live in societies free from stigma and discrimination.

References

Desjarlais R, Eisenberg L, Good B, Kleinman A (1995) World Mental Health: problems and priorities in low-income countries. OUP, Oxford

Drew N, Funk M, Tang S, Lamichhane J et al (2011) Human rights violations of people with mental and psychosocial disabilities: an unresolved global crisis. Lancet 378:1664–1675

Institute of Medicine (2001) Neurological, psychiatric, and developmental disorders: meeting the challenge in the developing world. IoM, Washington, DC

Lora A, Kohn R, Levav I et al (2012) Service availability and utilization and treatment gap for schizophrenic disorders: a survey in 50 low- and middle-income countries. Bull World Health Organ 90:47–54

Patel V, Thornicroft G (2009) Packages of care for mental, neurological, and substance use disorders in low- and middle-income countries: pLoS medicine series. PLoS Med 6(10):e1000160. doi:10.1371/journal.pmed.1000160

Prince M, Patel V, Saxena S, Maj M, Phillips MR et al (2007) No health without mental health. Lancet 370:859–877

Saxena S, Funk M, Chisholm D (2013) World health assembly adopts comprehensive mental health action plan 2013.2020. Lancet 381:1970–1971

WHO (2001) World health report: mental health: new understanding, new hope. WHO, Geneva

WHO (2010) mhGAP intervention guide for mental, neurological and substance use disorders in non-specialized health settings. WHO, Geneva

WHO (2013) Comprehensive mental health action plan 2013–2020. WHO, Geneva, Available at: apps.who.int/gb/ebwha/pdf_files/WHA66/A66_R8-en.pdf

WHO (2014) Mental health ATLAS 2014. WHO, Geneva

Erratum to: Chapter 32 of The Stigma of Mental Illness - End of the Story?

Wolfgang Gaebel, Wulf Rössler, and Norman Sartorius

Erratum to:
Chapter 32 in: W. Gaebel et al. (eds.), The Stigma of Mental Illness - End of the Story?, DOI 10.1007/978-3-319-27839-1

Erratum text:

There are two corrections on p. 574:

(1) the last line in Table 32.1 the abbreviation of Psychosis susceptibility syndrome (PPS) should be PSS instead of PPS

(2) in line 13 of the next paragraph it should be Klijn instead of Klijin

---

The updated original online version for this chapter can be found at
DOI 10.1007/978-3-319-27839-1_32

W. Gaebel (✉)
Department of Psychiatry and Psychotherapy, Medical Faculty,
Heinrich-Heine-University, LVR-Klinikum Düsseldorf,
Bergische Landstrasse 2, 40629 Düsseldorf, Germany
e-mail: Wolfgang.Gaebel@uni-duesseldorf.de

W. Rössler
Psychiatric University Hospital, University of Zurich,
Militärstrasse 8, Zurich, CH-8021, Switzerland
e-mail: wulf.roessler@uzh.ch

N. Sartorius
Association for the Improvement of Mental Health Programmes,
14 Chemin Colladon Geneva, 1209, Switzerland
e-mail: sartorius@normansartorius.com

© Springer International Publishing Switzerland 2017   E1
W. Gaebel et al. (eds.), *The Stigma of Mental Illness - End of the Story?*,
DOI 10.1007/978-3-319-27839-1_38

Conclusion and Recommendations for Future Action

Wolfgang Gaebel, Wulf Rössler, and Norman Sartorius

Over the past several millennia, people with mental illness have been rejected or mistreated in many societies – because of their illness-related behaviour and the fear that mental illness might be contagious or inheritable. At various points in history and in different countries, the mentally ill were executed, kept in chains, sent down the river in ships of fools, or beaten to death. This still happens but fortunately less and less frequently.

Advancements

In the more recent past – and in particular in the decades following the Second World War – things have begun to change. The notion that mentally ill people are the same as other people although they suffer from a mental illness gradually gained ground. The title of an article by Pope John Paul II in the 1990s "Mentally ill are also made in God's image" (Paul II 1996), summarized the notion for the church and the Roman Catholic parts of the population very succinctly. A similar discourse gradually emerged in other groups and among other developments resulting in the

W. Gaebel (✉)
Department of Psychiatry and Psychotherapy, Medical Faculty,
Heinrich-Heine-University, LVR-Klinikum Düsseldorf,
Bergische Landstrasse 2, 40629 Düsseldorf, Germany
e-mail: Wolfgang.Gaebel@uni-duesseldorf.de

W. Rössler
Psychiatric University Hospital, University of Zurich,
Militärstrasse 8, Zurich, CH-8021, Switzerland
e-mail: wulf.roessler@uzh.ch

N. Sartorius
Association for the Improvement of Mental Health Programmes,
14 Chemin Colladon Geneva, 1209, Switzerland
e-mail: sartorius@normansartorius.com

© Springer International Publishing Switzerland 2017
W. Gaebel et al. (eds.), *The Stigma of Mental Illness - End of the Story?*,
DOI 10.1007/978-3-319-27839-1

extraordinary UN 46/119 resolution, which stated that mentally ill must not be abused and that their treatment is a human right (United Nations. General Assembly 1991). This statement is unique: no other disease has ever been singled out for treatment in this way. The notion that treatment of mental disorders is a human right reflected the evidence that was presented to the representatives of the countries – evidence which showed that in many instances mentally ill people had no chance to receive treatment and that many were kept alive in institutions that did not offer anything but abuse, poor shelter, and miserable food.

The notion of stigma – close to what is today understood when it is mentioned – was also born at that time. Goffman's writing provided a basis for the modern understanding of stigma, stigmatization, and their relation to life of the stigmatized and those who surround them (Link and Stuart 2016; Finzen 2016). His work and the work of others who followed his line of thought led to what can be seen as the *first* and greatest advance in the fight against stigma in the past seven or eight decades – the growth of awareness of the central role that stigma plays in the development of mental health care, in the life of people with mental illness, and in the life of society in which the mentally ill have to live. The major steps forward in diagnostics, treatment, and care of mental illness have also contributed to the understanding of the importance of stigma, which was further underlined by estimates of the huge burden produced by mental illness – to a large extent related to the low priority given to mental health programmes and non-treatment due to stigma.

The growing awareness of the importance and pervasiveness of mental illness stigma was also reflected in the increasing numbers of scientific investigations (Sheehan et al. 2016; Henderson 2016; Loch and Rössler 2016; Zäske 2016; Schomerus and Angermeyer 2016) and made advocacy organizations take stigma as a chief target for their action (Montellano 2016; Johnson 2016).

The *second* major advance in the second half of the twentieth and the first decades of the twenty-first century is that work in many sites produced evidence about the effectiveness of the interventions that had been proposed as means to prevent or reduce stigmatization. Work described in Chaps. 13, 14, 15, 16, 17, 18, 19, 20, and 21 and reviewed by Stuart (2016) and Arboleda-Flórez (2016) offered opportunities to assess various approaches to problems related to stigma and made the choice of interventions for those who are starting to fight stigma easier. Their evaluation underlined the fact that the implementation of changes based on findings of research demands caution because of the ample demonstrations of difficulties and dangers of simply applying strategies that worked well in one setting than in another one that differs in its cultural, economic, or other characteristics (Koschorke et al. 2016, Stuart et al. 2012).

The *third* advance – that reflects a trend in the development of mental health care – is the gradual acceptance of the fact that everyone can contribute to stigmatization (Loch and Rössler 2016) and that everyone has opportunities to fight against it. Thus, the behaviour of health staff can contribute to the occurrence or strengthening of stigma; people with mental illness and their families may by their behaviour and by what they say strengthen stigma; decision makers in health services may by their decisions and in particular by the way in which they organize services contribute to stigma, strengthen or diminish it. The media, schools and other educational institutions, urban developers, industry, and other agents of the society can all influence the stigmatization and its development. The consequence of these facts is the still not quite accepted notion that the success of anti-stigma programmes depends on the active involvement of all those participating in the creation, maintenance, and destruction of stigma (Amering 2016).

A *fourth* advance that has yet to bear full benefits is that a number of governmental and non-governmental organizations have accepted the battle against stigma as one of their tasks. In addition to the World Health Organization – the world's chief medical authority which has included the introduction of measures against stigma in its programmes (Saxena 2016) – other political bodies have stepped forward as well. Thus, it was encouraging to see the European Union foster the development of a pact on mental health (European Commission 2008), which has the fight against stigma as one of its four major components and the ministerial action concerning Alzheimer's disease (European Commission 2009) which includes action against stigma related to the disease. Several non-governmental professional and non-professional organizations – such as the World Psychiatric Association (Stuart and Sartorius 2016), the European Psychiatric Association (Kastrup et al. 2016), and the World Federation for Mental Health (2013) – made the reduction of stigma as one of their targets and constitutional tasks. The engagement of these bodies has yet to be translated into specific and concrete action, but the first and most important step has been done.

Modern times also brought with them a technological development, which may play a major role in the work against stigma and be a *fifth* major advance in this respect: the communication revolution. The internet, telephone connections, computers, and all the other tools that have been developed recently offer numerous possibilities of linkage and communication among people and reduce the horrors of isolation that was the fate of many who suffered from chronic mental illness. The transmission of information with unprecedented speed and quantity makes it possible to transmit messages, knowledge, and information relevant to mental illness and to living with it. It is likely that the appropriate use of new communication technology will also help the work against stigma and it is important to make a maximum use of opportunities that it provides. If that is done appropriately, the fight against stigma will move to a new level of effectiveness.

Drawbacks

But, while these five advances are very encouraging, there are also serious drawbacks that might discourage those working in the field and those engaged in the acquisition of evidence and in training. *First*, the development of anti-stigma programmes still depends, to a large extent, on volunteer work. This is true for the organizations of patients (Montellano 2016) and their relatives (Johnson 2016) but also for many of the other organizations which have a lot of potential but very little money. Reliance on volunteer work depends on leaders who will entice others by their example and help development by wise choices and skilful management of problems. Leaders of that type are not easy to find, and the current education – at home and at school – seems to be contributing to a movement of young people and those already employed to professions which are likely to have a high income and protected work environments. Volunteer work also has its limits and is likely to abate unless fed by success and recognition by authorities and by those concerned as well as others. It would be of essential importance to make decision makers in the health service system understand that funds for work against stigma must be included in the normal service budget. Stigma cannot be beaten by occasional campaigns followed by long periods of inactivity, and it is the health services which should carry on with anti-stigma work once the campaigns are over.

Another problem that is unfortunately shared with many other undertakings is that results of scientific investigations are not finding their way to practical application. Components of anti-stigma programmes that have been shown to be ineffective are still applied (Bailey 2016). In many programmes, the measurement of success of anti-stigma work, for example, is still relying on the measurement of attitude change although there is good evidence that measuring attitudes has to be replaced by measuring changes of the behaviour of the target groups (Arboleda-Flórez 2016). A number of problems related to stigmatization could be approached by appropriate changes in the legislation and governmental procedures and rules: research and experience have clearly indicated what changes are necessary and how useful it is if they are implemented; yet, action in the legal field – with rare exceptions – is still feeble and without sufficient effects.

Difficulties of translation of evidence into practice are creating problems in two additional areas. The first is the use of anti-stigma programme activities in countries far from those in which they were developed (particularly if they are also at different levels of industrial development). Even within-country programmes have to be carefully adapted to the local situation and may therefore vary from one setting to another – in the choice of their goals, techniques, timetables of work, and in other ways. These difficulties are even more disturbing when work is carried out in another country, with different socio-cultural characteristics (Koschorke et al. 2016).

The *second* difficulty stems from differences in language, tradition, and history: work in anglophone countries, for example, is not necessarily considered as being acceptable nor is it likely to be taken as an example in francophone, lusophone, or Russian-speaking countries. The bridging of language and culture differences should be a major task of international governmental and non-governmental organizations: regrettably, until now, many of them have not been paying much attention to these issues. The fact that the language of communication in science is English may make it possible to have a conference at which the leading experts from various countries with different cultural and scientific traditions will attend symposia and discuss findings of recent research: what they have said or done during that time has often little similarity or congruence with their action in their home country. This fact is of particular importance in seeking ways to ensure that countries learn from each other in the area of fighting stigma, which is so intrinsically linked to culture and language.

Insufficient resources to support activities against stigma which are currently heavily dependent on volunteer work and the difficulties of translating scientific evidence into practice are joined by a *third* set of problems related to the difficulty of reducing self-stigmatization of all the participants – the persons with mental illness, their families or other carers, professionals dealing with mental illness, and even administrative support staff. There are few psychiatrists who are proudly announcing that they are the ones dealing with mentally ill people and telling students that the discipline of psychiatry is attractive, rewarding, interesting, and better than others. Patients are continuing to receive negative (sometimes faintly disguised) feedback from those to whom they disclose that they had a mental illness and are increasingly reluctant to even try to enter into the community, apply for jobs, or seek their rights. Family members who rarely receive recognition for the care that they provide are at increasingly high risk to end up in a burnout state which decreases their self-respect and diminishes their role as carers.

These three sets of problems should be seen as priority tasks for health services and all others involved in the prevention and management of mental illness. It is of essential importance – particularly in the context of current social development – to provide stable and continuing support for anti-stigma activities which should be seen as an essential part of health service provision. Professional and non-professional and governmental and non-governmental agencies should explore ways in which they could increase the application of the successful interventions and the application of results of research and experience in the construction and maintenance of anti-stigma activities. And, finally, self-stigmatization (Sheehan et al. 2016; Hankir et al. 2016; Gaebel et al. 2015; Sartorius et al. 2010) of all the partners in the process of care for people with mental illness should become a target of action programmes against stigmatization and its consequences.

Altogether, for the stigma of mental illness and all those who are associated with it, an "end of the story" – as provocatively formulated in the book's title – seems unlikely to appear soon, if at all: it may be more kind of a "never-ending story" requiring sustained programmes instead of short-lived campaigns. However, from what is known today and what has already been achieved so far as compiled in this book, a number of experience- and evidence-based recommendations can be extracted to further contribute to the ever challenging but steadily progressing endeavour of overcoming stigma and discrimination because of mental illness. The following paragraph organized around structural, public, and self-stigma, and based on the key conclusions of this book, may assist the readers in either examining or planning future actions.

A Synopsis of Core Recommendations

Structural Stigma

- *Legislative action* is effective for changing social structures and individual behaviours, even when an individual's attitude remains unchanged. Additionally, laws may facilitate protest mechanisms and give people, that had their rights violated, a meaningful voice. Finally, the consequences of laws on specific organizations may promote equality of opportunity and diminish mental illness stigma and discrimination (Stuart 2016).

- *Structural discrimination* may also be countered by comprehensive and long-term anti-stigma efforts, specifically addressing the disadvantages people with a mental illness encounter through mental health-care funding, legislative action, and health insurance policies (Rüsch and Xu 2016).
- Another example of legislative action designed to remove misconceptions, injustice, and discrimination is *employment equity legislation*. In order to make it work, strong advocacy is essential (Stuart 2016). Finally, inclusion legislation can support social participation and reduce prejudices through contact and a change in ones' attitude (Robertson 2016).
- The *human rights discourse* requires a change in perception, including a shift from its over-preoccupation on basic rights regarding the preservation of autonomy and freedom (i.e. negative rights) towards the protection of citizen entitlements that individuals diagnosed a mental illness are currently denied (Arboleda-Flórez 2016). We recommend a shift of emphasis to bring attention to the implementation of positive rights facilitating inclusion and enabling social participation (Stuart and Sartorius 2016).
- *Media guidelines* need substantial improvement and should include avoiding specific details, glamorizing, and giving undue prominence and sensationalism. Efforts should be made to make media take on an educative role and recognize the importance of providing specific contact details for support services for people with a mental illness. Practical advice by Stuart (2016) includes (1) considering whether suicide reports need to be broadcasted at all; (2) placing reports of critical incidents rather inside magazines and other printed goods; (3) taking into account how the story may impact on vulnerable persons; (4) leaving out detailed descriptions of methods used in suicide; (5) omitting specific information on the location of a critical incident; and (6) choosing the right words/terminology.
- *Terminology* and conceptual change by use of non-stigmatizing language (Harman and Heath 2016, Johnson 2016; Cunningham et al. 2016), including changes of stigmatized terms, for example, the renaming of "schizophrenia" in Japan (Maruta and Matsumoto 2016) and other Asian countries (Lasalvia et al, 2015), and talking about mental disorders than about "diseases/maladies" (Heinz 2016).

Public (Social) Stigma

- Action concerning social stigma includes advocacy, campaigns, and the facilitation of contact, education and protest.
- *Advocacy* covers education, mediation, counselling, dissemination of information, training, awareness raising, mutual help, defending, and denouncing. Engaging in such activities may remove barriers such as human rights violations, stigma, lack of mental health services, absence of mental health promotion, unemployment, and lack of housing (Stuart 2016).
- *Campaigning* includes well-organized long-term interventions (Krupchanka and Thornicroft 2016), incorporating a multifaceted strategy (Koschorke et al. 2016) combining the three most common approaches, including contact, education, and organization of protest activity.

Contact (an arranged meeting between mentally ill and non-ill citizens) to diminish prejudice and change attitudes towards mentally ill has the strongest level of evidence and may be implemented either by video (interviews/personal testimonies), but ideally in person with affected individuals, reporting their real life experiences (Chen et al. 2016) – talking openly about mental disorders (Johnson 2016) or in a trialogue with each other – an encounter of the three main parties dealing with psychiatric problems, mental disorders and with the mental health-care system (service users, family members and friends, and mental health workers) – on equal footing (Amering 2016).

Education should formulate realistic goals and take on a continuous long-term perspective (Zäske 2016). Actions must also have local relevance (Stuart and Sartorius 2016) and should challenge myths with facts (Bratbo and Vedelsby 2016). It should be planned strategically at the national level but equally support grassroots (Cunningham et al. 2016) and local programmes (Stuart and Sartorius 2016) utilizing evidence-based information (Harman and Heath 2016) and tailoring action according to local circumstances (Robertson 2016).

Protest to diminish ignorance and misinformation by stigmatized individuals or members of the general public who support them is often applied against stigmatizing public statements, such as media reports or advertisements (Rüsch and Xu 2016). Conflict and passion should not be feared (Cunningham et al. 2016) – different views and voices need to be heard.

A recommended procedure for anti-stigma activities in local communities should contain the following steps:

- Establish a local action committee
- Conduct a survey of sources of stigma (including information obtained from people with mental illness, their families and other carers, and health service staff)
- Select target groups
- Choose messages and media
- Evaluate the impact of interventions
- Continuously refine interventions

Interventions should contain *age-appropriate* information and should be provided at an early age (e.g. in schools). Interdisciplinary class lessons over a period of at least six months are recommended (e.g. German, history, biology, philosophy, ethics) (Bock et al. 2016).

• To address the three components of stigma (ignorance, prejudice, discrimination) the focus should be set on changing (Harman and Heath 2016):

- *Knowledge*: to counter ignorance/misinformation via education; and in the provision of knowledge the emphasis should be on providing facts and skills that will enable carers and others to deal with mental illness and help those affected
- *Attitudes*: to counter prejudice/stereotypes via contact
- *Behaviour*: to counter un-/intentional acts of discrimination through legislation, advocacy, and appropriate media guidelines

- According to the preference of multifaceted anti-stigma strategies (Koschorke et al. 2016), campaigns can also be embedded explicitly or implicitly in the action programmes of professional scientific organizations like the WPA or EPA (Stuart and Sartorius 2016; Kastrup et al. 2016) or like the WHO (Saxena 2016). The advantage of this kind of activities is that these organizations are acting also politically and in a network approach, targeting many potential recipients since most of them do have member or partner organizations on board which as distributors have access to many different forms of action.
- The focus of anti-stigma interventions should be on individual disorders than on "mental illness" in general (Harman and Heath 2016).
- *Regular evaluations* of the performed interventions (campaigns, programmes) are essential to ensure their adaptation and long-term success (Warner 2016). Success should hereby be determined in terms of reduced discriminatory behaviour (Rüsch and Xu 2016).
- Improving the options of available treatment, prevention, and rehabilitation by means of research and implementation (translational research) may decrease stigma because of better course or outcome of mental disorders (Gaebel et al. 2016).
- Health-care staff should be encouraged:

  - To stand up against the substandard treatment patients experience around the world (Link and Stuart 2016)
  - To keep an open mind, so as to learn from others (Link and Stuart 2016)
  - To take on a role modelling function ("The Wounded Healer") (Hankir et al. 2016)

Self-Stigma

- *Stigma management strategies* (Stuart 2016)
  - Disclosure has been considered an important first step in reducing self-stigmatization. An *empowerment model* (in contrast to a coping model) views stigmatized people as active individuals who work to achieve positive outcomes and consciously take control over their lives, rather than being passive targets of stigma and discrimination who try to conceal and avoid it.
  - *Interventions* vary from psychoeducational, occasionally accompanied by cognitive restructuring, to more complex multi-modal interventions.
  - Although evidence for self-stigma management interventions is limited, first results show promising effects for promoting empowerment and recovery.
- Another major strategy is to *support* the mentally ill, their relatives, and caregivers in their struggle with stigma. This requires mental health-care staff, who are well informed about the need to prevent discriminatory behaviour within their own professional field (and also in their own behaviour), and to provide full support for patients, relatives, and caregivers appropriately to cope with stigma (Zäske 2016).
- Effective treatment (including psychotherapy, cognitive behaviour therapy, psychoeducation, peer support groups, etc.) can reduce self-stigma and needs to be made widely accessible, including physical and financial availability (Montellano 2016).

References

Amering M (2016) Trialogue – an exercise in communication between consumers, carers and professional mental health workers beyond role stereotypes. In: Gaebel W, Rössler W, Sartorius N (eds) The stigma of mental illness – End of the story? 1st edn. Springer, Heidelberg, p581–590

Arboleda-Flórez J (2016) What has not been effective in reducing stigma? In: Gaebel W, Rössler W, Sartorius N (eds) The stigma of mental illness – End of the story? 1st edn. Springer, Heidelberg, p515–530

Bailey S (2016) Closing mental health gaps through tackling stigma and discrimination. In: Gaebel W, Rössler W, Sartorius N (eds) The stigma of mental illness – End of the story? 1st edn. Springer, Heidelberg, p531–534

Bock T, Urban A, Schulz G, Sielaff G, Kuby A, Mahlke C (2016) Irre menschlich Hamburg – an example of a bottom-up project. In: Gaebel W, Rössler W, Sartorius N (eds) The stigma of mental illness – End of the story? 1st edn. Springer, Heidelberg, p469–483

Bratbo J, Vedelsby A (2016) One of us – the national campaign for anti-stigma in Denmark. In: Gaebel W, Rössler W, Sartorius N (eds) The stigma of mental illness – End of the story? 1st edn. Springer, Heidelberg, p317–338

Chen SP, Dobson K, Kirsh B, Knaak S, Koller M, Krupa T, Lauria-Horner B, Luong D, Modgill G, Patten S, Pietrus M, Stuart H, Whitley R, Szeto A (2016) Fighting stigma in Canada – opening minds anti-stigma initiative. In: Gaebel W, Rössler W, Sartorius N (eds) The stigma of mental illness – End of the story? 1st edn. Springer, Heidelberg, p237–261

Cunningham R, Peterson D, Collings S (2016) Like Minds, like Mine – seventeen years of countering stigma and discrimination against people with experience of mental distress in New Zealand. In: Gaebel W, Rössler W, Sartorius N (eds) The stigma of mental illness – End of the story? 1st edn. Springer, Heidelberg, p263–287

European Commission (2008) European pact for mental health and well-being. In: EU Highlevel conference "Together for mental health and wellbeing", Brussels

European Commission (2009) Communication from the Commission to the European Parliament and the Council on a European initiative on Alzheimer's disease and other dementias. Available at: http://ec.europa.eu/health/archive/ph_information/dissemination/documents/com2009_380_en.pdf. Accessed 22 Oct 2015

Finzen A (2016) Stigma and stigmatization within and beyond psychiatry. In: Gaebel W, Rössler W, Sartorius N (eds) The stigma of mental illness – End of the story? 1st edn. Springer, Heidelberg, p29–42

Gaebel W, Zäske H, Zielasek J, Cleveland HR, Samjeske K, Stuart H, Arboleda-Florez J, Akiyama T, Baumann AE, Gureje O, Jorge MR, Kastrup M, Suzuki Y, Tasman A, Fidalgo TM, Jarema M, Johnson SB, Kola L, Krupchanka D, Larach V, Matthews L, Mellsop G, Ndetei DM, Okasha TA, Padalko E, Spurgeon JA, Tyszkowska M, Sartorius N (2015) Stigmatization of psychiatrists and general practitioners: results of an international survey. Eur Arch Psychiatry Clin Neurosci 265(3):189–197

Gaebel W, Riesbeck M, Siegert A, Zäske H, Zielasek J (2016) Improving treatment, Prevention and rehabilitation. In: Gaebel W, Rössler W, Sartorius N (eds) The stigma of mental illness – End of the story? 1st edn. Springer, Heidelberg, p537–549

Hankir A, Ventriglio A, Bhugra D (2016) Targeting the stigma of psychiatry and psychiatrists. In: Gaebel W, Rössler W, Sartorius N (eds) The stigma of mental illness – End of the story? 1st edn. Springer, Heidelberg, p613–625

Harman G, Heath J (2016) Australian country perspective – the work of beyond blue and SANE Australia. In: Gaebel W, Rössler W, Sartorius N (eds) The stigma of mental illness – End of the story? 1st edn. Springer, Heidelberg, p289–315

Heinz A (2016) Illness models and stigma. In: Gaebel W, Rössler W, Sartorius N (eds) The stigma of mental illness – End of the story? 1st edn. Springer, Heidelberg, p485–493

Henderson C (2016) Disorder-specific differences. In: Gaebel W, Rössler W, Sartorius N (eds) The stigma of mental illness – End of the story? 1st edn. Springer, Heidelberg, p83–109

Johnson B (2016) A EUFAMI viewpoint. In: Gaebel W, Rössler W, Sartorius N (eds) The stigma of mental illness – End of the story? 1st edn. Springer, Heidelberg, p191–207

Kastrup M, Heinz A, Wasserman D (2016) Exemplary contribution of professional scientific organizations – the European Psychiatric Association. In: Gaebel W, Rössler W, Sartorius N (eds) The stigma of mental illness – End of the story? 1st edn. Springer, Heidelberg, p627–633

Koschorke M, Evans-Lacko S, Sartorius N, Thornicroft G (2016) Stigma in different cultures. In: Gaebel W, Rössler W, Sartorius N (eds) The stigma of mental illness – End of the story? 1st edn. Springer, Heidelberg, p67–82

Krupchanka D, Thornicroft G (2016) Discrimination and stigma. In: Gaebel W, Rössler W, Sartorius N (eds) The stigma of mental illness – End of the story? 1st edn. Springer, Heidelberg, p123–139

Lasalvia A, Penta E, Sartorius N, Henderson S (2015) Should the label "schizophrenia" be abandoned? Schizophr Res 162(1–3):276–284

Link B, Stuart H (2016) On revisiting some origins of the stigma concept as it applies to mental illnesses. In: Gaebel W, Rössler W, Sartorius N (eds) The stigma of mental illness – End of the story? 1st edn. Springer, Heidelberg, p3–28

Loch A, Rössler W (2016) Who is contributing? In: Gaebel W, Rössler W, Sartorius N (eds) The stigma of mental illness – End of the story? 1st edn. Springer, Heidelberg, p111–121

Maruta T, Matsumoto C (2016) Stigma and the renaming of schizophrenia. In: Gaebel W, Rössler W, Sartorius N (eds) The stigma of mental illness – End of the story? 1st edn. Springer, Heidelberg, p571–579

Montellano P (2016) The viewpoint of GAMIAN-Europe. In: Gaebel W, Rössler W, Sartorius N (eds) The stigma of mental illness – End of the story? 1st edn. Springer, Heidelberg, p173–189

Paul PJ II (1996) Mentally ill are also made in God's image. Vatican City 11(30):3

Robertson J (2016) See me – Scotland case study. In: Gaebel W, Rössler W, Sartorius N (eds) The stigma of mental illness – End of the story? 1st edn. Springer, Heidelberg, p379–403

Rüsch N, Xu Z (2016) Strategies to reduce mental illness stigma. In: Gaebel W, Rössler W, Sartorius N (eds) The stigma of mental illness – End of the story? 1st edn. Springer, Heidelberg, p451–467

Sartorius N, Gaebel W, Cleveland HR, Stuart H, Akiyama T, Arboleda-Flòrez J, Baumann AE, Gureje O, Jorge MR, Kastrup M, Suzuki Y, Tasman A (2010) WPA guidance on how to combat stigmatization of psychiatry and psychiatrists. World Psychiatry 9(3):131–144

Saxena S (2016) Addressing stigma – the WHO comprehensive mental health action plan 2013–2020. In: Gaebel W, Rössler W, Sartorius N (eds) The stigma of mental illness – End of the story? 1st edn. Springer, Heidelberg, p635–640

Schomerus G, Angermeyer M (2016) Changes of stigma over time. In: Gaebel W, Rössler W, Sartorius N (eds) The stigma of mental illness – End of the story? 1st edn. Springer, Heidelberg, p157–172

Sheehan L, Nieweglowski K, Corrigan P (2016) Structures and types of stigma. In: Gaebel W, Rössler W, Sartorius N (eds) The stigma of mental illness – End of the story? 1st edn. Springer, Heidelberg, p43–66

Stuart H (2016) What has proven effective in anti-stigma programming? In: Gaebel W, Rössler W, Sartorius N (eds) The stigma of mental illness – End of the story? 1st edn. Springer, Heidelberg, p497–514

Stuart H, Sartorius N (2016) Opening doors – the global program to fight stigma and discrimination because of schizophrenia. In: Gaebel W, Rössler W, Sartorius N (eds) The stigma of mental illness – End of the story? 1st edn. Springer, Heidelberg, p227–235

Stuart H, Arboleda Florez J, Sartorius N (2012) Paradigms lost. Oxford University Press, Oxford, UK

United Nations. General Assembly (1991) A/Res/46/119. Principles for the protection of persons with mental illness and the improvement of mental health care. Available at: http://www.un.org/documents/ga/res/46/a46r119.htm. Accessed 24 Oct 2015

Warner R (2016) Fields of intervention. In: Gaebel W, Rössler W, Sartorius N (eds) The stigma of mental illness – End of the story? 1st edn. Springer, Heidelberg, p435–449

World Federation for Mental Health (2013) Action plan 2013–2015. Available at: http://wfmh.com/wp-content/uploads/2014/02/Action-Plan-2013-2015.pdf. Accessed 25 Oct 2015

Zäske H (2016) The influence of stigma on the course of illness. In: Gaebel W, Rössler W, Sartorius N (eds) The stigma of mental illness – End of the story? 1st edn. Springer, Heidelberg, p141–155

Index

A

Action committee, 91, 233, 437–438, 482, 647
Action groups, 231, 234
Action plans, 303, 320, 338, 396, 438, 599
Advocacy, 21, 203, 205, 268, 278, 311, 366,
    518, 525, 573–574, 631, 646
Advocacy groups, 445
    local, 445, 446
    national, 445
Ambassadors, 294, 323–325, 337, 370, 375
Anti-stigma programmes / interventions, 11,
    24, 41, 76–77, 90, 187, 197, 211, 213,
    216–218, 227, 237, 252, 263, 273, 289,
    317, 340, 343, 357, 367–371, 379, 388,
    394, 405, 407, 436, 453, 458–460, 462,
    470, 474, 475, 538, 544, 620, 630, 643,
    644, 647, 648
    contact, 12, 76, 91, 218, 248, 268–270,
        294, 295, 341, 352, 358, 375, 381,
        440, 452, 509, 620–624, 646, 647
    effectiveness, 243, 248-251, 293, 323,
        340, 454, 460, 497, 512, 593,
        608, 642
    evaluation, 91, 240, 246, 252, 267, 269,
        275, 278, 282, 396–402, 446, 648
    implementation, 217, 642
    mental health professionals / staff, 475
    procedure, 91, 360, 647
    protest, 273, 452–453, 502, 646, 647
    recommendations, 234, 381, 408,
        411, 415
    school programmes, 431, 438, 475
    volunteer programme, 369, 375
Attitudes, 7, 8, 24, 57, 89, 92, 157, 158, 162,
    216, 340, 358, 395, 421, 518, 537,
    544, 615
    change in attitudes, 8, 10, 12, 276, 361,
        382, 534

professional attitudes, 89, 95, 620
    public attitudes, 10–12, 22, 84, 87, 93,
        131, 238, 265, 273, 363, 524
Attributions, 85, 552, 556

B

Behaviour, 12, 33, 486, 552, 559
    deviating behaviour, 33–34, 39
Best practice, 71, 180, 312, 340, 426, 471, 588
beyondblue, 76, 93, 289–305, 341, 453

C

Carers
    expertise, 204
    needs, 205
    role, 195, 204
    support, 193, 206
Cognitive Restructuring, 456, 458, 648
Community mental health reforms, 191,
    520, 526
Community psychiatry, 161, 418–419,
    430, 637
Coping strategies, 148, 541, 542
Council of Europe, 628–631
Country activities, 211, 417
    Australia, 93, 289–315, 348, 507
    Austria, 91, 348, 418–419
    Canada, 227, 237–258, 575, 621
    China, 71, 134, 573
    Croatia, 420, 431
    Denmark, 317, 320, 334
    France, 588
    Germany, 8, 22, 91, 161, 405, 407, 426,
        585, 615
    Greece, 234, 516, 588
    Ireland, 357–377, 588

© Springer International Publishing Switzerland 2017
W. Gaebel et al. (eds.), *The Stigma of Mental Illness - End of the Story?*,
DOI 10.1007/978-3-319-27839-1

Country activities (*cont.*)
  Italy, 621
  Japan, 115, 571, 578, 646
  Korea, 573
  Lebanon, 621
  New Zealand, 232, 263, 272, 453
  Netherlands, 164, 574
  Norway, 421, 431
  Poland, 422, 588
  Portugal, 423, 621
  Romania, 424
  Scotland, 87, 341, 379, 389, 402
  Slovakia, 425
  Slovenia, 425, 621
  Sweden, 331, 427
  Switzerland, 585, 588
  Taiwan, 573
  Turkey, 229, 429
  UK, 348, 396, 615, 621
  USA, 7, 11, 93, 442, 621
Crisis Intervention Team (CIT), 442
Cultural influences on stigma, 67, 616
  concept of 'culture', 68
  cultural factors, 68
  cultural meanings, 70
  explanatory models, 70
  global patterns, 73

D

Diagnosis, 174, 192, 470, 492
  alcohol dependence, 84, 86
  anxiety, 472
  borderline personality disorder, 90,
    94, 474
  criteria, 491
  dementia, 86
  depression, 84, 92, 147, 158, 472
  eating disorder, 86
  panic attacks, 86
  psychosis, 147, 148, 473
  substance misuse disorders, 84, 86, 93, 95
  schizophrenia, 84, 86, 91, 147, 158, 197
Disabling environment, 126
Disclosure, 134, 203, 342, 456, 459, 510,
    588, 648
Discrimination, 40, 44, 48, 59, 84, 87,
    115–116, 123, 125, 141, 148, 157, 162,
    191, 196, 212, 214, 265, 283, 290, 296,
    320, 330, 499, 519, 543, 546, 552,
    583, 631
  anti-discrimination, 296, 383, 384, 422
  anticipated discrimination, 88, 125, 132,
    166, 347

  experiences, 131, 147, 166–167, 477
  individual discrimination, 127, 131,
    142, 462
  institutional discrimination, 126
  interactional discrimination, 50
  interpersonal discrimination, 125, 131
  levels of discrimination, 88, 125
  marginalization, 35–36, 38, 229, 502
  mechanisms, 125, 128
  prevalence, 344
  segregation, 48–50
  self-discrimination, 125, 132–133
  self-perception, 331–332, 408
  social exclusion, 50, 77, 141, 263, 614
  structural discrimination, 125, 133, 141,
    169, 340, 451, 461–462, 646
  systemic discrimination, 278
  victimisation, 339, 343, 532
  withdrawal, 48, 74
  work related, 129, 309, 394,
    405, 504, 520
Discrimination and Stigma Scale (DISC),
    88, 330
DSM-5, 485, 540, 545, 573
Duration of Untreated Illness (DUI), 143
Duration of Untreated Psychosis (DUP), 143

E

Education, 16, 77, 91, 95, 203, 212, 307, 308,
    341, 348, 381, 382, 430, 440, 452, 461,
    620, 644, 646, 647
  contact-based education, 238–247,
    250, 254
  press services, 409, 410
  schools, 308
  workplace, 298
Emotional reactions, 162, 164, 552, 558
Empowerment, 153, 279, 371, 383, 384, 396,
    413, 420, 457, 538, 542, 561, 592,
    595, 596, 607, 608, 648
  strategies, 420, 511
Employment, 342, 348
European Commission, 413, 643
European Committee for the Prevention of
    Torture and Inhuman or Degrading
    Treatment or Punishment (CPT), 629
European Federation of Associations of
    Families of People with Mental Illness
    (EUFAMI), 194–195, 587, 630
European Psychiatric Association (EPA), 575,
    623, 627, 628, 631, 643, 648
  guidance documents, 632, 633
Evidence, 67, 84, 162, 323, 498, 635

F

Families, 191, 192, 194, 197, 212
"Fighting" stigma. *See* Anti-stigma
    programmes/ interventions
Funding, 230, 313, 318–319, 337, 446, 461,
    476, 599
    the funding gap, 531

G

German Mental Health Alliance, 405–416
    the media project, 408, 409
    open face peer interview project, 411, 412
Global Alliance of Mental Illness Advocacy
    Networks-Europe (GAMIAN-Europe),
    173–188
Governmental organisations, 238, 643, 644
Grants, 389–390, 396
Grassroots activities, 153, 258, 368, 373, 614

H

Health-care provision, 128
    mental health-care, 128
    physical health-care, 129
Help seeking, 22, 92, 143, 295, 302, 366, 423,
    424, 537, 538, 545, 546, 614, 620
    barriers, 143, 503
History (of Stigma), xvi, 4, 16, 32, 515, 644
Human rights, xvii, 84, 187, 194, 209, 211,
    213–217, 222–223, 279, 344, 382, 491,
    499, 519, 523, 524, 526, 581, 631, 639,
    642, 646
    violations, 74, 127–128, 521, 583

I

ICD-10/11, 485, 573, 578
Illness Models, 158, 485–492
Image of Psychiatry, 160–162, 627, 633
Inclusion (social), 74, 188, 221, 263, 283, 320,
    358, 413, 528, 646
"Irre Menschlich Hamburg" initiative,
    469–482

K

Knowledge, 12, 84–89, 229, 294, 340, 376,
    381, 452, 461, 508, 647

L

Labelling, 4, 17, 19, 52, 69, 118, 215, 252, 339,
    490, 516, 545–546, 552–555, 571, 578

labelling theory, 17–18, 124
modified labelling theory / approach, 6,
    18–19, 148, 553
Labour market, 317–319, 334
Legislation, 127, 215, 221, 278, 342, 383, 384,
    396, 430, 461, 501, 524, 534, 630,
    644–646
    anti-discrimination legislation, 210, 213,
        215, 296, 342, 461, 502
    CRPD *see* (United Nations)
    disability, 209, 215, 219, 502
    Disability Discrimination Act,
        505, 601
    employment equity legislation, 309, 462,
        504, 646
    Equality Act, 351, 352, 533
    outpatient commitment legislation, 503
    UDHR *see* (United Nations)
Life expectancy, 129, 531
"Like Minds, Like Mine" campaign,
    263–285, 453
Low-and middle-income countries (LMICs),
    74, 127, 519, 635, 636

M

Media, 4, 17, 22, 37, 46, 86, 114, 119,
    130–131, 187, 203, 212, 255, 265,
    275, 309, 327, 370–371, 379, 392,
    408, 420, 439, 454, 461, 505, 616,
    642, 647
    (media) advocacy, 506
    educational activities, 408, 415
    fair media project, 411
    films / movies, 10, 616
    magazines, 37, 425, 426
    media guidelines, 505–507, 646
    media-watch group, 310, 445–446
    newspapers, 10, 37, 83, 86, 426, 430
    radio broadcasts, 10, 409
    reporting of suicides, 506–507
    sensationalism, 114, 505
    social media, 185, 239, 305, 326, 392
    stigmatizing representations, 184, 256,
        257, 309
Mental health, 532
    at the workplace, 251, 281–282, 298, 342,
        363–366, 413, 598
    foundation, (MHF), 381
    gaps, 531, 636
    service users, 245, 344, 533, 567–569
Mental health care, 90, 245, 642
    reform, 428, 520
    staff, 93, 94, 562–567, 642, 648

The Mental Health Commission
   Canada, 238, 503
   New Zealand, 264, 268
The Mental Health Foundation, 266, 381
Mental illness
   conceptualization, 9, 517, 572
   course, 141, 152
   prevention, 645
   Socioeconomic factors, 72
Mindfulness, 457
Mortality, 129, 531, 637

N
National Alliance for the Mentally Ill
      (NAMI), 445
Non-governmental organizations, (NGOs),
      xvii, 357, 380, 643, 644
   family members, xvii, 29, 191–207
   patients, xvii, 29, 173–188, 630

O
"ONE OF US" campaign, 317–338, 397
"Opening Minds" initiative, 237–258
"Open the Doors" programme, 24, 76, 90–92,
      227–235, 405, 419, 420, 436
Opinions About Mental Illness Scale (OMI),
      13–15, 75

P
Peer support, 456, 476, 481, 592–596
   cost effectiveness, 595, 596, 610
   dedicated peer support teams, 593
   department of health and peer support, 592
   effectiveness, 593, 595, 597–603
   myths and misperceptions, 604–606
   shared experiences, 592
Prevention, 475, 538–540, 544, 546
   indicated, 538–540
   primary, 538
   programmes, 538, 539
   secondary, 538–540
   selective, 538
   universal, 538, 539
Psychoeducation, 455, 458–460, 648

Q
Quality of life, 24, 192–194

R
Randomized controlled trials, 498
Recovery, 193, 270, 274, 279, 282, 518, 540,
      541, 546, 648
Rehabilitation, 542–544
Renaming terminology, 571–579, 646
   alternative terms, 575, 577
   principles, 572
   pros/ cons, 574
Research, xv, xvi, 4, 74, 117, 119, 187, 257,
      280, 341, 366, 421, 429, 586–587,
      642, 644
Resource allocation, 126, 127, 170

S
SANE Australia, 305–313
   "Change" programme, 357–377
   "Me" campaign, 76, 87, 164, 341, 343,
      360, 379–403, 453
Self-esteem, 150, 151, 180, 511, 528
Self-monitoring, 473
Self-support, 406, 409
Service-User Speakers' Bureau, 444
Shared decision-making, 593
Social cognitive model, 44, 124
Social context, 20, 71
Social distance, 8, 10–12, 36, 115, 117,
      162–164
Social Marketing, 349, 360, 379, 436
Social status, 55
Stakeholder, 393–395, 406, 463, 630
Status loss, 6, 339, 552–553
Stereotypes, 12, 15, 44, 45, 48, 84–86, 161,
      165, 212, 241, 339, 424, 451, 470
   stereotype agreement, 119, 151
   awareness, 152, 211–212, 218, 361, 379,
      383, 396
   dangerousness, 36, 45, 46, 84, 165, 552,
      555, 557
   incompetence, 43, 45, 46, 312
   internalized stereotypes, 119
   public, 51, 119
   unpredictability, 36, 84, 165,
      527, 555
Stigma, 239, 518–519, 614
   affiliate stigma, 134
   burden, 37, 132, 142, 173, 545
   changes of stigma, 22, 157–170
   components, 6, 9, 340
   concept, 3–5, 16, 30

courtesy stigma, 16, 50, 51, 54, 59–60, 118, 132, 134
double stigma, 50–51, 55
economic costs, 348–349
experiences, 538, 542, 545, 562, 568
external stigma, 607, 608
family stigma, 54, 118, 177, 188, 269, 578, 584, 587
health care staff / professionals, 50, 83, 88–89, 116, 117, 180, 245, 300, 331, 342, 520, 584, 587, 596, 607–609, 614, 620
ignorance, 67, 84, 185, 197, 647
institutional stigma, 115, 126, 538
internalized stigma, 51, 56, 87, 552
label avoidance, 44, 50, 52–53
origin, 3–5, 30, 142, 516
patients / service users, 614, 615
perceived, 158, 166–169, 537, 545
personal stigma, 141, 142, 150, 152
prejudice, 12, 36, 37, 40, 44, 45, 57, 59, 84, 112, 117, 185, 197, 212, 228, 469, 470, 500, 518, 555, 573, 613, 615, 647
psychiatrists, 23–24, 116, 117, 160, 161, 300, 613–616, 645
psychiatry, 17, 29–41, 160, 469–471, 613, 645
public stigma, 6, 8, 50, 53, 56, 59, 158, 162, 344, 345, 451, 452, 500, 538, 541, 646
reduction, 10, 41, 90, 92, 95, 228, 238–250, 293, 302, 343, 357–377, 380, 396, 435, 452, 486, 551, 573, 578, 579, 608–610, 623
research, 4, 11, 17, 21–22, 118, 197, 245, 552, 632
self-stigma, xv, 6, 41, 50, 51, 57, 111, 118, 124, 132–133, 151, 162, 174–175, 180, 187, 203, 280, 283, 311, 331, 426, 431, 451, 455, 458, 500, 520, 526, 537, 543, 544, 607–610, 645, 648
social stigma, 174, 177, 187, 646
structural stigma, xv, 25, 50, 53, 54, 95, 115, 158, 162, 169–170, 500, 645, 646
suicides, 58, 77, 92
types, 16, 31, 34, 40, 43, 50, 173
workplace stigma, 182, 252–255, 298
Stigma Management Strategies, 29, 510, 648
Stigmatization, 29, 32–34, 38, 470
cycle of stigmatization, 229–230
de-stigmatization, 29, 169

Subjective Impairment, 489
Suicidal ideation, 144–145
Support, 33, 38, 41, 203, 220, 376, 481, 648
Surveys, 73, 157, 176, 241, 330, 332, 363, 398, 477, 553, 574, 620
survey panel, 326

T
Target Groups, 233, 374, 407, 408, 437
educational institutions, 642–643
employers, 342, 358, 364, 379
health care staff / professionals, 217, 238, 245–251, 342, 620
media, 239, 255–257
schools, 379, 395, 430, 623, 642
students, 341, 430, 438, 617–623
workforce / workplaces, 239, 251–255
young people, 239–244, 334, 358, 366
Technological developments, 643
The "Time to Change" programme, 76, 164, 167, 182, 320, 335, 339–354, 360, 453, 532–534
The partnership Model / Framework, 245–246, 361–363, 368, 374
Therapeutic Community Movement, 591
Training, 270, 389, 480
community, 275, 306
health professionals, 306
attorneys, 443
judges, 443
police officers, 443, 480
probation officers, 443
employers, 371
managers, 413, 414
media representatives, 257, 371, 409
people working in self-support groups, 409
screenwriters, 409, 410
students, 277, 425
teachers, 475
Treatment, 23, 129, 203, 345, 537, 540, 541, 544–546, 551, 572, 615
Assertive Community Treatment (ACT), 57
barriers to treatment, 145, 307
inhumane treatment, 521
medication / drugs, 539–542
physical activity, 539, 540
psychological, 539, 540, 542, 543
Trialogue, 471, 475–476, 581–589

U

United Nations, 500, 522, 642
    Convention on the Rights of Persons with
        Disabilities (CRPD) 128, 209–223,
        582, 584
    The Universal Declaration of Human
        Rights (UDHR), 127, 382

V

Vicious circle of stigma, 118
Vignette descriptions, 7–8, 84–85
Vulnerability, 113, 132

W

World Federation for Mental Health (WFMH),
    414, 630, 643
World Health Organization (WHO), 413, 414,
    502, 521, 614, 629, 635, 636,
    643, 648
    Comprehensive Mental Health Action Plan
        2013–2020, 581, 635–640
World Psychiatric Association (WPA), 160,
    227, 405, 419, 420, 430, 435, 522, 572,
    574, 581, 588, 643, 648

Printed in the United States
By Bookmasters